G. Guglielmi · C. van Kuijk · H. K. Genant (Eds.)

Fundamentals of Hand and Wrist Imaging

Springer-Verlag Berlin Heidelberg GmbH

G. Guglielmi · C. van Kuijk · H. K. Genant (Eds.)

Fundamentals of Hand and Wrist Imaging

With Contributions by

S. Balzano · A. Barile · L. H. L. De Beuckeleer · J. Bittoun · J. L. Bloem
H. M. Bonél · O. Bottinelli · P. G. Bracke · M. Cammisa
R. Campani · A. Castriota Scanderbeg · A. Catalucci · A. Chevrot
L. F. Coenen · B. Dallapiccola · A. M. Davies · E. Dion · J.-L. Drapé
A. M. Dupont · J. Dutton · J. M. Elliott · C. Faletti · A. Feydy
F. Florio · I. Fogelman · M. Fuchsjäger · H. K. Genant · D. Godefroy
A. J. Grainger · G. Guglielmi · H. Imhof · F. Kainberger
D. de la Kethulle de Ryhove · C. van Kuijk · P. K. Lang · M. Maas
C. Masciocchi · M. Mastantuono · V. M. Metz · S. M. Metz-Schimmerl
M. Nardella · H. Nishimura · W. R. Obermann · R. Passariello
E. Pessis · T. Rand · M. Reiser · D. Resnick · R. R. van Rijn
M. P. J. F. Ritt · L. Satragno · A. M. De Schepper · A. De Serio
V. Strizzi · I. Sulzbacher · D. J. Theodorou · S. J. Theodorou
J. E. Vandevenne · H.-J. van der Woude

With 454 Figures in 794 Separate Illustrations

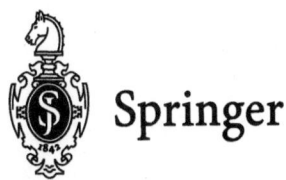 Springer

GIUSEPPE GUGLIELMI, MD
IRCCS Hospital "Casa Sollievo della Sofferenza"
Viale Cappuccini
71013 San Giovanni Rotondo
Italy

CORNELIS VAN KUIJK, MD, PhD
University of Amsterdam
Academic Medical Center
Department of Radiology
Meibergdreef 9
1105 AZ Amsterdam
The Netherlands

HARRY K. GENANT, MD
University of California at San Francisco
Department of Radiology
San Francisco, CA 94143-0628
USA

ISBN 978-3-642-63225-9

Library of Congress Cataloging-in-Publication Data
Fundamentals of hand and wrist imaging / Giuseppe Guglielmi, Cornelis van Kuijk,
Harry K. Genant (eds.).
    p.; cm.
    Includes bibliographical references and index.
    ISBN 978-3-642-63225-9   ISBN 978-3-642-56917-3 (eBook)
    DOI 10.1007/978-3-642-56917-3
    1. Hand--Imaging. 2. Wrist--Imaging. I. Guglielmi, G. (Giuseppe), 1957–
II. Van Kuijk, Cornelis 1962– III. Genant, Harry K.
    [DNLM: 1. Hand--radiography. 2. Wrist--radiography. WE 830 F981 2001]
    RC951.F86 2001
    617.5'750754--dc21   00-061190

http//www.springer.de

© Springer-Verlag Berlin Heidelberg 2001
Originally published by Springer-Verlag Berlin Heidelberg New York in 2001
Softcover reprint of the hardcover 1st edition 2001

Cover-Design: Erich Kirchner, Heidelberg
Typesetting: Verlagsservice Teichmann, Mauer

SPIN: 106 940 39   21/3135 – 5 4 3 2 1 0

To our families
HKG GG

To my father
CVK

Preface

An exceptional group of authors, renowned musculoskeletal radiologists and experts in their respective fields, have contributed to "Fundamentals of Hand and Wrist Imaging". We, the editors, asked the authors each to write a chapter that was readable, well illustrated and highly informative. The book is aimed at radiologists, hand surgeons, orthopedic and plastic surgeons as well as internist-endocrinologists and rheumatologists. It is intended as an aid in daily work for practicing physicians as well as for residents.

The book can be split into three parts. In the first part the different imaging modalities are discussed: from conventional radiography to magnetic resonance imaging and many more. The second part deals with different disease entities: from congenital dysplasias to degenerative disease and everything in between, including inflammatory and neoplastic disease. The third and last part covers specific topics such as the carpal tunnel syndrome and diseases of the nail bed.

All chapters are lavishly illustrated, on the principle that a picture is worth a thousand words.

We hope that we have achieved our goals in that readers will find in this book whatever they need to know about the fundamentals of hand and wrist imaging. Only readers can decide whether we have succeeded, and any suggestions for future editions will be welcomed.

We would like to thank all the participating authors for their efforts. We feel privileged to have worked with them.

San Giovanni Rotondo	GIUSEPPE GUGLIELMI
Amsterdam	CORNELIS VAN KUIJK
San Francisco	HARRY K. GENANT

Contents

22 Ungual and Subungual Disease
J.-L. Drapé, A. Chevrot, J. Bittoun

1 Radiography of the Wrist and Hand

V. M. METZ, M. FUCHSJÄGER, S. M. METZ-SCHIMMERL

1.1 Introduction

Although there are many imaging techniques available for evaluation of wrist and hand disorders, such as ultrasound, tomography, computed tomography and magnetic resonance imaging, the initial examination technique is and remains plain routine radiography. Routine radiographs should be performed carefully in a standardized way to avoid misdiagnosis and should be analyzed systematically. The number of radiographic positions depends on the clinical information and clinical questions. In cases of trauma, normally ipsilateral views of the injured wrist or hand are adequate. For inflammatory or systemic disorders, bilateral wrist and/or hand views have to be obtained. In this chapter the most important positions for routine radiography of the wrist and hand, criteria for an adequate examination, and a systematic approach for analysis are described.

1.2 Radiography of the Wrist: The Survey

The minimal survey examination of the wrist should consist of four views: posteroanterior (PA), lateral, semipronated oblique, and PA in ulnar deviation [1].

The *standard neutral PA view* should be performed with the patient sitting beside the table with the shoulder abducted 90° and the elbow flexed 90°. The elbow is at the same height as the shoulder (Fig. 1.1a). This is important because the various elbow and shoulder positions have an influence on the relationship between the distal radius and ulna [2, 3]. Only in this position can ulnar variance measurements be determined reliably. The hand – not the wrist – should be placed flat on the cassette without any radial or ulnar deviation (the third finger/third metacarpal bone collinear with the distal radius) and the fingers extended; the central beam is perpendicular to the cassette and is centered on the head of the capitate bone. A check for correct positioning can easily be performed by looking at the ulnar styloid process (Fig. 1.1b): if the shoulder and the elbow are at the same height, the ulnar styloid process is projected most laterally (projected free) and the entire groove of the extensor carpi ulnaris tendon is radial to the ulnar styloid process (no overlapping). A collinear alignment of the midaxis of the distal radius with the central axis of the third metacarpal indicates that there is no radial or ulnar deviation of the wrist. If the hand is placed flat on the cassette, the second

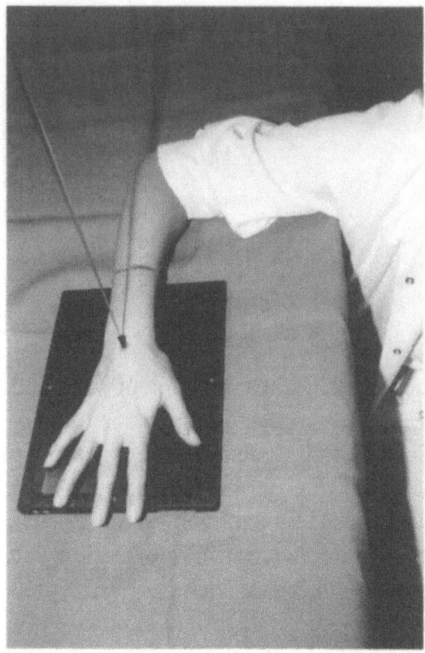
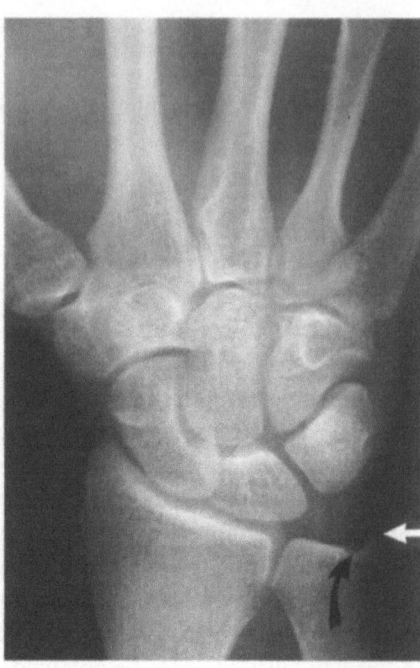

a   b

Fig. 1.1. a Position of the patient for obtaining a standard neutral posteroanterior (PA) view of the wrist. **b** Standard neutral PA radiograph of the wrist. The ulnar styloid process (*arrow*) is projected most laterally. The groove of the extensor carpi ulnaris tendon is seen (*curved arrow*)

through fifth carpometacarpal joints normally will show parallel articular surfaces. On the standard neutral PA view opposing cortices of the wrist will be profiled and should be parallel to each other. In most cases, on the PA view, there is a "normal" slight overlapping of the scaphoid and the lunate bone and the trapezio-trapezoideal joint space, which are not profiled. The joint space widths within the carpus are normally between 2 and 3 mm and all joint spaces should be of symmetrical width [4]. Three carpal arcs have been described [4] which should be evaluated on the PA view (Fig. 1.2): arc 1 joins the convexity of the proximal carpal row, arc 2 joins the concavity of the proximal carpal row, and arc 3 is created by the convexity of the distal carpal row (capitate and hamate bone). In general, loss of parallelism, overlapping of joint spaces, and abnormal or asymmetrical joint space width always indicate a pathologic condition (e.g., subluxation, dislocation, fracture).

On the neutral PA view one should be familiar with the shape and the position of the lunate bone. On the PA view, the lunate is a more trapezoidal shape. In radial deviation, under physiologic conditions, the lunate appears almost triangular, because it is flexed palmarly. If the lunate bone has a triangular shape on the true neutral radiograph, it indicates an abnormality (e.g., subluxation, dislocation, instability) [5, 6]. Normally, the lunate bone lies up to two thirds (and at least one half) over the radius on a neutral PA view. If it migrates more ulnarly, with or without widening of the radioscaphoid or scapholunate joint space, it may indicate an abnormality (e.g., ulnar translocation of the carpus).

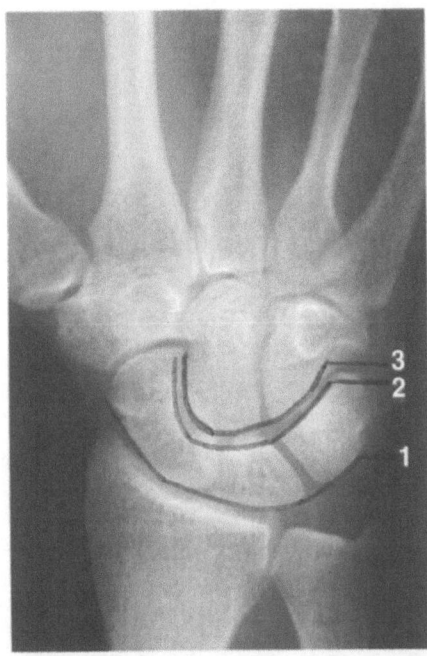

Fig. 1.2. Standard neutral PA view of the wrist. Three smooth carpal arcs can be drawn. Under normal conditions there is no step-off on the arcs

The *standard neutral lateral view* is obtained with the elbow flexed 90° and adduced against the trunk. The ulnar side of the wrist is placed on the cassette and the transverse axis of the wrist is perpendicular to the cassette (Fig. 1.3a). The dorsum of the wrist and hand should be parallel with the long axis of the radius without any flexion or extension and without any radial or ulnar deviation of the wrist. The central beam is centered to the region of the distal pole of the scaphoid and is perpendicular to the cassette. If the examination has been performed correctly the palmar surface of the pisiform bone is projected 2–3 mm dorsal to the palmar cortex of the distal pole of the scaphoid bone (Fig. 1.3b).The long axis of the third metacarpal bone should be nearly parallel with the long axis of the distal radius. In most cases, on a true lateral radiograph congruence of the distal radioulnar joint is shown by nearly complete overlap of the ulnar head and the distal radius, and dorsal or ventral dislocation of the distal radioulnar joint causes loss of this superimposition. Slight supination or pronation of the wrist from this neutral position (Fig. 1.4) and the wide range of normal variations render an analysis of incongruity of the distal radioulnar joint inadequate [7–9].The neutral lateral view has been described as an important view for determination of intercarpal angles for evaluation of carpal instabilities [5, 10–13].Two intercarpal angles are of most importance: the scapholunate (SL) angle and the capitolunate (CL) angle (Fig. 1.5). The scaphoid axis (S) can be obtained by drawing a line which joins the palmar distal and proximal cortex of the scaphoid bone. The line perpendicular to a line between the most distal dorsal and palmar pole of the lunate, and which runs through the center of the lunate head, is defined as the lunate axis (L). Similarly, the capitate axis (C) is drawn by joining a line which runs through the most distal

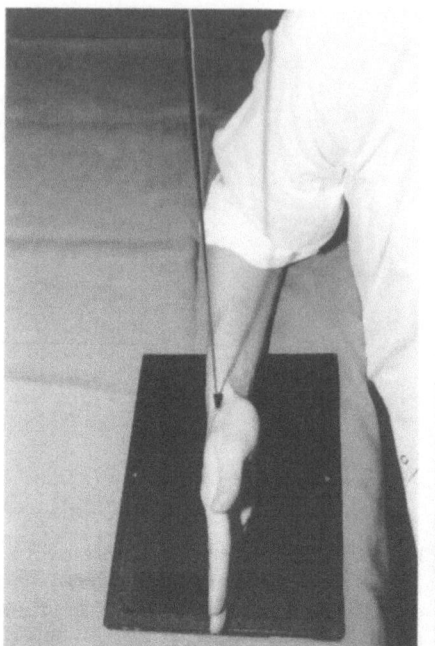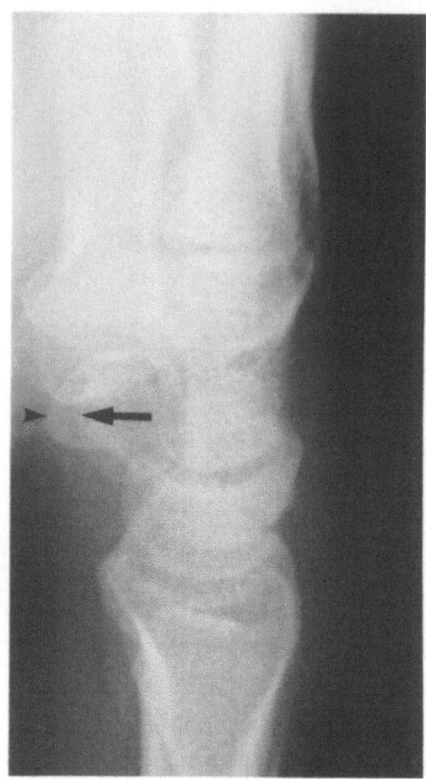

a

b

Fig. 1.3. a Position of the patient for obtaining a standard neutral lateral view of the wrist. b Standard neutral lateral radiograph of the wrist. The palmar cortex of the pisiform bone (*arrow*) is 2–3 mm dorsal to the cortex of the distal palmar pole of the scaphoid bone (*arrowhead*)

palmar and dorsal aspect of the capitate and a perpendicular line through the center of the head of the capitate bone. The SL angle is normally between 30° and 60°; it is questionably abnormal between 60° and 80°, and is definitely abnormal if it is more than 80°. The CL angle is normally between 0° and 30°.

The *PA semipronated oblique view* is obtained with the radial side of the wrist 45° off the cassette by using a sponge supporting the wrist and hand (Fig. 1.6a). The central beam is centered to the scaphocapitate junction and is perpendicular to the cassette. In this view the scapho-trapezio-trapezoidal and commonly the first carpometacarpal joints are profiled (Fig. 1.6b). In addition, this view is helpful to evaluate the distal pole of the scaphoid and the scaphoid tuberosity and waist.

For the *PA ulnar deviation view* (also a part of a motion study for determination of normal or abnormal motion between the radius and the carpus and between the proximal and distal carpal row) the hand is placed on the cassette with the hand and wrist in ulnar deviation (Fig. 1.7a). Again the central beam is centered to the head of the capitate bone and is perpendicular to the cassette. On the radiograph (Fig. 1.7b) adequate ulnar deviation can be observed by evaluation of the long axis of the third metacarpal bone; this is not perpendicular to the central

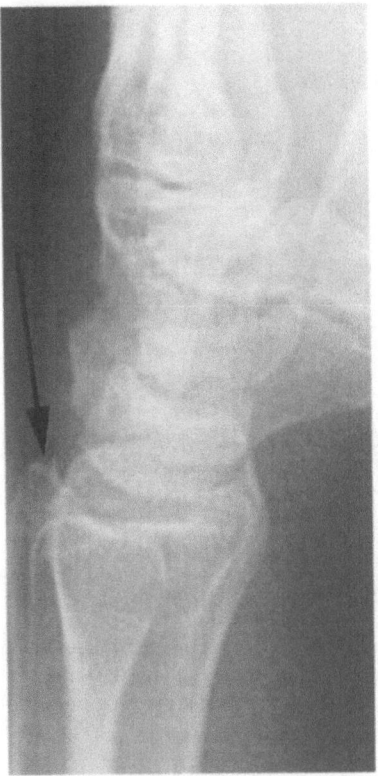

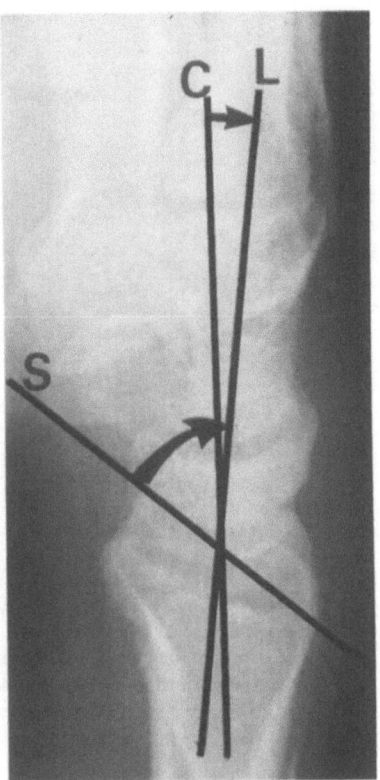

Fig. 1.4. Lateral view of the wrist with slight pronation of the wrist from the neutral position causes loss of superimposition of the distal radius and ulna (*arrow*)

Fig. 1.5. Standard neutral lateral radiograph of the wrist. *S* scaphoid axis, *L* lunate axis, *C* capitate axis. The SL angle is between 30° and 60° (*curved arrow*) and the CL angle is between 0° and 30° (*arrow*)

axis of the radius but the long axis of the scaphoid bone becomes nearly perpendicular to the radius axis. In this view the scaphoid is elongated because it tilts dorsally and the articular joint spaces between the scaphoid bone and the adjacent carpal bones are profiled better than on the routine neutral PA view [14]. The PA ulnar deviation view is helpful for detection of scaphoid fractures and fracture dislocations and for evaluation of normal or abnormal radiocarpal or midcarpal motion. In addition the scapholunate joint space becomes more profiled and scapholunate dissociation (abnormal widening) may become more evident.

1.2.1 Additional Views of the Wrist

The *anteroposterior (AP) view or palmodorsal view* (Fig. 1.8a) is performed by placing the dorsum of the hand and wrist flat on the cassette without any flexion or extension of the wrist [15]. The central beam enters palmarly at the head of the

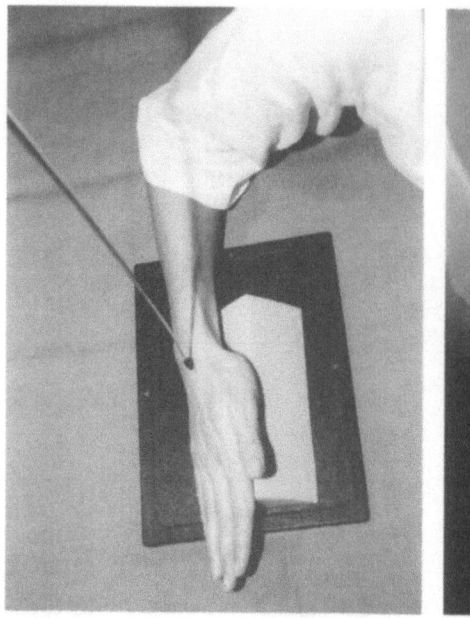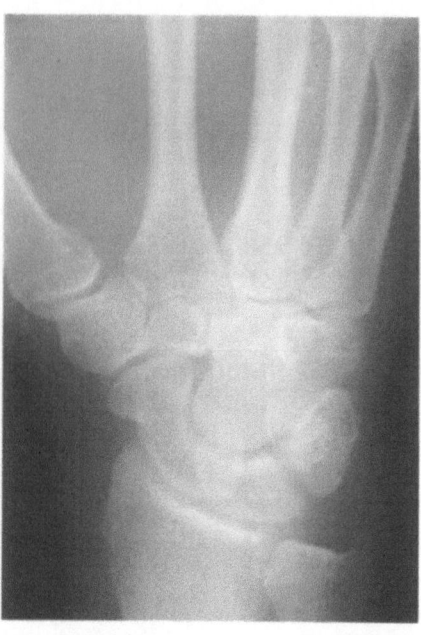

a   b

Fig. 1.6. a Position of the patient for obtaining a standard neutral 45° semipronated oblique view of the wrist. b On the standard neutral 45° semipronated oblique radiograph of the wrist the scapho-trapezio-trapezoidal joint spaces and the first carpometacarpal joint space are profiled

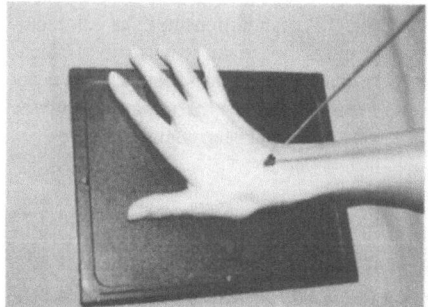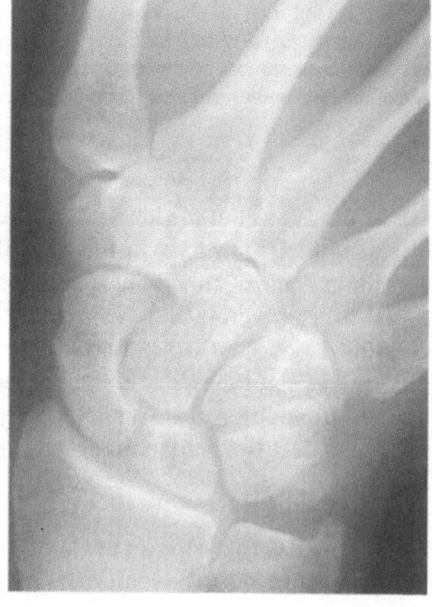

a   b

Fig. 1.7. a Wrist PA view with ulnar deviation. b Wrist PA radiograph with ulnar deviation. In ulnar deviation, the scaphoid bone elongates because it tilts dorsally. The long axis of the scaphoid bone becomes nearly parallel to the long axis of the radius. Compare this figure with Fig. 1b

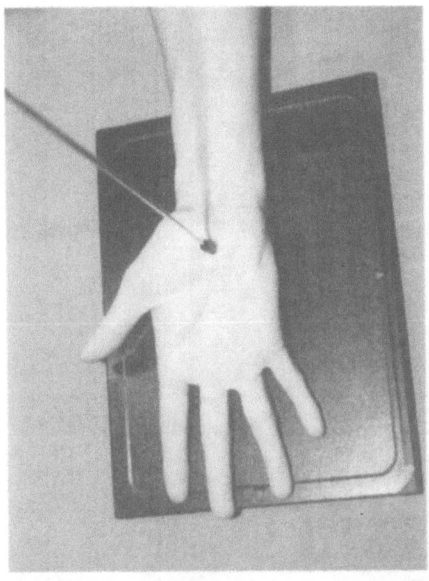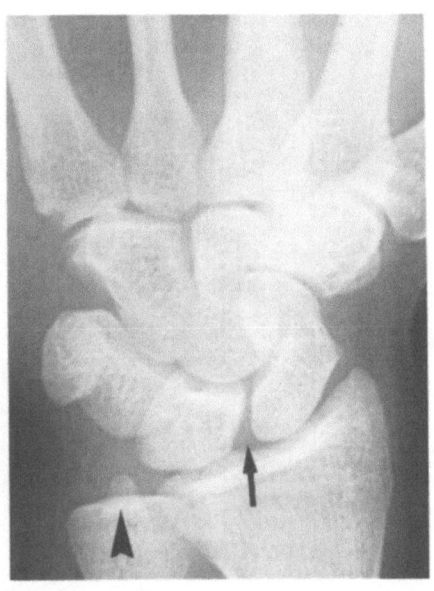

a b

Fig. 1.8. a Positioning for obtaining an anteroposterior (AP) view of the wrist. **b** AP view of the wrist. The scapholunate joint space is profiled (*arrow*) better than on the PA view (see Fig. 1.1b) and the ulnar styloid process projects over the ulnar head (*arrowhead*)

capitate bone and is perpendicular to the cassette. In contrast to the neutral PA view, in the AP view the ulnar styloid process projects over the ulnar head, which indicates to the viewer that this radiograph is obtained anteroposteriorly (Fig. 1.8b). On the AP view commonly the scapholunate joint space is better profiled than on the PA view. For evaluation of scapholunate diastases the AP view can be obtained with a clenched fist; this increases axial forces and scapholunate joint space abnormalities may become more evident [16].

The *PA view in radial deviation*, commonly part of a motion study (wrist instability series), is obtained by placing the wrist and hand as described for the standard PA view but with the wrist in maximal radial deviation (Fig. 1.9a). In this position the scaphoid bone foreshortens because it tilts palmarly and has the appearance of a "signet ring" (Fig. 1.9b). This finding is normal in radial deviation of the wrist. However, if a "signet ring" sign is recognized on a neutral PA view it indicates an abnormal position of the scaphoid bone (e.g., rotary subluxation of the scaphoid, volar intercalated segmental instability) [4, 17].

The *radiocarpal joint view* is designed to profile the articulation between the proximal carpal row and the dorsum of the distal radius, as the dorsal aspect of the distal radius overlaps the proximal carpal row due to the physiological volar tilt of the distal radius. This view is obtained by placing the wrist and hand in the same way as described for the routine PA view but the central beam is angled 25°–20° toward the elbow and centered to Lister's tubercle (Fig. 1.10a). On the radiograph, the radiocarpal joint is profiled (Fig. 1.10b), the scaphoid is elongated, and the capitate appears foreshortened allowing an additional view of those bones.

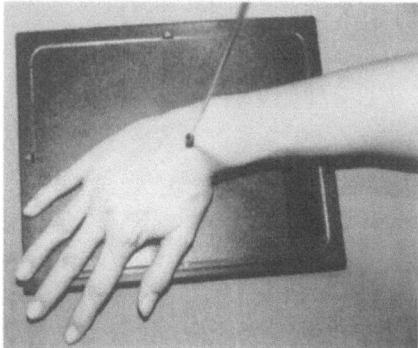

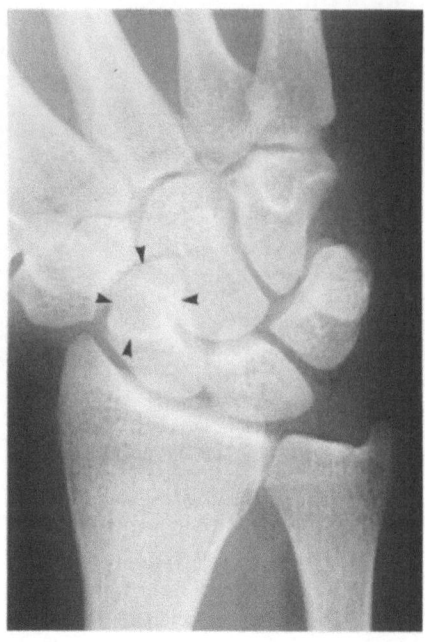

Fig. 1.9. a Positioning for obtaining a PA view of the wrist with maximal radial deviation. b PA view of the wrist with maximal radial deviation. The scaphoid foreshortens as it tilts palmarly, creating the "signet ring" sign (*arrowheads*). This is normal in radial deviation of the wrist

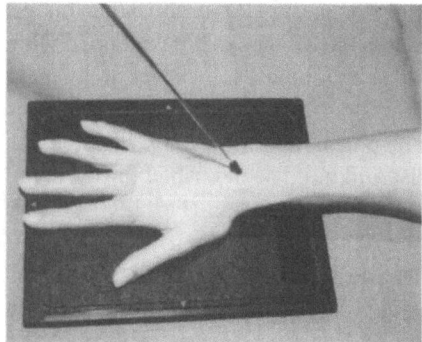

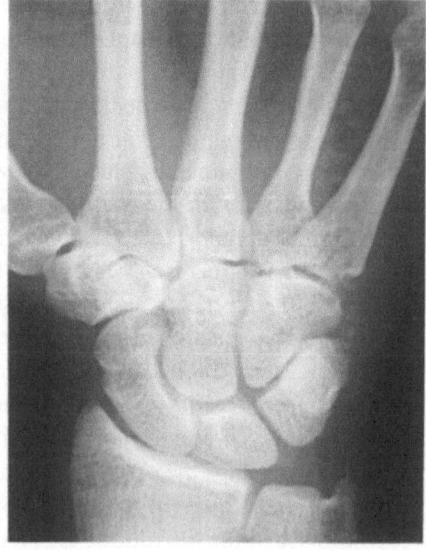

Fig. 1.10. a Examination technique for the radiocarpal joint view. b On the radiocarpal joint view the radiocarpal joint is profiled, the scaphoid is elongated, and the capitate is foreshortened. Compare it with Fig. 1.1b

For demonstration of the pisiform bone, the pisiotriquetral joint space, the palmar parts of the triquetrum and the ulnar surface of the hamate, the *semisupinated oblique view* is recommended [18]. For this view the ulnar side of the wrist and hand is placed on the cassette with 30°–45° supination (off-lateral) with the central beam perpendicular to the cassette and centered at the capitate head (Fig. 1.11).

Further to the standard views described above, additional views for more precise examination of the scaphoid are demanded [19, 20]. The *scaphoid oblique ulnar-deviated view* provides an oblique nonforeshortened view of the scaphoid because ulnar deviation elongates the scaphoid. Additionally, this view profiles the scapho-trapezio-trapezoidal joint (Fig. 1.12a). To obtain this view, the wrist is pronated 45° and is ulnar deviated with the ulnar side of the wrist placed on the cassette. The central beam is centered to the scaphoid waist and is perpendicular to the cassette (Fig. 1.12b). The *ulnar-deviated overpronated scaphoid view* is performed with the wrist in slight ulnar deviation and the radial side of the extended thumb and the radial side of the forearm placed on the cassette (Fig. 1.13a). The central beam is centered to the waist and perpendicular to the cassette. The scaphoid is overlapped by the capitate (distally) and by the lunate (proximally).

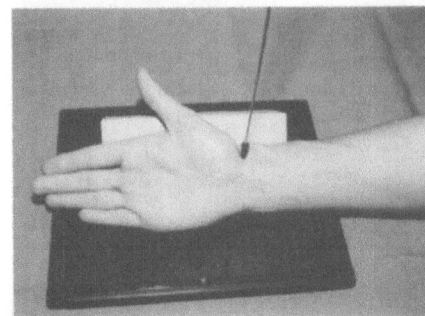
a

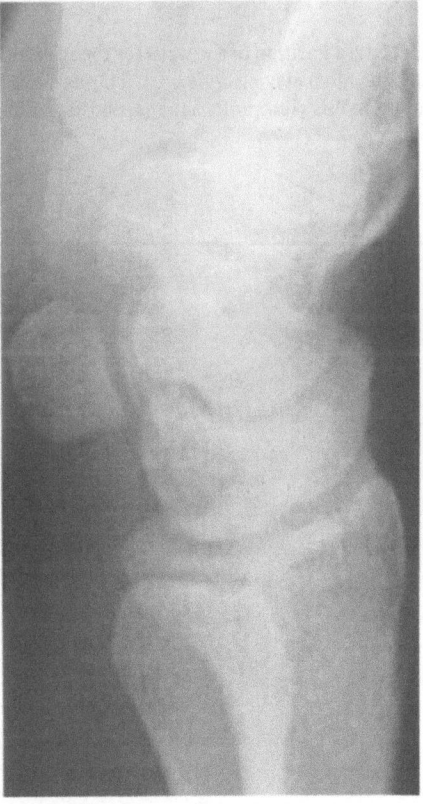
b

Fig. 1.11. a Positioning for the semisupinated oblique view of the wrist. b On the semisupinated oblique view the pisiotriquetral joint is profiled best

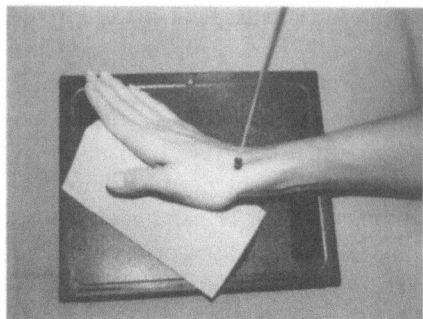
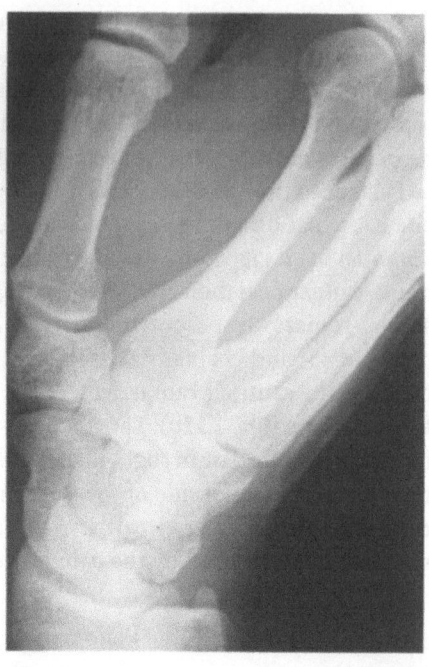

Fig. 1.12. a Position of the wrist for the scaphoid oblique ulnar-deviated view. **b** On the scaphoid oblique ulnar-deviated view an oblique, nonforeshortened view of the scaphoid is provided. In addition this view profiles the scapho-trapezio-trapezoidal joints

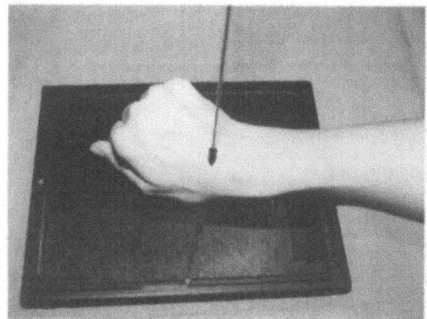
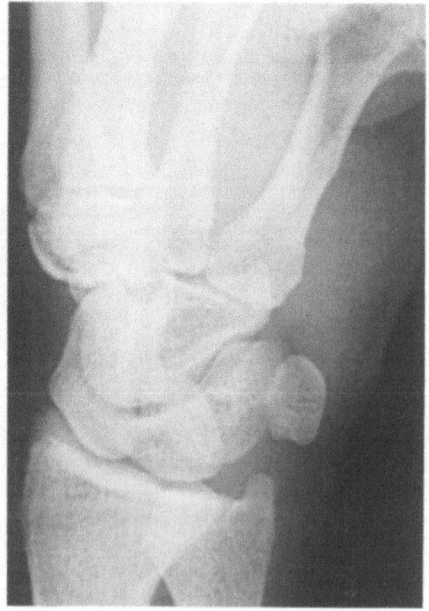

Fig. 1.13. a Positioning technique for obtaining the ulnar-deviated overpronated scaphoid view. **b** The scaphoid is overlapped by the capitate distally and by the lunate proximally; the pisiform is projected most laterally

The pisiform bone projects most laterally and the radioscaphoid joint space is profiled (Fig. 1.13b). This view is obtained to detect scaphoid lesions, especially chip fractures of the dorsal part of the waist of the scaphoid that are not clearly visible on routine views.

The *carpal boss view* has been described for evaluation of the nature (differential diagnosis: os styloideum, osteophytes, fracture, or normal dorsal bony structure) of a bony prominence at the junction of the second and third carpometacarpal joints [21]. For this view the ulnar side of the wrist is placed on the cassette with about 30° supination and the wrist is slightly ulnar-deviated (Fig. 1.14). The central beam passes the prominence tangentially.

Different techniques have been described for viewing the carpal tunnel [22–24]. For the inferosuperior *carpal tunnel view* the palmar side of the wrist is placed on the cassette, there is maximal dorsiflexion of the wrist maintained by the patient's contralateral hand, and the central beam is angled approximately 30° towards the elbow (Fig. 1.15a). This view allows evaluation of the hook of the hamate, the palmar site of the trapezium, the pisiform, the capitate and the tuberosity of the scaphoid (Fig. 1.15b).

The *lateral extension/lateral flexion views* are of major importance for evaluation of normal or abnormal movements (wrist instabilities, e.g., volar or dorsal intercalated segmental instabilities) of the carpal bones at the level of the radiocarpal and midcarpal joints [4, 17, 25]. These views are obtained with the wrist placed on the cassette just as it is for the true neutral lateral view (with the same criteria for an adequate examination) but with the wrist in maximal extension or

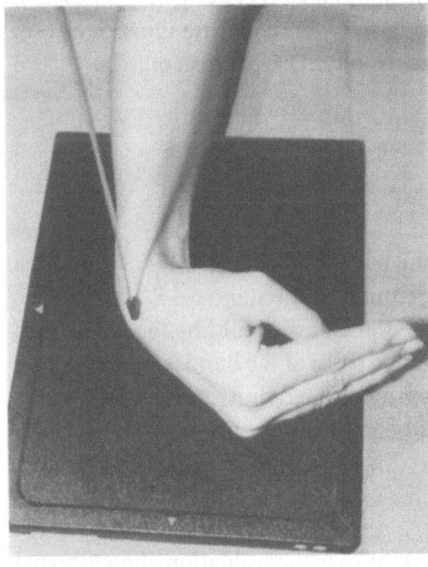

a

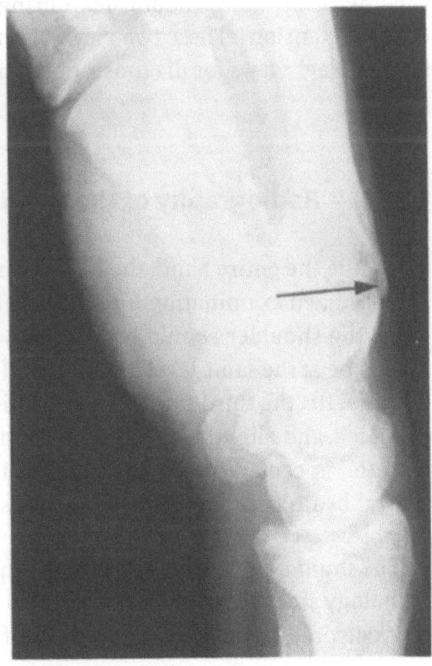

Fig. 1.14. a The carpal boss view position. b The carpal boss (*arrow*)

b

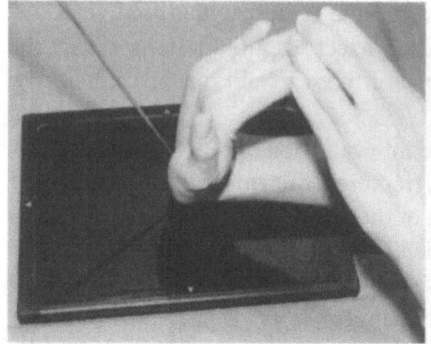
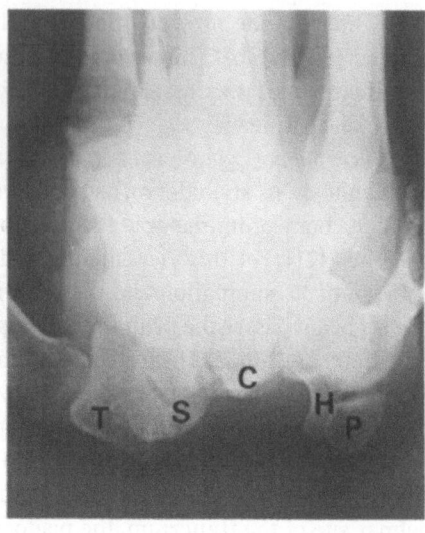

a

b

Fig. 1.15. a Position for obtaining the inferosuperior view of the carpal tunnel. **b** Inferosuperior view of the carpal tunnel. This view allows evaluation of the hook of the hamate (*H*), the palmar site of the trapezium (*T*), the pisiform (*P*), the capitate (*C*), and the tuberosity of the scaphoid (*S*)

flexion (Fig. 1.16). Failure of extension/flexion of the capitate axis (representing the distal carpal row) with respect to the lunate axis and/or failure of extension/flexion of the lunate axis (representing the proximal carpal row) with respect to the radius (representing the forearm) suggests the presence of an instability. In general: "everything should flex during flexion, and everything should extend during extension". These two views and the PA view in radial and ulnar deviation are the "key" views for diagnosis of the most common carpal instabilities.

1.3   Radiography of the Hand

To profile the entire hand, the *PA view* is the basic survey (Fig. 1.17). To obtain a standardized examination for all patients, similar to the standard PA view of the wrist, the shoulder should be abducted 90°, the elbow should be flexed 90° and should be at the same level as the shoulder. The palm of the hand is placed flat on the cassette, the third finger nearly collinear with the radius, and the fingers are extended and slightly spread. The central beam, which is perpendicular to the cassette, is centered over the head of the third metacarpal bone. Because the central beam is not centered to the wrist, measurement of ulnar variance is not reliable.

The *standard PA oblique view* is an important view for evaluation of metacarpal pathology since the metacarpals overlap each other in a true lateral view. It makes the ventroradial and dorsoulnar sides of the wrist and hand bones more evident.

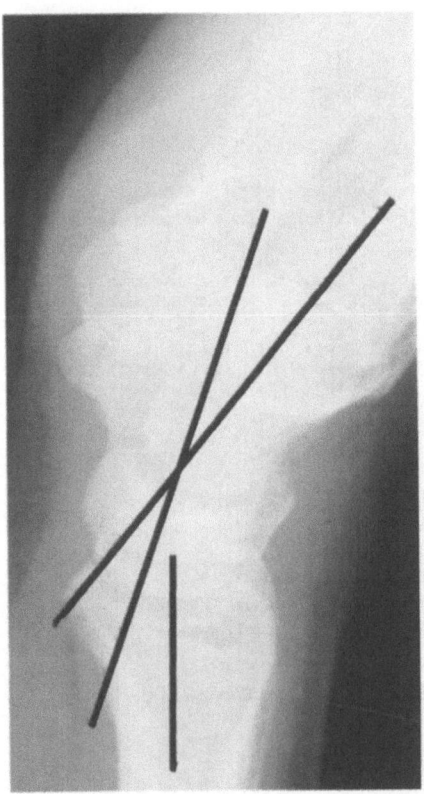
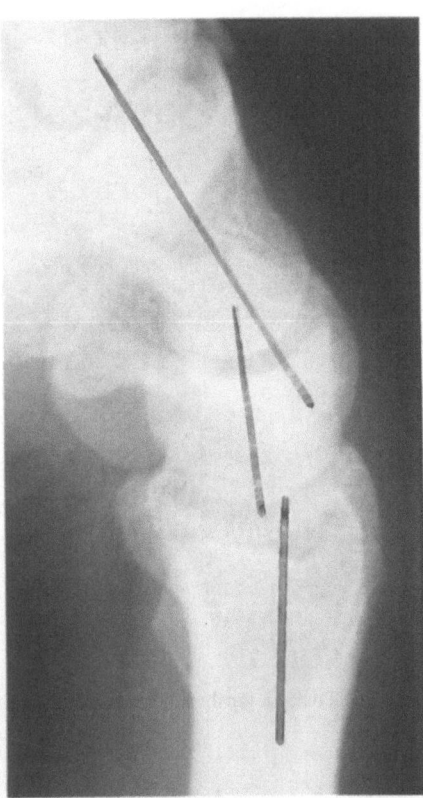

a

b

Fig. 1.16. a Lateral view of the wrist with maximal extension. All axes should normally extend during extension. **b** Lateral view of the wrist with maximal flexion. All axes should normally flex during flexion

To obtain this view (Fig. 1.18), the radial side of the hand is elevated 45° from the cassette, the fingers are extended, the central beam is centered over the head of the third metacarpal and is perpendicular to the cassette. The fingers should be extended and slightly separated which allows the interphalangeal joints to be profiled. The so-called "Zither Position" should be avoided because some metacarpophalangeal joints and the most interphalangeal joints are not profiled in this view (Fig. 1.19).

The *lateral view* of the hand allows excellent depiction of abnormalities located at the palmar or dorsal side of the hand (Fig. 1.20). The ulnar side of the hand is placed on the cassette and the hand is in neutral position (without any flexion or extension, ulnar or radial deviation, respectively). The fingers should be spread on a wedge sponge to avoid overlapping. The thumb is in an oblique position in this projection.

Specific metacarpal bones should be examined with three views: PA, semipronated oblique, and lateral. The position for the *PA view* is the same as for the position of the hand, but the field is collimated to the metacarpal(s), which is (are) of interest to reduce scatter and to improve image detail (Fig. 1.21). The central

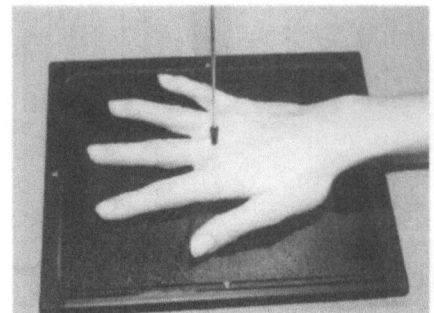
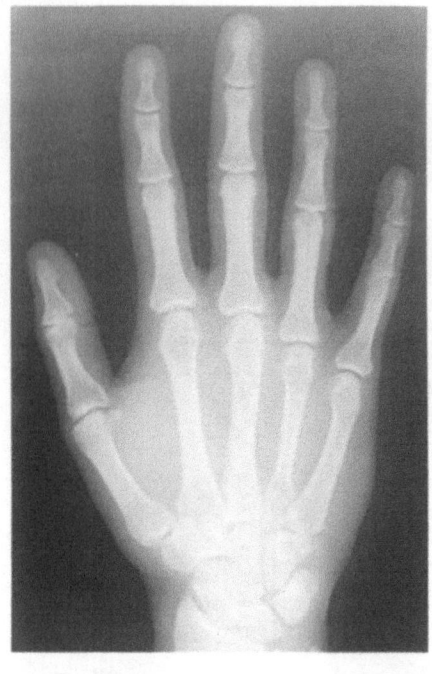

a

b

Fig. 1.17. a Position for the standard PA view of the hand. b Standard PA view of the hand

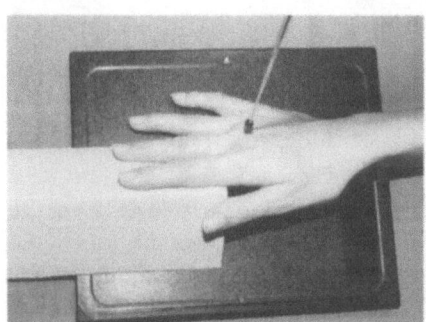
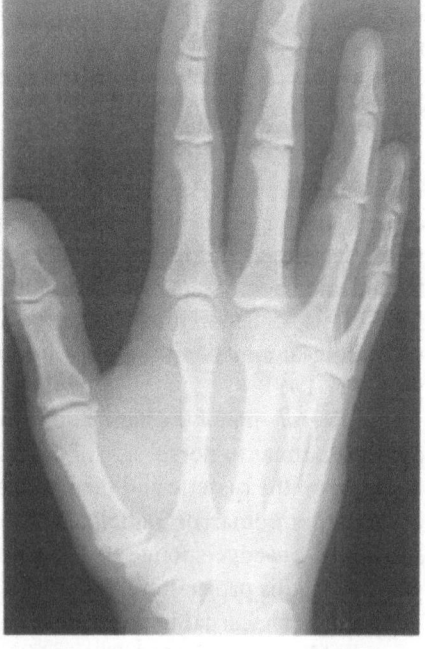

a

b

Fig. 1.18. a Position for the standard PA oblique view of the hand. b The oblique view of the hand allows better evaluation of the ventroradial and dorsoulnar sides of the hand. Extension and slight separation of the fingers allows the metacarpo- and interphalangeal joints to be profiled

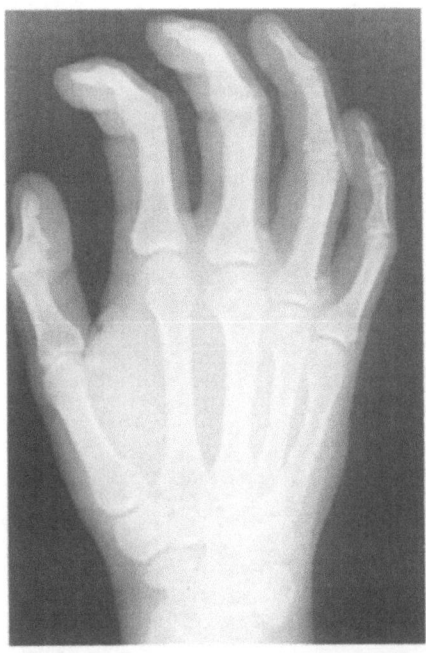

Fig. 1.19. The so-called "Zither Position". Compared with Fig. 1.18b, the interphalangeal joints are not profiled. This position should be avoided

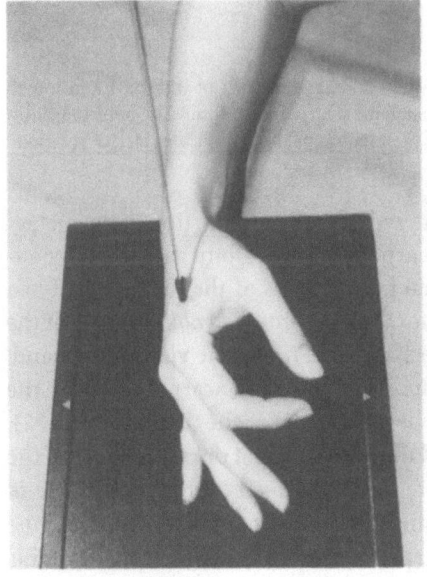

a

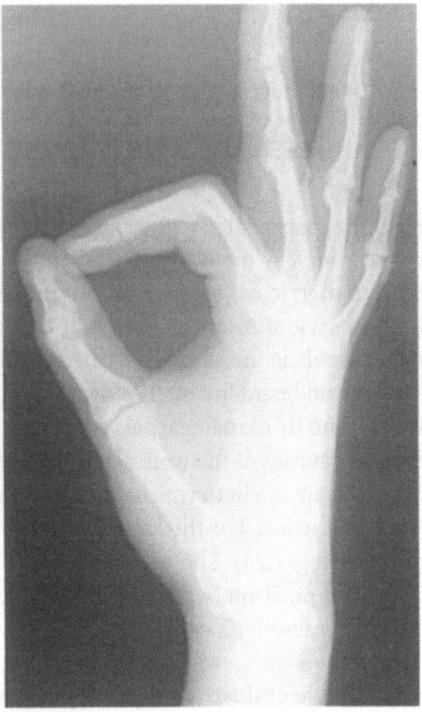

b

Fig. 1.20. a Position for the standard lateral view of the hand. b The lateral view of the hand allows excellent depiction of abnormalities located at the palmar or dorsal side of the hand

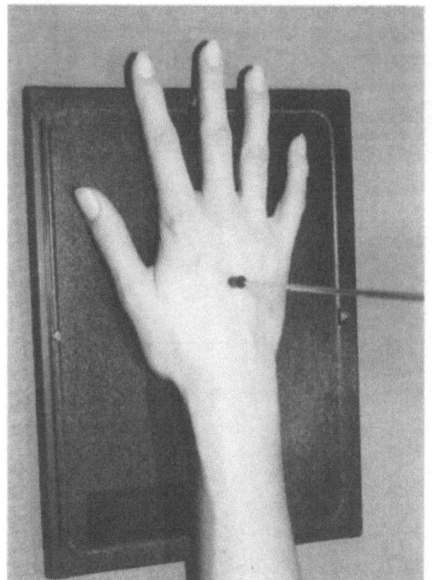

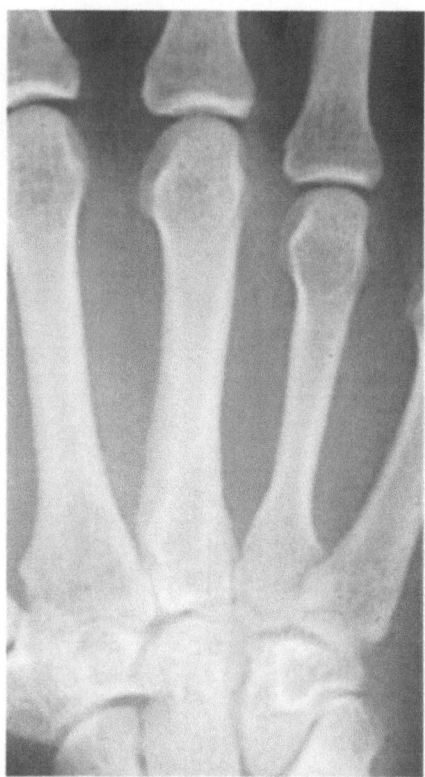

a

b

Fig. 1.21. a Positioning for specific metacarpal bones. **b** PA radiograph of the third and fourth metacarpal bones. The metacarpal head and the carpometacarpal joint should be depicted. Symmetric concavities on the radial and ulnar sides of the metacarpal bone indicates lack of rotation

beam, perpendicular to the cassette, is centered over the midportion of the metacarpal bone. The metacarpal head and the carpometacarpal joint should be depicted. Symmetric concavities on the radial and ulnar sides of the metacarpal bone indicate lack of rotation. The positioning for the *semipronated oblique view* of the metacarpals is the same described for the standard PA oblique view of the hand. The central beam is centered over the midportion of the metacarpals between the second and third metacarpals and again is perpendicular to the cassette (Fig. 1.22). The concavities of the ventral surfaces and the more straight dorsal surfaces of the metacarpals are better visualized and there is just minimal overlap at the base of the metacarpals. For the *lateral view* the ulnar side of the hand and wrist is on the cassette (Fig. 1.23). The axes of the metacarpals are collinear with the distal radius in neutral position (without flexion or extension). The central beam, perpendicular to the cassette, is centered over the midportion of the second metacarpal bone. This is the best view for demonstrating especially dorsal soft tissue swelling, allows reliable evaluation of palmar or dorsal displacement or angulation in case of a fracture, and permits accurate evaluation of subluxation or dislocations at the metacarpophalangeal and carpometacarpal joints.

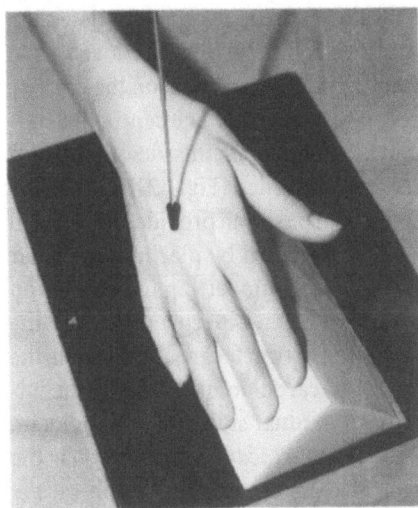 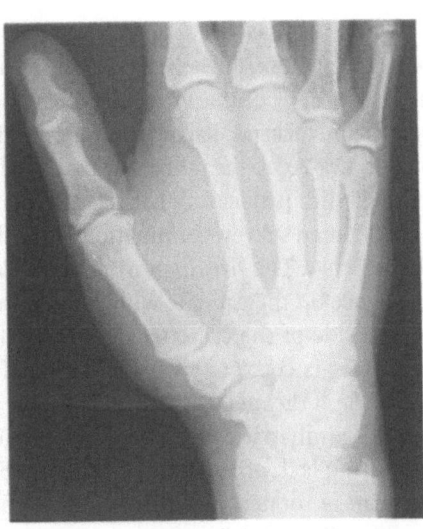

a   b

Fig. 1.22. a Positioning technique for the semipronated oblique view of the metacarpals. **b** Semipronated oblique view of the metacarpals. The concavities of the ventral surfaces and the more straight dorsal surfaces of the metacarpals are better visualized and there is only minimal overlap at the base of the metacarpals

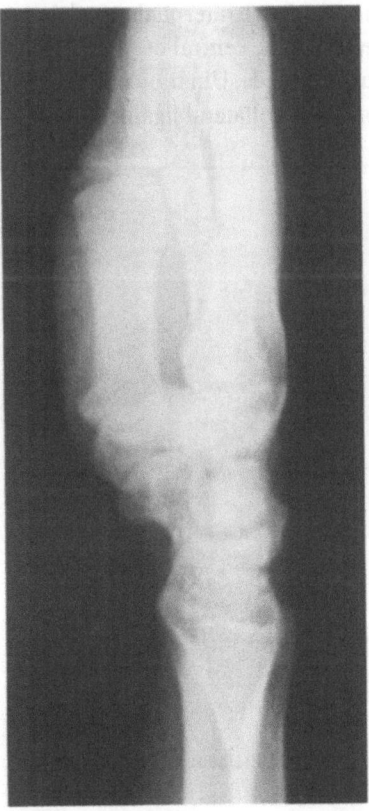

Fig. 1.23. Lateral view of the hand. For explanation see the text

The *metacarpal heads view (Brewerton view)* is a very sensitive view for detection of early erosions of the metacarpal heads and occult fractures of the metacarpal heads [26, 27]. For this view the dorsum of the fingers are placed flat on the cassette and the metacarpophalangeal joints are flexed 65° (Fig. 1.24a). The central beam is angled 15°–20° to the radial side and the thumb is extended. On this view the second through fifth metacarpophalangeal joints are exactly profiled (Fig. 1.24b).

A detailed survey examination of the first metacarpal bone provides the PA and the AP view. The *first metacarpal true PA view* is obtained by placing the thenar eminence on the cassette with abduction of the thumb and letting the palm drop off the side of the cassette (Fig. 1.25a). The central beam – perpendicular to the cassette – is centered over the midportion of the first metacarpal bone. On the radiograph the metacarpal head and the carpometacarpal joint should be included and symmetric concavities on both the radial and ulnar side should be evident, indicating lack of rotation (Fig. 1.25b). For the *first metacarpal true AP view* the forearm is rotated internally 180° to position the dorsum of the thumb on the cassette (Fig. 1.26). The fingers are extended. The central beam and the criteria for an adequate examination are the same as for the AP view.

For imaging of a specific finger the basic survey should include a PA view, an oblique view, and a lateral view. The positioning techniques are as described before. The finger of interest should be fully extended and the adjacent finger(s) separated from the affected finger to avoid overlapping. The central beam is perpendicular to the cassette and centered to the proximal interphalangeal joint. When finger extension is not possible, a PA view with the central beam angled to pass perpendicular to the joint of interest should be made. Ulnar or radial stress views may be required to demonstrate radial or ulnar collateral ligament or capsule abnormality (Fig. 1.27).

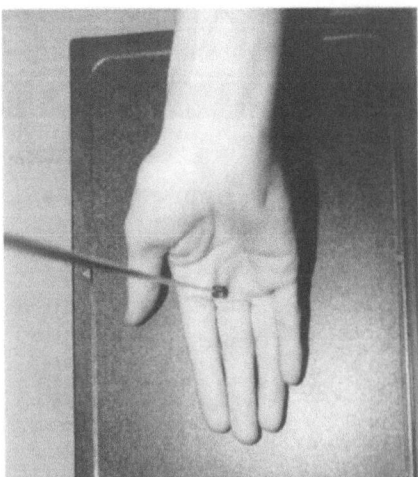
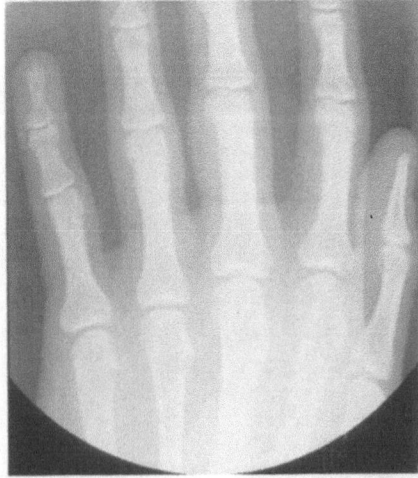

a   b

Fig. 1.24. a Technique for the metacarpal heads view. b On the metacarpal heads view carpometacarpal joints two to five are exactly profiled

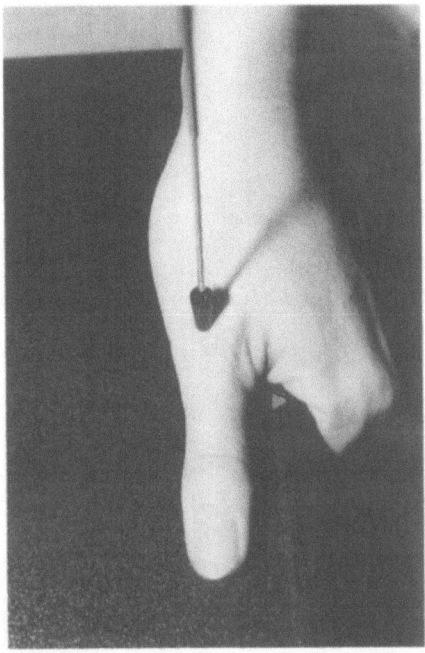

a

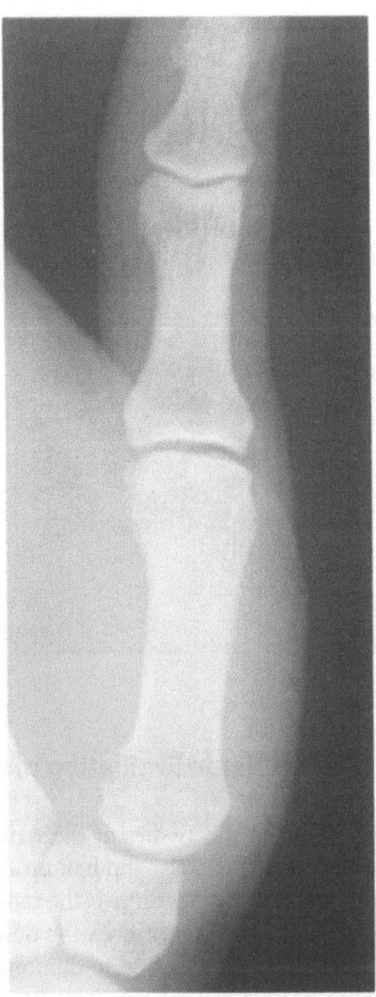

Fig. 1.25. a Technique for the first metacarpal true PA view. **b** First metacarpal true PA view. On the radiograph the metacarpal head and the carpometacarpal joint should be included and symmetric concavities on both the radial and ulnar side should be evident, indicating lack of rotation

b

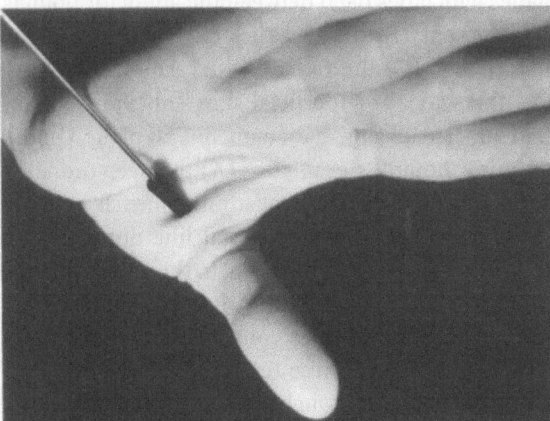

Fig. 1.26. Positioning for the first metacarpal AP view

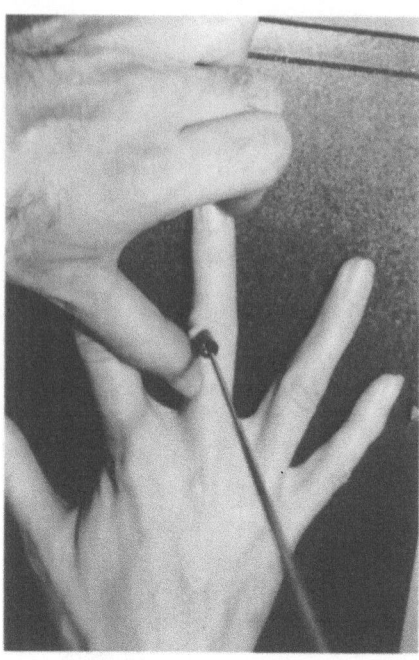

Fig. 1.27. Ulnar stress view of the finger

1.4   Soft tissue Evaluation of the Wrist and Hand

Evaluation of the soft tissues of the wrist and hand often is underestimated and ignored, especially in wrist and hand trauma with diagnosis depending mainly on bony lesions. However, swelling is the radiologic hallmark of trauma and soft tissue swelling may be the first or even the only sign of an underlying fracture [28–31]. Good film quality is required to demonstrate soft tissues adequately without diminishing bone detail. The neutral PA view and the neutral lateral view are the most important and mandatory views for soft tissue evaluation.

On the PA view of the wrist (Fig. 1.28) five fat planes are useful for analysis of trauma: (A) the scaphoid fat planes which lies deep between the abductor pollicis tendon and the radial collateral ligament, (B) the superficial skin–subcutaneous fat plane overlying the proximal thenar, (C) the radial styloid superficial skin–subcutaneous fat plane, (D) the ulnar styloid superficial skin–subcutaneous fat plane, and the (E) the hypothenar superficial skin–subcutaneous fat plane. On the lateral view (Fig. 1.29) four fat planes should be evaluated: (A) the deep pronator quadratus fat plane, which lies between the pronator quadratus muscle and the palmar flexor tendons, (B) the dorsal skin–subcutaneous fat line dorsal to the metacarpals, (C) the dorsal skin–subcutaneous fat line dorsal to the wrist, which is horizontal to convex towards the carpals, and (D) the dorsal skin–subcutaneous fat line dorsal the forearm. The latter three fat lines consist of three anatomic compartments and therefore swelling in any of these three regions is helpful in localizing the site of bony abnormality [32]. In conclusion, soft tissue swelling,

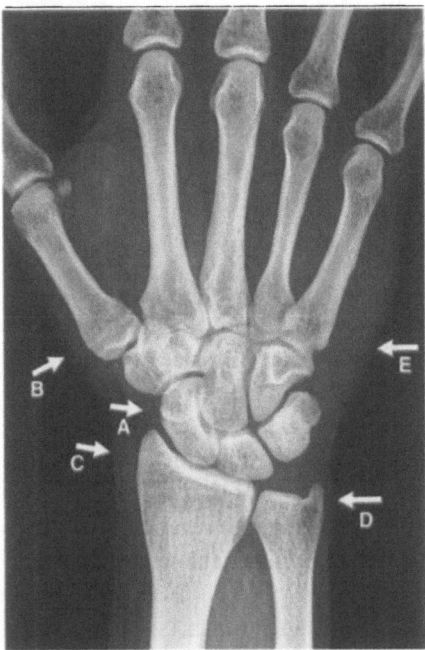

Fig. 1.28. Soft tissue evaluation of the wrist and hand on the PA view. *A* the scaphoid fat plane, *B* the superficial skin–subcutaneous fat plane overlying the proximal thenar, *C* the radial styloid superficial skin–subcutaneous fat plane, *D* the ulnar styloid superficial skin–subcutaneous fat plane, *E* the hypothenar superficial skin–subcutaneous fat plane

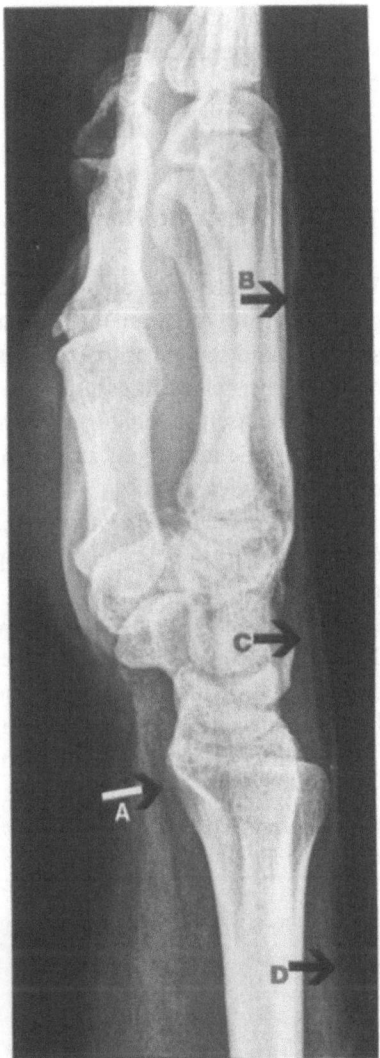

Fig. 1.29. Soft tissue evaluation of the wrist and hand on the lateral view. *A* the deep pronator quadratus fat plane, *B* the dorsal skin–subcutaneous fat line dorsal to the metacarpals, *C* the dorsal skin–subcutaneous fat line dorsal to the wrist, *D* the dorsal skin–subcutaneous fat line dorsal to the forearm

displacement of fat lines, and/or interruption of the fat lines mentioned above, strongly suggests occult fracture and additional views at the time of injury should be obtained for early diagnosis.

1.5   Wrist and Hand Measurements

Various measurements and classifications have been described for traumatic, degenerative, and inflammatory diseases of the wrist and hand. Not all these measurement and classification schemes can be discussed here because of space limitations. The following section is tailored to some of the most important measurements. It should be noted that measurements are only reliable and reproducible if the radiographs are performed in a standardized manner as described earlier in this chapter.

The *radial inclination angle* (syn.: radial deviation, ulnar inclination, radial tilt, radial angulation) describes the angulation of the distal articular surface of the radius in relation to the long axis of the radius on a PA view (Fig. 1.30). The radial inclination can be evaluated by drawing a line (R) through the distal radius shaft. The radial inclination angle is formed by a line (P) perpendicular to the radial line and the line (I) formed between the radial styloid and the distal sigmoid notch [33]. The mean radial inclination angle is 22° (±3°).

The *radial height* (syn.: radial length, length of the radial styloid) is defined as the distance between the two points A and B shown in Fig. 1.30 and is 13.5 (±3.8) mm in length.

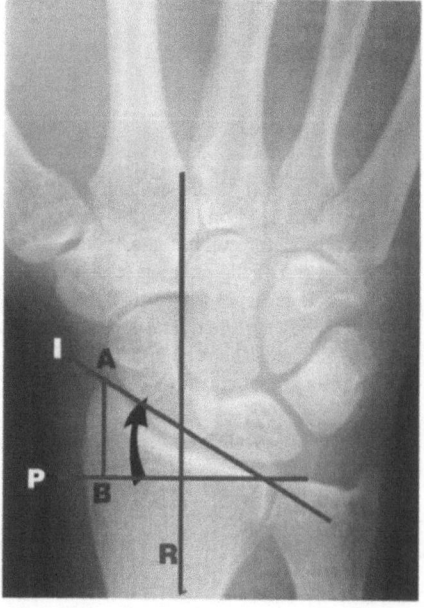

Fig. 1.30. Radial inclination angle and radial height. For explanation see the text

The *palmar tilt* (syn.: palmar slope, volar tilt) is determined by the line (T) running through the most distal dorsal and palmar rims of the distal radius on the lateral radiograph (Fig. 1.31). The degree of palmar tilt is the angle between the line of the palmar tilt and a line perpendicular to the long axis of the distal radius (R) [34]. Normal palmar tilt is on average 11°.

The *carpal angle* is the angle between a line tangential to the proximal edges of the lunate and scaphoid bones and one tangential to the triquetral bone (Fig. 1.32). The mean normal carpal angle is 131° [35]. A change in the carpal angle commonly reflects congenital abnormalities.

The *ulnar head inclination (UI)* and *radioulnar angle (RU)* have been reported to be altered by pathologic conditions of the wrist (congenital abnormalities), and malalignments in the distal radioulnar joint, respectively (Fig. 1.33). The UI is defined as the angle between the long axis of the ulna (U) in a PA view and a line drawn along the articular surface of the ulnar head facing the sigmoid notch (I). RU angle is defined as an angle between the latter line and a line which joins the radial and ulnar limits of the distal radius (R). The UI ranges from 11° to 27°; the RU ranges between 90° and 111° [36]. These two angles have been reported to compare with the opposite side in case of wrist injuries.

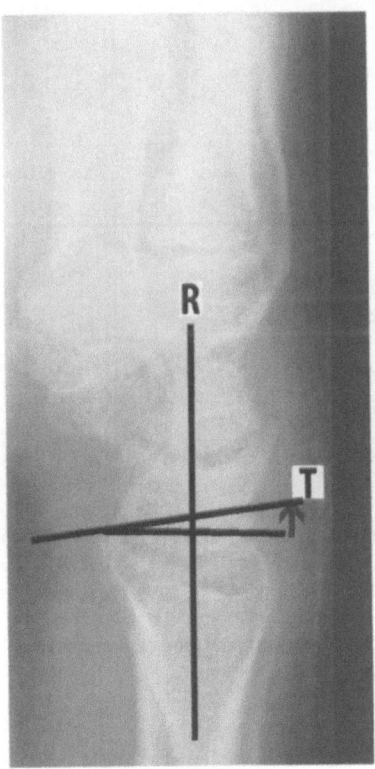

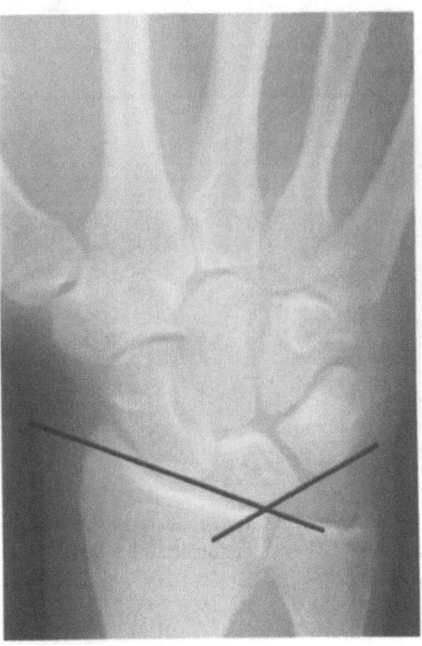

Fig. 1.31. Palmar tilt. For explanation see the text

Fig. 1.32. Carpal angle. For explanation see the text

The *ulnar variance* (syn.: radioulnar index) defines the relative positions of the distal articular surfaces of the radius and ulna. Ulnar variance (Fig. 1.34) can be measured by drawing a line from the carpal joint surface of the distal end of the radius toward the ulna and measuring the distance between this line and the carpal surface of the ulna [37]. With this technique the ulnar variance has a mean of 0.69 mm. In ulnar plus or in ulnar minus variance, the distal cortical surface of the ulna projects more distally or proximally than the distal articular surface of the radius, respectively. Several wrist problems are considered to be directly or indirectly related to relative differences in the length of the distal radius and ulna (e.g., Kienböck's disease, ulnar impingement, carpal instabilities). Standardized radiographic techniques are mandatory!

The *carpal height ratio* is defined as the ratio of the carpal height to the length of the third metacarpal bone measured on a neutral PA view (Fig. 1.35) [38]. The mean carpal height ratio is 0.54 (±4) mm. Carpal collapse may occur in Kienböck's disease, scapholunate advanced collapse, or in rheumatoid arthritis, and may result in a decrease in the carpal height ratio.

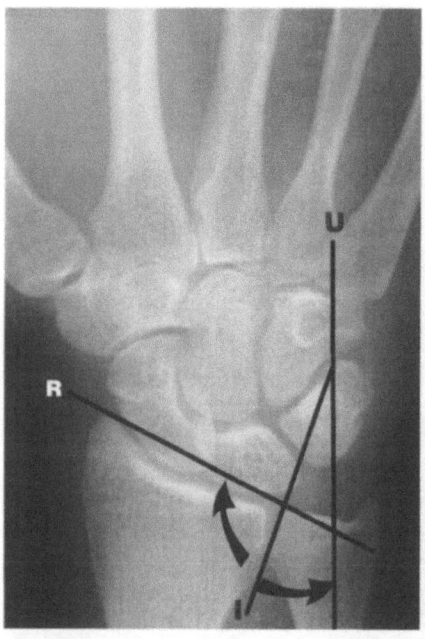

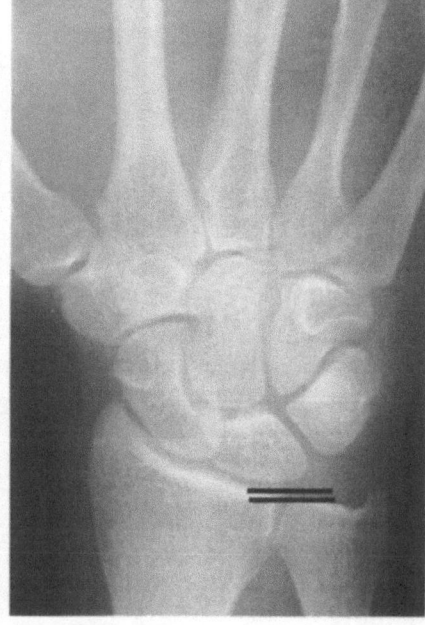

Fig. 1.33. Ulnar head inclination and radioulnar angle. For explanation see the text

Fig. 1.34. Ulnar variance. For explanation see the text

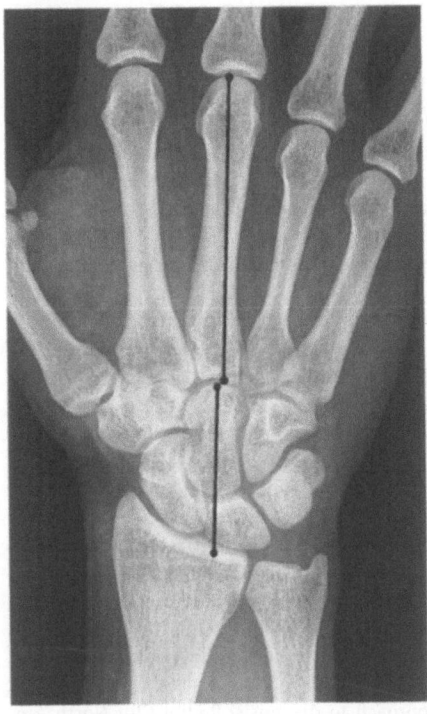

Fig. 1.35. Carpal height ratio. For explanation see the text

References

1. Yin Y et al (1994) Positions and techniques. In: Gilula LA, Yin Y (eds) Imaging of the wrist and hand. Saunders, Philadelphia, pp 93–158
2. Palmer AK et al (1982) Ulnar variance determination. J Hand Surg [Am] 7:376–379
3. Epner RA et al (1982) Ulnar variance: the effect of wrist positioning and roentgen film technique. J Hand Surg [Am] 7:298–305
4. Gilula LA (1979) Carpal injuries: analytic approach and case exercises. AJR 133:503–517
5. Linscheid RL et al (1972) Traumatic instability of the wrist: diagnosis, classification, and pathomechanics. J Bone Joint Surg Am 54:1612–1632
6. Taleisnik J (1984) Classification of carpal instability. Bull Hosp Joint Dis 3:135–140
7. Frahm R, Drescher E (1988) Radiologische Diagnostik nach komplizierter distaler Radiusfraktur unter besonderer Berücksichtigung der Computertomographie. Radiologe 148:295–300
8. Frahm R et al (1989) CT-Diagnostik bei Fehlstellung nach distaler Radiusfraktur. Radiologe 29:68–72
9. Mino DE et al (1983) The role of radiography and computerized tomography in the diagnosis of incongruity of the distal radioulnar joint: a prospective study. J Hand Surg 8:30–31
10. Nishikawa T et al (1985) Functional radiography of the wrist joint. J Jpn Hand Assoc 2:54–57
11. Gilula LA, Weeks PM (1978) Posttraumatic ligamentous instabilities of the wrist. Radiology 129:641–651
12. Taleisnik J (1988) Current concepts review: carpal instability. J Bone Joint Surg Am 70:1262–1268
13. Larsen CF et al (1991) Measurements of carpal bone angles on lateral wrist radiographs. J Hand Surg [Am] 16:888–893
14. Bontrager KL (1986) Radiographic positioning and related anatomy. In: Mosby-Yearbook, 1st edn. Mosby-Yearbook, St Louis, pp 111–126

15. Eisenberg RL et al (1989) Radiographic positioning, 1st edn. Little Brown, Boston, pp 42–63
16. Jones WA (1988) Beware the sprained wrist: the incidence and diagnosis os scapholunate instability. J Bone Joint Surg Br 70:293–297
17. Watson HK, Black DM (1987) Instabilities of the wrist. Hand Clin 3:103–111
18. Sartoris DJ, Resnick D (1988) Plain film radiography: routine and specialized techniques andprojections. In: Resnick D, Niwayama G (eds) Diagnosis of bone and joint disorders, vol 1. Saunders, Philadelphia, pp 3–54
19. Bernau A, Berquist TH (1983) Orthopaedic positioning, 1st edn. Urban and Schwarzenberg, Baltimore, pp 108–132
20. Ballinger PW (1986) Merrill's atlas of radiographic positions and radiologic procedures, vol 1. Mosby, St Louis, pp 50–74
21. Conway WF et al (1985) The carpal boss: an overview of radiographic evaluation. Radiology 156:29–31
22. Wilson JN (1954) Profiles of the carpal canal. J Bone Joint Surg Am 36:127–132
23. Hart VL, Ganyor V (1942) Radiography of the carpal canal. J Bone Joint Surg 23:382–383
24. Gruber L (1991) Practical approaches to obtaining hand radiographs and special techniques in hand radiology. Hand Clin 7:1–20
25. Schernberg F (1996) Radiography for wrist instabilities. In: Gliula LA, Yin Y (eds) Imaging of the wrist and hand. Saunders, Philadelphia, pp 169–188
26. Brewerton DA (1967) A tangential radiographic projection for demonstrating involvement of metacarpal heads in rheumatoid arthritis. Br J Radiol 40:233–234
27. Lane CS (1977) Detecting occult fractures of the metacarpal head: the Brewerton view. J Hand Surg 2:131–133
28. Curtis DJ et al (1984) Importance of soft-tissue evaluation in hand and wrist trauma: statistical evaluation. AJR 142:781–788
29. Curtis DJ (1981) Injuries of the wrist: an approach to diagnosis. Radiol Clin North Am 19:625–644
30. MacEwan DW (1964) Changes due to trauma in the fat plane overlying the quadratus muscle: a radiologic sign. Radiology 82:879–886
31. Curtis DJ (1994) Radiography of soft tissues in trauma to the wrist and hand. In: Gilula L, Yin Y (eds) Imaging of the wrist and hand. Saunders, Philadelphia, pp 159–167
32. Curtis DJ et al (1985) Compartmentalized swelling in hand and wrist trauma. AJR 145:195
33. DiBenedetto MR et al. (1991) Quantification of error in measurements of radial inclination and radial-carpal distance. J Hand Surg [Am] 16:399–400
34. Mann FA et al (1992) Normal palmar tilt: is dorsal tilting really normal? J Hand Surg [Br] 17:315–317
35. Harper HAS et al (1974) The carpal angle in American populations. Invest Radiol 9:217–221
36. Tornwall AH, et al (1986) Radiological examination and measurements of the wrist and distal radioulnar joint. Acta Radiol Diagn 27:581–588
37. Gelberman RH et al (1975) Ulnar variance in Kienböck's disease. J Bone Joint Surg Am 57:674–676
38. Stahelin A et al (1989) Determining carpal collapse: an improved method. J Bone Joint Surg Am 71:1400–1405

2 Conventional Arthrography

W. R. OBERMANN

2.1 Introduction

After the first applications of arthrography in the wrist joint in 1961 [1] this technique was mainly used for the diagnosis of rheumatoid arthritis. Only after 1979 [2, 3] did it become clear that this technique could, in combination with fluoroscopic spot filming and videofluoroscopy, properly evaluate the site of traumatic intra-articular ligament and disc ruptures. Later, with the aid of stress maneuvers, intra-articular ligament and disc ruptures could be easily diagnosed and even qualified [4], a technique also applicable to MR imaging [5]. This chapter will deal with an anatomical-radiological correlation study, arthrographic techniques and examples of variations and pathology shown by arthrography.

2.2 Anatomical-Radiological Correlation

In a previous study [4] an arthrogram in five fresh adult cadaver wrists was performed using a liquid silicone rubber compound mixed with barium sulfur powder and methylene blue. The injection was done in the radiocarpal joint. The liquid rubber became solid after catalyzation in about 3 h (setting time). The density of the compound was made equal to the density of 50% dilution of Hexabrix 320 (320 mg iodine per ml), which is the contrast medium usually used for arthrography [6]. Most of the following arthrographic anatomy is based on this study.

2.2.1 The Compartments of the Wrist

Functionally the wrist joint consists of the link between the forearm and the hand whereby motion takes place mainly at the radiocarpal and midcarpal joint. The motion between carpal and metacarpal bones is almost non-existent in the middle of the hand and increases toward the ulnar and radial directions, especially at the first carpometacarpal joint. The joint space of the wrist is divided into five compartments separated by interosseous ligaments or a triangular fibrocartilage (Fig. 2.1).

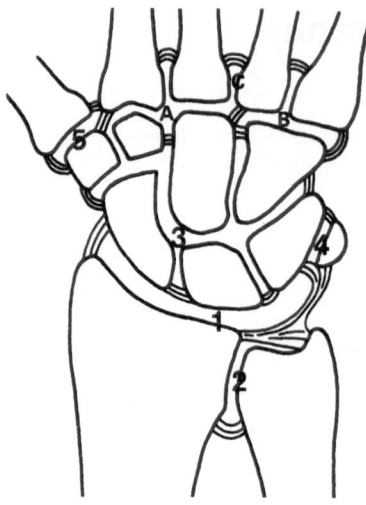

Fig. 2.1. Schematic drawing of the compartments of the wrist, showing the radiocarpal compartment (*1*), distal radioulnar joint compartment (*2*), midcarpal compartment (*3*) in connection with the common carpometacarpal compartment (*A, B*) and intermetacarpal compartments (*C*), pisotriquetral compartment (*4*) and first carpometacarpal compartment (*5*). The compartments are separated by interosseous ligaments and a disc. Sometimes the carpometacarpal compartment is divided into two (*A, B*). (Reprinted from [4], with kind permission from Elsevier Science)

2.2.1.1   The Radiocarpal Compartment

The radiocarpal compartment is formed proximally by the distal surface of the radius and the triangular fibrocartilage and distally by the proximal row of carpal bones excluding the pisiform. Interosseous ligaments extend between the carpal bones of the proximal row and prevent communication between this compartment and the midcarpal compartment (Fig. 2.2).

These interosseous ligaments run from dorsally to volarly, the scapholunate interosseous ligament being large and strong and the lunotriquetral interosseous ligament being much smaller and more convex (Fig. 2.3). The articular disc or triangular fibrocartilage (Fig. 2.3) prevents communication between the radiocarpal and distal radioulnar compartments (Fig. 2.2), whereas a part of the triangular fibrocartilage complex, sometimes called the meniscus, is attached to the triquetrum preventing communication between the radiocarpal and pisiform-triquetral compartments.

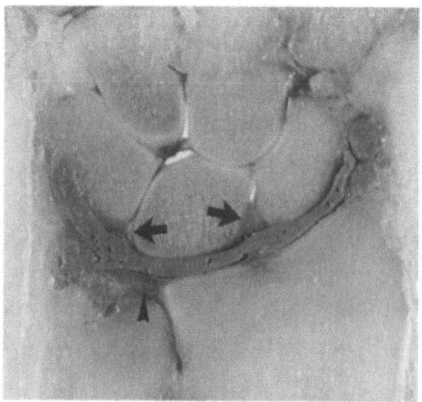

Fig. 2.2. Coronal cryosection specimen (*dark*) showing contrast (rubber compound) in the radiocarpal joint. The interosseous ligaments (*arrows*) and articular disc (*arrowhead*) prevent penetration of the contrast into the midcarpal joint and distal radioulnar joint

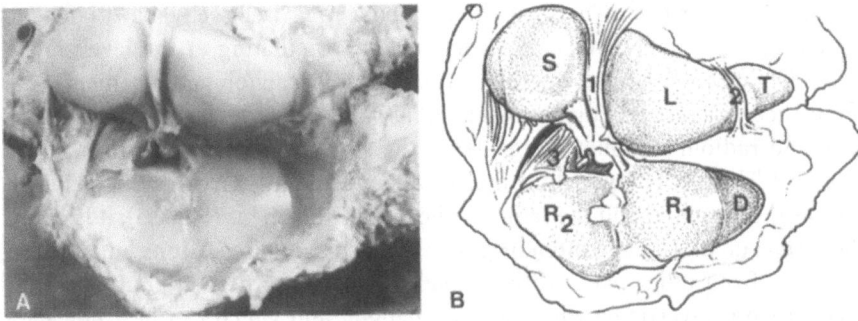

Fig. 2.3. Photograph of a dissection of a fixed specimen (*A*) and a schematic representation (*B*). Right hand. The dorsal side of the radiocarpal joint is widely opened as the hand is strongly volar-flexed. Note the large scapholunate interosseous ligament (*1*) compared with the much smaller lunotriquetral interosseous ligament (*2*) which runs along a short and more convex circumference of the bones. Note also the very convex proximal surface of the triquetrum (*T*) opposite the disc (*D*). Scaphoid (*S*), lunate (*L*), radial facets (*R1, R2*) and radiolunotriquetral ligament (*3*) are also seen. (Reprinted from [4], with kind permission from Elsevier Science)

The radiocarpal compartment shows a prestyloid recess (Fig. 2.2) at the region of the triangular fibrocartilage which approaches the ulnar styloid process. The capsule at the dorsal side of the radiocarpal compartment or radiocarpal joint attaches rather distally at the scaphoid and lunate (Fig. 2.4) providing a lot of space when injecting the radiocarpal joint from dorsally.

Sometimes there is a local outpouching of this dorsal capsule near the scaphoid and radius called the dorsal recess. At the volar side of the radiocarpal joint, the

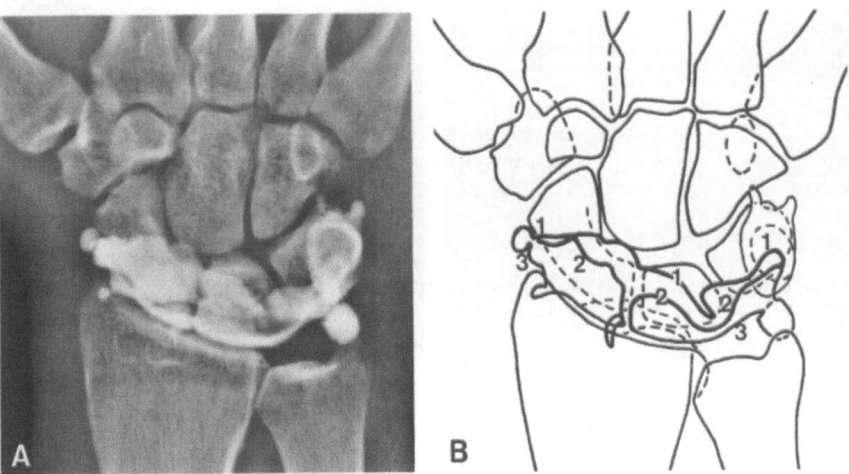

Fig. 2.4. Posteroanterior arthrogram (*A*) and schematic representation (*B*). The dorsal and volar distal borders are projected free from each other and, hence, can be appreciated, the normal configuration being well known. The distal border of the dorsal side is indicated by thick line *1*, the distal border of volar side is indicated by thick line *2* and the proximal border at the deepest point of the radial facets and the disc is indicated by thick line *3*. (Reprinted from [4], with kind permission from Elsevier Science)

joint is much narrower. There are three outpouchings well seen on a 70° oblique view (Fig. 2.5). First there is the volar recess, originating at the level of the scapholunate interval and laterally near the radioscapholunate ligament. Secondly there is a recess in the form of a sulcus running along the radioscaphocapitate and radiolunotriquetral ligaments, the so-called interligamentous sulcus (Fig. 2.5). The third outpouching is also like a sulcus and runs between the distal pole of the scaphoid and the radioscaphocapitate ligament (Fig. 2.5); it is called the distal sulcus. Ganglia often originate from sulci and recessions but can also originate from other parts of the capsule. Sometimes there are outpouchings formed from diverticula which are not ganglia and which can best be called diverticles (Fig. 2.4).

There can be a connection with the pisotriquetral joint (Fig. 2.6), and in a group of 70 patients in whom a radiocarpal arthrogram was performed [4] this was found in two thirds (64%).

The pisotriquetral joint has a proximal (larger) and a distal outpouching best called the proximal and distal recesses (Fig. 2.7). The proximal recess is mostly larger to accommodate the motion of the pisiform bone during flexion-extension motion (sesame bone).

The triangular fibrocartilage or disc often shows a slit-like perforation running from dorsally to volarly at the thinnest (radial) portion of the disc (Fig. 2.8). This was seen in a young cadaver specimen and in 18 of a group of 65 patients without

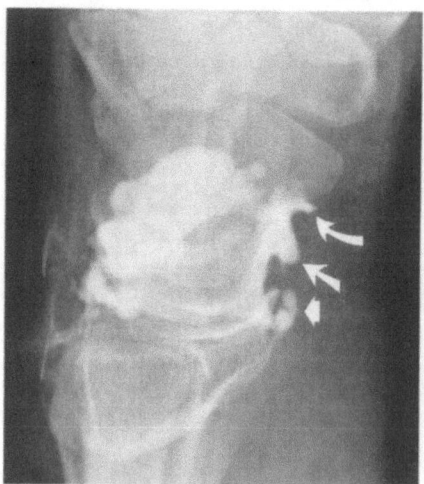
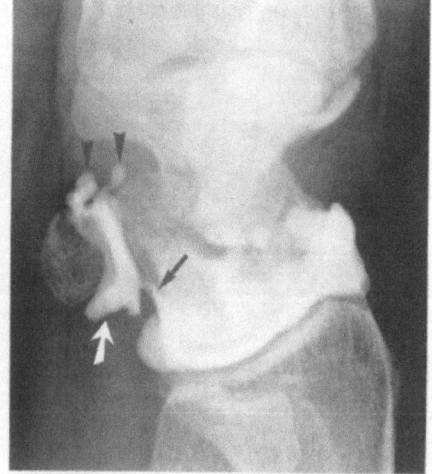

Fig. 2.5. Radiograph of the 70° oblique view. There is good demonstration of the volar recess (*short arrow*), the interligamentous sulcus (*arrow*) and the distal sulcus (*curved arrow*). (Reprinted from [4], with kind permission from Elsevier Science)

Fig. 2.6. Reversed 70° oblique view radiograph showing the small connection between the radiocarpal joint and the pisotriquetral (*PT*) joint (*arrow*). The proximal recess of the PT joint (*white arrow*) and diverticular outpouchings at the distal recess of the PT joint (*arrowheads*) are also seen. (Reprinted from [4], with kind permission from Elsevier Science)

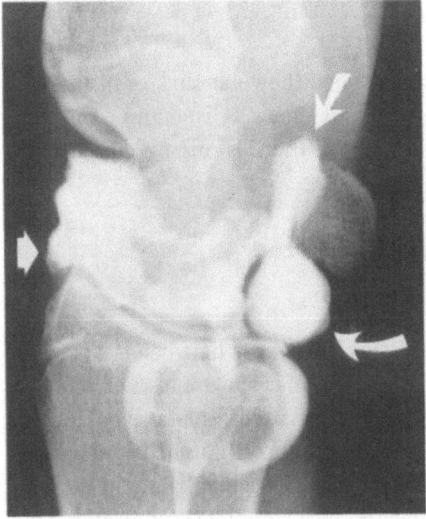 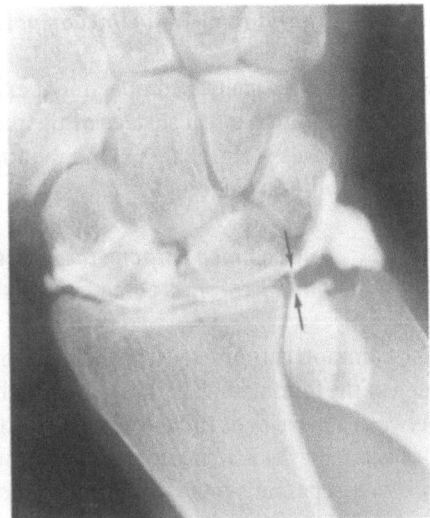

Fig. 2.7. Reversed oblique radiograph showing the large proximal recess (*arrow*) and small distal recess (*curved arrow*) of the pisotriquetral joint, and the small dorsal recess (*short arrow*). (Reprinted from [4], with kind permission from Elsevier Science)

Fig. 2.8. Posteroanterior radiograph showing a slit-like disc perforation (*arrows*). (Reprinted from [4], with kind permission from Elsevier Science)

previous radius or ulna fracture (28%). It was independent of ulnar length and age and bore no relation to complaints [4]; when arthrograms were made bilaterally the perforation was usually bilateral. Probably these slit-like perforations have no clinical significance.

2.2.1.2 The Distal Radioulnar Compartment

The distal radioulnar compartment or joint is the compartment where the cartilage-covered ulnar head articulates with the cartilage-covered ulnar notch of the radius and with the triangular fibrocartilage (Fig. 2.1). The articular disc forms the barrier to the radiocarpal joint. The triangular fibrocartilage or articular disc can be regarded as a ligament complex with a slide function.

2.2.1.3 The Midcarpal Compartment

The midcarpal compartment (Fig. 2.1) extends between the proximal and distal carpal rows and communicates with the common carpometacarpal compartment along the articulation between trapezium and trapezoid. This compartment is bordered proximally by the interosseous ligaments between scaphoid and lunate and between lunate and triquetrum, and distally by the interosseous ligaments between hamate and capitate and between capitate and trapezoid. The latter two ligaments usually do not seal off the articulation completely because they mostly do not run completely dorsally.

2.2.1.4   The Pisiform-Triquetral Compartment

The pisiform-triquetral compartment exists between the volar surface of the tri-quetrum and the dorsal surface of the pisiform and shows a distal and a (larger) proximal recess (Figs. 2.6, 2.7). As mentioned above there is often a connection with the radiocarpal joint.

2.2.1.5   The Common Carpometacarpal Compartment and
Intermetacarpal Compartments

The common carpometacarpal compartment (Fig. 2.1) exists between the base of each of the four medial metacarpals and the distal row of carpal bones, and distally between the bases of the metacarpals, to form three small intermetacarpal joints. Occasionally the articulation between the hamate and fourth and fifth metacar-pals is a separate synovial cavity produced by an interosseous ligament attach-ment between capitate and fourth metacarpal and by a complete seal provided by the capitate-hamate interosseous ligament.

2.2.1.6   The First Carpometacarpal Compartment

The first carpometacarpal compartment is a separate cavity between the trapezi-um and the base of the first metacarpal (Fig. 2.1).

2.3   Arthrographic Technique

There are six joints in the hand and wrist region that are regularly injected. These are the distal radioulnar joint, the radiocarpal joint, the midcarpal joint, the pisot-riquetral joint, the carpometacarpal I joint and the metacarpophalangeal I joint. The patient is best positioned prone on the X-ray table with the arm alongside the head and toward the end of the table. The examiner can be seated at the end of the table. The fluoroscopic unit can be a conventional unit with the tube under the table or a C-arc also with the tube under the table.

The puncture site should be marked under fluoroscopy and, after sterile skin preparation of the whole hand, the hand should be placed on a sterile wrap. Subse-quently, under fluoroscopic control, a 23G short needle connected to a preloaded extension tube and syringe containing Hexabrix 320 mixed with xylocaine 2% (1:1) can be directed to the particular joint. The needle is in the joint cavity if the contrast medium runs quickly away from the needle tip. The mixture containing 2% anesthetic is useful for pain-testing (see later) and the density of the contrast medium is adequate for good images.

In the case of injecting corticosteroids (see later) the position of the needle is also controlled by the same contrast medium, after which the corticosteroid can be injected.

2.3.1   The Radiocarpal Joint

The puncture can be done from dorsally, obliquely directed to the radiocarpal joint with the hand in a lateral position and somewhat volar-flexed. The puncture can be done at the region of the lunate or scaphoid. When using the dorsal puncture between lunate and radius a line can be drawn at the dorsal side of the wrist under fluoroscopic control, connecting the proximal border of the hamate with the middle of the lunate and towards proximal, crossing the radiolunate space (Fig. 2.9).

Thereafter the wrist should be positioned laterally with the hand in some flexion. At the site just distal to the overhanging dorsal lip of the radius, a vertical line should be drawn crossing the other line. The point at which the two lines intersect is the puncture point. The puncture should be performed with the hand in a lateral position. When the needle enters the joint space (Fig. 2.10) the hand should be rotated back to a frontal position (Fig. 2.10) with the palm flat on the tabletop and the joint spaces between scaphoid and lunate and between lunate and triquetrum profiled as much as possible. Thereafter some contrast should be injected to determine whether the needle is intra-articular. If not, the needle has to be repositioned slightly to achieve such a position. Two to five milliliters should be injected depending on the joint capacity and the connections with other joints. The connection site with other joints should be imaged (Fig. 2.11).

After injection the wrist should be gently moved and thereafter more vigorously in radial and ulnar deviation directions in order to open perforations which were sealed of in neutral position. The standard series of images consists of a

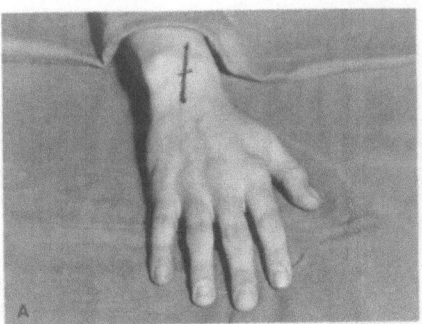

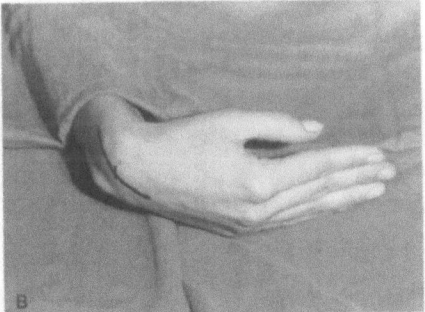

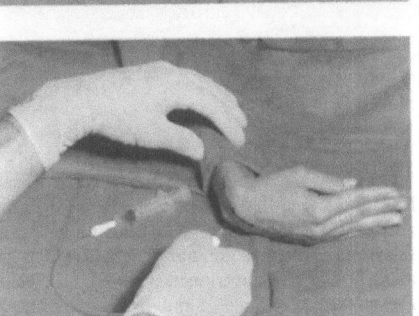

Fig. 2.9. A, B Photographs of the puncture site marking and needle position. The proximodistal line courses over the proximal border of the hamate and the middle of the lunate. The *short transverse line* represents the level of the space between the dorsal lip of the radius and the lunate in a lateral position and with some volar flexion of the hand. **C** Photograph of the needle puncture at the point of intersection of the two skin lines towards the radiolunate joint space. The needle is advanced into the joint under fluoroscopic control. (Reprinted from [4], with kind permission from Elsevier Science)

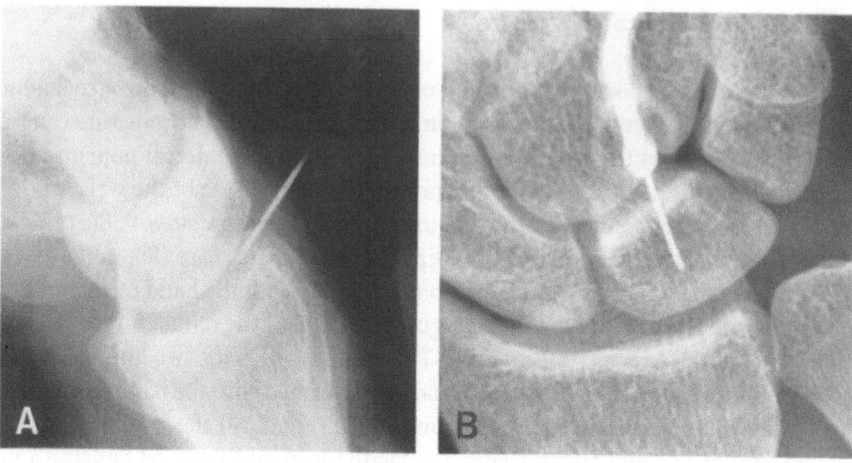

Fig. 2.10. A Lateral radiograph of needle position at the joint space between the radius and lunate. **B** Posteroanterior radiograph after rotating and extending the hand to a posteroanterior position. The needle maintains its close relation with the radiolunate joint and is near the dorsal lip of the radius. The joint spaces between lunate and scaphoid and between lunate and triquetrum are projected as freely as possible. (Reprinted from [4], with kind permission from Elsevier Science)

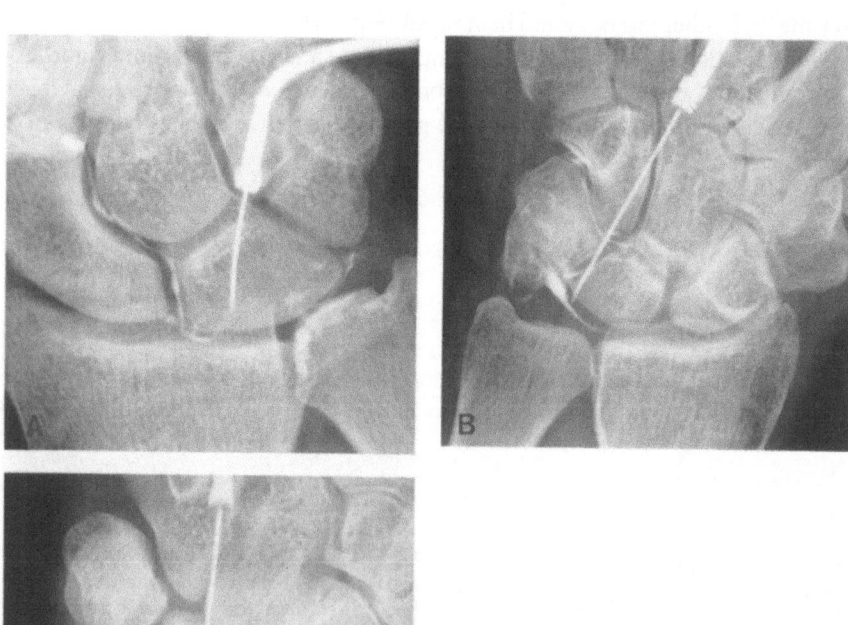

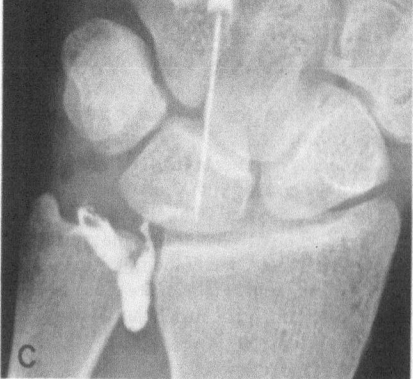

Fig. 2.11A–C. Posteroanterior radiographs. **A** Fast leakage during injection at the level of the scapholunate joint. Note also the simultaneous filling of the distal radioulnar joint. **B** Fast leakage at the level of the lunotriquetral joint. **C** Fast leakage at the lateral side of the discus. (Reprinted from [4], with kind permission from Elsevier Science)

posteroanterior (Fig. 2.4) and lateral view, a 70° oblique and reversed oblique view (Figs. 2.5, 2.6), a distraction view (Fig. 2.12) and radial and ulnar deviation stress view (Figs. 2.13, 2.14).

Interosseous ligament ruptures are best viewed and qualified on the last three views. In the case of a disc perforation or rupture an additional disc profiled view can be taken (Fig. 2.15). In the case of abnormalities at a particular part of the joint additional appropriate views can be taken. Sometimes, because of passing a tendon sheath, after removal of the needle some tendon sheath filling is seen because of back leakage from the joint.

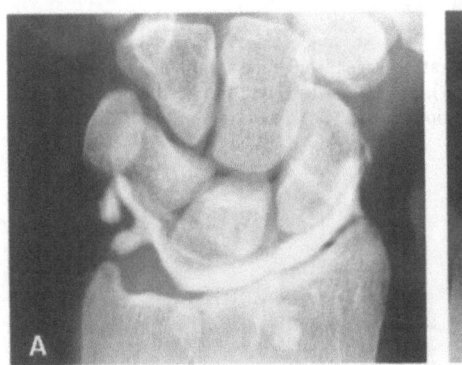
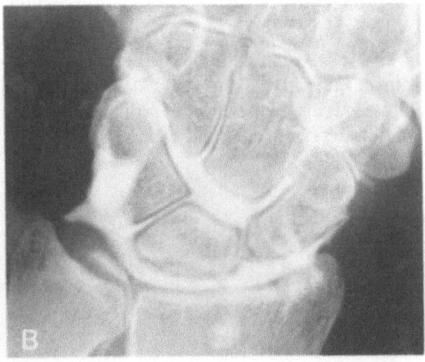

Fig. 2.12A, B. Posteroanterior radiographs. **A** Distraction view with contrast only in the radiocarpal joint. **B** Distraction view with contrast in all three compartments through a lunotriquetral interosseous ligament and a disc rupture. (Reprinted from [4], with kind permission from Elsevier Science)

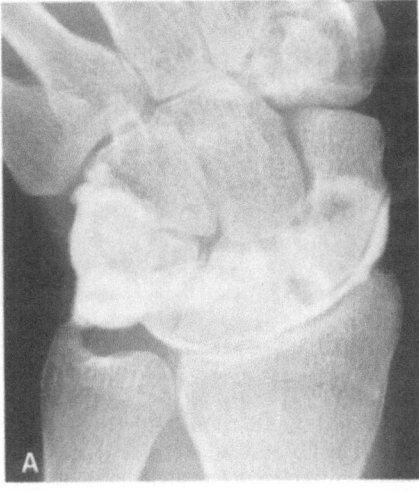
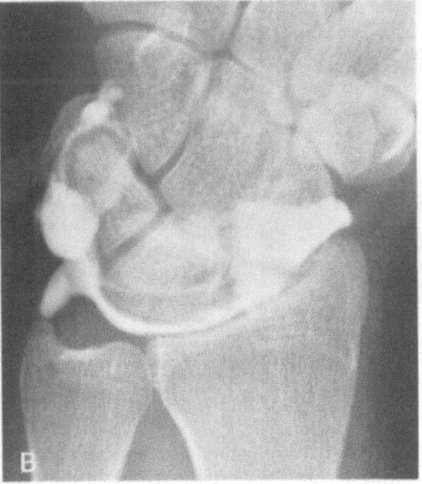

Fig. 2.13A, B. Posteroanterior radiographs. **A** Ulnar deviation with stress. **B** Radial deviation with stress. Note the smoothly curved scapholunate contrast-bordered junction on ulnar deviation and the lunotriquetral junction on radial deviation. (Reprinted from [4], with kind permission from Elsevier Science)

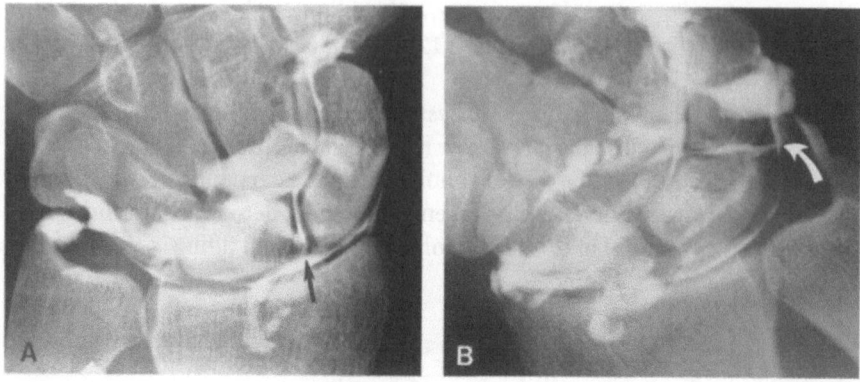

Fig. 2.14A, B. Posteroanterior radiographs. **A** Contrast leakage through the scapholunate interosseous ligament only after ulnar stress deviation (*arrow*). **B** Contrast leakage through the lunotriquetral interosseous ligament only after radial stress deviation (*arrow*). (Reprinted from [4], with kind permission from Elsevier Science)

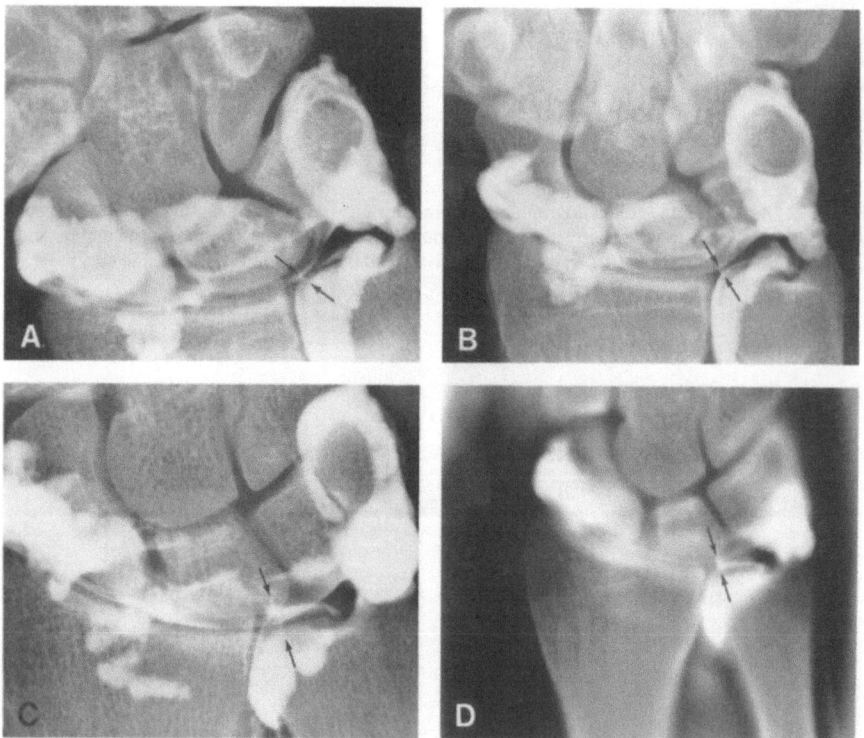

Fig. 2.15A–D. Posteroanterior radiographs and tomogram. **A** Slit-like perforation of the disc filled with contrast (*arrows*) and projected over the ulnar head and lunate cartilage. **B** Free projection of the slit-like disc perforation (*arrows*) by elevating the hand from the table-top. **C** Disc perforation (*arrows*) with more substantial overprojection of ulnar head and lunate cartilage. **D** Tomography of example C with clear delineation of the disc with the slit-like perforation (*arrows*) at the thinnest portion (TFCC I type perforation). (Reprinted from [4], with kind permission from Elsevier Science)

2.3.2   The Midcarpal Joint

The midcarpal joint can best be punctured from dorsally at the junction of the scaphoid, capitate and trapezoid (Fig. 2.16) in a perpendicular direction. On entering the joint a diminished resistance is felt. Injected contrast should run away from the needle tip if it is intra-articular; if it does not the needle tip should be repositioned.

The standard views are approximately the same as those for the radiocarpal joint. The same stress maneuvers are again useful for assessment of the interosseous ligament. In this joint about 2 ml contrast medium can be injected too.

2.3.3   The Distal Radioulnar Joint

The distal radioulnar joint should also be punctured from dorsally, not directed to the joint space between ulnar head and radial notch but more to the lateral side of the ulnar head, somewhat proximal (Fig. 2.17).

When meeting the cartilage of the head the needle should be intra-articular. When the contrast medium runs away from the needle tip the needle position is correct. About 1 ml contrast medium can be injected. Often there is some back-leakage to the extensor digiti minimi tendon sheath, which is often passed by the needle.

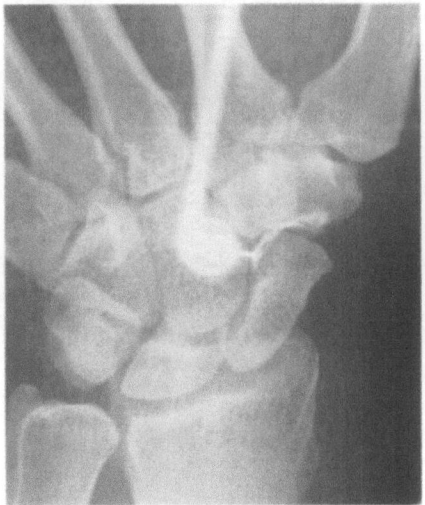

Fig. 2.16. Injection of the midcarpal joint from dorsally at the junction of scaphoid, trapezoid and capitate. The contrast medium runs quickly away from the needle tip

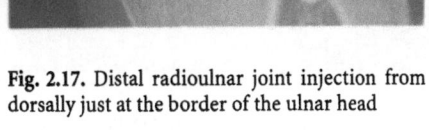

Fig. 2.17. Distal radioulnar joint injection from dorsally just at the border of the ulnar head

2.3.4 The Pisotriquetral Joint

The pisotriquetral joint should be injected from ulnarly when the joint space between pisiform and triquetrum is projected free (Fig. 2.18). The depth is rather difficult to judge and one can easily pass the joint because it is flat. One should therefore start trying to inject when the needle is about 0.5 cm deep.

2.3.5 The Carpometacarpal I Joint

The carpometacarpal joint is saddle-shaped and rather difficult to inject. One can try injecting from dorsally or laterally pointing to the joint space. When performing the injection, some traction at the thumb can help to improve the chances of getting the needle in the joint.

2.3.6 The Metacarpophalangeal I Joint

The metacarpophalangeal I joint can best be punctured dorsally in an oblique manner toward the joint space (Fig. 2.19). Applying some traction when puncturing improves the chances of a successful puncture.

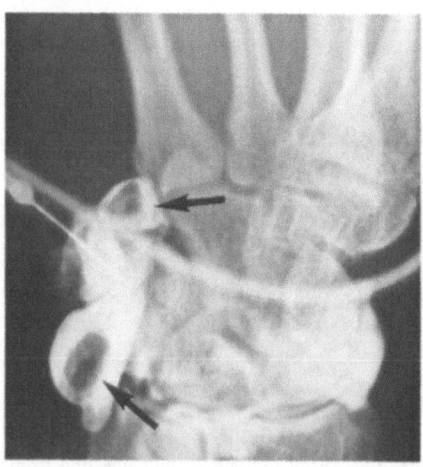

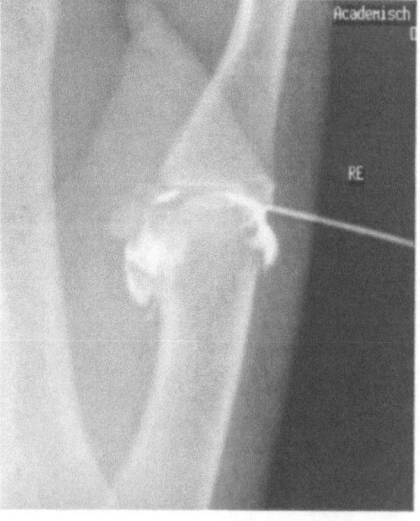

Fig. 2.18. Selective pisotriquetral (*PT*) joint injection after a radiocarpal arthrogram. Injection in a reversed oblique position. Notice two free bodies in the PT joint (*arrows*)

Fig. 2.19. Metacarpophalangeal I joint injection from dorsally

2.4 Indications

2.4.1 The Radiocarpal Joint

The main indication for arthrography of the radiocarpal joint is to search for interosseous ligament and disc rupture (Fig. 2.20) and to correlate it with the patient's complaints. The site of the pain can best be marked by a lead marker. The size of a ligament rupture can be imaged by stress maneuvers (Figs. 2.14, 2.21).

In the case of a wide scapholunate joint space, these stress maneuvers can also distinguish between rupture of the scapholunate interosseous ligament and a lax or elongated ligament (Fig. 2.22). Correlation between the abnormalities found and the complaints can be tested by adding an anesthetic (2%) to the contrast medium (1:1) [7]. In general, adding an anesthetic to the contrast medium allows one to test whether pain is originating from a joint (pain-testing). In a damaged joint it is probably the reactive synovitis that generates the pain, and this can be blocked by an anesthetic.

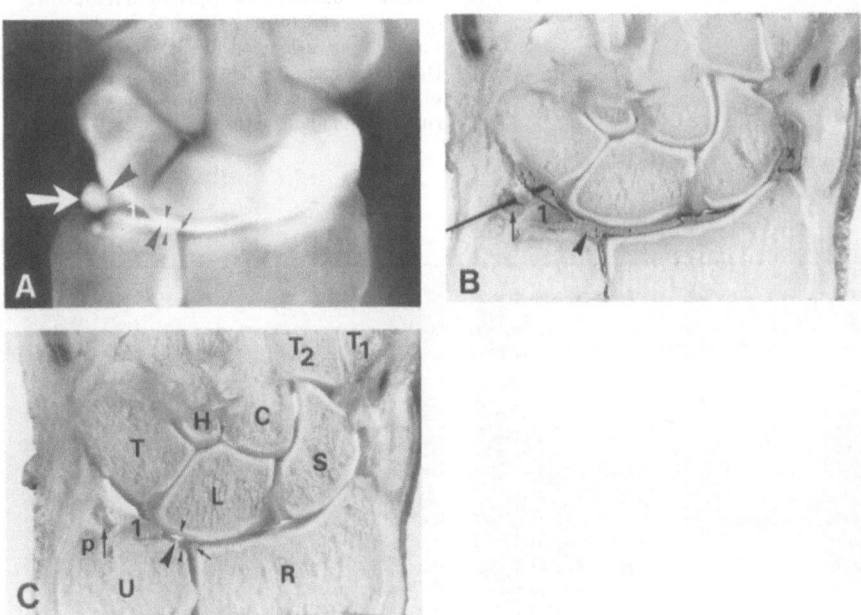

Fig. 2.20A–C. Posteroanterior tomogram and photographs of corresponding coronal cryosections of the same specimen before (**B**) and after removal of the silicon barium compound (**C**). The round prestyloid recess (*black and white arrows*) near the ulnar styloid process (*p*), and the neck-like connection with the radiocarpal joint (*large arrowhead and probe*) are seen. Note also the extensive disc rupture (*arrowhead*) with chondropathy of the lunate and ulnar head at that site (*small arrowheads*) and disc remnant at the medial distal border of the radius (*small arrow*). The disc rupture allowed filling of the distal radioulnar joint. Section through trapezium (*T1*), trapezoid (*T2*), scaphoid (*S*), lunate (*L*), capitate (*C*), hamate (*H*), triquetrum (*T*), radius (*R*), ulnar head (*U*), ulnar styloid process (*p*) and disc (*1*). (Reprinted from [4], with kind permission from Elsevier Science)

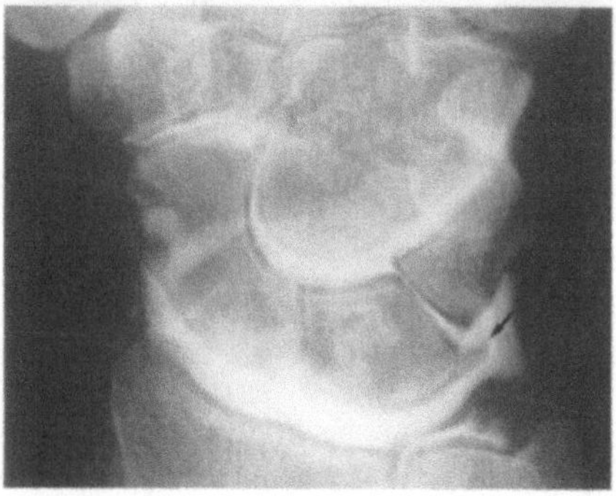

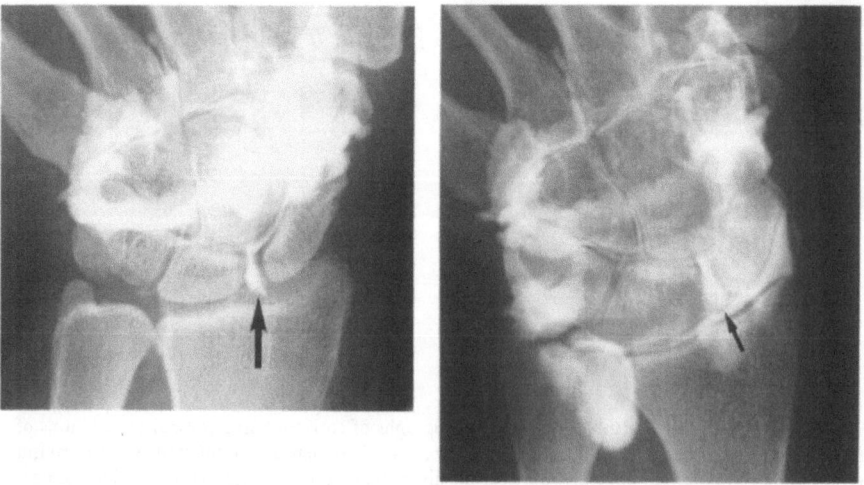

Fig. 2.21A–C. Stress maneuvers at arthrography. **A** Forced ulnar deviation opening the scapholunate interval in a case of scapholunate dissociation. Remnant of the interosseous ligament is seen (*arrow*). There is perforation of the disc (*arrowhead*). **B** Forced radial deviation. Opening of the lunotriquetral interval (*arrow*) showing complete rupture of the lunotriquetral interosseous ligament. **C** Distraction maneuver. There is good visualization of complete lunotriquetral interosseous ligament rupture with remnant (*arrow*)

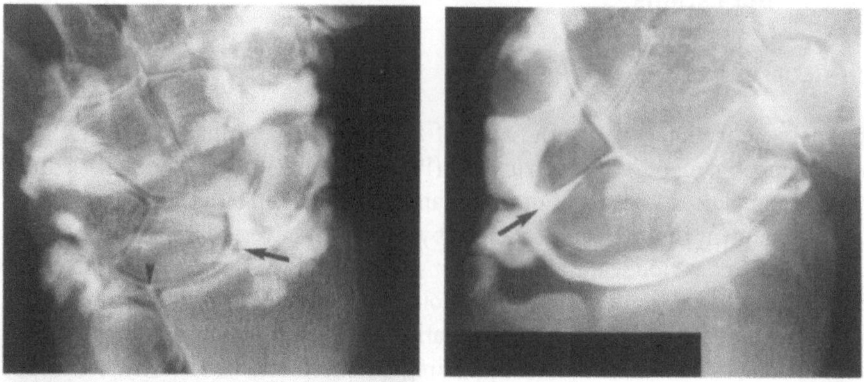

Fig. 2.22A, B. Two examples of scapholunate interosseous ligament laxity without rupture. **A** After midcarpal injection there is pooling of contrast medium between scaphoid and lunate (*arrow*). The ligament is intact. **B** After tricompartment arthrography there is pooling of contrast between scaphoid and lunate. The ligament is intact but elongated (*arrow*). Both patients showed a wide scapholunate joint space on plain film

Other indications are adhesive capsulitis (Fig. 2.23), free bodies, synovitis, ganglia (Fig. 2.24), pain-testing and therapeutic corticosteroid injections. When there is no filling of a ganglion or stalk of a ganglion in a patient with a ganglion recurrence, one can also inject the ganglion directly after the wrist arthrography to demonstrate the origin of the ganglion.

Occasionally one will be confronted with variations (Fig. 2.25) [8].

2.4.2   The Midcarpal Joint

The main indication for a midcarpal joint arthrogram is the search for an interosseous ligament rupture in combination with pain located at the region of the midcarpal compartment. Other indications are adhesive capsulitis, free bodies, synovitis, ganglia, pain-testing and corticosteroid injections.

2.4.3   The Distal Radioulnar Joint

The main indication for a distal radioulnar joint arthrogram is to judge the proximal side of the triangular fibrocartilage in the case of partial tears, together with correlating abnormalities with pain complaints. Other indications are adhesive capsulitis, free bodies, synovitis, pain-testing and therapeutic corticosteroid injections.

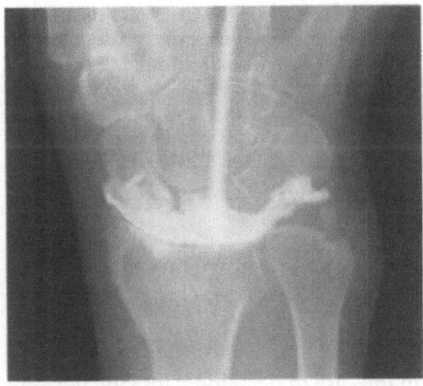

Fig. 2.23. Adhesive capsulitis in a patient with a malunion of a Colles' fracture and pseudoarthrosis of the ulnar styloid process

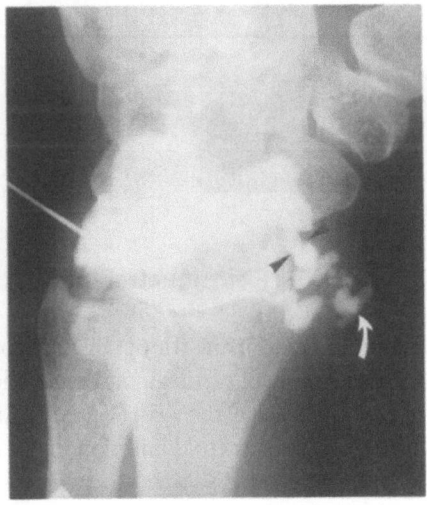

Fig. 2.24. Arthrogram of the radiocarpal joint. A residual ganglion is present at the volar side of the wrist. The ganglion (*arrow*) originates from the radiocarpal joint, in particular from the sulcus interligamentum (*arrowheads*)

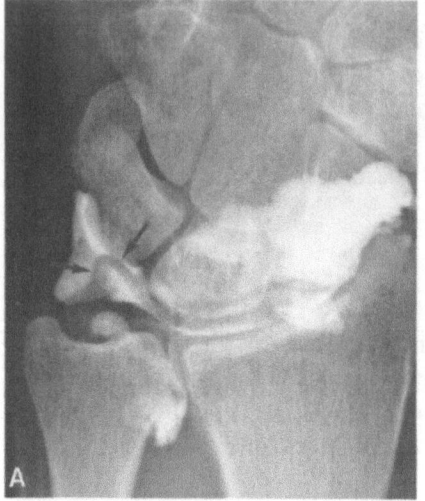
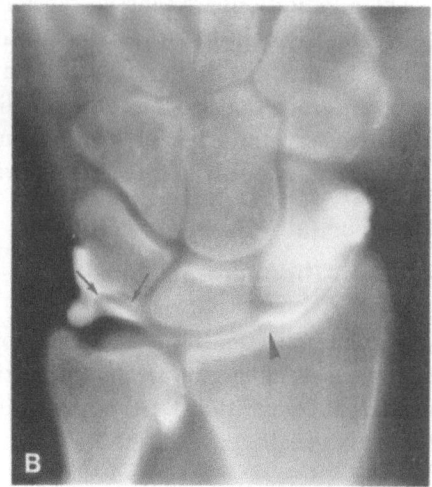
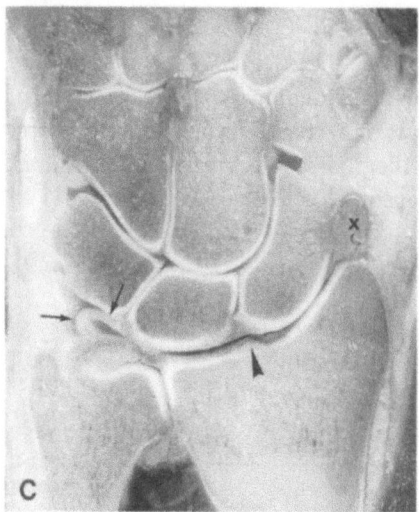

Fig. 2.25. Posteroanterior radiograph (A), tomogram (B) and photograph (C) of a corresponding
coronal cryosection of the same specimen. This
variant has a cartilaginous connection between
the lunotriquetral interosseous ligament and the
articular disc (*arrows*). Note the cartilaginous in-
terfacet ridge (*arrowhead*) which fits into the depression at the scapholunate junction formed by
the interosseous ligament. In C at the medial side
the silicon barium compound (*X*) has been removed. (Reprinted from [4], with kind permission
from Elsevier Science)

2.4.4   The Pisotriquetral Joint

The indications for an arthrogram of the pisotriquetral joint are free bodies (Fig. 2.26)
or the suspicion of cartilaginous free bodies in the case of occasional locking flexion-
extension motion of the wrist (Fig. 2.27). Another indication is pain-testing in osteoarthritis and corticosteroid injection.

2.4.5   The Carpometacarpal I Joint and the Metacarpophalangeal I Joint

The main indications for an arthrogram of the carpometacarpal I joint and the metacarpophalangeal I joint are pain-testing in osteoarthritis and corticosteroid injections.

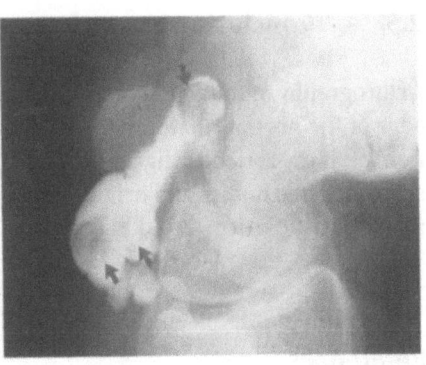

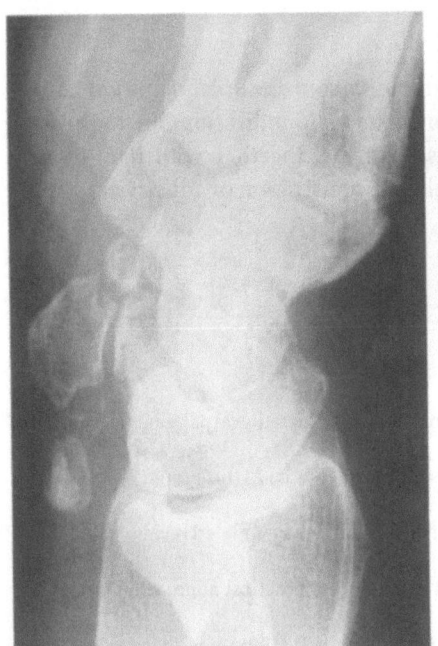

A

B

Fig. 2.26. Plain oblique film (**A**) and arthrogram (**B**) of the pisotriquetral joint. The patient had locking symptoms of the wrist. Free bodies are seen in the pisotriquetral joint (*arrows*)

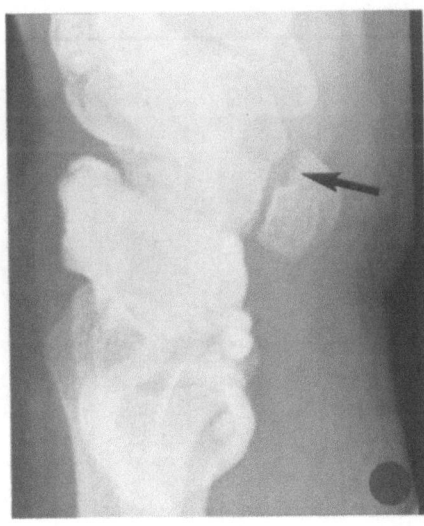

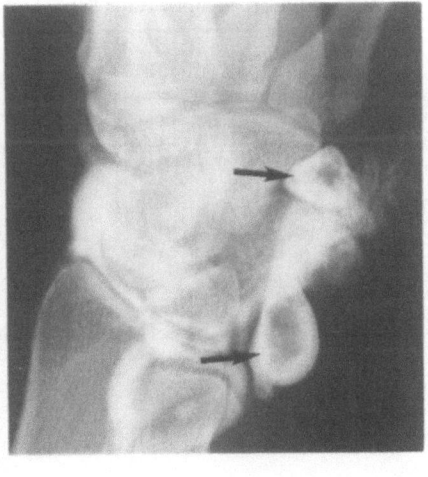

A

B

Fig. 2.27. Oblique radiocarpal arthrogram (**A**) and arthrogram (**B**) of the pisotriquetral joint in a patient with locking symptoms. There is no contrast in the pisotriquetral joint and no radio-opaque free bodies. The only sign of synovial chondromatosis is an erosion at the pisiform bone (*arrow*). **B** After selective injection of the pisotriquetral joint large cartilaginous free bodies are seen (*arrows*)

2.5   Conclusions

Arthrography of the wrist compartments requires some technical skill and knowledge of the normal anatomy and variations. The main indications are the evaluation of intra-articular ligament and disc damage, together with pain-testing,
search for free bodies and origins of ganglia, demonstration of adhesive capsulitis
and to assist corticosteroid injections.

References

1. Kessler L, Silberman Z (1961) An experimental study of the radiocarpal joint by arthrography. Surg Gynecol Obstet 112:33–40
2. Goldman AB (1979) The wrist. In: Freiberger RH, Kaye JJ (eds) Arthrography. Apple-Centu-
   ry-Crofts, New York, pp 277–290
3. Gilula LA, Hardy DC, Totty WG (1998) Wrist arthrography: an updated review. J Med Imaging 2:251–266
4. Obermann WR (1994) Radiology of carpal instability: a practical approach. Elsevier Science, Amsterdam
5. Tjin A, Ton ER, Pattynama PMT, Bloem JL, Obermann WR (1995) Interosseous ligaments:
   device for applying stress in wrist MR imaging. Radiology 196:863–864
6. Obermann WR, Kieft GJ (1987) Knee arthrography: a comparison of iohexol, ioxaglate
   sodium meglumine, and metrizoate. Radiology 162:729–733
7. Tjin A Ton ER, Schweitzer ME, Zwinderman AH, Obermann WR, Pattynama PM (1997)
   Value of intra-articular lidocaine in conventional wrist arthrography in differentiating
   symptomatic tears from asymptomatic perforation. Radiology 205(P):365
8. Ono H, Gilula LA, Marzke MW, Tempe AZ, Obermann WR (1996) Bicompartmentalization
   of the radiocarpal joint. J Hand Surg [Am] 21:788–793

3 Computed Tomography

A. Chevrot, J.-L. Drapé, E. Pessis, A. Feydy, D. Godefroy, A. M. Dupont

3.1 Introduction

In the examination of the wrist, computed tomography (CT) often reveals additional findings to the plain films, even now when magnetic resonance imaging (MRI) has become an important modality for musculoskeletal imaging. The availability of systems; the speed of imaging and the possibility of providing tomographic thin slices with high resolution make CT an interesting modality for hand and wrist imaging. The good image contrast and the optimization of contrast by intra-articular injection are another advantage. Furthermore, the amount of radiation to the wrist is minimal. Therefore, it is even possible to obtain scans in different positions, i.e., to image radioulnar dislocation. This chapter reviews the techniques and applications of spiral CT in wrist pathologies.

3.2 Technique

Scanning technique depends on patient history, on the clinical question to be answered and on the capabilities of the CT scanner available. For the wrist, the use of high-resolution imaging with thin slices is warranted. It is necessary to obtain slices that are approximately 1 mm thick. Slices of 2 or 3 mm thick could be sufficient in cases of trauma with an obvious fracture, in order to assess the relationship between different fragments, but thinner slices are necessary to detect a fracture that is suspected clinically but is occult on plain films. Also, thin slices are needed to study the interosseous ligaments (after intra-articular injection). With our system 0.5 mm slices are possible with a helical acquisition, which allows for image reconstruction every 0.3 mm with very good reformatting possibilities in differently oriented planes.

We routinely use the ultrahigh-resolution algorithm with the following parameters:

Scan time:	60–90 s
Pitch:	0.7
Slice thickness:	0.5–1 mm
Table speed:	0.3–1 mm/s
Reconstruction interval:	0.5
Matrix:	1024+1024

Field of view:	180 mm
kVp:	120
mAs:	‘135

A single helical acquisition with native axial slices of the wrist and secondary multiplanar reformations can replace more complex direct tailored oblique series [1, 8, 19].

The patient lies prone on the CT table, the arm elevated to place the hand in pronation, palm on the table. To prevent the "target artifact", it is possible to elevate the wrist with a 5–10 cm cushion.

For CT arthrography (arthro CT) contrast is injected intra-articularly. This technique allows excellent imaging of the interosseous ligaments (Figs. 3.1, 3.2) and is used when tears of interosseous ligaments (DISI, dorsal intercalated segment instability; or VISI, volar intercalated segment instability) are suspected.

Intravenous contrast injection is generally not required for spiral CT of the wrist. Moreover with such thin slices it is difficult to detect any enhancement. If the visualization of the vascular content of a lesion is required, we recommend MRI, as it is more sensitive.

We routinely use multiplanar reformatting techniques (MPR) (Fig. 3.3) or three-dimensional (3D) reconstructions as they can influence the management of wrist trauma. Maximum intensity projections (MIP) can also be used. (Figs. 3.4, 3.5).

3.3 Use of CT in Wrist Pathology

Spiral CT can be used to diagnose different diseases or to enhance information in different clinical symptoms. In this chapter we will discus the use of CT in:

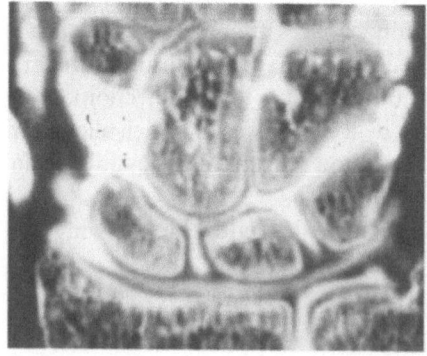 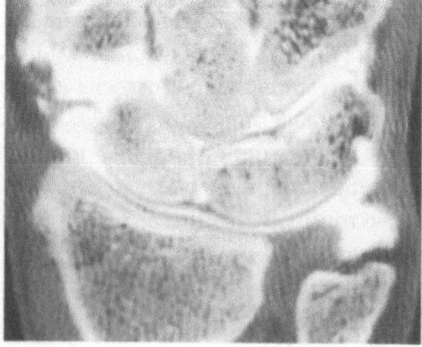

Fig. 3.1. Arthro CT of the wrist (0.5 mm thick slice, coronal reformation). The three compartments are injected. Note the normal appearance of the scapholunate and lunotriquetral ligaments

Fig. 3.2. Arthro CT of the wrist (0.5 mm thick slice, coronal reformation). Mediocarpal and radiocarpal compartments are injected. This is a case of complete lunotriquetral coalition

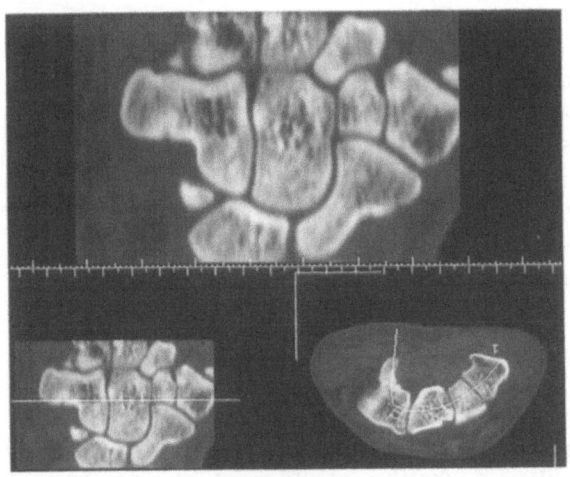

Fig. 3.3. CT of the wrist (0.5 mm thick slice, curve reformation). Note the pattern of the hook of the hamate

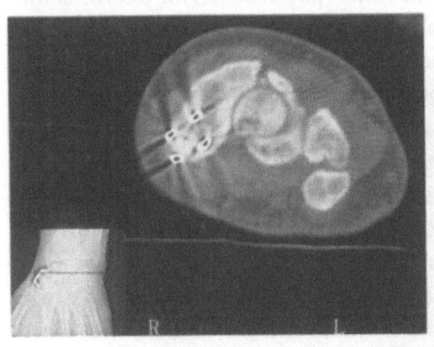

a

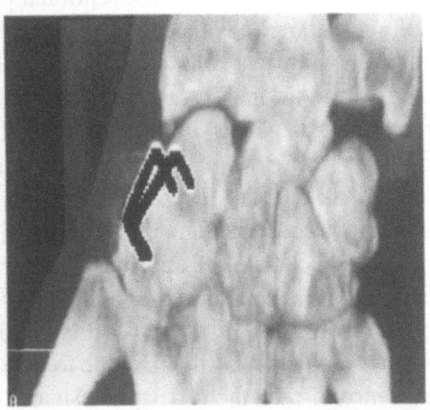

b

Fig. 3.4a, b. CT of the wrist (1 mm thick slice, MIP imaging). **a** Direct reconstruction artifacts due to metallic devices. **b** MIP demonstrating the positions of the metallic devices

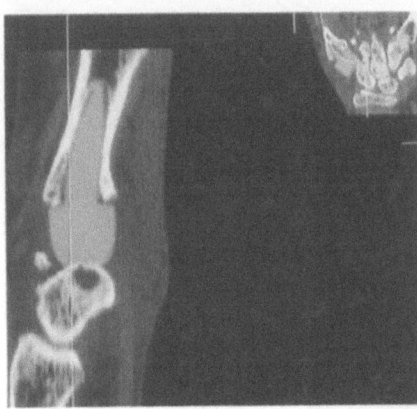

a

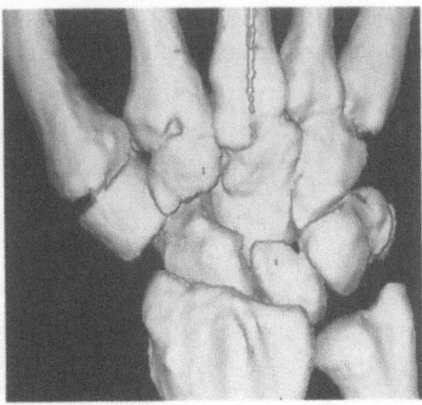

b

Fig. 3.5a, b. Metacarpal implants. CT of the wrist (1 mm thick slice). **a** Frontal reformation. **b** Three-dimensional reconstruction

1 carpal fractures and trauma
2 radioulnar lesion (dislocation of the distal radioulnar joint)
3 ulnar impaction syndrome
4 lesions of the triangular fibrocartilage complex
5 carpal instability
6 carpal tunnel syndrome, ulnar tunnel syndrome
7 tendinitis, tenosynovitis
8 ganglion cysts
9 other and miscellaneous lesions

3.3.1   Carpal Fractures and Trauma

The scaphoid (or os naviculare) is the most frequent fractured bone in the wrist. The fracture occurs mostly in the waist (65%) and in the proximal aspect. Most of the fractures are seen on conventional plain films (posteroanterior and/or semi-oblique radiographs). However, nondisplaced scaphoid fractures can be invisible at the first X-ray examination. It is well known that, in the case of clinical suspicion, an additional X-ray examination performed 5–10 days after trauma will reveal the diagnosis, due to the visibility of bone resorption surrounding the fracture line. However, a more rapid diagnosis can be accomplished using an immediate CT or MRI examination. CT is the best tool to delineate the fracture line and associated bone displacement [2, 5] (Figs. 3.6–3.8). With spiral CT, it is possible to choose the appropriate reformation plane able to demonstrate these findings. CT also allows the follow-up of the fracture line and of the intensity of bone resorption [10]. With CT it is possible to monitor the evolution after treatment, even with a cast. CT is able to detect delayed union or non-union [17]. The presence of metallic osteosynthesis material produces artifacts on the acquired and directly reconstructed slices. It is interesting to notice that these artifacts can be minimized on reformatted images.

CT is also an excellent tool to demonstrate nondisplaced fractures of other carpal bones (Fig. 3.9) that are occult on conventional images. The fracture of the hook of the hamate is often not diagnosed due to the difficulty of obtaining a

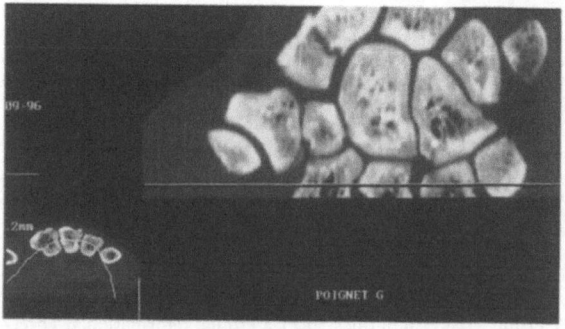

Fig. 3.6. Transverse nondisplaced fracture of the neck of the scaphoid. CT of the wrist (0.5 mm thick slice, curve frontal reformation)

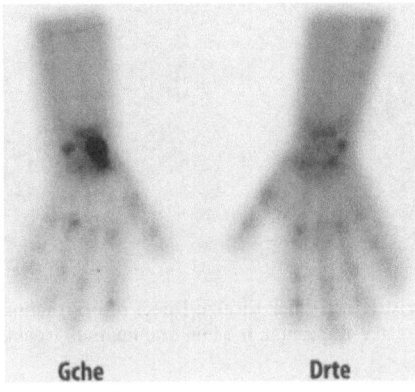

Gche   Drte

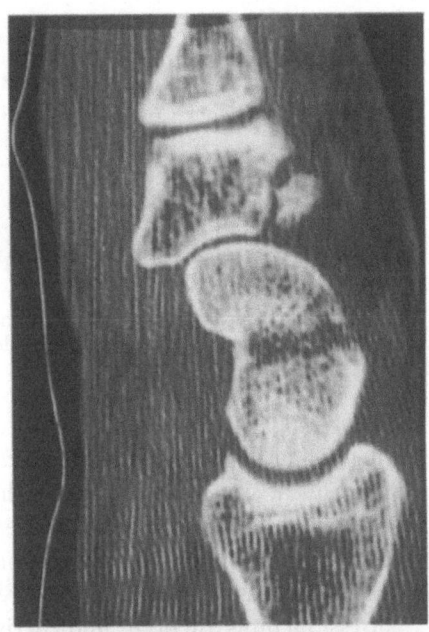

Fig. 3.7a–c. Fracture of the scaphoid. Subtle fracture unseen on plain film. **a** Bone scintigraphy.
There is a hot spot in the area of the scaphoid. **b**
CT of the wrist (1 mm thick slice, sagittal reformation). A linear radiolucency is seen crossing the
neck of the scaphoid. **c** Same examination, frontal
reformation. A fracture of the neck of the
scaphoid is demonstrated

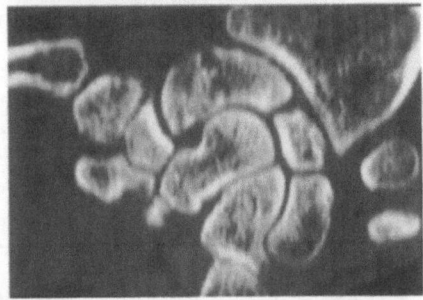

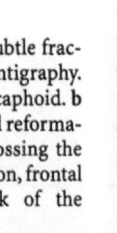

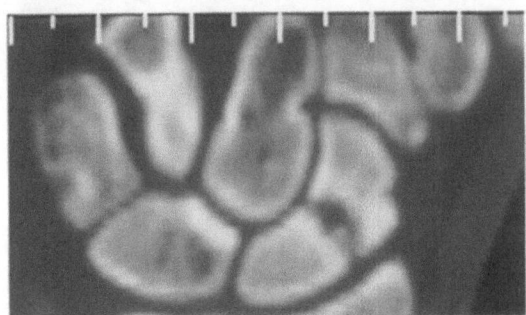

Fig. 3.8. Non-union of a scaphoid fracture. CT of the wrist (1 mm thick slice,
frontal reformation). Note the wide radiolucent line featuring the non-unit-
ed fracture line

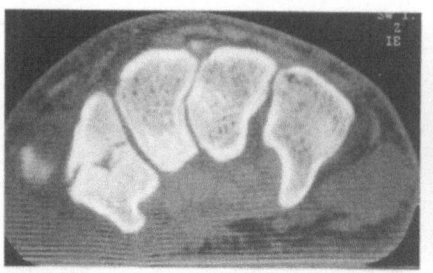
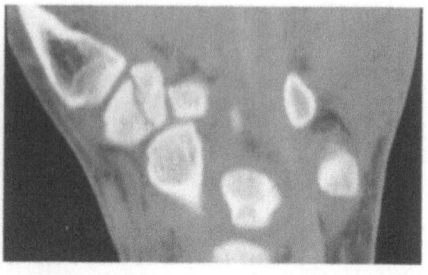

a   b

Fig. 3.9a, b. Fracture of the trapezium. CT of the wrist (1 mm thick slice). **a** Direct reconstruction showing a radiolucent fracture line in the middle of the trapezium. **b** Same examination, frontal reformation

radiograph of this small bone. CT gives an obvious finding (Figs. 3.10, 3.11). The fracture line is situated at the base of the hamate hook [11, 16].

Fracture dislocations of the wrist are usually obvious on plain films. CT demonstrates clearly the perilunate dislocation, allowing a precise evaluation of the displacement and associated bone fractures [9, 13] (Fig. 3.12).

Stress fractures can occur in the wrist. The diagnosis is difficult on plain films due to the lack of displacement and poor delineation of the fracture line. CT is able

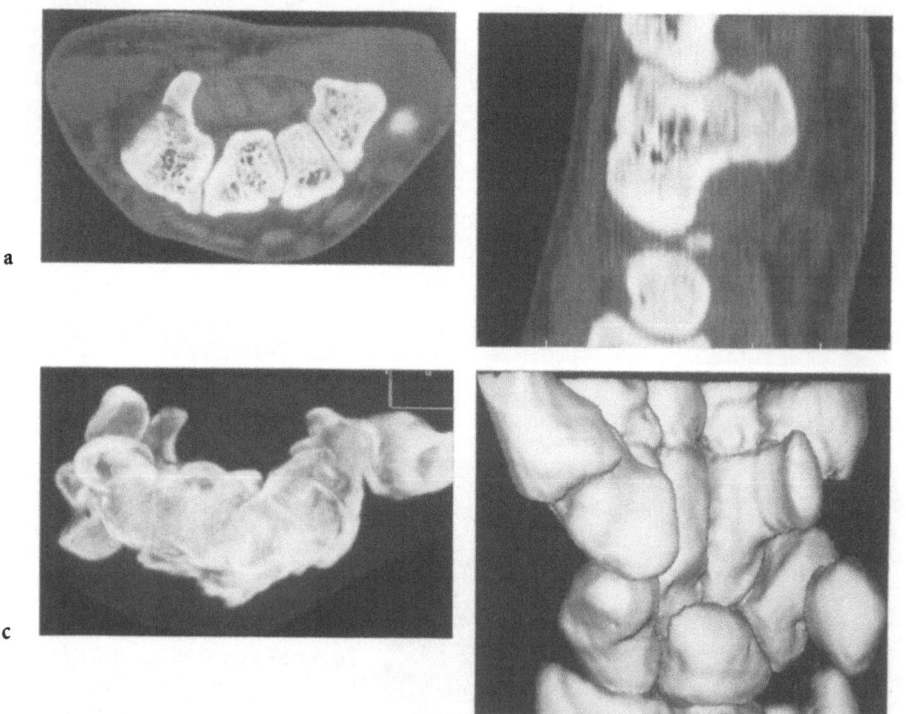

a

b

c

d

Fig. 3.10a–d. Fracture of the hook of the hamate. CT of the wrist (0.5 mm thick slice). **a** Direct reconstruction. **b** Sagittal reformation. **c** MIP representation. **d** Three-dimensional representation

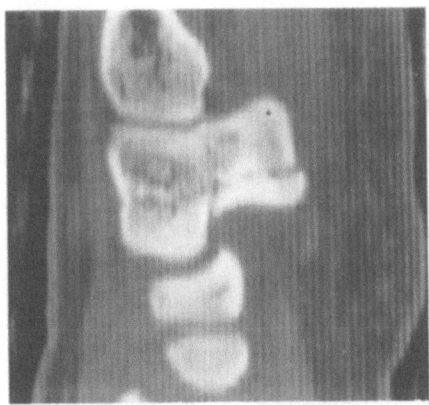

Fig. 3.11. Subtle fracture of the hook of the hamate. CT of the wrist (0.5 mm thick slice, sagittal reformation). This is an avulsion fracture of the insertion of the pisohamate ligament

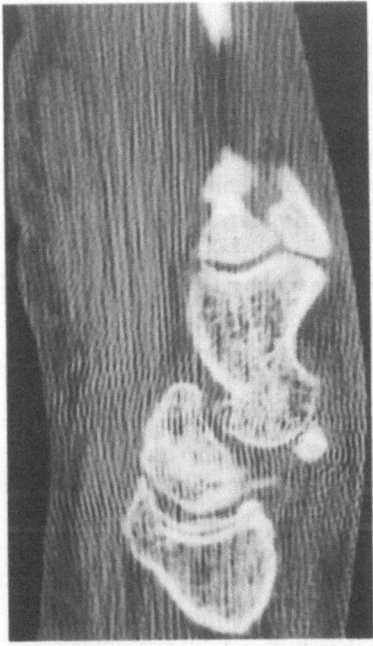

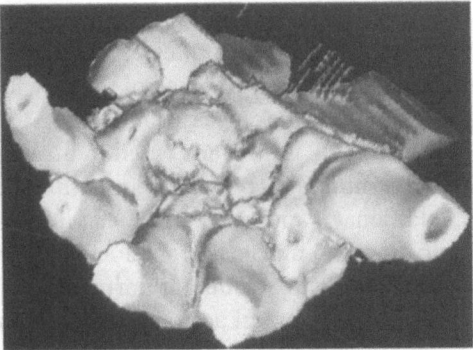

b

Fig. 3.12a, b. Perilunate dislocation of the wrist. CT of the wrist (1 mm thick slice). a Sagittal reformation. Note the posterior position of the head of the capitum behind the lunate. b Three-dimensional imaging. Note the bulging of the lunate in the middle of the carpal canal

a

to detect these lesions. MRI is also a good diagnostic choice, based on the alterations in relaxation times and therefore the bone signal in fractured bone. Diffuse bone marrow edema and low signal intensity of the fracture line can be seen.

In addition several supernumerary bones can be studied with CT (Fig. 3.13).

3.3.2 Radioulnar Lesion (Dislocation of the Distal Radioulnar Joint)

To permit pronation and supination, the head of the ulna rotates in the sigmoid notch of the radius, maintained by the anterior and posterior ligaments and by the

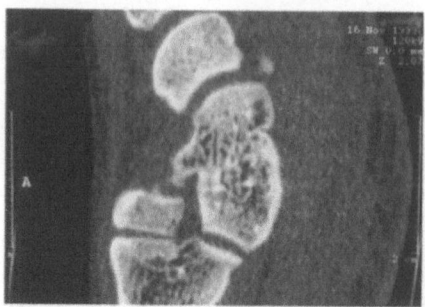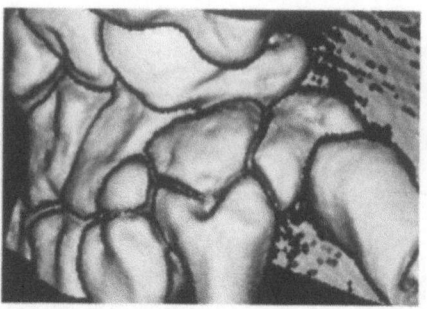

a   b

Fig. 3.13a, b. Hunchback wrist. This frequent abnormality is due to fragmentation of the posterior aspect of the base of the second metacarpal bone (old fracture or supernumerary bone). This creates a bulge at the posterior aspect of the wrist, sometimes associated with pain. CT of the wrist (1 mm thick slice). a Sagittal reformation. b Three-dimensional imaging

triangular fibrocartilage complex (TFCC). Injuries to those structures can cause dysfunction between the head of the ulna and the radius. Radiographic findings are absent or subtle and easily missed.

A special CT technique is used to diagnose distal radioulnar joint (DRUJ) lesions. It is unnecessary to obtain very thin slices: a 2–3 mm thick slice is sufficient. In addition, CT must be performed with the wrist in neutral position, maximal supination and maximal pronation. It is sometimes useful to study both wrists simultaneously to account for normal anatomical variations. A slight dorsal subluxation, in the neutral position to maximum pronation, is considered normal.

Several methods of assessing DRUJ subluxation have been proposed [7, 13] (Fig. 3.14):

- Radioulnar lines method: the ulnar head lies between the DRU and VRU lines when the DRUJ is congruent. Subluxation is diagnosed when the maximal width of the dorsally or ventrally subluxed ulna is larger than one fourth of the sigmoid notch diameter.
- Congruity method: Congruence between the arch of the sigmoid notch and the arch of the ulnar head (Fig. 3.15).
- Epicenter method: the center of rotation of the ulna (which is between the center of the ulnar head and the center of the ulnar styloid) stays in front of the middle of the sigmoid notch.

These assessments may also be obtained with MRI, but acquisition of images in the different positions is more time-consuming (Fig. 3.16).

3.3.3   Ulnar Impaction Syndrome

In the case of positive ulnar variance (ulnar length exceeding radial length), microtrauma can occur between the ulnar head, the TFCC and the lunate. This condition leads to a tear of the TFCC and to chondral and subchondral bone lesions of

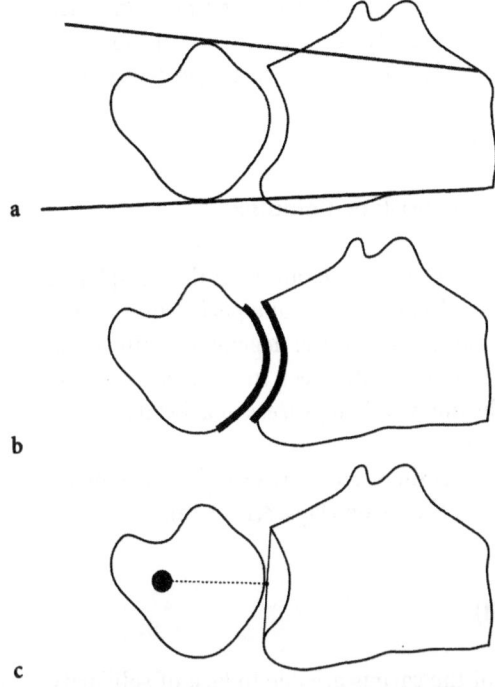

Fig. 3.14a–c. Methods of measuring distal radioulnar joint position. **a** Radioulnar lines method. **b** Congruity method. **c** Epicenter method (see text for details)

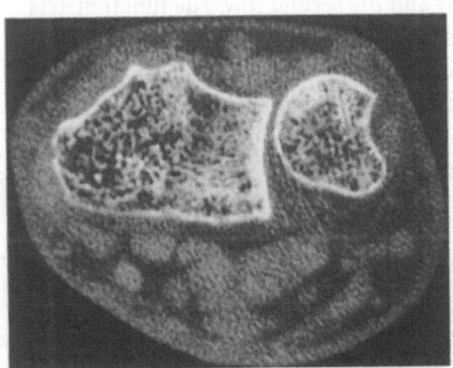

Fig. 3.15. Posterior subluxation of the ulna. CT of the wrist (1 mm thick slice). A little posterior subluxation is normally possible, but in this case it is a narrowing of the posterior joint space

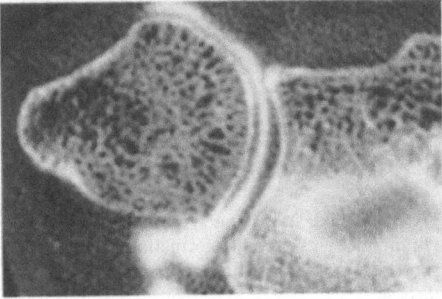

Fig. 3.16. Normal distal radioulnar joint cartilage. Arthro CT (1 mm thick slice, frontal reformation). Note the thickness of the cartilage

the lunate. The performance of CT is less spectacular than the findings with MRI. The latter demonstrates changes in signal intensity of the lunate [6, 20]. However, arthro CT can effectively show the TFCC lesion and the cartilage defect. This condition leads to Kienböck's disease. (Figs. 3.17, 3.18).

3.3.4   Lesions of the Triangular Fibrocartilage Complex

The pathology of the TFCC is complex and the correlation with the complaints and symptoms of the patient is not always obvious. Lesion and perforations of the TFCC are caused by trauma but also occur due to natural degeneration in aging. CT is useful to demonstrate associated fractures, often seen in cases of traumatic lesions. A fracture through the base of the ulnar styloid process or a distal fracture of the radius can be invisible on plain films.

Arthro CT is able to distinguish between the various patterns of a traumatic TFCC tear, indicating with detail the site of the lesion (Figs. 3.19, 3.20).

3.3.5   Carpal Instability (DISI, VISI)

Abnormal motions of the small bones of the carpus are due to lack of solidarity caused by tears of intracarpal ligaments. The normal carpus shows harmonic motions of the small bones of the first row and the second row. The function acts like a camshaft, allowing lateral motions of the wrist without lateral shifting. This function is used in different types of action such as the use of a hammer or in very delicate movements (like painting or writing). The scapholunate and the lunotri-quetral ligaments play an important role in this function. Lesions of these ligaments occur after rotatory traumatic luxation of the lunate and the scaphoid.

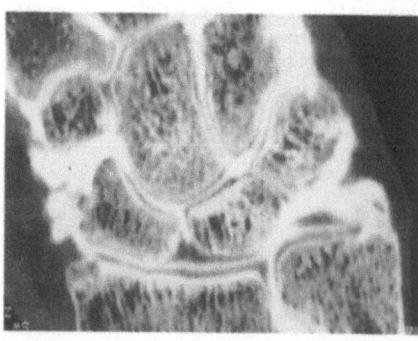

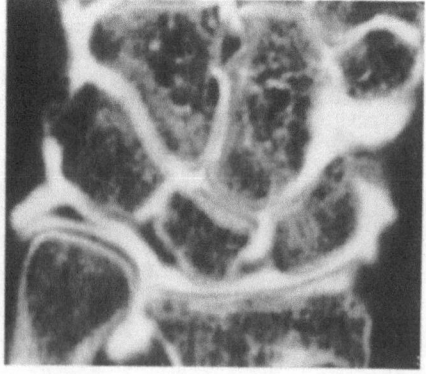

Fig. 3.17. Ulnar impaction syndrome. Arthro CT (1 mm thick slice, frontal reformation). Note the ulnar-lunate contact and disappearance of the cartilage

Fig. 3.18. Ulnar impaction syndrome. Arthro CT (1 mm thick slice, frontal reformation). The lunate shows dystrophic structure leading to Kienböck's disease

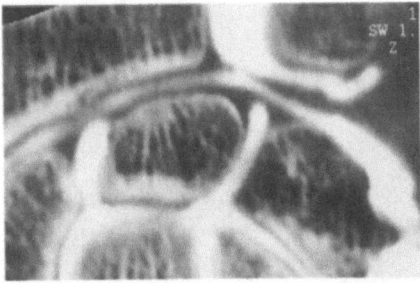

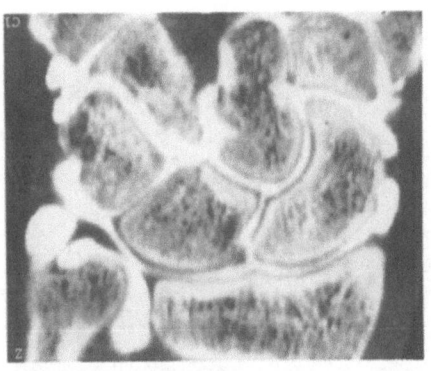

Fig. 3.19. Small lesion of the triangular fibrocartilage complex. Arthro CT (0.5 mm thick slice, frontal reformation). The scapholunate and lunotriquetral ligaments are normal; there is lack of continuity in the triangular ligament

Fig. 3.20. Lesion of the triangular fibrocartilage complex and ulnar impaction syndrome. Arthro CT (0.5 mm thick slice, frontal reformation). Note the long ulna and lack of continuity in the triangular ligament. The scapholunate and lunotriquetral ligaments are also torn

- Dorsal instability (DISI) is the most frequent midcarpal instability. It is accompanied by (or due to) a complete tear of the scapholunate ligament. This creates an increase in the scapholunate angle (Figs. 3.21, 3.22).
- Palmar or volar instability (VISI) is characterized by a posterior subluxation of both scaphoid and lunate that remain interdependent. It is due to lack of union with the triquetrum, because of a lunotriquetral ligament tear. The scapholunate angle is normal (Figs. 3.23, 3.24).

These instabilities are usually clearly observed on plain films. But CT demonstrates very well the malpositioning, due to its ability to reformat images in several different sagittal planes.

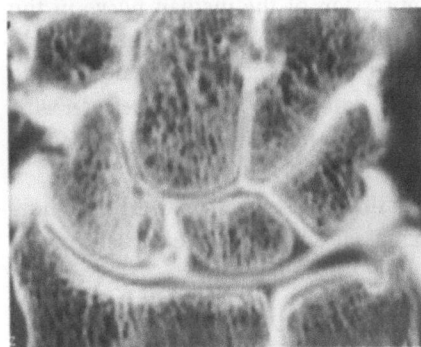

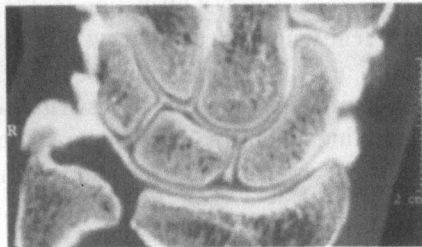

Fig. 3.21. Tear of the scapholunate ligament. Arthro CT (1 mm thick slice, frontal reformation). There is discontinuity in the scapholunate ligament. The head of the scaphoid is dystrophic. The lunotriquetral ligament is also torn. The triangular fibrocartilage complex is normal

Fig. 3.22. Isolated torn lunotriquetral ligament. Arthro CT (0.5 mm thick slice, frontal reformation). Note the lack of continuity in the lunotriquetral ligament

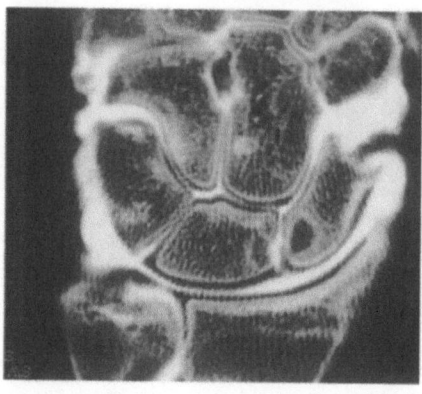

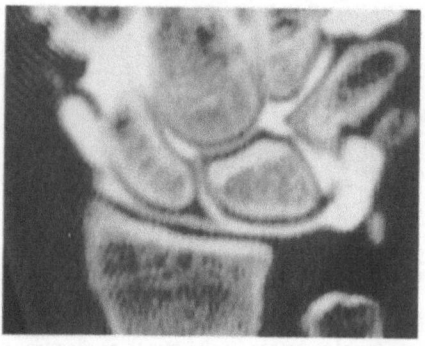

Fig. 3.24. Lunotriquetral and scapholunate ligament tears. Arthro CT (0.5 mm thick slice, frontal reformation)

Fig. 3.23. Isolated torn lunotriquetral ligament. Arthro CT (0.5 mm thick slice, frontal reformation). There are also dystrophic cystic lesions on both sides of the scapholunate joint, in spite of an intact scapholunate ligament

Arthro CT is also used to analyze damage to the interosseous ligaments. It is necessary to use imaging parameters that allow high-resolution imaging [3].

Instability may lead to painful degenerative arthritis, such as degenerative scaphoradial arthritis. This late-occurring disease is known as a scapholunate advanced collapse (SLAC). It is well depicted by CT or arthro CT [21] (Figs. 3.25–3.27). Radiologists must be aware of the increased frequency of asymptomatic ligamentous tears with aging [15].

3.3.6   Carpal Tunnel Syndrome, Ulnar Tunnel Syndrome

Carpal tunnel syndrome is caused by compression of the median nerve in the wrist. Electromyography is recommended. Diagnostic imaging is not routinely used. The use of CT can demonstrate tunnel calcification, bony avulsions, bone displacement and cyst formation [4, 12]. These pathologies can also be seen with MRI. Tenosynovitis, ganglion cysts, bowing of the retinaculum and sometimes the medial nerve itself can be also visualized by ultrasound (Figs. 3.28, 3.29).

Compression of the ulnar nerve is also possible in Guyon's canal. CT can show interesting findings causing compression: a mass lesion, a fracture, muscle hypertrophy, an accessory muscle or an abnormality of the ulnar artery.

3.3.7   Tendinitis, Tenosynovitis

Tendinitis and tenosynovitis are very frequent causes of wrist discomfort or pain. Cross-sectional imaging such as CT or MRI can provide good images of the following lesions:

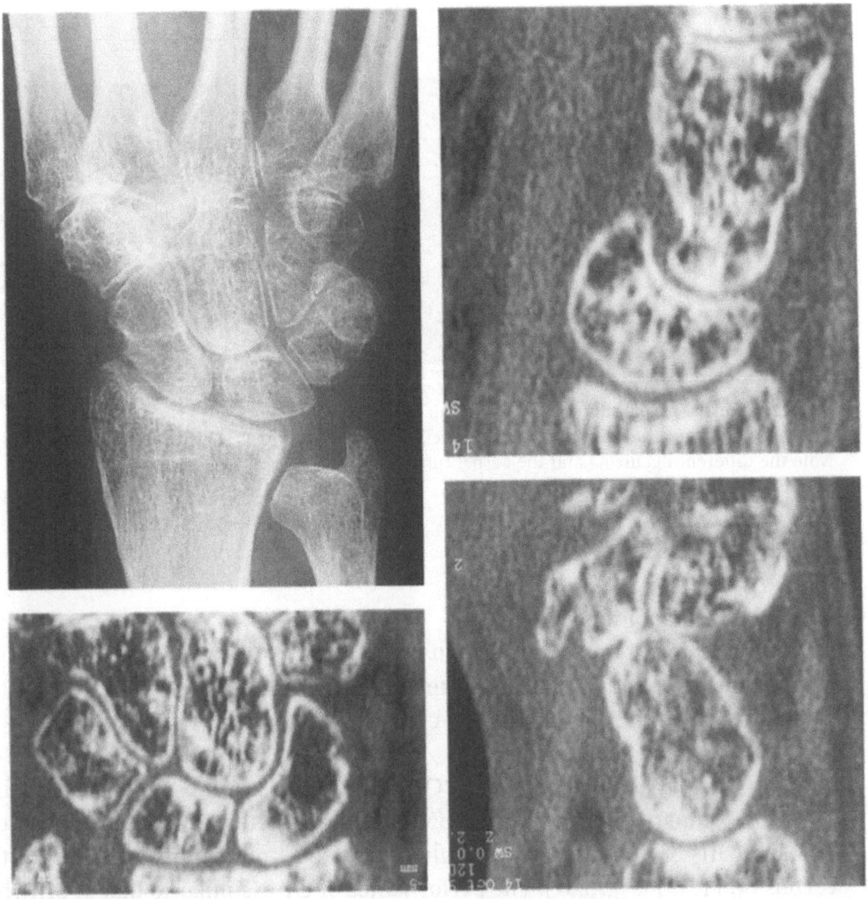

Fig. 3.25a–d. Scapholunate advanced collapse (SLAC), early stages. **a** Plain film. There is demineralization and narrowing of the radioscaphoid joint space. **b–d** CT of the wrist (0.5 mm thick slice). **b** Sagittal reformation. DISI. **c** Sagittal reformation increases the density of the reaction of the subchondral bone of the scaphoid and the radius. **d** Frontal reformation shows narrowing of the radioscaphoid joint space. There is dystrophic condensation of the head of the scaphoid

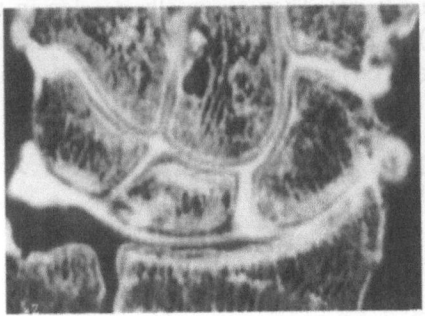

Fig. 3.26. SLAC lesion, more advanced stage. Arthro CT (0.5 mm thick slice, frontal reformation). There is a tear of the scapholunate ligament and disappearance of the radius and scaphoid cartilages

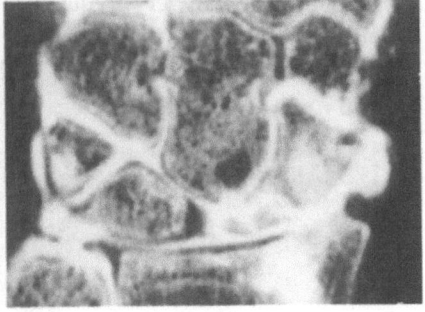

Fig. 3.27. SLAC, more advanced stage. Arthro CT (0.5 mm thick slice, frontal reformation). There is a scapholunate ligament tear, collapse of the head of the scaphoid, radial erosion and a dystrophic appearance of the lunate and the head of the capitate

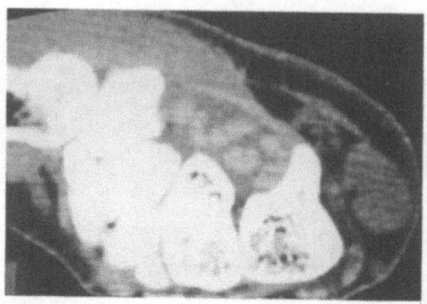
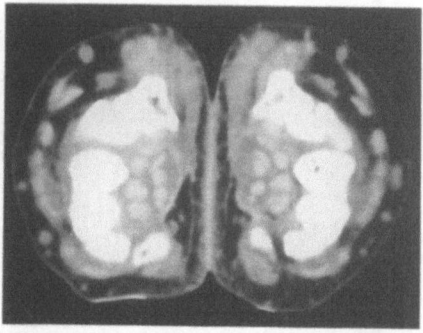

Fig. 3.28. Normal carpal tunnel. CT (1 mm thick slice, crossing the lower aspect of the tunnel). Note the different ligaments and the carpal tunnel; also the flexor retinaculum

Fig. 3.29. Carpal tunnel. CT (1 mm thick slice, middle aspect of the tunnel). Both sides are shown; the left side had surgery. Note the lack of visibility of the flexor retinaculum

- thickening of the tendon
- thickening of the tendon sheath
- luxation or subluxation of the tendon
- absence of the tendon due to a complete tendon tear (Fig. 3.30)

CT can help in the diagnosis of de Quervain's disease (tenosynovitis of the first extensor compartment – abductor pollicis longus, extensor pollicis brevis), the tenosynovitis of the extensor carpi ulnaris tendon, and the other tendons of the carpus [4, 11, 19] (Fig. 3.31). The performance of CT is similar to that of MRI, but MRI can demonstrate subperiosteal bone reactions. Suspected tenosynovitis is a common indication for an ultrasound examination.

3.3.8   Ganglion Cysts

Ganglion cysts are very frequent in the wrist. They essentially develop in the dorsum of the wrist (54–68% of cases). Ganglion cysts of the tendon sheaths are less frequent. Symptoms due to ganglion cysts vary according to the cyst location

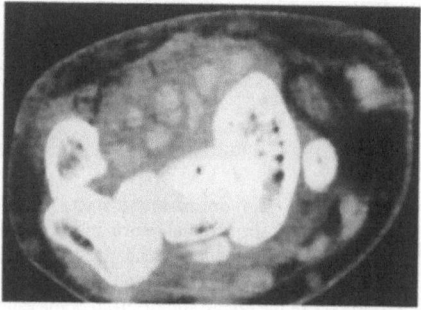

Fig. 3.30. Tenosynovitis of the flexor tendon. CT of the wrist (1 mm thick slice crossing the upper aspect of the carpal tunnel, soft tissue window). Note the dense pattern of the flexor ligament surrounded by lower-density tissues

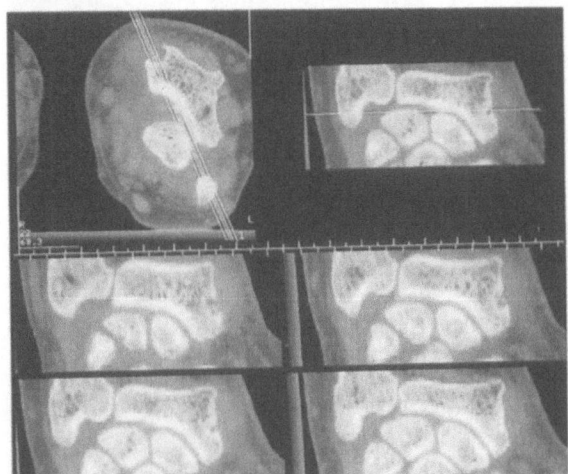

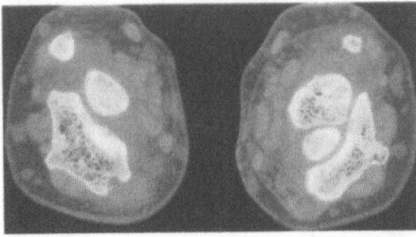

Fig. 3.31a,b. De Quervain's disease. CT of the wrist (1 mm thick slice). **a** Slice. **b** Reformation in the frontal plane . There is swelling of the soft tissue surrounding the radial styloid. The cystic formation in the radial styloid itself is due to inflammatory granuloma

and size. The main clinical sign is the presence of a painful mass. Cyst in the carpal canal or Guyon's canal can produce nerve (median nerve or ulnar nerve) compression.

Radiographs are often normal. Ultrasound is helpful to delineate the cyst, but CT and MRI give more precise analysis of the relation between the cyst and adjacent structures and of its extent. CT and arthro CT demonstrate fluid content, wall (capsule) and septa, and sometimes the communicating channel with the joint (Figs. 3.32, 3.33). CT features are characteristic with a pattern of several interconnecting cavities. Moreover, CT is an excellent tool for detecting recurrences after treatment.

3.3.9 Other and Miscellaneous Lesions

Bone and soft tissue lesions are well analyzed by CT. Degenerative bone lesions (Fig. 3.34) or avascular bone necrosis or dystrophy (Fig. 3.35) are well seen. CT also is able to detect small bone lesions, such as osteoid osteoma, that are otherwise difficult to visualize (Fig. 3.36). Foreign bodies in the soft tissues are better seen with CT than with other techniques.

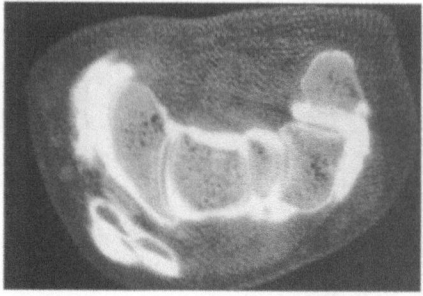 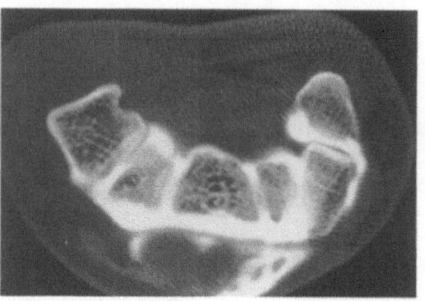

Fig. 3.32. Dorsal ganglion cyst. Arthro CT of the wrist (1 mm thick slice, crossing the upper aspect of the wrist: note the pisotriquetral joint). The radial tendon sheaths are injected. There is swelling of soft tissue behind the lunate, featuring the injected ganglion cyst

Fig. 3.33. Dorsal ganglion cyst. Arthro CT of the wrist (1 mm thick slice, crossing the upper aspect of the wrist). The contrast includes the posterior synovial and surrounds the posterior cyst

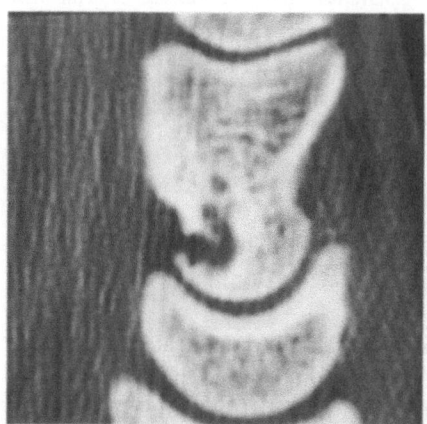 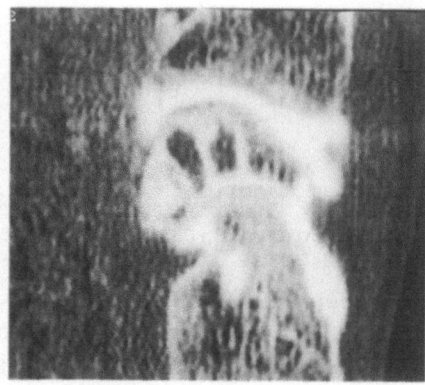

Fig. 3.34. Dystrophic cyst of the capitate. CT of the wrist (1 mm thick slice, sagittal reformation). There is a posterior round radiolucency of the head of the hamate

Fig. 3.35. Kienböck's disease. Arthro CT of the wrist (0.5 thick slice, sagittal reformation). Several radiolucencies are in the lunate. One of them takes the contrast featuring the cystic formation

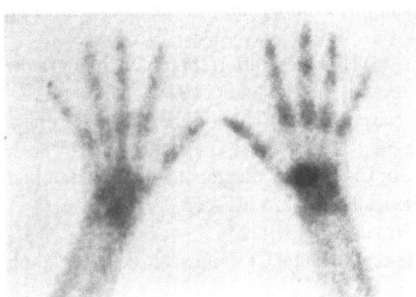
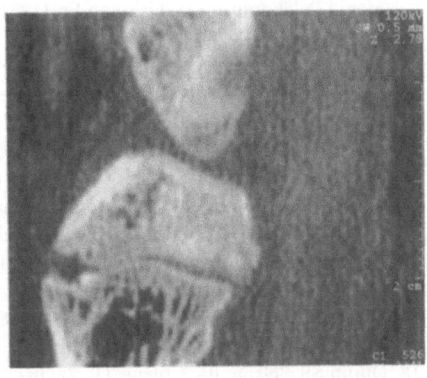

a

b

Fig. 3.36a, b. Osteoid osteoma of the trapezoid: **a** Bone scintigraphy. There is a hot spot at the level of the trapezoid. **b** CT of the wrist (0.5 mm thick slice, sagittal reformation). There is visualization of the nidus at the posterior aspect of the trapezoid

3.4   Conclusion

Despite the capabilities of MRI, spiral CT remains a powerful modality for the evaluation of wrist trauma and disease. Its potential for high-resolution imaging and ultrathin slices associated with the ability to obtain multiplanar reformations and three-dimensional images represent an excellent tool for detailed analysis of wrist lesions. The use of arthro CT remains an imaging method to depict ligamentous lesions.

References

1. Biondetti PR, Vannier MW, Gilula LA, Kapp R (1987) Wrist: coronal and transaxial CT scanning. Radiology 163:149–151
2. Bush CH, Gillepsy T III, Dell PC (1987) High-resolution CT of the wrist: initial experience with scaphoid disorders and surgical fusions. AJR 149:757–760
3. Chevrot A (1998) Imagerie clinique du poignet et de la main. Collection d'imagerie radiologique. Masson, Paris
4. Cone RO, Szabo R, Resnick D, Gelberman R, Taleisnik J, Gilula LA (1983) Computed tomography of the normal soft tissues of the wrist. Invest Radiol 18:546–551
5. Friedman L, Johnston GH, Young-Hing K (1990) Computed tomography of wrist trauma. Can Assoc Radiol J 41:141–145
6. Imaeda T, Nakamura R, Shionoya K, Makino N (1996) Ulnar impaction syndrome: MR imaging findings. Radiology 201:495–500
7. Kerr R, Kingston S (1997) Imaging of sports injuries of the wrist and hand. Semin Musc Skeletal Radiol 1:5–27
8. Kuszyk BS, Fishman EK (1996) Direct coronal CT of the wrist: helical acquisition with simplified patient positioning. AJR 166:419–420
9. James SE, Richards R, McGrouther DA (1992) Three-dimensional CT imaging of the wrist. A practical system. J Hand Surg [Br] 17:504–506
10. Jonsson K, Jonsson A, Sloth M, Kopylov P, Wingstrand H (1992) CT of the wrist in suspected scaphoid fracture. Acta Radiol 33:500–511

11. Magid D, Thompson JS, Fishman EK (1991) Computed tomography of the hand and wrist. Hand Clin 7:219–233
12. Merhar GL, Clark RA, Schneider HJ, Stern PJ (1986) High-resolution computed tomography of the wrist in patients with carpal tunnel syndrome. Skeletal Radiol 15:549–552
13. Nakamura R, Horii E, Tanaka Y, Imaeda T, Hayakawa N (1989) Three-dimensional CT imaging for wrist disorders. J Hand Surg [Br] 14:53–58
14. Nakamura R, Horii E, Imaeda T, Nakao E (1996) Criteria for diagnosing distal radioulnar joint subluxation by computed tomography. Skeletal Radiol 25:649–653
15. Pierce ME (1990) CT of the wrist: what is abnormal? AJR 154:1127
16. Pretorius ES, Fishman EK (1999) Spiral T and tridimensional CT of musculoskeletal pathology. Radiol Clin North Am 37:953–974
17. Quinn SF, Murray W, Watkins T, Kloss J (1987) CT for determining the results of treatment of fractures of the wrist. AJR 149:109–111
18. Quinn SF, Belsole RS, Greene TL, Rayhack JM (1989) Work in progress: postarthrography computed tomography of the wrist: evaluation of the triangular fibrocartilage complex. Skeletal Radiol 17:565–569
19. Stewart NR, Gilula LA (1992) CT of the wrist: a tailored approach. Radiology 183:13–20
20. Tomaino MM (1998) Ulnar impaction syndrome in the ulnar negative and neutral wrist. Diagnosis and pathoanatomy. J Hand Surg [Br] 23:754–757
21. Watson HK, Ballet FL (1984) The SLAC wrist: scapholunate advanced collapse pattern of degenerative arthritis. J Hand Surg [Am] 9:358–365

4 Ultrasound of the Hand

Olivia Bottinelli, Rodolfo Campani

4.1 Introduction

Perfect knowledge of the complex anatomy of the structures involved and high-frequency probes are necessary for the application of ultrasound (US) in musculoskeletal imaging. Thanks to the introduction of "small parts" or "superficial soft tissue" probes with high frequency (over 7.5 MHz), the US study of small structures in very superficial sites is increasingly used in clinical practice because it provides answers to very specific diagnostic queries.

Other imaging methods, such as computed tomography (CT) and magnetic resonance imaging (MRI), have the advantage of better tomographic and volumetric views and better image contrast resolution, but on the other hand these methods are very complex techniques requiring long imaging and/or reconstruction times and scanning planes. US can presently depict most periskeletal soft tissues in the hand and US anatomy is well studied and described. US provides not only morphological but also functional information. The latter is provided by dynamic studies, and has recently benefited from the introduction of color and power Doppler modes, which are particularly important in depicting the vascularization of tumors.

US studies should be considered an indispensable tool for preliminary clinical assessment and, whenever possible, should be performed in close cooperation with the referring physician targeted to specific diagnostic queries.

4.2 Technique and Method

For correct execution of the examination, linear probes with high frequency (in any case >7.5 MHz) should be used. Small-sized broadband probes are now available, which provide the further advantage of limited surface contact with the skin. Nevertheless, the first part of the examination should be carried out with larger and more panoramic probes. Smaller probes with higher frequency should be used once the region of interest has been located. The US beam must be positioned perpendicular to the long axis of the structure of interest to avoid artifacts caused by an acute reflection angle, with consequent hypoechogenicity in the structure under examination.

Transverse scans are performed first, for best identification of single structures and their relationships. Transverse scans on the palm show the hyperechoic profiles of carpal, metacarpal and phalangeal bones, giving fundamental landmarks, with the individual tendons and the small muscles dividing them shown ventrally. Subsequent longitudinal scans allow the various tendons, nerves and vessels to be followed along their whole course.

After the static and morphological assessment, we perform a dynamic study for real-time depiction of preserved continuity of tendon and muscle fibers and of normal function. Real-time dynamic studies are unquestionably one of the main advantages of US over the other imaging modalities.

In our opinion, comparative assessment of homologous contralateral structures is fundamental to permit immediate and easier detection of any abnormal finding.

Finally color Doppler, with adequate settings using the low-velocity scale, permits the assessment of the course and patency of all arterial and venous branches from the larger ones in the wrist to the smaller ones in the fingers and phalanges. It is very useful to detect flow changes (e.g. in Raynaud's syndrome), inflammation-related hyperemia, and abnormal and anarchic vascularization in neoplasms (particularly malignant ones) and vascular malformations.

4.3   Anatomical–US Correlations

For correct interpretation of the numerous diseases that can affect the hand, it is necessary to review the basics of US anatomy.

US permits the study of:

- Carpal, metacarpal and phalangeal bones.
- Muscles, which are subdivided into three groups, namely: muscles of the thenar eminence (long flexor, opponent, short abductor and adductor of the thumb) at the thumb base; muscles of the hypothenar eminence (short abductor and short flexor) at the base of the fifth finger; and finally intermediate muscles (the four lumbricales, more superficial, and the three interosseous volar and the four interosseous dorsal). These muscles have a typical echostructure characterized by neatly arranged hypoechoic fibers and thin hyperechoic bands.
- Tendons, grouped as superficial and deep flexor tendons, coursing on the palmar aspect, and the thinner and more superficial extensor tendons, coursing dorsally. US clearly shows the typical regular and echogenic fibrillar structure common to all tendons (Fig. 4.1). Peritendinous synovial sheaths, where present, are clearly depicted as hypoechoic bands surrounding the individual tendons or tendon bundles.
- Vessels, which can be followed along their whole course. Spectral studies permit the differentiation of arteries from veins.
- Nerves. The excellent resolution of current available probes the study of even the inner structure of median and ulnar nerves (distinguishing them from surrounding tendons), which are characterized by hypoechoic round lacunae making the small secondary nerve bundles (Fig. 4.2).
- The articular capsules, their thickness and the integrity of periarticular ligaments (collateral ligaments).

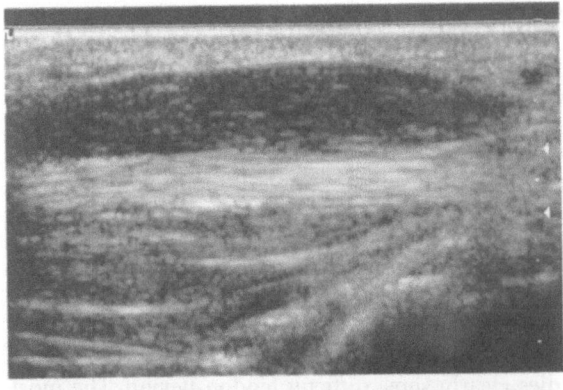

a

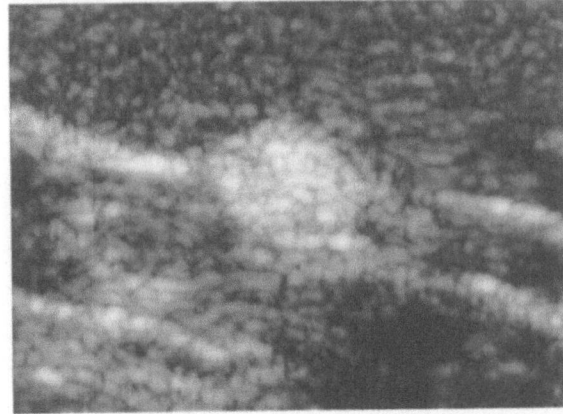

b

Fig. 4.1. Longitudinal (**a**) and transverse (**b**) scans of the flexor tendon of the first finger of the right hand clearly show the typical echogenic fibrillar structure

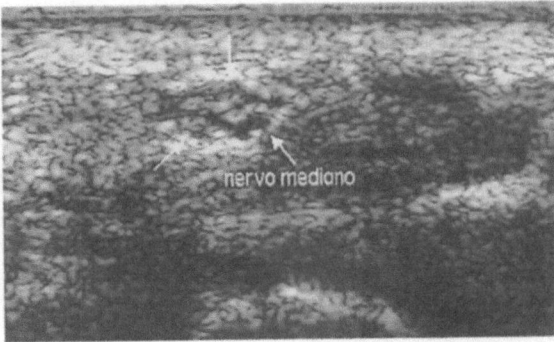

Fig. 4.2. Transverse scan of a median nerve (*arrows*) of the left hand shows the typical microlacunar structure of the secondary nerve bundles forming the nerve. *nervo mediano* median nerve

4.4   Abnormal Patterns

4.4.1   Tendons

Inflammation is certainly the most frequent disease found at US. It is called tenosynovitis as it involves mainly or exclusively the peritendinous synovial sheets
covering the tendons. There are two subtypes of inflammation:
- Stenosing tenosynovitis, which affects only the tendons with a synovial sheath
  where they course in osteofibrotic channels. Indeed, the inflammation mainly
  affects the peritendinous fibrous sheath that thickens because of hyperplasia
  and thus compresses and impresses the tendon preventing normal sliding
  (Fig. 4.3). Dynamic studies clearly show difficult tendon flexion. The most
  frequent type of stenosing tenosynovitis is called De Quervain disease and
  involves the long abductor and short extensor tendons of the first finger.
- Hypertrophic-exudative tenosynovitis, where inflammation involves the true
  synovial sheath. The main findings are serous exudation or hyperplasia of the
  sheath, which is thickened and distended by hypoechoic effusion (Fig. 4.4).

In these cases US is a very sensitive tool in showing even very little effusion in
the sheath. Dynamic studies are fundamental too, for direct demonstration of
normal sliding of tendon fibers.

Bacterial and tubercular tenosynovitis are uncommon forms of the disease
characterized by massive distention of all peritendinous synovial sheaths in the
region involved, with markedly heterogeneous hypoechoic granular material inside (Fig. 4.5). In these pathological conditions the tendon fiber, which is usually
preserved in nonspecific inflammatory tenosynovitis, appears markedly heterogeneous and irregular because of degeneration (Fig. 4.5a).

Rupture of flexor and extensor tendons of the hand is not an uncommon event.
It may result from trauma, causing partial or complete tear of the fibers, or from
degeneration phenomena that weaken the tendon resistance to functional stress
and thus predispose to fiber rupture.

US permits prompt diagnosis of this condition because it can easily and accurately demonstrate the site and severity of damage as well as perilesional blood
effusion, which is not abundant because tendons are poorly vascularized. Tendon

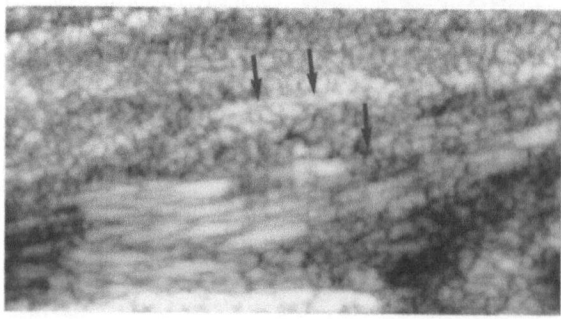

Fig. 4.3. Tendon inflammation.
Stenosing tenosynovitis with apparent fibrous compression on
the tendon (*arrows*)

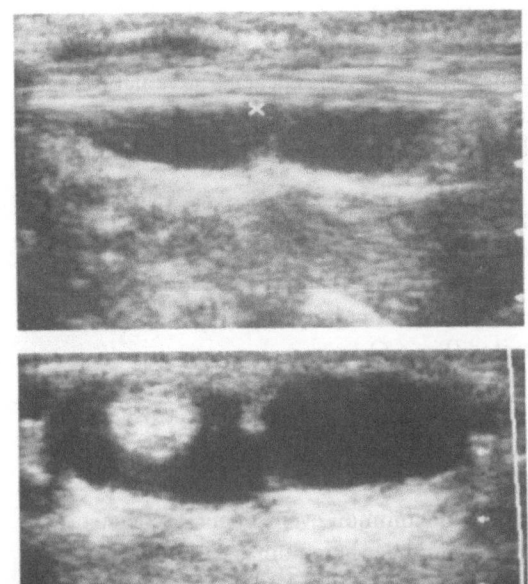

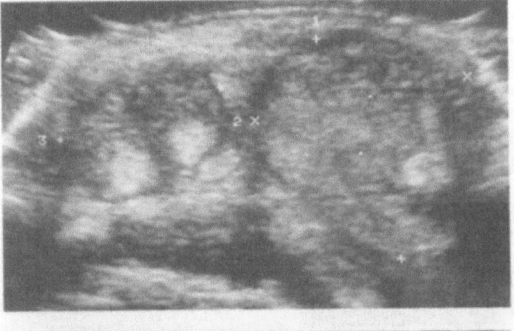

Fig. 4.4. Tendon inflammation: longitudinal (**a**) (calipers) and transverse (**b**) scans. In the exudative form the sheath is distended and occupied by hypo- or anechoic effusion

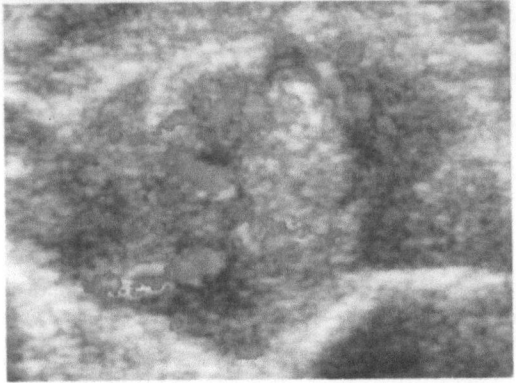

Fig. 4.5a, b. Tendon inflammation. Bacterial tenosynovitis involves the whole sheath, with abundant heterogeneous material (**a**) (calipers, numbers) and important vascularization with color Doppler (**b**)

rupture from major trauma is usually associated with damage to adjacent muscular structures, skin and subcutaneous tissue.

Cysts are round or oval, echo-free and closely related to the synovial sheath of the tendons they originate from. They are usually of a degenerative nature. Integration of conventional with dynamic studies is extremely important in this case too because dynamic US can easily show the close continuity between tendon and cyst during fiber sliding.

Tumors are a rare event, but giant cell tumor is typical of the tendons with a synovial sheath and solely localized in tendons of the hand and feet. US shows a solid mass with fairly homogeneous hypoechoic structure and poor vascularization, which develops and grows eccentric to the tendon, usually spared by the mass and neither compressed nor infiltrated (Fig. 4.6).

4.4.2 Muscles and Subcutaneous Tissue

Trauma to the hand muscles is a rather uncommon event. When associated with fiber damage it is characterized by intramuscular hematomas with different echostructure according to the evolutionary stage.

Granulomatous reactions from a foreign body are a more frequent finding that can occur both in muscles and in subcutaneous tissue. US shows hypoecho-

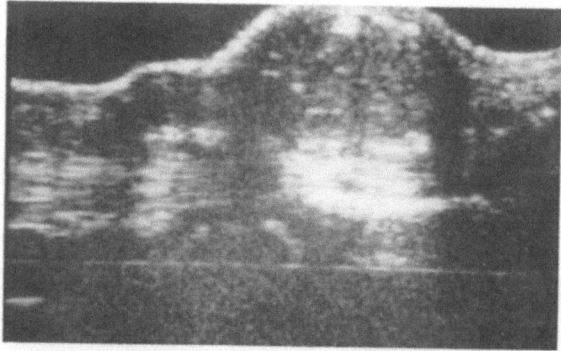

a

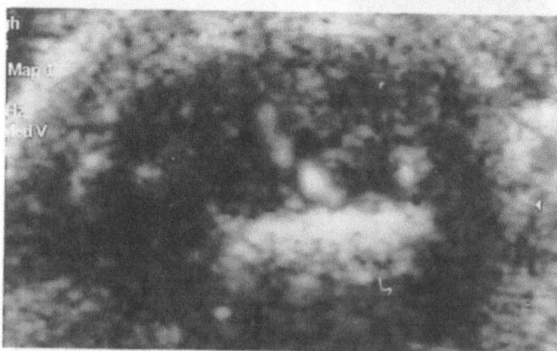

b

Fig. 4.6a, b. Giant cell tumor in the fourth finger of the right hand. The round hypoechoic mass develops eccentric to the course of the tendon, which is spared (a). Power Doppler shows a single afference inside the tumor (b)

ic masses with very irregular margins usually containing hyperechoic foreign bodies (Fig. 4.7).

Another condition localized in the hand is Dupuytren disease, which is related to pseudonodules and to palmar aponeurosis thickening. US shows typical fusiform solid nodules originating from the superficial palmar fascia.

Tumors, which can involve both the subcutaneous tissue and muscle, are mainly benign. The most frequent ones are lipoma, fibroma, angioma and neuroma. US findings are rather nonspecific and range from homogeneous hypoechogenicity to marked hyperechogenicity, but always with a mass with clear-cut and regular outline, often with a capsule and no major vessels at color or power Doppler (Fig. 4.8).

On the contrary, malignant lesions have totally different and pathognomonic color and power Doppler patterns. They are usually hypoechoic masses with blurred and irregular margins indicating infiltration of surrounding regions; the echostructure is heterogeneous (Fig. 4.9) and color Doppler depicts rich vascularization both around and inside the mass, with smaller and bigger vascular branches. Doppler sampling shows very different flows inside these masses, which testifies to their anarchic growth. The glomus tumor has a typical richly vascularized pattern. Its usual location is at the base of the nail (Fig. 4.10).

Finally, US can demonstrate amyloid deposits, which are particularly frequent in dialysis patients, in both para-articular sites and subcutaneous tissue. Amyloid deposits appear as oval masses with irregular margins and markedly heterogeneous echostructure, partly hyper- and partly hypoechoic.

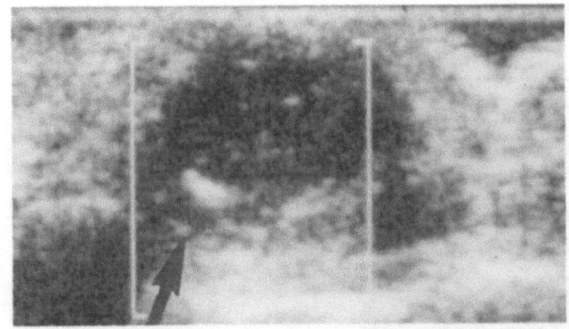

Fig. 4.7. A hyperechoic foreign body (wood splinter; *arrow*) in the soft tissues of a finger is surrounded by hypoechoic granulomatous reaction

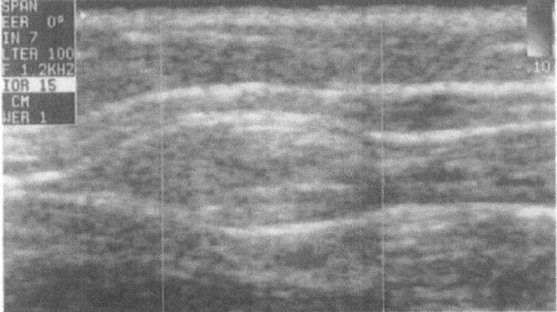

Fig. 4.8. Lipoma of the thenar eminence (diameter 15.0 mm) with no vascularization and homogeneous echogenic appearance

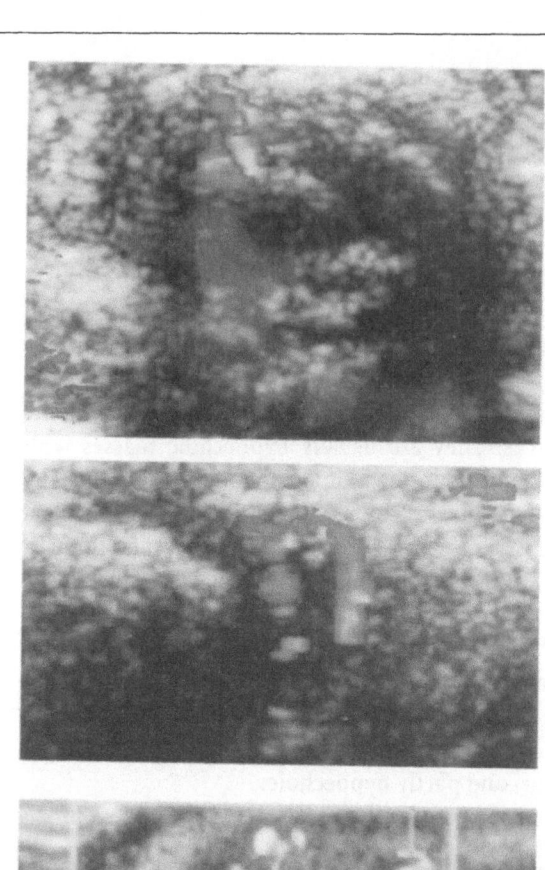

Fig. 4.9a, b. Synovial sarcoma. (a) Transverse scan shows a heterogeneous hypoechoic mass with blurred and irregular margins with infiltration of surrounding regions and large feeding vessels, clearly depicted even on a longitudinal scan (b)

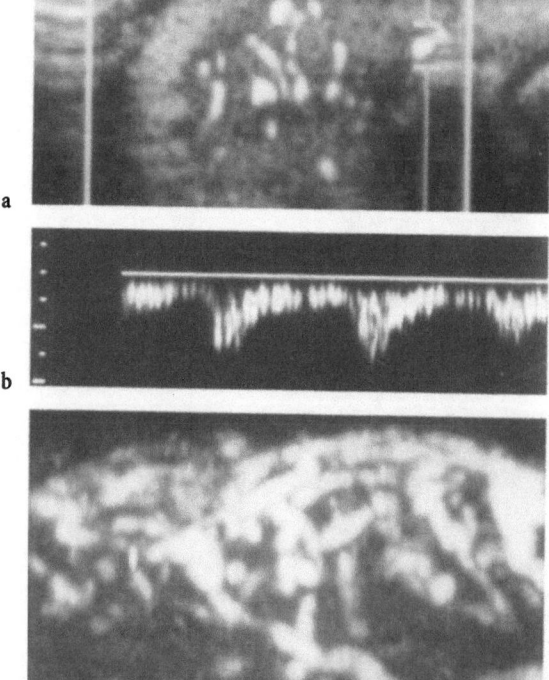

Fig. 4.10a–c. Glomus tumor around the nail of the first finger of the right hand. Power Doppler (a) with spectral analysis (b): typical hypervascularization with tangled vessels, better seen on the three-dimensional reconstruction (c)

4.4.3   Joints

The so-called arthrogenous ganglia, or cystic hygromas, are cystic masses that originate from the joint and communicate with it through a connection that is usually very thin but clearly depicted sonographically (Fig. 4.11). Ganglia have a homogeneous liquid content and regular walls.

Trauma to the joint capsule and periarticular ligaments, e.g., collateral ligaments, is usually characterized by effusion, which is often of a hemorrhagic nature, in the joint involved.

In addition, rheumatoid arthritis localizes in joints, particularly the interphalangeal joints of the hand. High-frequency probes permit depiction of early involvement of the synovial membranes of the joint and of the synovial sheaths of the tendon. Besides effusion, US can also demonstrate degenerative changes in the tendon, which are typical of the disease, appearing as hypoechoic/echo-free cyst-like nodules (Fig. 4.12). Finally, in advanced disease US can show the most frequent complication of synovitis, that is rupture of tendon fibers.

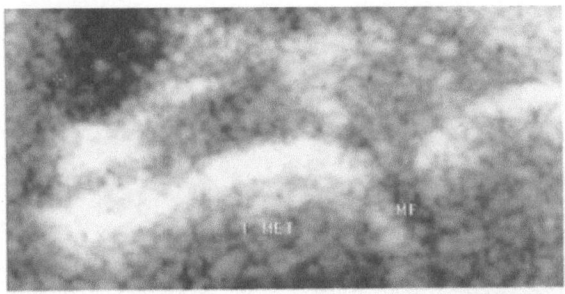

Fig. 4.11. Small arthrogenic ganglion (calipers=1.26 cm.) where US clearly shows the communication with the underlying metacarpophalangeal joint. *I MET* first metacarpal bone, *MF* metacarpophalangeal joint

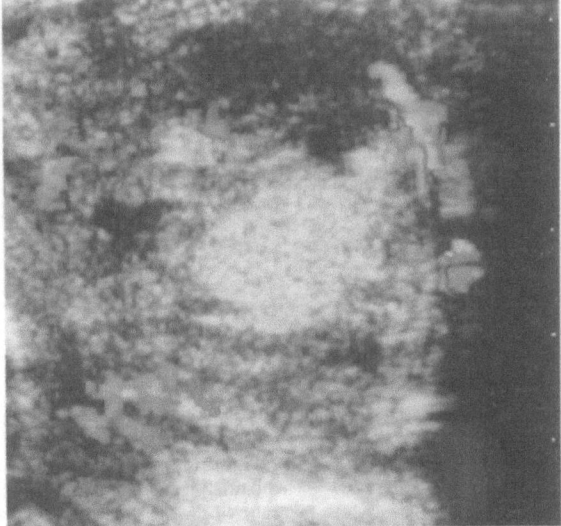

Fig. 4.12. Rheumatoid arthritis in the hand. Note the presence of hypervascularized synovial pannus

4.4.4   Nerves and Vessels

Carpal tunnel syndrome is certainly the most frequent and best known tunnel syndrome. Guyon's channel syndrome is less frequent (Fig. 4.13). US plays a very important role in defining the nature of the syndrome, such as tenosynovitis with sheath thickening, abnormal muscles, cysts, tumors occupying the channel, and conditions resulting from fractures.

Impairment is often demonstrated in the fibers of the involved nerve, which exhibits thickening above the extrinsic compression, reduced echogenicity of the constituent nerve bundles and finely irregular margins.

Benign and malignant tumors originating from median and ulnar nerves have different morphology and echostructure depending on whether they are neurofibromas or schwannomas. Thus neurofibromas are fusiform, hypoechoic and poorly vascularized, while schwannomas are round, sometimes nearly echo-free and more vascularized (Fig. 4.14).

Finally, among the vascular diseases arteriovenous malformations are a not infrequent finding (Fig. 4.15). Color Doppler and power Doppler are of fundamental importance in the diagnosis of these malformation and of Raynaud's disease.

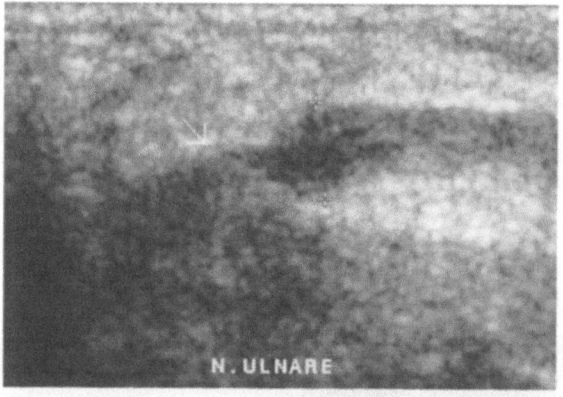

a

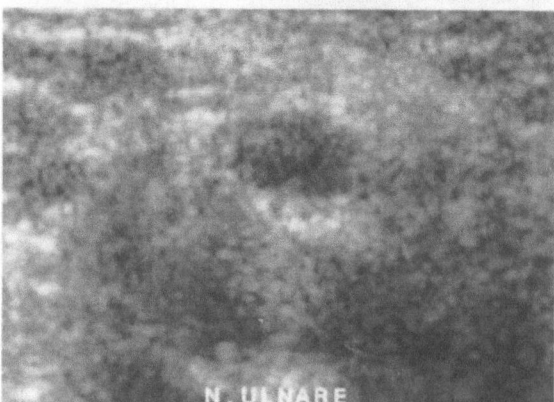

b

Fig. 4.13. Guyon's channel syndrome: longitudinal (a) and transverse (b) scans. The ulnar nerve is deformed and thickened, with finely irregular margins (*arrow*). *N ULNARE* ulnar nerve

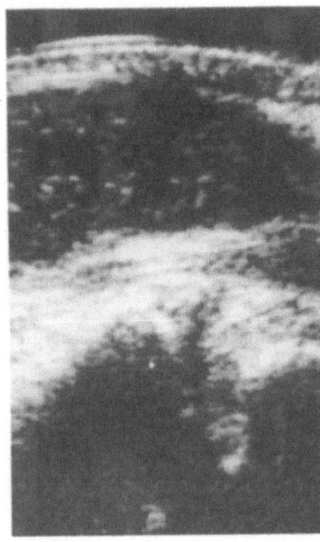

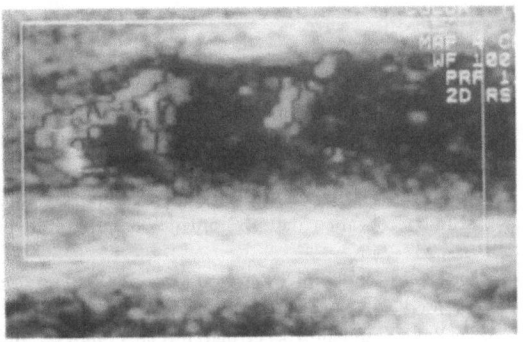

a

b

Fig. 4.14. Uncommon malignant schwannoma of the median nerve (**a**) with rich vascularization (**b**)

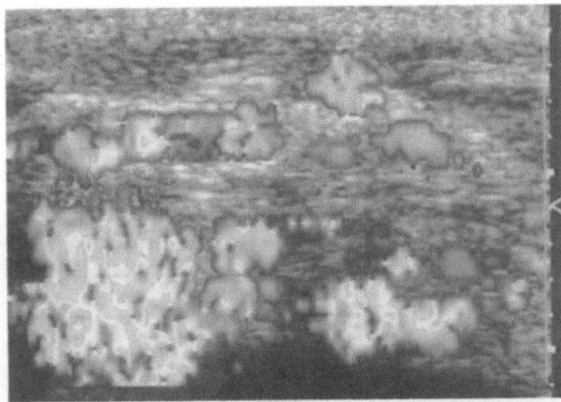

a

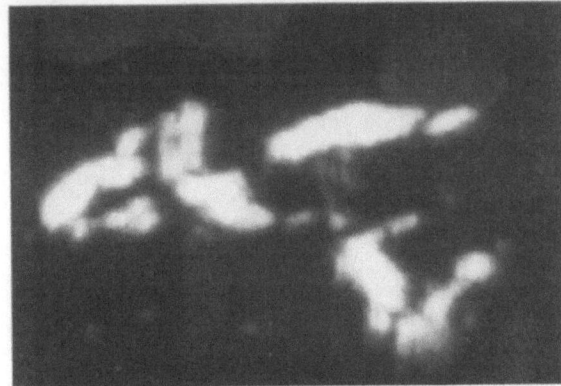

b

Fig. 4.15a, b. Arteriovenous malformation of the hand palm in a young patient. Color (**a**) and power Doppler with three-dimensional reconstruction (**b**) clearly show the typical serpiginous appearance of the vessels

References

1. Bottinelli O, Campani R, Bozzini A, La Fianza A, Calliada F (1993) Studio ecografico della mano: anatomia normale e quadri patologici. Radiol Med 85 [Suppl. 1.5]:227-236
2. Campani R, Bottinelli O, Bozzini A, et al (1990) Ecotomografia. In: Ziviello M, Biggi E, Ferrari F (eds). Idelson, Naples, pp 468-494
3. Caprotti P, Campani R, Bottinelli O, Genovese E, Caprotti C (1993) Artrite reumatoide: studio ecografico delle lesioni dei tessuti molli perischeletrici. Radiol Med 85 [Suppl. 1.5]:237-246
4. De Pra L, Gandellini S, Petrolati M, et al (1986) Lo studio ecografico della mano. I. Anatomia. US Med 7:53-60
5. De Pra L, Gandellini S, Petrolati M, et al (1986) Lo studio ecografico della mano. II. Patologia. US Med 7:133-139
6. Fornage BD, Schernberg FL, Rifkin MD (1985) Ultrasound examination of the hand. Radiology 155:785-788
7. Höglund M (1997) Ultrasound diagnosis of soft-tissue tumours in the hand and forearm. Acta Radiol 38:508-513
8. Höglund M, Tordai P, Muren C (1994) Diagnosis of ganglions in the hand and wrist by sonography. Acta Radiol 35:35-39
9. Höglund M, Muren C, Engkvist O (1997) Ultrasound characteristics of five common soft-tissue tumours in the hand and forearm. Acta Radiol 38:348-355
10. Miquel A, Frouge C, Adrien C, Hibou I, Bittoun J, Bisson M, Bléry M (1995) Ténosynovite tuberculeuse du poignet: diagnostic échographique et apport de l'IRM. J Radiol 76:285-288
11. Perugia L, Postacchini F, Ippolito E (1981) I tendini: biologia, patologia, clinica. Masson, Milan
12. Riehl J, Schmitt H, Bergmann D, Sieberth HG (1997) Tuberculous tenosynovitis of the hand: evaluation with B-mode ultrasonography. J Ultrasound Med 16:369-372
13. Souissi M, Ebelin M, Rigot J, Lemerle JP, Moreau JF (1989) Exploration ultrasonographique des parties molles de la main. III. Pathologie traumatique et inflammatoire des tendons flechisseurs des doigts de la main. J Radiol 70:352-355
14. Trentanni C, Galli A, Melucci G, Stasi G (1997) Diagnosi ecografia della tenosinovite stenosante di De Quervain. Radiol Med 93:194-198

5   Magnetic Resonance Imaging

HARALD MARCEL BONÉL, MAXIMILIAN REISER

5.1   Introduction

The fine anatomic detail of the hand and wrist presents a challenge for even the newest imaging technologies, and tests the magnetic resonance imaging (MRI) capabilities of even the most advanced MR imaging systems. Much of the anatomic and functional knowledge of the wrist is derived from hand surgery literature and was obtained by anatomic dissection or surgical and arthroscopic exploration.

The interlocking bones of the wrist are stabilized by multiple intrinsic and extrinsic ligaments and form a functional unit that allows both complex movement and great flexibility, while providing high stability at the same time. Concise anatomic and functional knowledge is therefore required for MR protocol planning as well as reporting of MRI examinations [22]. This chapter is intended to assist in protocol planning of MR imaging of the hand and wrist.

5.2   Technical Considerations

In order to present the anatomic detail necessary for MR examinations of the hand and wrist, sufficient spatial resolution as well as tissue contrast are essential. The wrist is usually imaged in the periphery of the main magnetic field, where the overall signal-to-noise ratios are less. Therefore, it is critical to employ a local or surface coil, which matches the volume of the hand or wrist, to gain sufficient signal-to-noise levels (Fig. 5.1). Small cylindrical transmit–receive coils that provide adequate signal-to-noise ratios and radiofrequency homogeneity to adequately visualize the entire cross-section of the wrist and hand are available from most MR equipment manufacturers. Powerful gradient coils and amplifiers capable of providing strong and more rapidly varying gradient fields are the basis for the spatial information that forms the MR image. They allow the most rapid acquisition of images with high in-plane resolution in thin section thickness.

Assuming that all other technical factors are equal, high-field MRI scanners have a distinct advantage in image quality over low-field units. However, the availability of appropriate surface coils as well as the knowledge and skill of the radiologist overseeing and reporting the study may well compensate for the intrinsic advantage of higher field strength systems. Recent technical advances may further

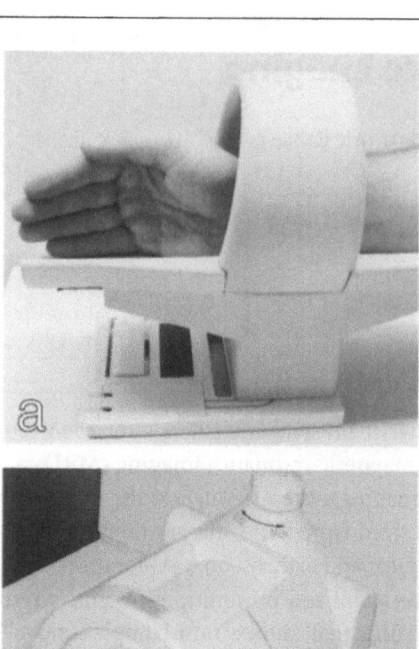
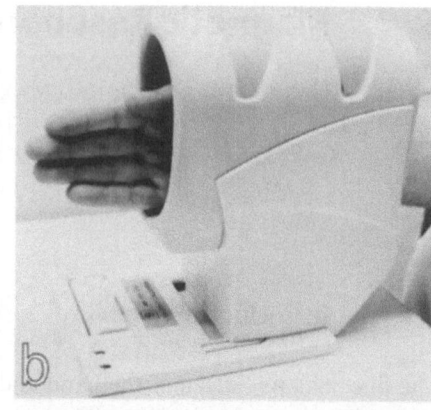
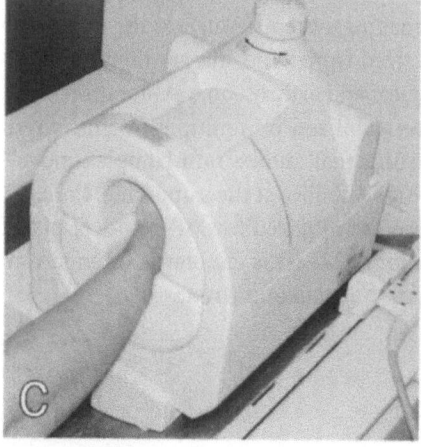
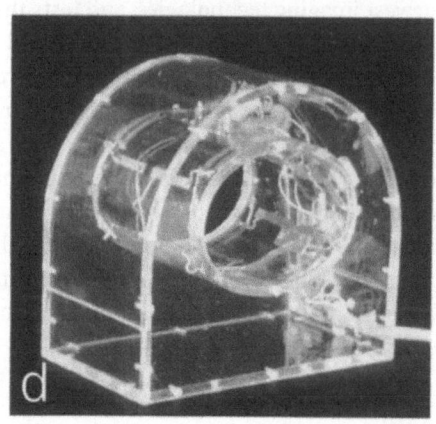
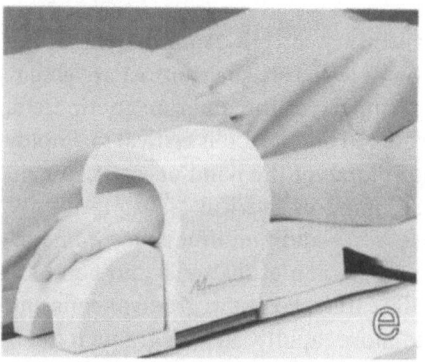

Fig. 5.1. a The standard wrist coil of a dedicated low-field MRI system. This send and receive coil uses a solenoidal unpolarized design; the internal diameter is about 9 cm to suit even very large wrists. **b** To increase coil load this wrist coil has an oval diameter. Two receivers are combined to gain about 40% more signal and reduce image noise (phased-array design with two channels). This coil provides sufficient signal for diagnostic imaging even at 0.2 T (Esaote Artoscan, Genoa, Italy). **c** The standard send and receive extremity coil of a 1.5 T system (Siemens Magnetom Vision, Erlangen, Germany) suits knees as well as wrists. Because of its large volume in the limited space of the gantry of the MR scanner, the patient has to raise the arm above the head to be examined in a prone position. This "Superman" position is increasingly painful during long imaging times, especially in elderly patients with shoulder problems. **d** The prototype of a dedicated wrist coil of a high-field system is shown (four-channel phased-array coil designed for a 1.5 T scanner). Again, the diameter is oval to suit the wrist or hand, and the four receiver units can be recognized (courtesy of PD Dr. T. Link, Munich, Germany; reprinted with permission). **e** A commercially available quadrature wrist coil (courtesy of ICG Medical Advances, Milwaukee, Wis., USA; reprinted with permission). Both the phased-array and quadrature coils (**d**, **e**) are especially suitable for high-resolution imaging at high field strength

nullify the fact that certain pulse sequences such as fat-suppressed T1-weighted sequences are not yet available at low field strength. Low-field systems using optimized protocols can serve very well as a means of excluding specific diagnoses [7], but do not deliver the diagnostic detail provided by advanced high-field scanners using elaborate and thorough protocols. Nevertheless, for selected indications, such as occult fractures of the scaphoid and similarly well-defined entities, low-field scanners could be the first choice if availability is greater.

5.3 Patient Considerations

5.3.1 Patients at Risk

Magnetic fields used in medical imaging are very strong. For example, a 1.5 T scanner has a magnetic field which is 3000 times stronger than the magnetic field of the earth. Technical implants, such as cardiac pacemakers, ear implants or subcutaneous insulin pumps, can be influenced by these magnetic fields or even cease to function. Therefore, it is critical to obtain information from the manufacturer of these devices prior to the examination to determine the threshold field strength for the device operation. Usually cardiac pacemakers do not function in a high-field scanner. A recent in vitro study has shown that in dedicated low-field scanners the magnetic stray fields are so small that cardiac pacemakers still work even if they are very close to the gantry [51]. These results, however, should be backed up by clinical data before being applied in routine imaging.

5.3.2 Patient Preparation

Even small motion artifacts can have devastating effects on the image quality at this level of spatial resolution. It is therefore especially important to take the time to inform the patient beforehand of the nature of the MR imaging study to allay any fear and ensure the comfort of the patient during the procedure. Premedication is essential in patients with claustrophobia. In children, the presence of a parent near the head of the child in the examination room might be an alternative or of additional help. Otherwise, the use of a dedicated open MR scanner might be indicated. In claustrophobic patients, the dedicated scanner has several advantages: it allows personal contact of the technician in the same room with the patient, noise levels are much lower and the patient can read to pass the time while being scanned.

5.3.3 Markers

It is extremely important to use a marker, such as a capsule containing vitamin D or nitroglycerin (as used for medication), to indicate the localization of the most painful area of the wrist. The marker can be attached to the skin with adhesive tape prior to the positioning. In the case of superficial pathologies, the markers should be used to indicate the proximal and distal or lateral and medial border of the region in question. In this way a compression of the pathology, which could obscure it, is avoided.

For MR imaging of fingers, a pill could already compress the anatomy too much if used in a dedicated coil. In this case, a thick film of Vaseline applied to the skin is an efficient marker, as it shows up with high signal intensity on T1-weighted images.

5.3.4   Positioning

In dedicated low-field systems, the patient can sit beside the main magnet and place the wrist inside the receiver coil of the magnetic gantry. In high-field systems, the patient is usually placed in either of two positions: prone with the wrist overhead in the isocenter of the magnet or supine with the wrist at the side of the body. While it is generally beneficial to use the isocenter of the magnet for high signal and image contrast, many patients cannot tolerate this position for 10 min, which is less than half the time of a standard imaging protocol, and movement artifacts are likely to result in any repeated or additional sequences.

Passive restraints, such as foam rubber pads, tape and sandbags are appropriate aids to immobilize the wrist and hand during image acquisition and avoid involuntary movement. Proper padding of the forearm, elbow and shoulder are further measures to ensure patient comfort and at the same time reduce the potential of motion artifacts during the examination.

For imaging of the wrist, a foam rubber cylinder can be placed in the hand to form a fist. Also the back of the wrist and metacarpus should be padded to avoid undesirable dorsiflexion of the wrist, which produces an oblique orientation of the capsular ligaments, especially in coronal planes.

5.3.5   Slice Orientation

5.3.5.1   Wrist

The wrist is usually imaged in pronation. An axial localizer covering the distal radioulnar joint as well as the proximal and distal row of the carpal bones is a very useful anatomic basis for selecting the coronal and sagittal orientation and the extent of imaging slices.

The most proximal of these axial planes displaying the carpal bones, which displays the scaphoid, lunate and pisiform bones at the same time, is most reliable for positioning of coronal planes. A typically positioned utmost palmar coronal plane will display the distal scaphoid and the volar pisiform bone at the same time.

If aligned with the distal radioulnar joint, a completely different view would result, which deviates to the dorsal direction on the ulnar side mimicking a supinated view of the wrist. The range of coronal planes should include the extensor tendons and the major part of the flexor tendons in the carpal tunnel, covering all bony structures of the wrist.

Axial planes are preferably planned using coronal planes, which show the capitate bone. The planes are oriented perpendicular to the longitudinal axis of the capitate bone. This allows a slight radial or ulnar abduction to be compensated. For imaging of the complete wrist, the distal radioulnar joint and the bases of the second to fifth metacarpal bones are used.

Sagittal planes are planned using either axial or coronal planes or both. Depending on the clinical question, sagittal planes can be used to examine the midsection only (e.g., in the case of carpal instability), the lateral aspect of the wrist to display the triangular fibrocartilage complex and its attachments or the medial part of the wrist to evaluate the region of the scaphoid bone.

5.3.5.2   Fingers

For imaging of the fingers, an entirely stretched position of the fingers is most desirable. While this aspect matters little for sagittal planes, it is important for images in coronal and axial planes, which would otherwise have less diagnostic value due to pronounced partial volume effects.

Axial planes are positioned perpendicular to the respective finger. Sagittal images are preferably planned on both coronal and axial localizers to eliminate significant partial volume effects. Coronal planes are positioned perpendicular to true axial images.

Imaging of the thumb requires a very careful and dedicated technique. Usually multiple localizers must be performed to allow exact positioning, as the other fingers cannot be used as an indicator of the orientation of the thumb.

5.4   Spatial Resolution

Spatial resolution defines the ability to view closely spaced anatomic detail. The smaller the voxel dimensions the better the resolution of fine detail. Figure 5.2 illustrates the definitions and terms used for defining the field-of-view, voxel size and in-plane resolution. Generally, it is advisable to calculate the voxel size for easier comparison of protocols.

In hand and wrist imaging, a slice thickness of 3 mm or less combined with an in-plane resolution of at least 1 mm^2 is generally recommended to present sufficient anatomic detail. For the detection of fine anatomic detail, such as the triangular fibrocartilage complex (TFCC), an in-plane resolution of 0.3×0.3 mm^2 may be necessary [59, 61].

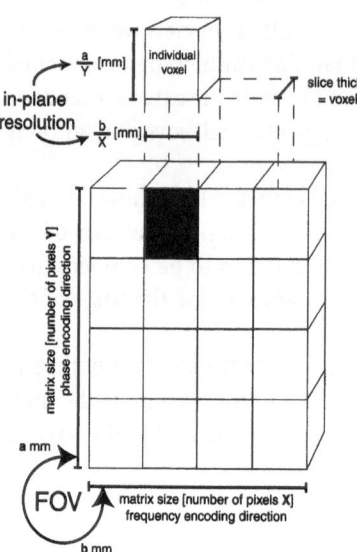

Fig. 5.2. This scheme illustrates the definitions of field-of-view, voxel size and in-plane resolution. In order to simplify the scheme, a very coarse matrix of 4×4 pixels is shown. For the examination of the wrist, usually a matrix of 192×256 pixels or more is applied

5.5 Image Contrast and Tissue Composition

Along with the spatial resolution, image contrast is a major determinant of diagnostic image quality. In MRI sequences image contrast usually decreases with increased spatial resolution and vice versa, and the radiologist has to find a compromise between the two.

Image contrast in MRI is a complex function of many factors, such as the proton density of the sample, its molecular environment and the resulting T1 and T2 relaxation times and the magnetic susceptibility of the nuclei, which can be explained as a tendency to resist magnetization. Non-mobile protons in solids, such as in cortical bone or dense fibrous tissue, have very long T1 and very short T2 relaxation times and therefore do not contribute to the measurable MR signal intensity. By comparison, tissues with a high density of mobile protons, such as fat, water and muscle, contribute considerably to the MR signal. However, a high density of protons does not necessarily guarantee a high signal in the MR image.

By definition, T2-weighted images are characterized by a very high signal of water, whereas in T1-weighted images fat appears brightest. Table 5.1 provides information about the appearance of fat and water in T1- and T2-weighted images. Proton density weighted images are generally less suitable to differentiate the chemical composition of the various tissues. However, anatomic detail is as good or even better than in T1-weighted images, but proton density weighted images depict collagen fibers better.

MR imaging of collagen is also essential in imaging of the hand and wrist. Usually at least one T1- and one T2-weighted sequence are used to visualize the tendon, ligament or triangular fibrocartilage in question. Table 5.2 details the appearance of collagen in various degrees of degeneration and rupture in T1- and T2-weighted sequences.

Table 5.1. T1 and T2-weighted image contrast

	Fat	Water
T1-weighted	Bright	Intermediate
T2-weighted	Low	High
Proton density	Intermediate	Low

Table 5.2. Appearance of collagen fibers in various degrees of degeneration or when interrupted in SE and TSE sequences. This scheme can be applied to many diagnoses of the triangular fibrocartilage complex

Intact	Mild degeneration	Severe degeneration	Tear
Water tightly bound	Water loosely bound	Some free water	Water in tear
Intact collagen fibers	Mostly intact collagen fibers	Some intact collagen fibers	Collagen remnants
Black on all sequences	Gray on short TE images	Bright gray on short TE images	Bright gray on short TE images
	Black on long TE images	Gray on long TE images	Bright gray or white on long TE images

5.6 Pulse Sequences

Pulse sequences are measurement programs applied to the MR scanner to acquire image signal. Image contrast, spatial resolution and measurement times are the result of parameter adjustments of these pulse sequences.

5.6.1 Spin-Echo Sequence

The spin-echo (SE) sequence is most commonly used for the evaluation of the hand and wrist. Simple manipulation of the timing parameters results in T1-weighted, T2-weighted and proton density weighted image contrast (Table 5.3). Usually this sequence is implemented as a two-dimensional multisection technique. Typically SE imaging yields a minimal slice thickness of 2–3 mm. SE sequences are suitable for hand and wrist imaging because they depict anatomic structures very well with high contrast. Long acquisition times, especially for T2-weighted sequences, are the major drawback of this sequence type.

Table 5.3. Image appearance as a function of the repetition time and echo time for SE images. The numbers give an overview of a 1.5 T system and may differ by manufacturer

	Short echo time (TE) (20 ms)	Long echo time (TE) (80 ms)
Short repetition time (TR) (600 ms)	T1-weighted	(Mixed contrast not a common setting)
Long repetition time (TR) (2000 ms)	Proton density weighted	T2-weighted

5.6.2   Fast Spin-Echo Sequence

Fast-spin-echo (FSE) sequences are also referred as turbo-spin-echo (TSE) sequences and were originally developed to speed up image acquisition by obtaining multiple echoes. This is achieved by refocusing impulses, which are the characteristic feature of the FSE sequence scheme. Usually, imaging time is greatly shortened. FSE sequences are most commonly implemented as a two-dimensional multisection technique. The number of echoes obtained is called an "echo train". The longer the echo train the more data can be acquired, but the fewer sections obtained in a given repetition time. Hence, the major value of FSE imaging lies in T2-weighted imaging, where more images with the same spatial resolution can be obtained in a shorter time or the same number of planes with a better resolution result in a comparable time. The appearance of FSE images is very similar to that of SE images; however, two important differences must be pointed out:

- Using comparable imaging parameters, fat appears brighter on T2-weighted FSE sequences than on SE sequences. This effect is even more striking if longer echo trains are used [20, 64]. As this may obscure bone marrow disease, chemical shift fat suppression is frequently necessary to differentiate the high signal from fat and bone marrow changes. A robust alternative, also available at low field strength, is short tau inversion recovery (STIR) imaging, which is explained below.
- In addition, fine anatomic detail is slightly more blurred in FSE images compared with SE images acquired with similar sequence parameters. Short, effective echo times, a small in-plane resolution and long echo trains further aggravate this blurring. This problem, however, can be solved with a finer in-plane resolution, e.g., a matrix of 256+256 instead of 256+192 pixels using the same field-of-view. Modern FSE sequence designs applied in advanced high-field scanners acquire the information on fine detail at a time in the sequence cycle when signal is still abundant, and therefore blurring is usually less significant.

The parameter setting, especially of the echo-time, resembles that of a comparable SE sequence.

5.6.3   Gradient Recalled Echo Sequences

Gradient recalled echo (GRE) sequences can be implemented as two-dimensional sequences, comparable to SE sequences, or as three-dimensional sequences, which gain more signal and have therefore the potential for even thinner slice reconstructions. The thinner slice thickness combined with a high in-plane resolution theoretically permit the detection of smaller abnormalities, provided there is sufficient signal-to-noise ratio in the image. This great potential, however, is often nullified by the small contrast between the anatomic structures in the image, and often does not demonstrate a greater sensitivity towards the presence of disease. An advantageous use of three-dimensional GRE sequences for wrist pathologies, including those of the TFCC and various ligaments of the wrist, has been described by Totterman and Miller [59, 61].

Three-dimensional GRE sequences are the method of choice for cartilage imaging, especially if acquisition time matters in a routine imaging setting [23, 39, 57, 62]. Fast GRE sequences are also the method of choice for kinematic studies of the wrist. Steady-state GRE sequences have shown superb image quality in MR presentation of cortical and spongy bone [57] (Fig. 5.3). Table 5.4 lists the typical sequence parameters applied in two-dimensional GRE imaging.

5.6.4. Short Tau Inversion Recovery Sequence

In short tau inversion recovery (STIR) imaging prepulses can be executed in conjunction with either GRE, SE or FSE sequences. An inversion recovery prepulse can be applied to generate images that are generally dependent on T1 relaxation effects as a part of presaturation protocols. An inversion recovery impulse inverts the net magnetization and flips it 180° from its original orientation. When this impulse ceases, the spins relax, and the magnitude recovers, passing from a maxi-

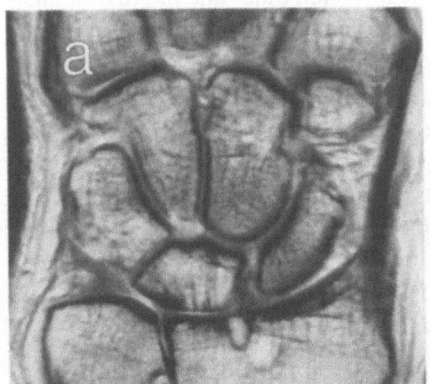
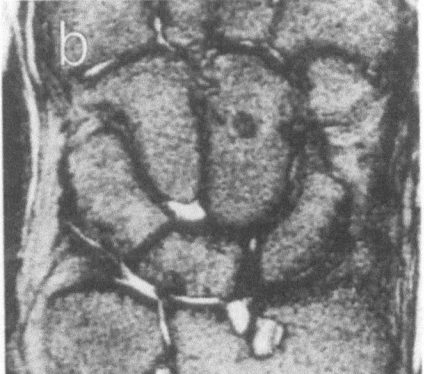
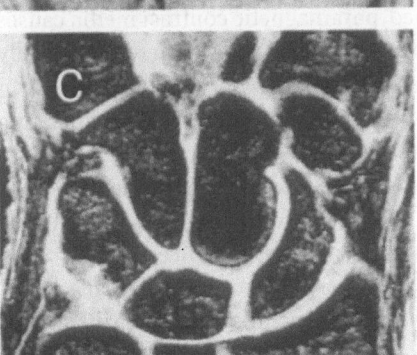

Fig. 5.3a–c. The same slice was acquired using three different sequences. a The steady-state-GRE sequence (CISS: constructive interference in steady state) shows the cortical and trabecular structures very well. While the STIR sequence (b) still provides some structural information on the spongy bone, the fat-suppressed gradient-spoiled GRE sequence (c) (FLASH: fast low angle shot) nullifies all trabecular structures. Cartilage appears dark in the CISS (a) and STIR (b) sequences but of bright signal intensity in the FLASH sequence (c). Water is best recognized in the STIR sequence (b)

Table 5.4. Image appearance as a function of the repetition time, echo time and flip angle for GRE images. The numbers give an impression of values used typically on a 1.5 T system with a repetition time of 200–500 ms and may differ for different manufacturers. T2-weighted image contrast in GRE sequences gives a slightly different image impression compared with SE imaging. This is because the MR physics is slightly different and GRE sequences giving high water signal are therefore labeled as T2*-weighted

Image contrast	Echo time TE (ms)	Flip angle (deg)
T1-weighted	Short (10–15)	Large (55–90°)
T2*-weighted	Long (30–50)	Small (5–20°)
Proton-density weighted	Short (8–15)	Small (5–15°)

mum negative value through zero, and then builds up in the positive direction. Tissues with a short T1 relaxation time, such as fat, reach the longitudinal magnetization faster than protons in water. This time difference can be used to exclude signal from fat in the MR signal (Fig. 5.4).

To generate a detectable MR signal, a signal generation scheme is then applied. While a combination with a SE scheme can be performed at any field strength, it is used less frequently because of its long sequence duration. On mid- and high-field systems, turbo-inversion-recovery sequences with a varying length of the echo train are used most often. A combination with a GRE sequence scheme may be beneficial on low-field MR scanners [8]. The inversion time "tau" has to be adjusted according to the strength of the main field. The smaller the field strength, the shorter the inversion time ideal for fat suppression.

STIR sequences are especially useful in the detection of bone marrow abnormalities in the hand and wrist, as found in occult fractures [10, 24]. Also in STIR sequences, intrinsic ligaments and the TFCC are easily delineated [50]. If the contrast with free water is required, such as in imaging of cysts or to contrast the TFCC, proton-density fat-saturated TSE and STIR sequences are an appropriate choice [57].

5.6.5   Fat-Suppressed T1- and T2-Weighted Sequences

Local accumulation of intravenously applied, paramagnetic contrast media causes a shortening of the T1 relaxation time in the enhancing tissue. Therefore, usually T1-weighted sequences are applied to detect enhancing tissues. In the presence of fatty tissues, which are very bright on T1-weighted sequences, slightly enhancing tissues may not be recognized easily due to rescaling effects. For image presentations, the raw signal intensities have to be transformed to a gray scale of usually 256 gray levels. In a non-fat-suppressed T1-weighted sequence, the brightest gray level is matched with fat, if none of the other structures enhances very strongly with paramagnetic contrast. If fat is suppressed, usually strongly enhancing structures are brightest in the image, while tissues enhancing much less will still be recognized as the full scale is applied on the smaller range of signal intensities representing mostly enhancing tissues.

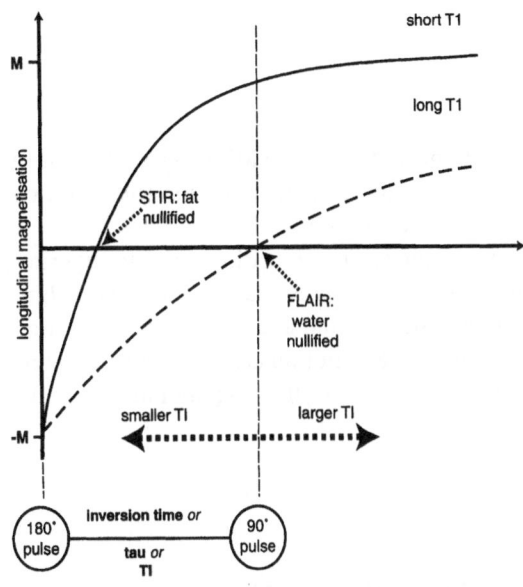

Fig. 5.4. Inversion recovery sequences. When the inversion pulse ceases, the longitudinal magnetization of the hand increases. Tissues with a shorter T1, such as fat, return faster to the equilibrium than tissues with a longer T1, such as water. In STIR imaging, the TI is set to nullify the signal from fat. For comparison, signal from water is nullified in FLAIR imaging (fluid attenuated inversion recovery). FLAIR imaging is, however, not commonly used in musculoskeletal MRI

Especially in T2-weighted FSE sequences, signal from fat is represented by a middle range of signal intensities, which is considerably higher compared with only slightly edematous tissues. Therefore, the detection of these pathologic structures is made easier by fat suppression, which presents these structures with a higher level of gray in comparison with fat.

The most common technique for fat suppression is frequency selective presaturation, which can be combined with a variety of sequence schemes such as GRE, SE and TSE sequences. This method is based on the chemical shift difference between protons bound to fat or water. A frequency selective presaturation pulse is applied prior to the excitation in order to eliminate longitudinal magnetization for a specific tissue, usually fat. This technique relies on the capability to spectrally resolve the two proton pools and selectively spoil one resonance without significantly attenuating the other. Because the separation between fat and water increases in proportion to the main magnetic field strength, this technique can only be applied at higher field strength and in uniform magnetic fields. Frequency selective presaturation pulses are not applicable in an open MR unit at low or mid-field strength, where spectral separations are too small to allow selective excitation of a single resonance.

Frequency selective fat suppression techniques are especially difficult in off-center regions or for any situations that distort the uniformity of the magnetic field. Therefore, the fat suppression is often not uniform. The efficacy of fat suppression is checked most conveniently by comparison with a non-fat-suppressed image in the same plane or by matching a STIR sequence, which works more reliably in this situation because it relies on a different technique.

5.7   Artifacts

5.7.1   Movement Artifacts

Motion artifacts usually appear as blurring or ghosting in MR images. There are a variety of causes for motion of the wrist and fingers. Patient motion and pulsation artifacts from the blood vessels are the most common.

Ghost images usually appear along the phase-encoding direction and superimpose with slight signal intensity over the anatomic presentation. From the technical point of view, signal averaging, flow compensation and regional presaturation techniques are most commonly used to decrease motion artifacts. Short imaging times, maximal patient comfort and passive restraints limiting motion are equally important.

5.7.2   Backfolding

Backfolding artifacts are also referred to as aliasing, fold-over or wrap-around artifacts. They occur if the dimension of the wrist in the preparation direction is larger than the field-of-view in this direction. Structures from outside the field-of-view are then shown in the image at the opposite side (Fig. 5.5).

Aliasing can be suppressed by oversampling. Oversampling describes a technique in which the field-of-view in the preparation direction is doubled, so it contains the unwanted parts, which are then ignored for the image reconstruction.

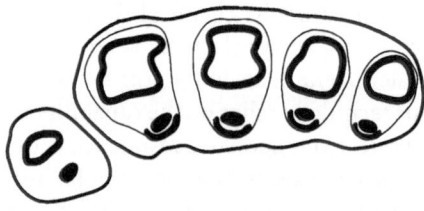

correct field of view

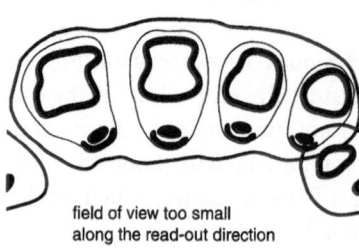

field of view too small
along the read-out direction

Fig. 5.5. Schematic explanation of the backfolding artifact. In this example, axial slices of the wrist are acquired using a field-of-view (FOV) which is too small for the radioulnar extent of the wrist. The part of the wrist that is too large for the FOV setting is therefore overlaid over the anatomic structures at the opposite side, and the region with overlays cannot be evaluated for this reason

5.7.3   Chemical Shift

In clinical MR imaging, chemical shift phenomena are usually observed at water-fat interfaces. The underlying cause for this artifact is found in the different molecular environments of the protons in fat and water, which causes differences in the resonant (Larmor) frequency. This non-uniformity in the local magnetic field is more pronounced at high field strength and results in frequency shifts along the read-out gradient, which the MR system cannot recognize as such. Hypointense and hyperintense lines result along the read-out gradient, which are caused by pixel displacement (5 to 6 pixels at 1.5 T, 1 to 2 pixels for 0.5 T) (Fig. 5.6). Chemical shift is more significant if a small spatial resolution is used, and can occur in any sequence type.

5.8   MR Presentation of the Anatomic Structures of the Hand and Wrist

Specific questions based on a thorough patient history and clinical examination are essential for planning an MR imaging protocol which provides all necessary detail but does not exceed a reasonable imaging time tolerable for the patient.

Anatomy: fat stripe in water

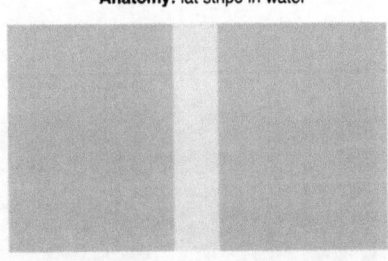

Image: dark line at water-fat interface, bright line at fat-water interface

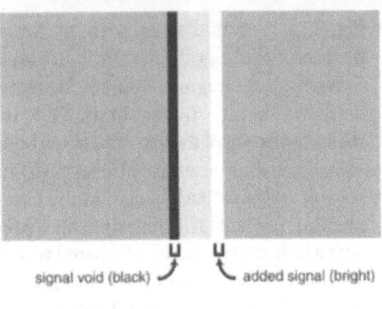

signal void (black)   added signal (bright)

read-out direction

Fig. 5.6. Schematic explanation of the chemical shift artifact. In this example, a water-fat shift is illustrated. At the water-fat interface a dark line results, while a bright line marks the fat-water transition

T1-weighted SE sequences are usually part of most MR imaging protocols. Axial T1-weighted coronal images are acquired with 3 mm sections, using a field-of-view of than 12+12 cm^2 or less and 256+256 or higher matrix [28]. A fat-suppressed coronal sequence, such as a proton-density fat-saturated FSE sequence, is a fast and effective way to depict all clinically relevant structures of the wrist with reasonable quality [57].

5.8.1   Osseous Structures of the Wrist

T1-weighted images provide sufficient anatomic detail of the osseous structures of the wrist, and coronal planes are probably most helpful. Coronal planes must be aligned parallel to the proximal carpal row consisting of the scaphoid, lunate and triquetral bones on axial scout views. The orientation of the distal radioulnar joint correlates poorly with the proximal carpal row, and therefore should not be used for planning coronal images. Osseous alignment of the distal radius with the lunate and capitate bones is best visualized in sagittal planes aligned in the midline of the wrist. The articulation of the radius and ulna in the distal radioulnar joint is best seen in axial planes. The finger joints are very difficult to assess, and frequently images in all three planes are needed.

STIR sequences or fat-suppressed T2-weighted sequences depict well the medullary changes in the course of post-traumatic or avascular disease (Figs. 5.7, 5.8).

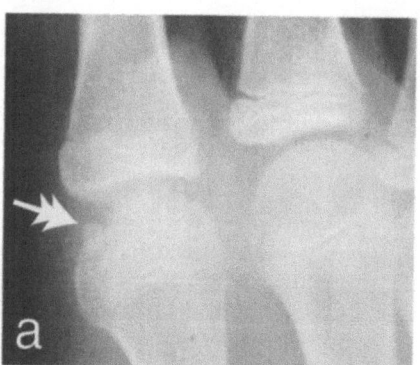
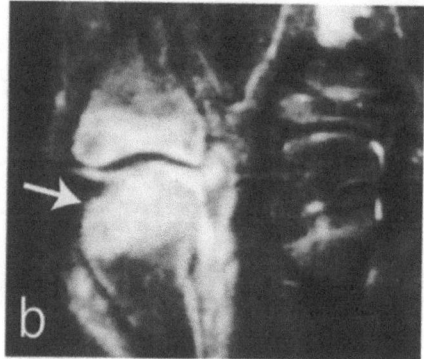
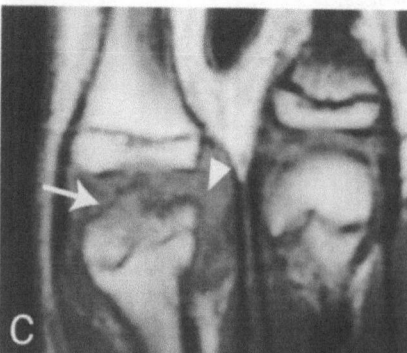

Fig. 5.7a–c. Avascular necrosis of the second metacarpophalangeal joint. In the conventional radiograph the fragmentation of the metacarpal head can be seen (*arrow* in **a**). STIR imaging shows the extent of the accompanying bone marrow edema more accurately (*arrow* in **b**) and displays also edematous changes in the base of the proximal phalanx. The bone marrow changes appear a little exaggerated if compared with the T1-weighted SE sequence (*arrow* in **c**). In this sequence, the bone marrow edema appears as of intermediate signal intensity (*arrowhead*)

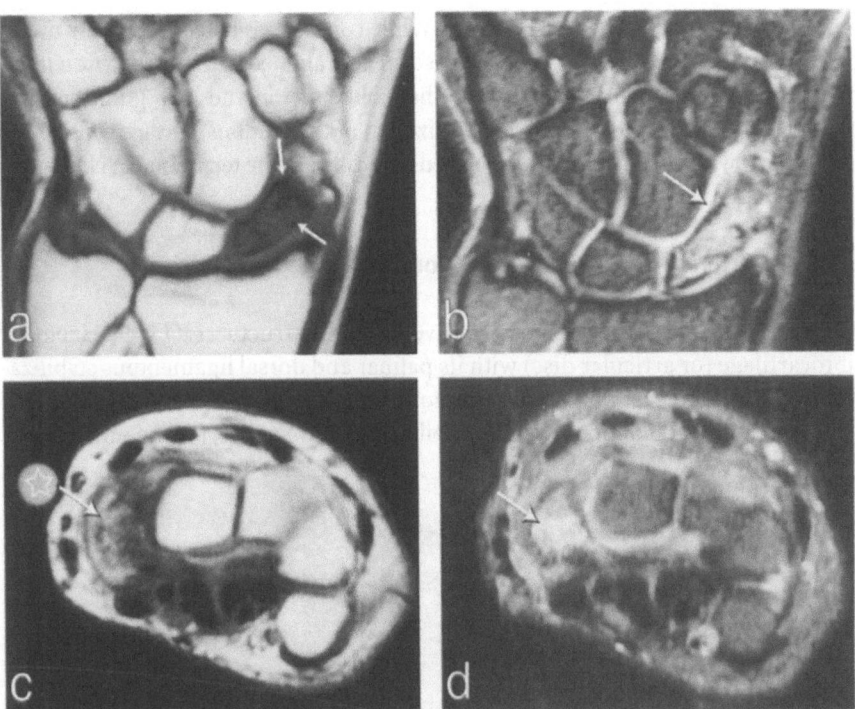

Fig. 5.8a–d. Non-displaced fracture through the waist of the scaphoid bone (follow-up study after 6 months). Coronal and axial T1-weighted SE (**a, c**) and fat-suppressed T2-weighted (**b, d**) images. The bone marrow signal is very low in T1-weighted images, which is consistent with an avascular necrosis of the scaphoid bone (*arrows* in **a**). The major part of the proximal scaphoid pole is markedly edematous. The irregular bone marrow space of the proximal scaphoid is consistent with an initial collapse of the spongy bone. The two *arrows* in **c** and **d** indicate the fracture line of the scaphoid. The site of the fracture line is also identified in corresponding coronal images (*arrow* in **b**)

MRI is the method of choice for the detection of radiographically occult fractures [10, 11, 13, 24]. Functional aspects such as the cause of bone marrow changes can be the leading observation in many diagnoses dealing with inadequate weight-bearing of the wrist. For example, focal signal intensity change in the ulnar part of the lunate is the most conspicuous finding in patients with ulnar impaction syndrome [25].

Scapholunate advanced collapse (SLAC) and scaphoid nonunion advanced collapse (SNAC) are characteristic degeneration patterns of the proximal carpal row and represent the degeneration mechanisms in scapholunate insufficiency and nonunion of the scaphoid [56]. Protocols including coronal and axial sequences usually show the typical appearance of SLAC and SNAC injuries.

5.8.2   Extensor and Flexor Tendons

Both proton-density and T2-weighted sequences in axial planes yield all information necessary concerning the intrinsic signal characteristics of the tendons and any associated fluid [21] (Figs. 5.9, 5.10). While coronal sequences are rarely useful due to partial volume effects, parasagittal sequences aligned with the specific tendon may provide additional information to the hand surgeon and help guide surgical planning. Because of the superficial localization of the tendons, surface coils covering the area where the rupture is suspected clinically are the technique of choice [6].

5.8.3   Triangular Fibrocartilage Complex

The TFCC is defined as a composite of five anatomic structures: (1) the triangular fibrocartilage (or articular disc) with its palmar and dorsal ligamentous stabilizations; (2) the ulnocarpal meniscus homologue adjacent to the prestyloid recess; (3) the ulnocarpal ligaments, which stabilize the mid-carpus, (4) the ulnar collat-

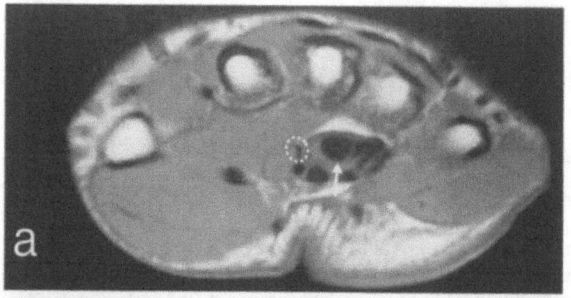
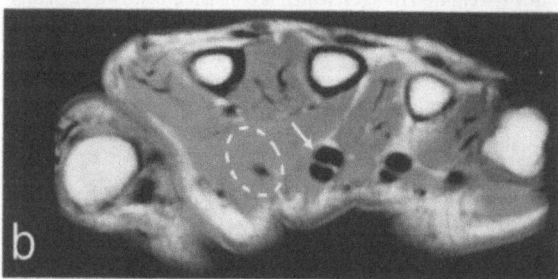
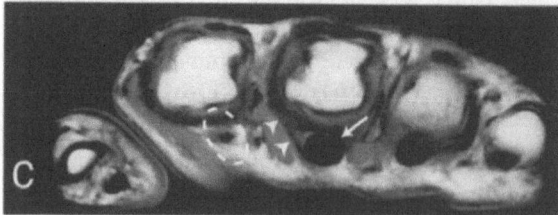
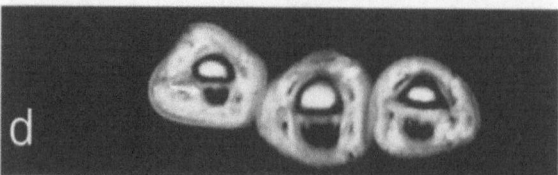

Fig. 5.9a–d. Rupture of the profound flexor tendon of the second digit. Intact collagen fibers appear as high signal intensity throughout all four axial proton density-weighted planes (*arrows* in a–d). In the proximal mid-carpus, the most distal end of the proximal stump of the tendon can be identified (*dotted circle* in a). The tendon is interrupted in the distal mid-carpus (b) and at the metacarpophalangeal joint (c). The annular pulley can well be appreciated in the third phalanx (*arrowheads*) but is indistinct at the second digit. The distal stump is again identified at the height of the middle phalanx (d)

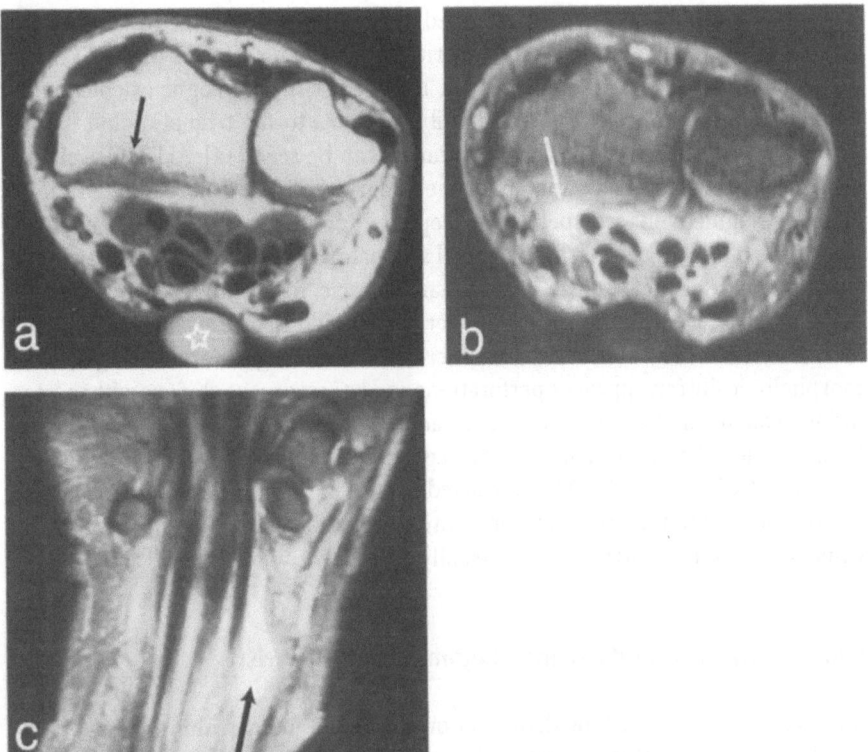

Fig. 5.10a–c. Traumatic tenosynovitis of the flexor tendons proximal to and in the carpal tunnel. Axial T1-weighted SE (**a**) and axial and coronal fat-suppressed FSE T2 weighted sequences (**b, c**). The bone marrow edema in the distal radius (*black arrow* in **a**) is consistent with a trabecular injury and there is no sign of a cortical fracture. The maximal pain is localized on the palmar side and was marked with an oil pill (*white star* in **a**). A large amount of fluid surrounds the flexor pollicis muscles and the flexor digitorum profundus muscles (*white arrow* in **b**). *Arrows* indicate the corresponding fluid collections in **b** and **c**. Note that the flexor tendons are intact and of low signal intensity in **b**, but appear of intermediate signal intensity in the proximal regions in **c**, because partial volume effects of the synovial fluid and the tendons are averaged in the coronal plane

eral ligament and (5) the sheath of the extensor ulnaris tendon, which inserts on the base of the fifth metacarpal and exchanges collagen fibers with the TFCC [38].

The essential anatomic components of the TFCC are revealed using coronal planes with very thin slice thickness and a high spatial resolution (typically 8×8 cm^2 field-of-view and a matrix of 256×256 pixels). Thickness, integrity and signal characteristics of the TFCC can be assessed. If severe degeneration of the TFCC is present, assessment of additional traumatic lesions can be very difficult [30]. High-resolution SE, TSE and GRE sequences have been successfully applied in MRI of the TFCC, but a diagnostic superiority of any of these sequences has not been shown [36, 42, 60, 67]. A combination of fat-saturated T1-weighted or T2-weighted GRE sequences depicts lesions very clearly compared with the other sequences, but has not been tested in vivo [35].

Sagittal proton-density or T2-weighted images aligned with the distal ulna provide additional information on the anterior to posterior diameter of the TFCC, its dorsal and palmar height and its signal. The meniscus homologue extends on the palmar side in coronal planes and its fibrotic links to the triquetral and hamate bones and to the base of the fifth metacarpal can be seen [14]. Axial T1-weighted sequences provide information about the congruity of the distal radioulnar joint, and T2-weighted images specifically depict its joint-space. Adjacent stabilizing structures of the wrist, such as the dorsal and palmar radioulnar ligaments and the tendon sheath of the extensor carpi ulnaris muscle, frequently exchange collagen fibers or even fuse with the TFCC and therefore should also be evaluated. Traumatic lesions of the TFCC are often hard to differentiate from degenerative changes, which morphologically can appear as perforations and become more obvious with increasing age, starting in the third or fourth decade [33]. The most important classification to assist the differential diagnosis of degeneration and lesions of the TFCC was published by Palmer in 1989 [37]. Isolated central perforations of the articular disc are usually asymptomatic, and consecutive tears usually of degenerative origin, while peripheral eccentric tears are usually caused by trauma (Fig. 5.11).

5.8.4   Intrinsic and Extrinsic Ligaments of the Wrist

Intrinsic ligaments, which by definition originate and insert within the wrist, serve stabilizing functions. Palmar intrinsic ligaments are usually thicker and stronger than their dorsal counterparts. Generally they are of low signal intensity but most conspicuously visualized anatomically by proton-density sequences. Zlatkin et al. [67] proposed three criteria for diagnosing tears of the interosseous ligaments: (1) non-visualization of the ligament in its usual anatomic position; (2) fluid signal in T2-weighted

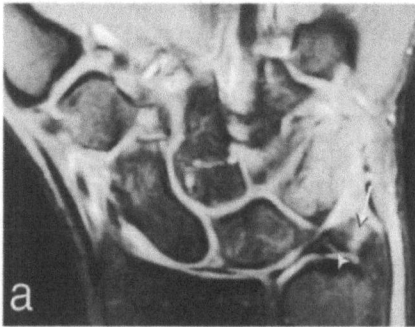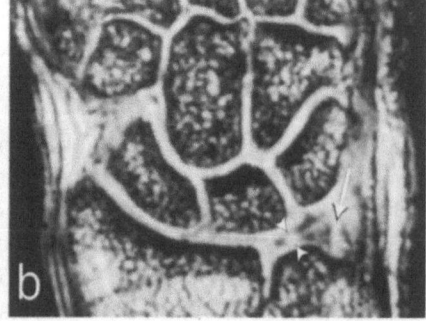

Fig. 5.11. Partial (a) and complete (b) tear of the triangular fibrocartilage complex (TFCC) in two different patients. a The fat-saturated T2-weighted FSE sequence shows a marked regional increase in signal intensity at the ulnar attachment of the TFCC (*arrow*). In addition, linear signal intensity (*arrowhead*) extends from the proximal central part but does not reach the carpal surface. b The complete rupture of the ulnar attachment is clearly delineated by the GRE sequence (*arrow*). Diffuse signal changes throughout the fibrocartilage are a sign of degeneration, while the linear bright line in the center (*arrowheads*) represents a traumatic tear

images traversing the ligament and (3) morphologic distortion of the ligamentous structure (Quelle). It may be very difficult to differentiate a normal from a torn ligament on the basis of signal changes alone. The interindividual variation is quite large, and perforations of the central segment of the interosseous ligaments are part of the aging process and usually do not produce any instability or symptoms.

The radioscapholunate (RSL) ligament is best shown on coronal planes and its palmar radiolunate part by parasagittal planes [54]. The scapholunate part of the ligament is frequently displayed in high-resolution images. Despite the fact that three-dimensional GRE sequences provide more signal than TSE and SE sequences and encourage high-resolution imaging, a definite decision on the preferred sequence type has not been made, and all three are used in routine imaging [50, 65, 67]. In addition, the role of MR arthrography for imaging the RSL and lunotriquetral ligaments is still controversial [18]. The dorsal part of the scapholunate ligament provides biomechanical stability and has been identified as a potential origin of wrist ganglia [17]. The central part of the scapholunate ligament is less important and shows age-related degenerative changes (Fig. 5.12).

The triquetroscaphoid ligament is most frequently shown in paraxial planes, the ulnolunate in paracoronal and parasagittal planes, the ulnotriquetral in paracoronal and parasagittal planes and the palmar radiolunotriquetral ligaments in paracoronal and paraxial planes following their anatomic orientation. The configuration of these ligaments, however, varies between individuals, and they are therefore infrequently identified.

Multiple classification and nomenclature schemes have been published for the palmar extrinsic ligaments of the wrist. These typically describe the V-shaped arches inserting at the distal radius and lunate bones [53]. The dorsal extrinsic ligaments are anatomically far less consistent. The major structure is the radiocarpal ligament [1], which can be characterized as a thickening of the dorsal capsule and extends from the styloid of the radius to the lunate and triquetral bones. Three-dimensional acquisitions that allow for free reconstruction of planes are advantageous for the assessment of the extrinsic ligaments of the wrist [53, 55].

5.8.5   Carpal Tunnel

The flexor retinaculum is a thick band of collagen fibers that extends laterally from the pisiform bone and the hook of the hamate to its medial attachments formed by the trapezoid and distal scaphoid bones. The median nerve takes its course along the volar forearm and wrist deep to the flexor digitorum superficialis. In the distal forearm, the nerve is located deep to the tendon of the palmaris longus tendon and volar to the superficialis tendons.

Axial T2-weighted sequences are the basis of evaluation in patients with carpal tunnel syndrome, because the size and the intrinsic signal characteristics of the median nerve are usually shown with superior contrast. A double-echo sequence, which provides an additional proton-density or T1-weighted image, is especially

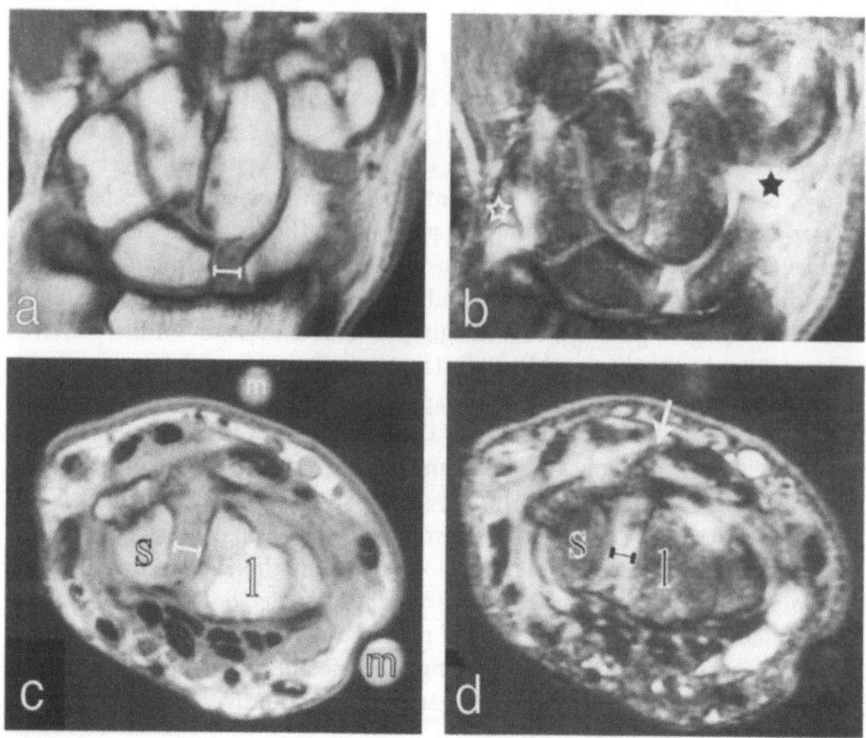

Fig. 5.12. Tear of the scapholunate ligament, presented in axial and coronal SE T1 (**a, c**) and fat-suppressed T2-weighted (**b, d**) images. The lunoscaphoid distance is increased in both axial and coronal images (*bar* in **a, c** and **d**). Bone marrow changes in the proximal poles of the capitate and lunate bones are conspicuous and indicate that this is a chronic rupture with secondary mild degenerative changes (**a, b**). The scaphoid bone tilts dorsally, giving space for a focal joint effusion (*black asterisk* in **b**). The meniscus homologue is well depicted (*white asterisk* in **b**), as degenerative synovitis fills the prestyloid recess. Because of tenosynovial thickening, the extensor tendons are lifted from the dorsal capsule (**c, d**). The dorsal radial ligament is markedly irregular (*arrow* in **d**). The two markers (*m* in **c**) indicate the most painful spots on the wrist (note the fluid interface inside the capsules). *S* scaphoid, *L* lunate

useful to study tissue composition and should be correlated with the T2-weighted images. Concomitant pathologies might require additional coronal or sagittal planes.

The carpal tunnel is best displayed using true axial T2-weighted images that are aligned perpendicular to the longitudinal axis of the hamate bone (Fig. 5.13). As there is usually very little fat in the carpal tunnel, fat-suppressed or STIR sequences are usually not necessary. A slice thickness of 3 mm combined with an in-plane resolution of 0.5 mm^2 or less usually suffices.

For reporting on carpal tunnel variations, a good understanding of normal anatomic variations is helpful [40]. Despite the fact that MRI is capable of describing distinct signs of carpal tunnel syndrome [27, 32], its use to diagnose carpal tunnel syndrome is frequently challenged [43] and is recommended mostly for

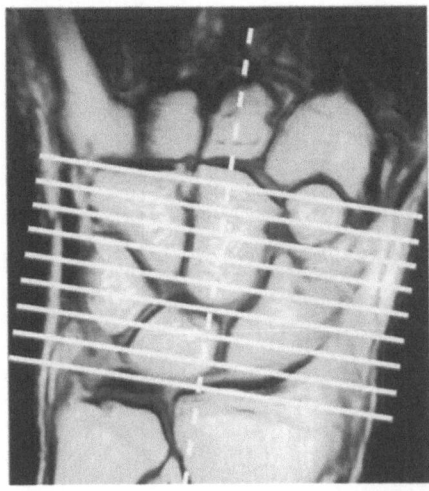

Fig. 5.13. Planning of axial slices for imaging of the carpal tunnel. On the coronal image a radial tilt of the carpal bones can be observed and is indicated by the *dashed* line aligned with the longitudinal axis of the capitate bone. In order to compensate for the radial tilt, it is necessary to orient the planes perpendicular to the capitate bone

clinically unclear cases and postoperative recurrence [41]. Recent studies have focused on the volume of the carpal tunnel during kinematic studies [3, 9, 12, 41] and have shown a compression of the nerve during flexion.

5.8.6   Neurovascular Structures

Peripheral nerves other than the median nerve are rarely diagnosed in MR imaging [19, 45, 63]. The ulnar nerve, traveling medially to the ulnar artery in Guyon's canal, is more superficial than the carpal tunnel. Usually it can be visualized quite easily near the volar process of the hamate bone [31]. Ulnar nerve entrapment in Guyon's canal secondary to anomalous muscles or calcifications has been diagnosed in selected cases [47, 58, 66]. The radial nerve branches proximally to the wrist. At the level of the wrist the small branches of the radial nerve are only infrequently identified on MR images. Despite its high quality in the diagnosis of the major arteries [46], MR angiography is still used quite rarely (Fig. 5.14).

5.8.7   Fingers and Thumb

Local coils and positioning in the center of magnetic uniformity are essential for imaging of the fingers and thumb. Axial and sagittal planes visualize the flexor and extensor tendons (and aponeuroses). The fine anatomic detail of the annular segments requires especially thin axial sections to be detected (Fig. 5.15). Coronal and sagittal sequences are best for evaluating osseous and cartilaginous structures of the small finger joints. MR arthrography has been found to be very sensitive for imaging of game-keeper's thumb; however, its performance in comparison with other imaging techniques, such as ultrasound, is yet to be examined [2].

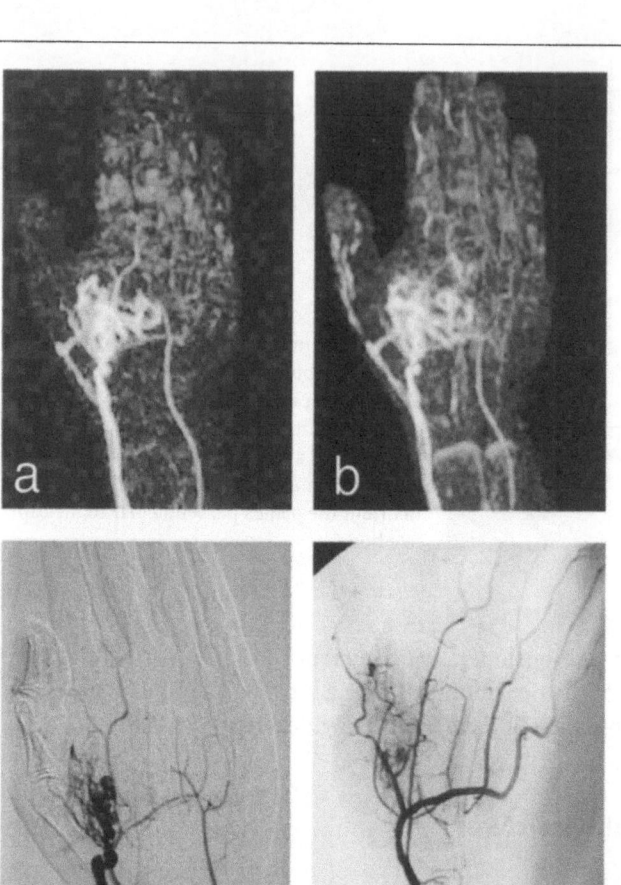

Fig. 5.14a–d. Arteriovenous malformation (AVM) of the hand (9-year-old patient). The MR images in the arterial and venous phase (a, b) were the basis to indicate an interventional approach. The angiograms (c, d) were acquired prior to successful coiling of the AVM. In both the arterial (c) and venous phases (d), conventional angiography provides more anatomic detail than MR angiography

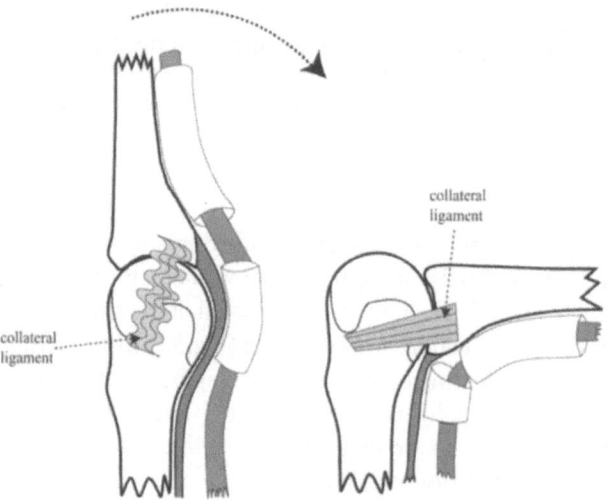

Fig. 5.15. Schematic drawing of the anatomy of the pulleys of the index. During flexion, the collateral ligaments are straightened

5.8.8   Synovia

The normal synovium is a very thin structure, which usually cannot be identified in MR images in the absence of synovial fluid and paramagnetic contrast media. Hypertrophic (or proliferative) changes, which accompany synovitis, enhance conspicuously after intravenous contrast on T1-weighted images. On T2-weighted images, these synovial proliferations frequently present as villous structures of intermediate signal intensity compared with the free joint fluid. Severe synovitis can additionally present with bone erosions.

5.9   Paramagnetic Contrast

5.9.1   Intravenous Application

Intravenous contrast facilitates the diagnosis of rheumatoid disease by allowing direct presentation of the inflammatory tissue and increasing the diagnostic sensitivity of MRI [5]. In fact, of all diagnostic imaging modalities, MRI has the best histopathologic correlation to display inflammatory pannus [15]. Fat-suppressed gadolinium-enhanced T1-weighted SE images can clearly demonstrate most of the essential lesions in rheumatoid arthritis including the proliferative synovium, bone erosion, bone marrow inflammatory change and tenosynovitis [34].

In the diagnostic investigation of tumors, intravenous contrast frequently improves the differentiation of necrotic or scarred parts of the tumor from viable tissues [4], and aids in the assessment of their maximal size and invasion of neurovascular bundles [26, 29, 44].

Muscular lesions are usually detected in T2-weighted and STIR sequences. However, intravenous contrast results in localized enhancement even in muscle tears that are occult to conventional MRI examinations and is recommended in an otherwise inconspicuous examination [16].

In the case of a strong synovial reaction and assisted by exertion, the joint space enhances as a result of diffused contrast medium ("indirect arthrography"). If only a little paramagnetic contrast medium diffuses into the joint space, however, the contrast effect is very small. Indirect arthrography has therefore rarely been used in imaging of the hand and wrist.

5.9.2   MR Arthrography

Distension of the joint capsule and the high contrast of the joint space in T1-weighted MR sequences are the main advantages of MR arthrography of the wrist. Several studies have shown the superiority of MR arthrography over non-enhanced MRI in the clinical settings of chronic wrist pain and detection of intrinsic and extrinsic ligaments [48–50]. The diagnostic performance of MRI in suspected lesions of the TFCC is also improved by adding MR arthrography to the standard examination [52, 65].

MR arthrograms of the wrist are very comprehensive. The TFCC and the intrinsic ligaments, for example, are shown with high image contrast. However, because MR arthrography is static and does not document the subsequent filling of the different joint spaces indicating ligamentous lesions, conventional images are still of great interest to the radiologist for reporting. Furthermore, inflammatory changes might be overlooked, as hypervascularized structures are not contrasted intravenously. Proliferative synovial changes do not contrast as well against the joint effusion, as they would do after intravenous injection of paramagnetic contrast media.

5.10   Design of the Wrist Protocol

The design of the imaging protocol largely depends on the clinical question and to some extent on the personal preferences of the reporting radiologist. As a rule, smaller and rarer pathologies are more likely to be detected if clinical information is more precise and specific regions can be focused on.

Imaging protocols on a specific MR scanner improve tremendously when they are worked on in mid-term time intervals. By designing the protocol to ensure optimal scanner use, even less advanced MR imaging systems can provide sufficient image quality for routine imaging.

5.10.1   Localizer

A localizer (or "scout") is a set of fast sequences in multiple planes that gives sufficient anatomic coverage to plan the set of diagnostic imaging planes of high image quality. Usually the scout has a field-of-view (FOV) 2 or 3 times larger than the final FOV for the diagnostic sequences. In MRI of tumors, a larger scout might also be useful to show potential skip metastases, which might otherwise not be shown completely. For imaging of the hand and wrist, localizers in all imaging planes are preferable. Usually SE or GRE sequences are used with a large FOV and a large voxel size to shorten imaging time. In most diagnostic centers, image contrast is of lesser concern than scanning time and anatomic coverage.

If the treating physician does not identify an anatomic region to focus on, a T2-weighted scout can often show an edematous region or joint effusion as a sequela of the underlying pathology, and indicates a possible region to target. Fast STIR sequences are a proper choice, as they also show bone marrow changes with high conspicuity. A T2-weighted scout is also well suited to MRI centers where technologists are sometimes on their own when no radiologist is available, because it again indicates the site of pathology in most cases. Proper planning of the examination is often the key to short examination times, as it helps to avoid the repetition of scans and unnecessary scans.

5.10.2 Sample Protocol

Table 5.5 gives an overview of the sequence types and parameters that could be used with a 1.5 T system. The number of excitations depends largely on the manufacturer of the MR system and is therefore omitted. Sequence parameters, especially the TE of T2-weighted GRE or TSE sequences, also vary with the MR system used and different parameter settings should be tested for routine use. Flow compensation should be used wherever applicable.

A screening protocol includes, for example, a coronal fat-suppressed sequence (T2 or STIR) accompanied by a high-resolution T1-weighted sequence (GRE or SE) and an axial multi-echo sequence delivering proton-density and T2-weighted images. On the basis of the images obtained, further high-resolution images with and without contrast injection might be indicated. It is wise to obtain contrast-enhanced images in a plane orientation in which both T2 and T1-weighted pre-contrast sequences are already available. If the fat saturation of the post-contrast image is not perfect, an additional T1-weighted sequence should be obtained without fat suppression and with exactly the same parameters as the pre-contrast acquisition.

5.10.3 Reducing the Imaging Time

5.10.3.1 Sequence Type

Because of its superb anatomic detail, SE imaging should be part of all routine protocols. If very thin sections are necessary, for example for evaluation of the TFCC or of carpal ligaments, three-dimensional GRE sequences can be applied to advantage. TSE sequences are the sequence of choice if many slices are needed, for example along the axial orientation of the wrist. For fat-suppressed inversion recovery imaging, turbo-inversion-recovery or GRE sequences can be beneficial, as they deliver a similar image contrast and quality in a shorter time.

5.10.3.2 Rectangular Field-of-View

In the middle hand and for imaging the fingers, an especially high spatial resolution might be necessary. The use of a rectangular FOV is a very suitable way to compensate for the increased imaging time (Fig. 5.16). The number of phase-encoding steps is reduced, while the spatial resolution is unchanged. If only half the lines are measured, the scan time is cut by half and the FOV is also reduced to 50% of its original size along the preparation direction. While the voxel size remains unchanged, signal-to-noise ratio is reduced proportionally to the square root of the fraction of lines measured.

Table 5.5. Parameters and sequences for a standard wrist protocol

Description (cm)	FOV	Matrix (no. of pixels)	Slice thickness (mm)/ gap (mm)	TR (ms)/ TE (ms)	Flip angle (deg) or TI (ms)	Remarks
1. Coronal STIR (turbo-STIR if available)	8×12	192×256	3/0.3		120 ms	
2. Coronal fat-saturated TSE T2-weighted	8×12	256×256	3/0.3	3600/60–90		Higher resolution than STIR to avoid blurred images. A smaller TE will greatly increase the image signal, but will gain proton density contrast if less than 60 ms
3. Coronal SE T1-weighted high spatial resolution	8×12	512×384	3/0.3	400 to 600/12 or less		No phase wrap
4. Coronal 3D GRE T2-weighted	10×13	192×256	1 (no gap)	30/15 or less	15°	
5. Axial FSE multiecho proton density and T2-weighted	8×8	256×256	3 to 4/0.3 to 1	4000/20 and 80		Gap depends on the total coverage needed
6. Sagittal fat-saturated FSE	10×10	256×256	3/0.3 to 1	3200/60 to 80		Displays synovitis, ganglia, TFCC, etc. Substitute for T1-weighted sequence for paramagnetic contrast
7. Sagittal SE	10×10	256×256	3/0.3 to 1	400 to 600 12 or less		Preferable for bone imaging, shorter than T2-weighted sequence

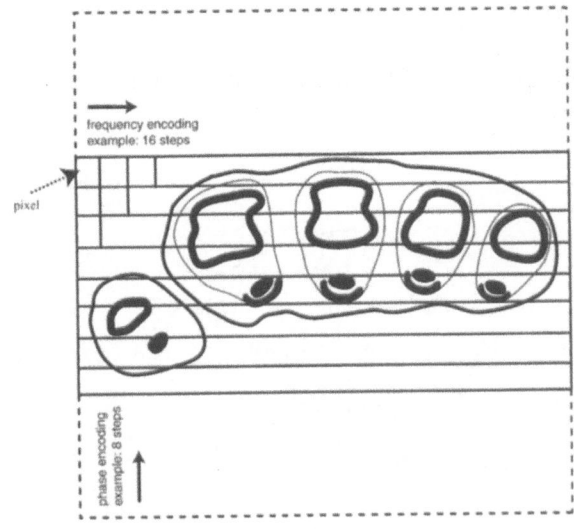

Fig. 5.16. Rectangular field-of-view (FOV). Theoretical setting of MRI of the pulleys, where high-resolution imaging is needed. For a complete coverage of the middle hand, a square (FOV) is not needed, as the complete anatomy can be covered with a rectangular FOV. In this case, only half as many phase-encoding steps are used for a FOV of half the size in one direction. The imaging time is not prolonged

5.10.3.3 Unnecessary Anatomic Coverage

If the clinical question is well defined, such as in follow-up studies or well-documented trauma mechanisms, limited protocols can dramatically decrease the imaging time. Focusing on the anatomy of interest can be a very efficient way to achieve short examination times, as fewer slices require a shorter TR and imaging time decreases linearly with the TR used.

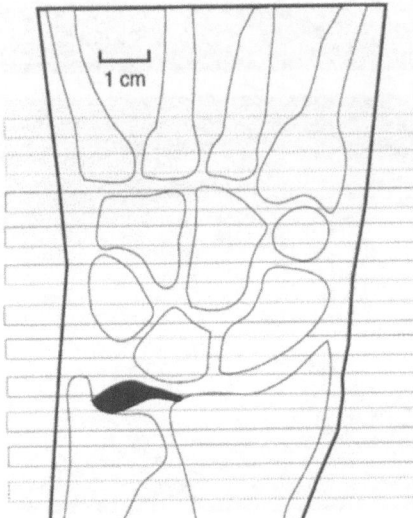

Fig. 5.17. Unnecessary anatomic coverage in a clinical example of carpal tunnel syndrome. The two distal and the most proximal slices are not needed to depict the complete carpal tunnel, and may therefore be eliminated to shorten imaging time

5.11   Anatomy of the Wrist

The most important anatomic structures of the wrist are identified in Fig. 5.18 using axial and coronal planes.

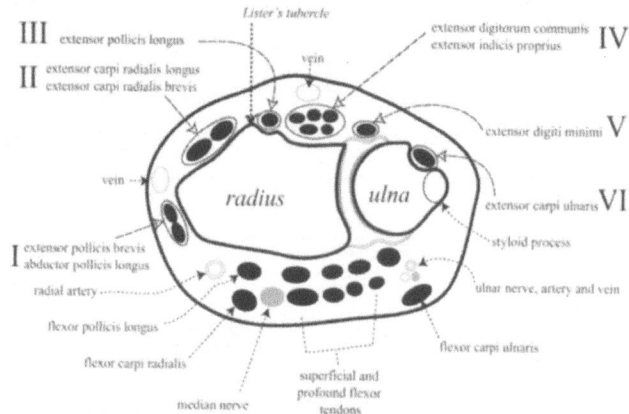

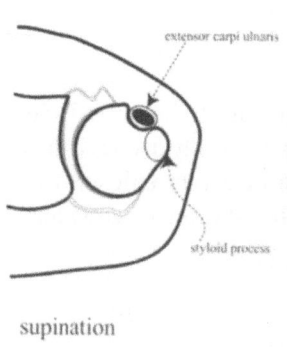

supination

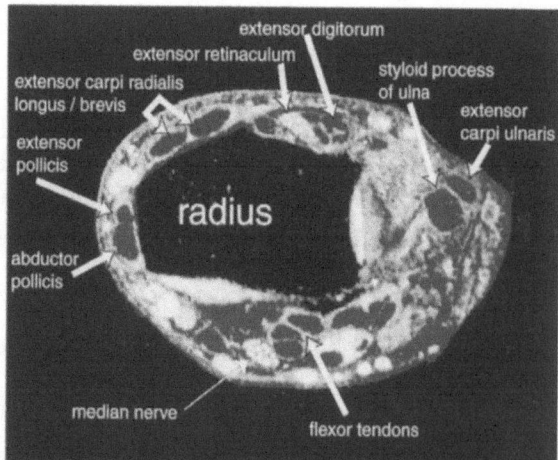

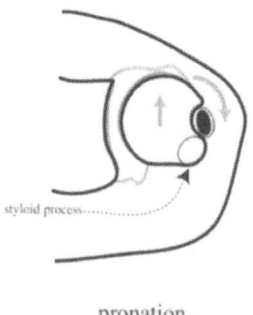

pronation

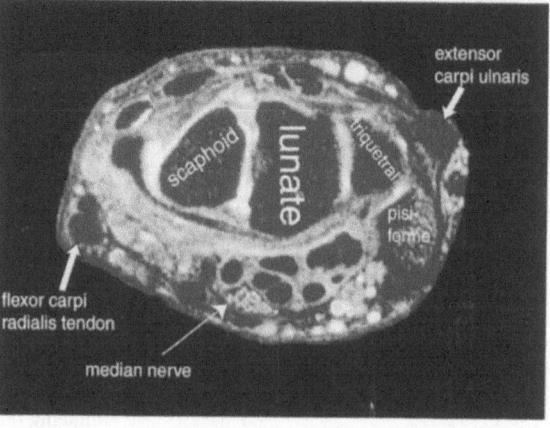

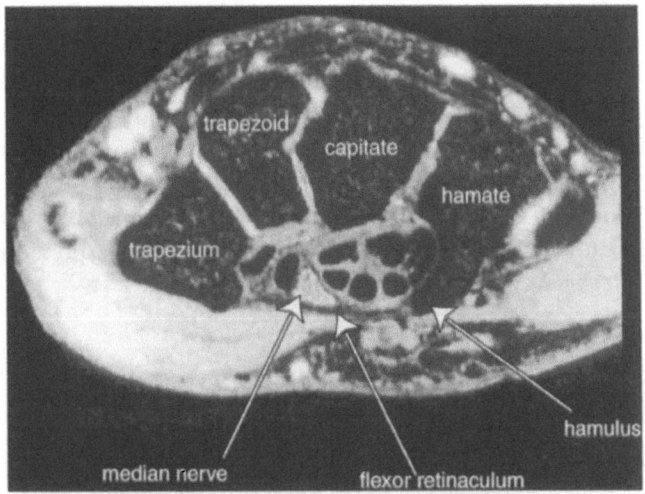

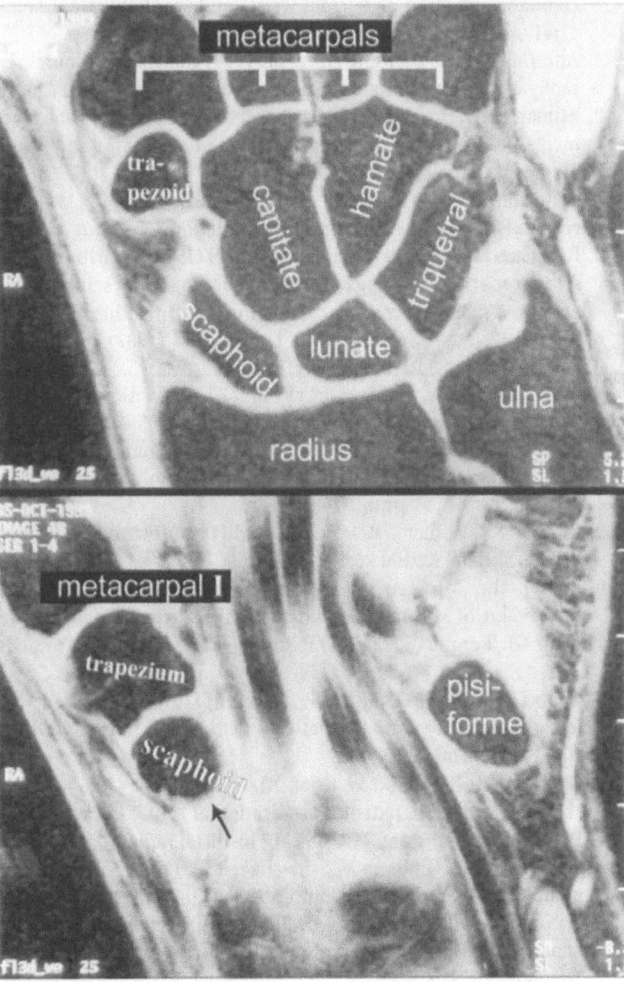

Fig. 5.18. A fast water-excitation fat-saturated gradient-echo sequences was the basis for these anatomic images. All coronal and axial views were acquired using the four-channel phased-array coil shown in Fig. 1d on the wrist of a healthy volunteer

Acknowledgements. The authors would like to thank Dr. Phillip F. J. Tirman (San Francisco, California, USA) and Dr. Oliver Cvitanic (Oklahoma City, Oklahoma, USA) very much for providing some of the figures used in this chapter. Many thanks also to PD Dr. Thomas Link (Technical University of Munich, Germany) and ICG Medical Advances (10437 Innovation Drive, Milwaukee, Wisconsin, USA) for permission to reprint Fig.5.1d and e. The support of PD Dr. Axel Stäbler (LMU, Munich, Germany) and Dr. Thomas Helmberger (LMU, Munich, Germany) is also greatly appreciated. Finally, the authors wish to express their special thanks to Victoria Vandenberg for the final review of this text.

References

1. Adler BD, Logan PM, Janzen DL, et al (1996) Extrinsic radiocarpal ligaments: magnetic resonance imaging of normal wrists and scapholunate dissociation. Can Assoc Radiol J 47:417–422
2. Ahn JM, Sartoris DJ, Kang HS, et al (1998) Gamekeeper thumb: comparison of MR arthrography with conventional arthrography and MR imaging in cadavers. Radiology 206:737–744
3. Allmann KH, Horch R, Gabelmann A, et al (1996) Morphology of the carpal tunnel. Movement studies in patients with constriction symptoms and healthy probands using MR tomography. Unfallchirurgie 22:5–11
4. Azouz EM, Babyn PS, Mascia AT, Tuuha SE, Daecarie JC (1998) MRI of the abnormal pediatric hand and wrist with plain film correlation. J Comput Assist Tomogr 22:252–261
5. Backhaus M, Kamradt T, Sandrock D, et al (1999)Arthritis of the finger joints: a comprehensive approach comparing conventional radiography, scintigraphy, ultrasound, and contrast-enhanced magnetic resonance imaging. Arthritis Rheum 42:1232–1245
6. Beltran J, Noto AM, Herman LJ, Lubbers LM (1987) Tendons: high-field-strength, surface coil MR imaging. Radiology 162:735–740
7. Bonel H, Frick A, Sittek H, et al (1997) Examination of the hand and wrist joints with a dedicated low-field MRI device. Radiologe 37:785–793
8. Bonel H, Helmberger T, Geiss HC, et al (1998) Comparison of sequences for depicting bone marrow alterations in osteomyelitis applied in a low field strength magnetic resonance imaging system. Magma 7:1–8
9. Brahme SK, Hodler J, Braun RM, et al (1997)Dynamic MR imaging of carpal tunnel syndrome. Skeletal Radiol 26:482–487
10. Breitenseher MJ, Metz VM, Gilula LA, et al (1997) Radiographically occult scaphoid fractures: value of MR imaging in detection (see comments). Radiology 203:245–250
11. Byers GE, Berquist TH (1996) Radiology of sports-related injuries. Curr Probl Diagn Radiol 25:1–49
12. Cobb TK, Bond JR, Cooney WP, Metcalf BJ (1997) Assessment of the ratio of carpal contents to carpal tunnel volume in patients with carpal tunnel syndrome: a preliminary report. J Hand Surg [Am] 22:635–639
13. Cook PA, Yu JS, Wiand W, Cook AJ, Coleman CR (1997) Suspected scaphoid fractures in skeletally immature patients: application of MRI. J Comput Assist Tomogr 21:511–515
14. Drobner WS, Hausman MR (1992) The distal radioulnar joint. Hand Clin 8:631–644
15. el Noueam KI, Giuliano V, Schweitzer ME, O'Hara BJ (1997) Rheumatoid nodules: MR/pathological correlation. J Comput Assist Tomogr 21:796–799
16. el Noueam KI, Schweitzer ME, Bhatia M, Bartolozzi AR (1997) The utility of contrast-enhanced MRI in diagnosis of muscle injuries occult to conventional MRI. J Comput Assist Tomogr 21:965–968

17. el Noueam KI, Schweitzer ME, Blasbalg R, et al (1999) Is a subset of wrist ganglia the sequela of internal derangements of the wrist joint? MR imaging findings. Radiology 212:537-540

18. Farooki S, Seeger LL (1999) Magnetic resonance imaging in the evaluation of ligament injuries. Skeletal Radiol 28:61-74

19. Gumucio CA, Lund H, Young VL, Young AE (1992) Diagnosis and management of ulnar nerve entrapment. Mo Med 89:231-240

20. Henkelman RM, Hardy PA, Bishop JE, Poon CS, Plewes DB (1992) Why fat is bright in RARE and fast spin-echo imaging. J Magn Reson Imaging 2:533-540

21. Heuck A, Bonel H, Staebler A, Schmitt R (1997) Imaging in sports medicine: hand and wrist. Eur J Radiol 26:2-15

22. Heuck A, Steinbach L, Neumann C, Stoller D, Genant H (1989) Possibilities of MR tomography of diseases of the hand and wrist. Radiologe 29:53-60

23. Hodgson RJ, Barry MA, Carpenter TA, et al (1995) Magnetic resonance imaging protocol optimization for evaluation of hyaline cartilage in the distal interphalangeal joint of fingers. Invest Radiol 30:522-531

24. Hunter JC, Escobedo EM, Wilson AJ, et al (1997) MR imaging of clinically suspected scaphoid fractures. AJR 168:1287-1293

25. Imaeda T, Nakamura R, Shionoya K, Makino N (1996) Ulnar impaction syndrome: MR imaging findings. Radiology 201:495-500

26. Karasick D, Karasick S (1992) Giant cell tumor of tendon sheath: spectrum of radiologic findings. Skeletal Radiol. 21, 219-224

27. Kleindienst A, Hamm B, Hildebrandt G, Klug N (1996) Diagnosis and staging of carpal tunnel syndrome: comparison of magnetic resonance imaging and intra-operative findings. Acta Neurochir (Wien) 138:228-233

28. Kneeland JB (1995) Technical considerations for MR imaging of the hand and wrist. Magn Reson Imaging Clin North Am 3:191-196

29. Kransdorf MJ, Murphey MD (1995) MR imaging of musculoskeletal tumors of the hand and wrist. Magn Reson Imaging Clin North Am 3:327-344

30. Melone CP Jr, Nathan R (1992) Traumatic disruption of the triangular fibrocartilage complex. Pathoanat Clin Orthop 65-73

31. Meuller LP, Kreitner KF, Seidl C, Degreif J (1997) Traumatic thrombosis of the distal ulnar artery (hypothenar hammer syndrome) in a golf player with an accessory muscle loop around Guyon's canal. Case report. Handchir Mikrochir Plast Chir 29:183-186

32. Middleton WD, Kneeland JB, Kellman GM, et al (1987) MR imaging of the carpal tunnel: normal anatomy and preliminary findings in the carpal tunnel syndrome. AJR 148:307-316

33. Mikic ZD (1978) Age changes in the triangular fibrocartilage of the wrist joint. J Anat 126:367-384

34. Nakahara N, Uetani M, Hayashi K, et al (1996) Gadolinium-enhanced MR imaging of the wrist in rheumatoid arthritis: value of fat suppression pulse sequences. Skeletal Radiol 25:639-647

35. Nakamura T, Yabe Y, Horiuchi Y (1999) Fat suppression magnetic resonance imaging of the triangular fibrocartilage complex. Comparison with spin echo, gradient echo pulse sequences and histology. J Hand Surg [Br] 24:22-26

36. Oneson SR, Timins ME, Scales LM, Erickson SJ, Chamoy L (1997) MR imaging diagnosis of triangular fibrocartilage pathology with arthroscopic correlation. AJR 168:1513-1518

37. Palmer AK (1989) Triangular fibrocartilage complex lesions: a classification. J Hand Surg [Am] 14:594-606

38. Palmer AK, Werner FW (1981) The triangular fibrocartilage complex of the wrist: anatomy and function. J Hand Surg [Am] 6:153-162

39. Peterfy CG, van Dijke CF, Lu Y, et al (1995) Quantification of the volume of articular cartilage in the metacarpophalangeal joints of the hand: accuracy and precision of three-dimensional MR imaging. AJR 165:371-375

40. Pierre-Jerome C, Bekkelund SI, Husby G, et al (1996) MRI of anatomical variants of the wrist in women. Surg Radiol Anat 18:37-41

41. Pierre-Jerome C, Bekkelund SI, Mellgren SI, Nordstrom R (1997) Bilateral fast magnetic resonance imaging of the operated carpal tunnel. Scand J Plast Reconstr Surg Hand Surg 31:171–177

42. Potter HG, Asnis-Ernberg L, Weiland AJ, et al (1997) The utility of high-resolution magnetic resonance imaging in the evaluation of the triangular fibrocartilage complex of the wrist. J Bone Joint Surg Am 79:1675–1684

43. Radack DM, Schweitzer ME, Taras J (1997)Carpal tunnel syndrome: are the MR findings a result of population selection bias? AJR 169:1649–1653

44. Rafecas JC, Daube JR, Ehman RL (1988) Deep branch ulnar neuropathy due to giant cell tumor: report of a case. Neurology 38:327–329

45. Rettig AC (1990) Neurovascular injuries in the wrists and hands of athletes. Clin Sports Med 9:389–417

46. Rofsky NM (1995) MR angiography of the hand and wrist. Magn Reson Imaging Clin North Am 3:345–359

47. Ruocco MJ, Walsh JJ, Jackson JP (1998) MR imaging of ulnar nerve entrapment secondary to an anomalous wrist muscle. Skeletal Radiol 27:218–221

48. Scheck RJ, Kubitzek C, Hierner R, et al (1997) The scapholunate interosseous ligament in MR arthrography of the wrist: correlation with non-enhanced MRI and wrist arthroscopy. Skeletal Radiol 26:263–271

49. Scheck RJ, Romagnolo A, Hierner R, et al (1999) The carpal ligaments in MR arthrography of the wrist: correlation with standard MRI and wrist arthroscopy. J Magn Reson Imaging 9:468–474

50. Schweitzer ME, Brahme SK, Hodler J, et al (1992) Chronic wrist pain: spin-echo and short tau inversion recovery MR imaging and conventional and MR arthrography. Radiology 182:205–211

51. Shellock FG, FG, O'Neil M, Ivans V, et al (1999) Cardiac pacemakers and implantable cardioverter defibrillators are unaffected by operation of an extremity MR imaging system. AJR 172:165–170

52. Shionova K, Nakamura R, Imaeda T, Makino N (1998) Arthrography is superior to magnetic resonance imaging for diagnosing injuries of the triangular fibrocartilage. J Hand Surg [Br] 23:402–405

53. Smith DK (1993) Volar carpal ligaments of the wrist: normal appearance on multiplanar reconstructions of three-dimensional Fourier transform MR imaging. AJR 161:353–357

54. Smith DK (1994) Scapholunate interosseous ligament of the wrist: MR appearances in asymptomatic volunteers and arthrographically normal wrists. Radiology 192:217–221

55. Smith DK (1995) MR imaging of normal and injured wrist ligaments. Magn Reson Imaging Clin North Am 3:229–248

56. Staebler A, Heuck A, Reiser M (1997) Imaging of the hand: degeneration, impingement and overuse. Eur J Radiol 25:118–128

57. Staebler A, Spieker A, Bonel H, et al (2000) MRI of the wrist: comparison of high resolution pulse sequences and different fat suppression techniques. Rofo Fortschr Geb Rontgenstr Neuen Bildgeb Verfahr 172:168–174

58. Thurman RT, Jindal P, Wolff TW (1991) Ulnar nerve compression in Guyon's canal caused by calcinosis in scleroderma. J Hand Surg [Am] 16:739–741

59. Totterman SM, Miller RJ (1995) Triangular fibrocartilage complex: normal appearance on coronal three-dimensional gradient-recalled-echo MR images. Radiology 195:521–527

60. Totterman SM, Miller RJ, McCance SE, Meyers SP (1996) Lesions of the triangular fibrocartilage complex: MR findings with a three-dimensional gradient-recalled-echo sequence. Radiology 199:227–232

61. Totterman SMS, Miller RJ, McCance SE, Meyers SP (1996) Lesions of the triangular fibrocartilage complex: MR findings with a three-dimensional gradient-recalled-echo sequence. Radiology 199:227–232

62. Uhl M, Ihling C, Allmann KH, et al (1998) Human articular cartilage: in vitro correlation of MRI and histologic findings. Eur Radiol 8:1123–1129

63. Weinstein SM, Herring SA (1992) Nerve problems and compartment syndromes in the hand, wrist, and forearm. Clin Sports Med 11:161–188

64. Williamson DS, Mulken RV, Jakab PD, Jolesz FA (1996) Coherence transfer by isotropic mixing in Carr-Purcell-Meiboom-Gill imaging: implications for the bright fat phenomenon in fast spin-echo imaging. Magn Reson Med 35:506–513

65. Zanetti M, Bream J, Hodler J (1997) Triangular fibrocartilage and intercarpal ligaments of the wrist: does MR arthrography improve standard MRI? J Magn Reson Imaging 7:590–594

66. Zeiss J, Jakab E (1995) MR demonstration of an anomalous muscle in a patient with coexistent carpal and ulnar tunnel syndrome. Case report and literature summary. Clin Imaging 19:102–105

67. Zlatkin MB, Chao PC, Osterman AL, et al (1989) Chronic wrist pain: evaluation with high-resolution MR imaging. Radiology 173:723–729

6 Dynamic Magnetic Resonance Imaging of the Hand and Wrist

R. Passariello, M. Mastantuono, L. Satragno

6.1 Introduction

High-resolution static-view magnetic resonance imaging (MRI) of the wrist has proved to be an effective technique in the study of this complex area and provides information that (generally) permits differentiation among the various conditions that are responsible for wrist pain. However, insufficiency of ligamentous structures and the related subtle alteration of carpal motion are often unrecognized and frequently misdiagnosed in static-view MRI. Altered radiocarpal and intracarpal biomechanics due to ligamentous insufficiency or fractures may result in pain, instability and early degeneration.

The diagnostic advantages of dynamic studies of wrist kinetics are reported in the scientific literature and as far as these particular cases are concerned, over the last few years kinematic MRI has been suggested for examining the function of the wrist (Fig. 6.1).

6.2 Kinematic MRI

Kinematic MRI improves the diagnostic accuracy of MRI, especially in detecting dynamic instability patterns, transitory subluxation and bony or soft tissue im-

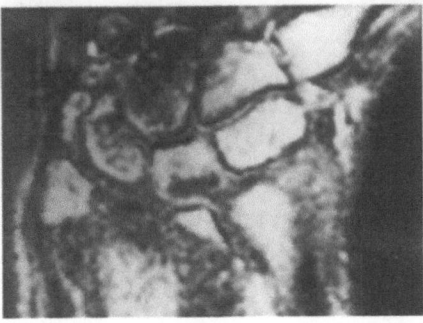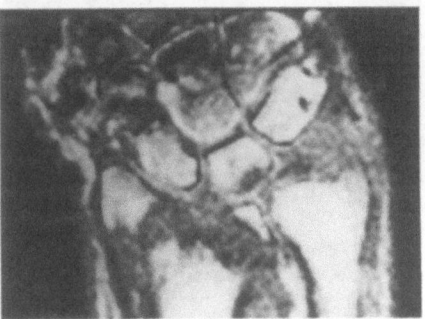

a   b

Fig. 6.1a, b. Lunatomalacia in a patient with post-traumatic ulna plus relationship (foreshortening of the radius secondary to impaction). Kinematic MR images obtained in the coronal plane images show a bony impingement with concentration of forces on the proximal surface of the lunate during radial deviation (**b**) due to a prominent ulna. Overload with repeated compression pattern is an unfavorable prognostic factor

pingement syndromes that affect the wrist and are not often sufficiently characterized using static-view MR techniques. Dynamic MRI may passively and actively
test the joint. Although (compared with the passive technique) active movement
dynamic MRI studies generally provide a more physiological examination of the
joint, many difficulties are encountered caused by the dimensions and complex
interrelationship of carpal anatomical structures in the wrist.

Provocative maneuvers (acquisitions performed under load or against stress) may
also be helpful (Fig. 6.2). However, at present only the incremental passive positioning
technique (with or without muscular tension) offers the possibility of evaluating the
complex relationship between carpal bones during movement in daily clinical routine.

6.3   Incremental Passive Kinematic MRI

The simplest kinematic MRI is the incremental passive positioning technique. It is
performed by obtaining multiple coronal plane images at different locations as the
wrist joint is passively and incrementally moved from ulnar to radial deviation. An
operator-activated, nonferromagnetic positioning device is used (Fig. 6.3). This
device incorporates a mechanism that allows measurable steps. In an alternative
method kinematic MRI may also be obtained in sagittal plane images with the
wrist in flexion, a neutral position and extension (Fig. 6.4), and furthermore in
pronation and supination (for the evaluation of the distal radioulnar joint and
subluxation of the extensor carpi ulnaris tendon) (Fig. 6.5).

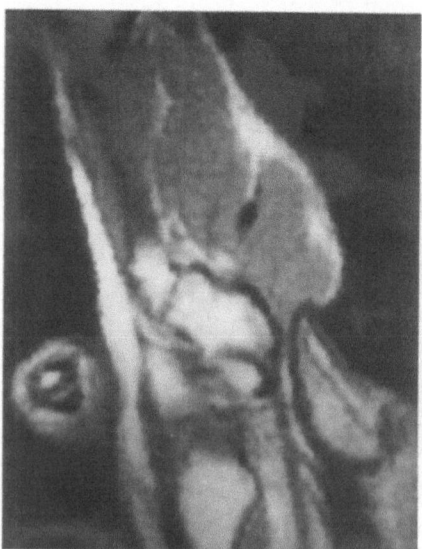
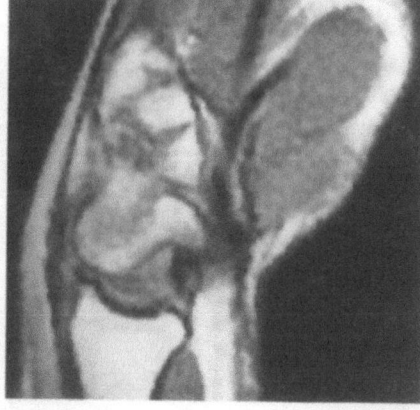

a   b

Fig. 6.2. Provocative test acquisition performed while pressure is applied by the operator's finger
on the distal pole of the scaphoid (**a**). A dorsal luxation of the proximal pole of the scaphoid out
of the radial fossa is evident on the contiguous sagittal image (**b**)

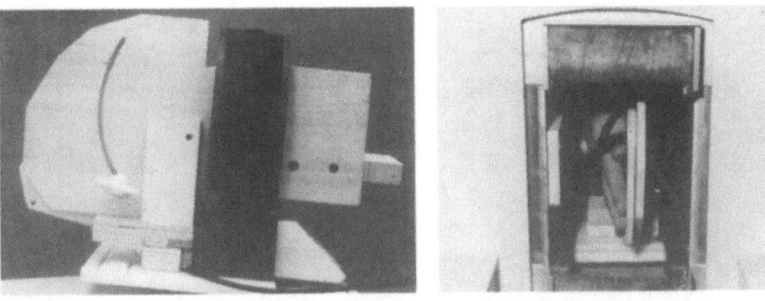

a

b

Fig. 6.3a, b. Operator-activated, nonferromagnetic positioning devices used in the dynamic examination for evaluation of movement from ulnar to radial deviation

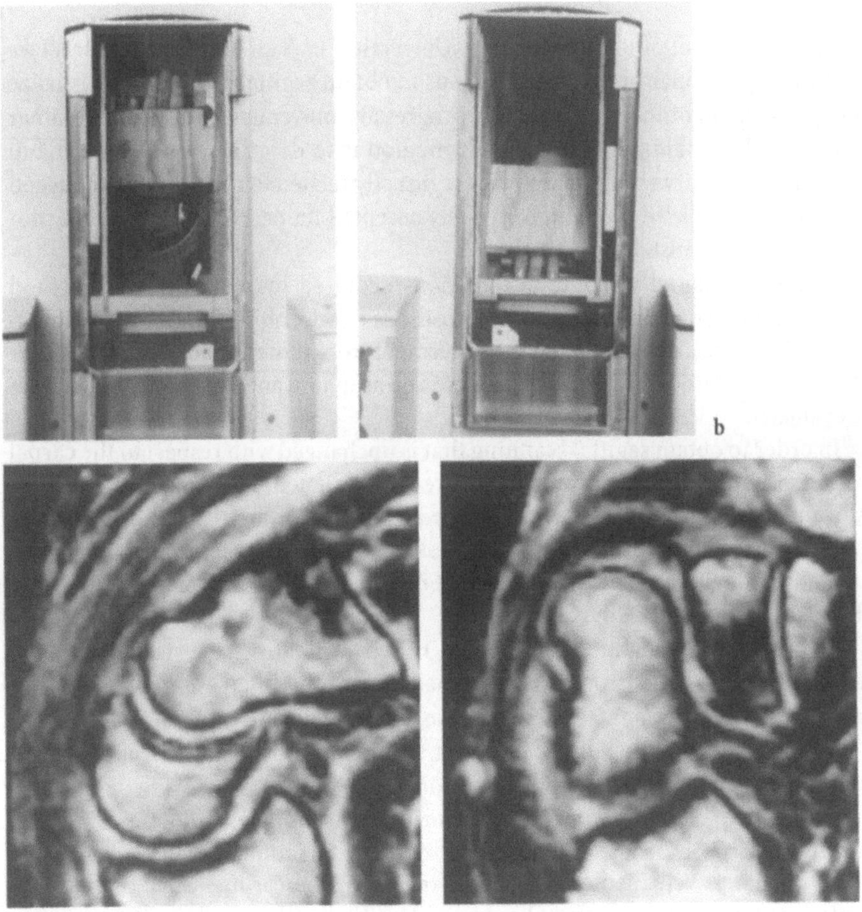

a

b

c

d

Fig. 6.4. Nonferromagnetic positioning devices used for dynamic evaluation in extension (**a**), flexion (**b**) and neutral position; sagittal GE images acquired in extension depict the normal dynamic relationship between the central (**c**) and lateral (**d**) carpal column relative to the radius in this position

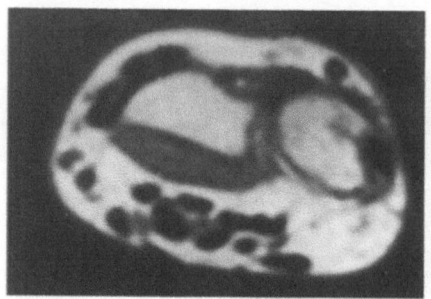 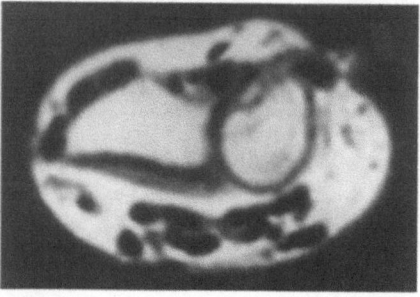

a   b

Fig. 6.5. Biomechanics of the distal radioulnar joint: the extensor carpi ulnaris tendon is located within its ulnar groove in pronation (**a**) and appears subluxated in extreme pronation (**b**)

6.4   Imaging Protocol

In the Department of Radiology of the University "La Sapienza" (Rome, Italy) we perform a particular protocol allowing us to obtain sagittal scans which visualize the same region of the carpus during progressive movement from radial to ulnar deviation. The main advantage of this method is to describe carpal motion and dynamic instability with images that are directly related to the columnar concept. This concept is based on the most widely accepted models of interpretation proposed for carpal instability.

Moreover sagittal tomographic sections acquired by means of this method allow simultaneous assessment of interosseous relationships for every position in which the wrist is placed during the movement from ulnar to radial deviation. For all positions, the degree of lunate, capitate and scaphoid angulation can be precisely evaluated.

In order to obtain sagittal scanning that is unchanged with respect to the carpal column (with which the scanning plane remains aligned) in the various phases of movement; the protocol incorporates the acquisition of multislice coronal scans. Each scan is acquired after every successive incremental step in the degree of radioulnar deviation. The coronal sets of images are used as a reference to orient the sagittal scans correctly.

To carry out a dynamic examination, 12 sets of multislice scans are normally acquired: six of them are acquired coronally after every increase in the degree of ulnar deviation (these images are used, as mentioned above, for correct orientation of the sagittal scan planes); the other six are multislice sagittal scans that will be reconstructed afterwards in cinemotion (Fig. 6 6).

In practice, it is very simple to perform our technique: from a set of scans acquired in coronal view of the carpus in ulnar deviation, we choose an image that adequately represents the median region of the carpus. Once the coronal section to be used for reference has been identified, orthogonal sagittal scans are placed upon the carpal joint side, taking care to match the scan with the tangent at the interarticular spaces between the columns. Having acquired the sagittal

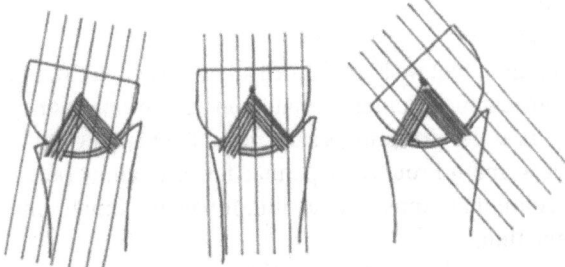

Fig. 6.6. Multislice scans acquired at a sagittal level are orientated by the operator with reference to the position of the carpus visualized at the coronal level, taking care to match the scan with the tangent at the interarticular spaces between the columns. Sagittal scan planes will be reconstructed afterwards in cinemotion

scans, one proceeds (after the first step in radial deviation movement) with the acquisition of a new set of coronal images, maintaining the position that was chosen for the acquisition of the previous set of coronal scans. Among the coronal images that are acquired (after the step), a new coronal image is chosen for reference, picking out the image that represents the same morphological coronal section of the carpus that was used as a reference for the first acquisition. Thus it is possible to continue the examination placing new sagittal images following precise carpal references.

The total acquisition time required for a dynamic evaluation of the wrist is mainly related to the number of positions acquired for the representation of the joint movement; in our experience, six different positions are the minimum required for homogeneous motion effect in the reconstruction. Other extrinsic operator-controlled parameters affect scan time and signal-to-noise ratio and some of these can be modified by the user to reduce the total acquisition time and to optimize either the image quality or the appearance of the reconstructed MR images.

Thin slices and a small field of view (FOV) are needed in the wrist due to the small size of the anatomical structures of the carpus. These parameters obviously affect signal-to-noise ratio and scan time.

Signal-to-noise ratio and image appearance can be improved by applying more than one excitation in sagittal images; a compromise to maintain an acceptable total scan time is to increase the number of excitations only in images acquired in full ulnar and radial deviation and in neutral position.

Using dedicated low-field equipment and a T1-weighted spin-echo sequence with a 192×192 matrix the examination takes almost 20 min.

The TR that we use in the sagittal acquisitions is 500 ms or the minimum that is sufficient to include the whole carpus in the volume in which the multislice representation is required. The TR required for the coronal scans is generally lower, about 300 ms, since the coronal study is carried out in thicker slices and in most cases it is sufficient to visualize only the central portion of the carpus.

6.5   Kinematic Results

The result obtained using the method that we have defined allows easier analysis of radiocarpal and intracarpal biomechanics. Conjunct rotation in flexion extension of the proximal row normally occurs as the wrist moves from radial to ulnar deviation.

During radial deviation, the scaphoid rotates or palmar-flexes to allow radiocarpal shortening and the scapholunate interosseous link forces the lunate into volar-flexion during radial deviation.

In ulnar deviation the triquetrum slides in relation to the hamate and due to the orientation of triquetrohamate facets the movement induces a dorsiflexion and volar displacement of the triquetrum and the entire proximal carpal row.

The counteracting forces upon the lunate (dorsiflexion influence of the triquetrum and volarflexion influence of the scaphoid) are responsible for the complex twisting movement of the lunate with volar to dorsal shift and progressive dorsal tilt of the lunate when the wrist moves from radial to ulnar deviation (in full radial deviation lunate flexes approximately 15° and in full ulnar deviation it extends around 20°). The analysis of this physiological "twist" of the lunate is easy and accurately obtained in sagittal dynamic reconstruction of the central column acquired during the movement from radial to ulnar deviation.

A normal relationship among the bones of the lateral column and the integrity of the scapholunate ligament controls the lunate. When the scaphoid does not counteract the dorsiflexion influence of the triquetrum upon the lunate, because of an elongation or a complete tear of scapholunate ligament, we observe a dorsal tilt and a volar shift of the lunate.

On the other hand lunate dorsiflexion is controlled by the medial column and usually lunotriquetral and triquetrohamate dissociation are responsible for the VISI instability pattern (Fig. 6.7).

The pattern of articular relationship alteration is clearly demonstrated in static MRI images only if the ligaments are completely torn or in the case of a specific associated lesion.

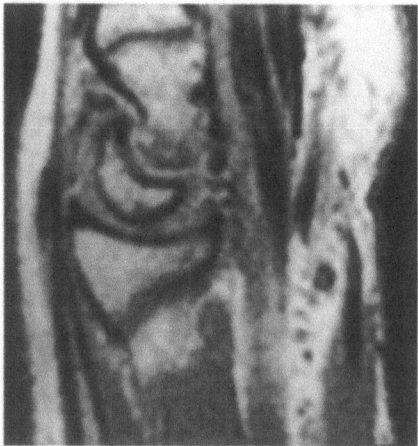

Fig. 6.7. Sagittal MR image show volar tilting of the lunate (VISI pattern)

Even in presence of complete tears of interosseous ligaments of carpus, diastase among the bones may be not evident in the static MRI examination, where neither widening of the interosseous interval nor abnormal rotation of the carpal bones can be recognized. For example, in a complete tear of the scapholunate, diastase, rotation or subluxation of the scaphoid may be absent, especially if the radiocarpal ligaments are normal. This kind of alteration is clearly depicted by performing dynamic scans (Fig. 6.8).

In minor sprains (partial tears with elongation) or in the presence of a single ligamentous tear we observe a minor derangement of carpal biomechanics that is evident only during the motion in which the lunate or part of the proximal carpal row remain in abnormal flexion or extension (Figs. 6.9–6.12).

Almost always the accentuated dorsal tilt of lunate related to the position of the hand and especially its reduced mobility during radial deviation are a sign of ligamentous incompetence or of dynamic instability, even if the dorsal shift of capitate and volar rotation of scaphoid are not evident.

Particular attention must be paid to detecting dynamic instability by means of volar tilt of the lunate that is evident only if it is strongly elicited due to the dorsiflexion bias of the lunate itself.

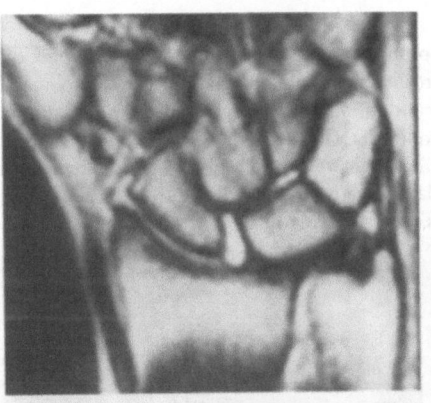

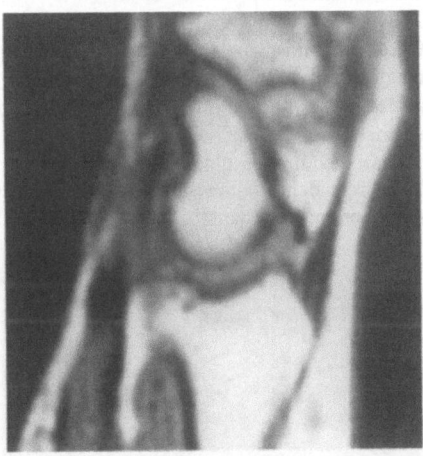

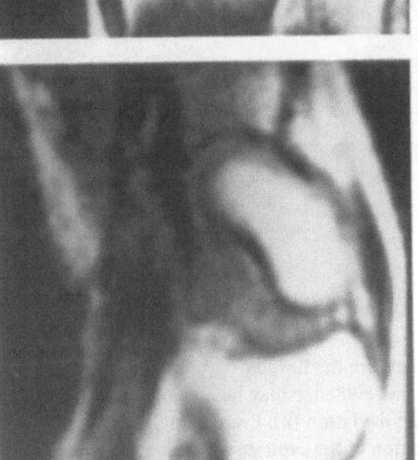

a

b

c

Fig. 6.8. Routine static MRI study only shows fluid in the scapholunate space (a). The subluxation of proximal pole of scaphoid is not evident in the sagittal plane in neutral position (b); it is well depicted in the images obtained with the wrist in partial flexion (c)

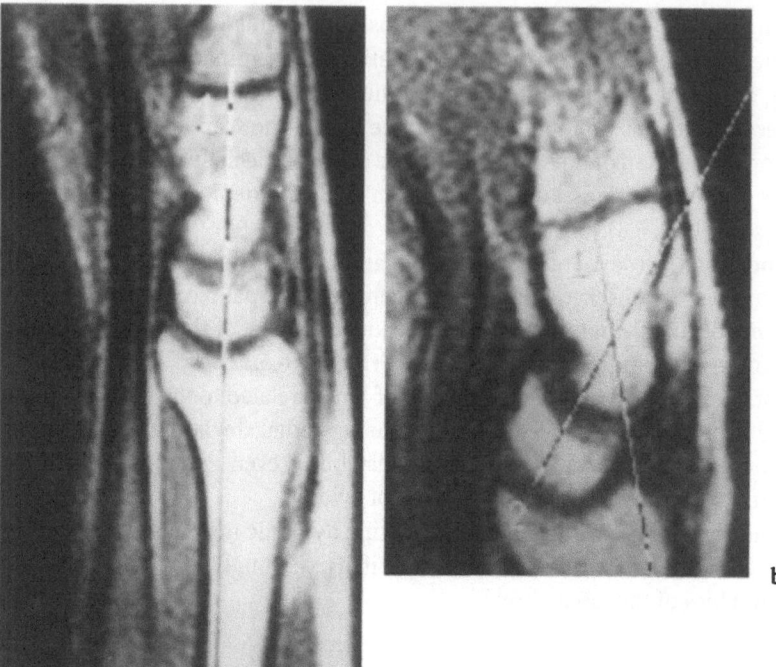

Fig. 6.9a, b. Mid-carpal instability: derangement of the normal conjunct rotation of the bones of the proximal carpal row when the wrist moves from radial to ulnar deviation. The capitolunate angle appears normal on the static radiographs and on MRI in neutral position (a) (as in the normal wrist, the capitate and radius remain collinear). On the sagittal image of the central column (acquired in ulnar deviation after the painful snap) subluxation between capitate and lunate is evident (b); the capitate is dorsally displaced relative to the radius due to the abnormal movement of the lunate that tilts dorsally but does not shift volarly

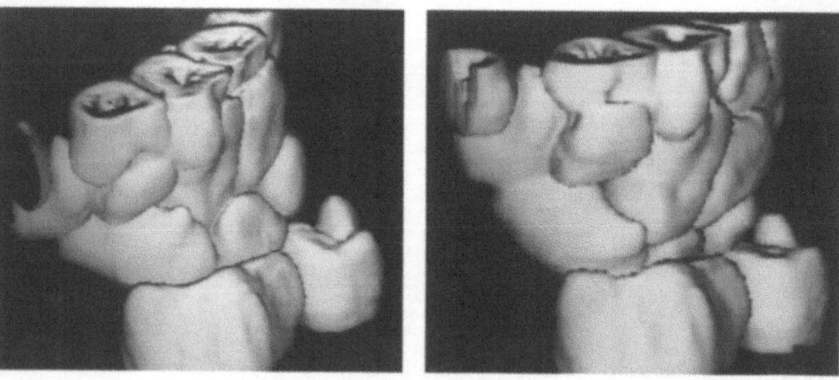

Fig. 6.10a, b. During ulnar deviation the lunate flips from the flexed to extended position, with a painful "clunk", and leaves behind the scaphoid; this evidence may be also obtained using CT. Images reconstructed from data obtained in radial deviation (a). Even a small degree of ulnar deviation may be responsible for a sudden subluxation of the capitate and hamate relative to the lunate and triquetrum (b)

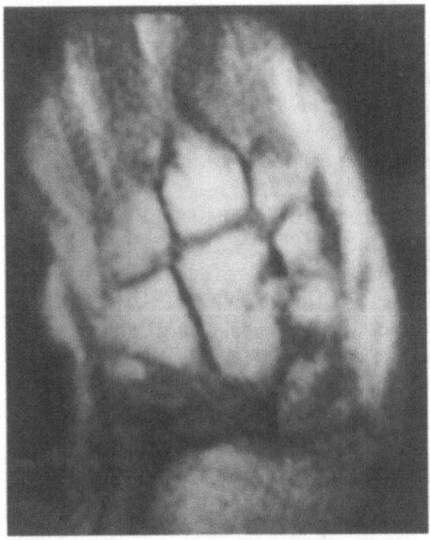
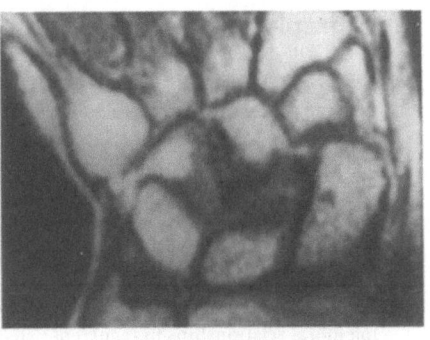

b

a

Fig. 6.11. Coronal MRI multislice tomographic view images clearly demonstrate the dorsal subluxation of the capitate and hamate relative to the lunate and triquetrum: dorsal slice (**a**), volar slice (**b**)

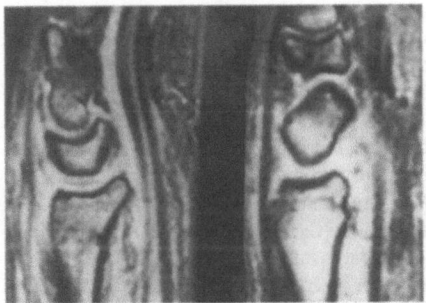
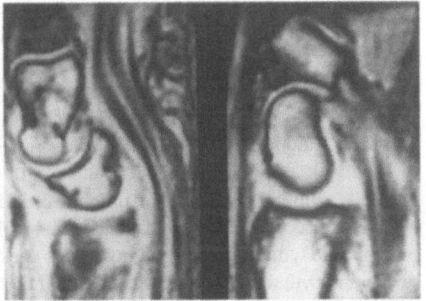

a

b

Fig. 6.12. In a different case from Fig. 6.11 sagittal tomographic sections allow simultaneous assessment of interosseous relationships for every position in which the wrist is placed during the movement from radial (**a**) to ulnar (**b**) deviation. Dorsal luxation of the capitate is evident only in full ulnar deviation (**b**)

In conclusion, dynamic MRI offers a tomographic view and simultaneously depicts abnormal relationships between the carpal bones during movement, disclosing carpal ligamentous abnormalities that predispose to dynamic carpal instabilities. In our experience sagittal MR images have been demonstrated to be the most useful in the assessment of carpal alignment. Especially if acquired during lateral deviation movements of the wrist, the images offer the possibility to evaluate the intracolumn derangement.

Bibliography

1. Bergey PD, Zlatkin MB, Dalinka M, Osterman AL, Machek J, Dolinar J (1989) Dynamic MR imaging of the wrist: early results with a specially designed positioning device. Radiology 173:26
2. Brossman J, Muhle C, Bull C, et al (1993) Evaluation of patellar tracking in patients with suspected patellar malalignment: cine MR imaging vs. arthroscopy. AJR 162:361
3. Culver JE (1986) Instabilities of the wrist. Clin Sports Med 5:725
4. Fulmer JM, Harms SE, Flamig DP, Guerdon G, Machek J, Dolinar J (1989) High-resolution cine MR imaging of the wrist. Radiology 173:26
5. Gilula LA (1977) Carpal injuries: analytic approach and case exercises. AJR 133:503
6. Kujala UM, Osterman K, Kormano M, Nelimarkka O, Hurme M, Taimela S (1989) Patellofemoral relationships in recurrent patellar dislocation. J Bone Joint Surg Br 71:788
7. Kujala UM, Osterman K, Kormano M, Komu M, Schlenzka D (1989) Patellar motion analyzed by magnetic resonance imaging. Acta Orthop Scand 60:13
8. Lichtman DM, Noble WH, Alexander CE (1984) Dynamic triquetrolunate instability. J Hand Surg [Am] 9:185
9. Linscheid RL, Dobyns H, Beabout JW, Bryan RS (1972) Traumatic instability of the wrist. J Bone Joint Surg Am 54:1612
10. Mastantuono M, Argento G, Larciprete M, Bassetti E, Capanna G, Morricone I, Passariello R (1995) MRI of the limbs with low-field dedicated equipment: 30 months of clinical studies in articular and musculo-skeletal pathology. Med Imaging Int Germ BPA 3(199):12
11. Mastantuono M, Larciprete M, Argento G, Palombi D, De Bac S, Bassetti E, Passariello R (1995) Wrist dynamic MR imaging with a dedicated magnet in the study of carpal instability: a new technique. Proceedings of the Society of Magnetic Resonance 3rd scientific meeting and exhibition and the European Society for Magnetic Resonance in Medicine and Biology, 12th annual meeting and exhibition, Nice, France, 19–25 Aug 1995, vol 3, ISSN 1065–9889, p 1530
12. Mastantuono M, Larciprete M, Bassetti E, Argento G, Satragno L, Passariello R (1997) Advances in kinematic of the patella: a new method of dynamic acquisition to evaluate the extensor complex of the knee. European Congress of Radiology ECR 1997, Vienna, Austria, 2–7 March 1997, p 160. Eur Radiol [Suppl] 7:160
13. Mastantuono M, Larciprete M, Bassetti E, Satragno L, Passariello R (1997) A new protocol of dynamic acquisition for the evaluation of the extensor complex of the knee with MRI. 2nd international symposium on musculoskeletal MRI. San Francisco, California USA, 1–5 June 1997
14. Mastantuono M, Argento G, Larciprete M, Bassetti E, Di Carlo VCV, Ascarelli A, Passariello R (1997) Dynamic MRI imaging in the study of carpal instability: a new technique. Instructional course on "Stiffness of the joints of the upper limb". Fourth congress of FESSH, June 1997, Bologna, 15–18 June 1997. J Hand Surg [Br] 22 [Suppl 1]:6
15. Mastantuono M, Argento G, Larciprete M, Bassetti E, Di Carlo VCV, Ascarelli A, Passariello R (1997) The importance of MR evaluation in the study of rheumatic pathology of the hand. Fourth congress of FESSH, June 1997, Bologna, 15–18 June 1997. J Hand Surg [Br] 22 [Suppl 1]:9
16. Mastantuono M, Larciprete M, Argento G, Bassetti E, DiCarloV, Tancioni V, Satragno L, Passariello R (1998) Nuove prospettive nella valutazione con Risonanza Magnetica dinamica del complesso estensore del ginocchio. Radiol Med 95(5):430–436
17. Mastantuono M, Bassetti E, Tancioni V, Di Giorgio L, Larciprete M, Di Carlo VCV, Satragno L, Passariello R (1998) Valutazione della biomeccanica carpale con Cine RM. Quadri normali e condizioni di instabilita. 38 Congresso Nazionale SIRM, Maggio 1998, Milano. Radiol Med 95 [Suppl 1]:140
18. Mastantuono M, Bassetti E, Trenta F, Arata FM, Iachelli M, Passariello R (1998) MRI evaluation of the wrist with dynamic studying. Fifth annual meeting of the European Society of Muscoskeletal Radiology, Bled (Slovenia), 30–31 Oct 1998, abstracts book, p 151
19. Mastantuono M, Bassetti E, Di Giorgio L, Manganaro F, Francone L, Moneta MR, Passariello R (1999) Midcarpal instability: evaluation with dynamic MRI. European Society of Musculoskeletal Radiology (ESSR); 6th annual meeting, Edinburgh, Scotland, 8–9 Oct 1999

20. Nordin M, Frankel VH (1989) Basic biomechanics of the musculoskeletal system, 2nd edn. Lea and Febiger, Philadelphia
21. Reicher MA, Kellerhouse LE (1990) Normal wrist anatomy, biomechanics, basic imaging protocol, and normal multiplanar MRI of the wrist. In: Reicher MA, Kellerhouse LE (eds) MRI of the hand and wrist. Raven Press, New York
22. Shellock FG, Mandelbaum B (1990) Kinematic MRI of the joints. In: Mink JH, Deutsch AL (eds) MRI of the musculoskeletal system: a teaching file. Raven Press, New York
23. Shellock FG, Pressman BD (1989) MR imaging of the temporomandibular joint: improvements in the imaging protocol. AJNR 10:595
24. Shellock FG, Mink JH, Deutsch AL, Fox JM (1989) Evaluation of patellar tracking abnormalities using kinematic MR imaging: clinical experience in 130 patients. Radiology 172:799
25. Shellock FG, Mink JH, Deutsch AL, Fox JM (1989) Kinematic magnetic resonance imaging for evaluation of patellar tracking. Physician Sports Med 17:99
26. Shellock FG, Mink JH, Fox JM (1988) Patellofemoral joint: kinematic MR imaging to assess tracking abnormalities. Radiology 168:551
27. Shellock FG, Mink JH, Deutsch AL, Fox JM, Ferkel RD (1990) Evaluation of patients with persistent symptoms after lateral retinacular release by kinematic magnetic resonance imaging of the patellofemoral joint. Arthroscopy 6:226
28. Shellock FG (1993) Kinematic MRI evaluation of the joints. In: Stoller DW (ed) Magnetic resonance imaging in orthopaedics and rheumatology. Lippincott, Philadelphia
29. Tjin A, Ton ER, Pattynama PMT, Bloem JL, Obermann WR (1995) Interosseous ligaments: device for applying stress in wrist MR imaging. Radiology 196:863

7 Bone Scintigraphy

J. Dutton, I. Fogelman

7.1 Introduction

Bone is a living tissue with a vascular supply and constantly undergoes modelling and remodelling throughout life as a result of physical stresses and strains. This is particularly true in the hands, which are subjected to repetitive minor trauma as a result of everyday living. In the immature skeleton there is non-pathological increased metabolic activity at the growth plates until fusion occurs. In pathological conditions there will be changes in vascularity and localised abnormalities of osteoclastic and osteoblastic activity. Radionuclide bone scans, which provide a functional display of skeletal metabolism, can detect abnormal vascularity and assess the level of bone turnover in the hand and wrist, thus providing useful information in the evaluation of suspected pathology (Fig.7.1).

7.2 Techniques

Nuclear medicine techniques have been available in the clinical setting for approximately 50 years, and although technical advances have resulted in dramatic improvement in image appearances, the basic principles of the technique remain unchanged. In essence, radionuclide imaging is an investigation in which a radio-isotope is introduced into the body (usually by intravenous injection) and the body, or body part, is positioned close to a gamma camera which can detect radioactivity. The radioisotopes administered may be salts of rare elements from the far end of the periodic table, such as gallium-67 citrate, or more often are specific compounds that have been tagged chemically to a radioactive element

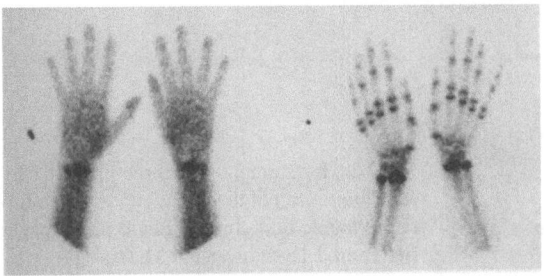

Fig. 7.1. Normal bone scan of the hands in the immature skeleton. Early blood pool (*left*) and 2-h images (*right*) of the hands and wrist (see text). Note the increased signal from the growth plates and the symmetry between the hands

which acts as a marker to identify the distribution of the compound, such as ^{99m}Tc-MDP (methylene diphosphonate linked to radioactive technetium). Common to all radioisotopes, however, is their ability to emit radioactivity (gamma rays) which can be detected by nuclear medicine cameras.

A small amount of the radioactivity emitted from the radioisotope is absorbed by the patient. The radiation dose to the patient varies with different types of radioisotopes but generally the doses from nuclear medicine techniques are higher than those from radiographic techniques when limited to the hand [1, 2]:

Bone scan (400 MBq ^{99m}Tc-MDP)   = 2.3 mSv
Extremity radiograph   = 0.01 mSv

By far the commonest radionuclide scan performed to assess the hands and wrists is a bone scan using ^{99m}Tc-MDP. Similar agents are ^{99m}Tc-hydroxyethylidene diphosphonate and ^{99m}Tc-hydroxymethylene diphosphonate. ^{99m}Tc-MDP has bone-seeking properties and although the precise mechanism of its chemical reaction with bone has not been elucidated, it is believed to bind to bone matrix by a process known as chemi-adsorption [3]. For imaging the hand or wrist ^{99m}Tc-MDP is administered by bolus intravenous injection in the limb contralateral to that which is symptomatic, or preferably as a pedal injection which allows direct comparison between the upper limbs.

If information regarding vascularity of the hand or wrist is required then a three-phase bone scan can be performed which involves three distinct stages of image acquisition with an initial phase using a bolus injection (radionuclide angiogram) to assess vascularity of the site of interest, an early blood pool phase (at 5 min) to assess vascular and extravascular distribution of tracer, and finally delayed imaging at approximately 2–4 h after tracer injection to assess the uptake of tracer in bone (Fig. 7.2). Imaging at 24 h may occasionally be useful as there is improved ratio of bone to soft tissue uptake at this time; however, with such delayed imaging count rates are low and prolonged scanning times are required to produce useful images.

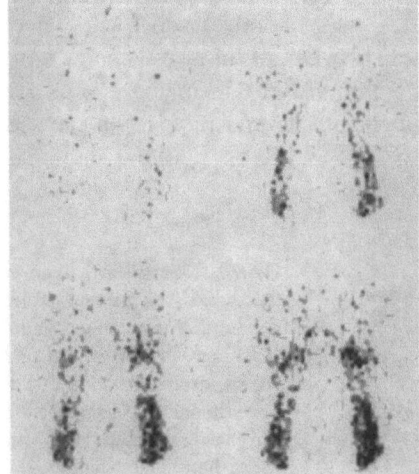

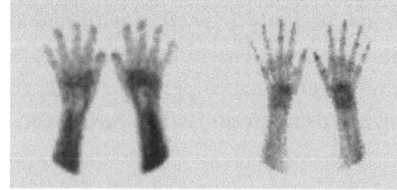

b

Fig. 7.2a, b. Example of a three-phase ^{99m}Tc-MDP bone scan of the hands and wrists. a Initial dynamic flow study. b Blood pool images (*left*) and delayed images at 3 h (*right*)

a

Bone scan images of the hands and wrists have a spatial resolution in the region of 6–10 mm. Image quality deteriorates with movement of the limb and with increasing distance from the gamma camera. In hand and wrist imaging these problems rarely arise as the limbs can usually be immobilised to prevent movement artefact and there is little soft tissue overlying the bony structures so the gamma camera face is very close to the structures of interest. A pinhole collimator, providing image magnification, can improve image resolution. Thus, good-quality images can be produced, even when reduced amounts of activity are administered. The standard amount of activity administered to adults for ^{99m}Tc-MDP bone scans is 555–750 MBq, giving an effective dose equivalent of 3–5 mSv [1]. Acceptable bone scans of the hands and wrists can be obtained with reduced amounts of activity (e.g. 400 MBq) with proportionately increased scanning times. The activity administered is reduced in the child and this can be scaled according to body weight using the formula:

Activity to administer (MBq)=X factor × 750 MBq

Published lists of the X factor are available [4]. There is a minimum activity of 40 MBq below which image quality is unsatisfactory.

Both limbs should be imaged to allow comparisons between the normal and the affected limb. Care should be taken to ensure that the limbs are positioned symmetrically. The standard technique is to place the hands, palms facing downwards with the wrists in neutral position, in the centre of the field of view of the gamma camera (Fig. 7.3). A low-energy, high-resolution collimator is employed. The dynamic sequence can be acquired as sixty, 1-s frames; the early blood pool image follows as a 2-min image commencing 2 min after tracer injection; and finally the delayed image is acquired for 5 min (or 800,000 counts, whichever is longer). It should be noted that there is considerable local variation in protocol details. It is conventional to place a radioactive marker (seen as a hot spot on the final image) adjacent to the right-sided limb. Some institutions advocate the use of alternative positions of the limbs including palmar views of the wrist in ulnar or radial deviation and sometimes lateral views.

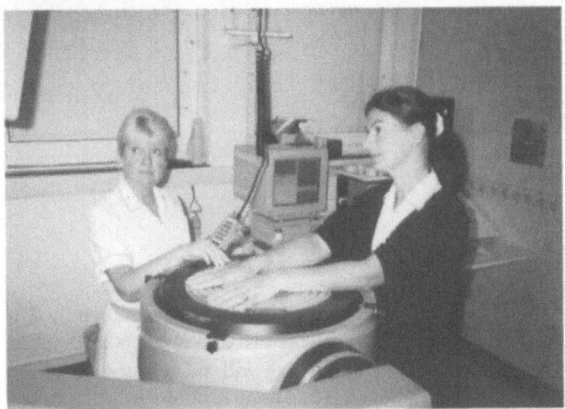

Fig. 7.3. Our technologists demonstrate the standard positioning for hand and wrist scans with the palms facing downwards in the centre of the field of view of the gamma camera

Despite the sensitivity of hand and wrist bone scans, they are relatively non-specific, with different pathologies often producing similar appearances. Furthermore, the proximity of the carpal bones to each other and the presence of tendons and ligaments means that precise localisation of abnormalities in the carpus can be difficult. The co-registered bone scan may improve localisation of bone scan abnormalities by directly superimposing bone scan images on radiographs. This has been attempted in different ways.

In one technique the hand and wrist are immobilised in a customised cast that is made from heat flexible polypropylene [5] (Fig. 7.4). Three markers are applied to the cast at the level of the first and third digits and the distal forearm. The markers are metallic and therefore visible on radiographs (Fig. 7.5). They have a central tiny hole over which a radioactive source can be placed so that the central point of the markers is visualised as a dot on the scintigram. The bone scan image is acquired and following this a conventional radiograph is performed without removal of the cast or markers. The markers aid alignment of the bone scan and radiograph images. This technique has been shown to be advantageous over non-registered bone scans in assessing carpal abnormalities [5].

Alternative techniques for co-registration exist. In another method, the hand is positioned on a customised X-ray film cassette that rests on the face of the gamma camera [6] (Fig. 7.6). The film cassette can be loaded with standard X-ray film and exposed with a mobile X-ray unit. Thus there is no change in positioning between the nuclear medicine and radiographic acquisition. As in the previous method, markers are used on the images for precise alignment during the registration process, but in this case, the markers are on the film cassette and not on the patient.

More difficult to overcome is the problem of non-specificity of bone scan findings. The same characteristics can be associated with different pathologies; for

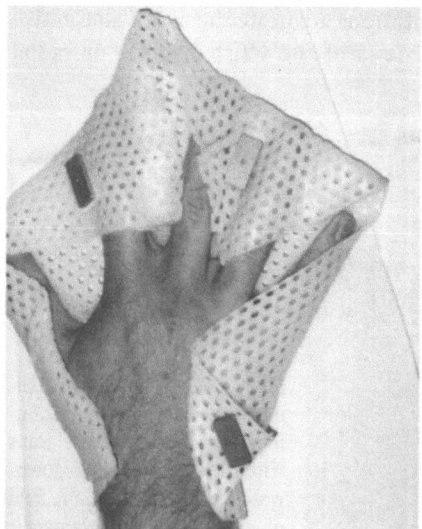

Fig. 7.4. The hand and wrist are immobilised in a polypropylene cast and markers are applied to the cast which will aid registration of the radiograph and bone scan images

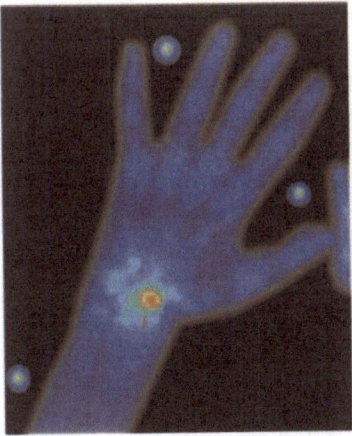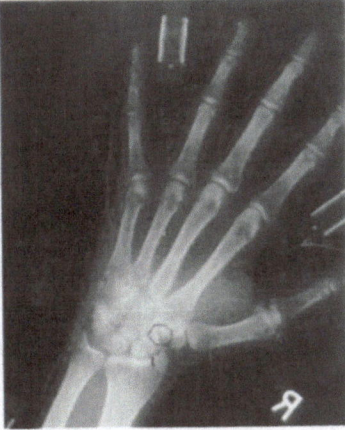

Fig. 7.5. Example of registration images. *Left*: The bone scan shows markedly increased tracer uptake at the radial aspect of the carpus. The three hot spots external to the patient represent the radioactive markers for image alignment. *Right*: Radiograph of the same hand. The red marker demonstrates that the intense bone scan activity is localised to the articulation of the scaphoid and trapezium

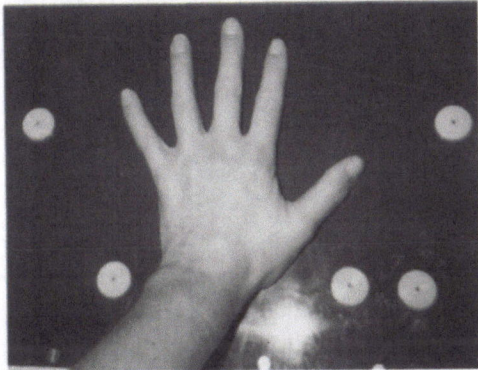

Fig. 7.6. The hand is positioned, palm facing downwards, on a customised X-ray film cassette. The round discs represent the markers used for alignment of the radiograph and bone scan images

example, increased tracer uptake at a joint may appear identical in different forms of arthritis. Alternatively a vascular bone tumour could be mistaken for an acute traumatic fracture. The clinical scenario or the distribution of bone scan abnormalities may help to specify the disease entity.

As mentioned earlier, bone scans form the large majority of all nuclear medicine imaging studies of the hands and wrists, although sometimes other tracers are useful, for example, radioactive labelled leucocytes may be used for suspected infection [7] and HIG (polyclonal human immunoglobulin) [8] or labelled anti-E-selectin monoclonal antibody [9] may be used in imaging arthritis. The choice of tracer depends on the clinical question posed. Most frequently nuclear medicine hand and wrist imaging is requested by orthopaedic surgeons, rheumatologists and casualty departments, and the commonest reasons for referral include suspected fracture, reflex sympathetic dystrophy (RSD), unexplained hand and wrist pain, or assessment of arthritis.

7.3   Unexplained Hand and Wrist Pain

The number of people taking time off work through illness has risen dramatically in the past few years and in Britain this figure is about 1.3 million people each year of whom approximately 27,000 are forced to give up work. Despite the lack of objective evidence that a direct relationship exists between work activities and the onset of musculoskeletal disorders, repetitive activities and cumulative trauma is thought to cause or exaggerate several types of injury, including carpal tunnel syndrome, tenosynovitis and degenerative joint disease [10]. Although nuclear medicine has no direct role in diagnosis of a cumulative trauma disorder, bone scan images of the hands and wrists may be performed as part of an algorithm for evaluation of hand and wrist pain to help exclude other pathology such as fractures, infection, avascular necrosis, tumours or arthritis. The timing of the bone scan in relation to other investigations depends on the clinical problem and, to a lesser extent, on local expertise, experience and the accessibility of nuclear medicine techniques. When radionuclide imaging is undertaken, almost all scans are performed with bone-seeking agents such as ^{99m}Tc-MDP. In only a very small number of cases would an alternative tracer be use. Lesions in the cervical spine, upper arm, elbow or forearm may be responsible for producing hand or wrist pain and in some circumstances, such as unexplained hand and wrist pain, it might be prudent to include these areas in the bone scan.

7.4   Fractures

Bone scintigraphy has an important role in patients in whom standard radiographs fail to demonstrate a lesion following trauma but clinical symptoms are suggestive of a fracture [11–13]. It is particularly useful in identification of scaphoid fractures where failure to treat may have serious consequences, both from the increased risk of non-union, mal-union or avascular necrosis and with the potential for medical litigation [14]. Negative scintigraphy is equally as useful as positive findings because exclusion of a fracture will shorten the period of immobilisation and allow earlier return to work.

Fractures produce focal increase in uptake of bone-seeking radioisotopes and in the hands and wrists, positive scans will usually be seen within 12–24 h of injury (Fig. 7.7). Bone scans are expensive by comparison with plain film radiography and should not be used routinely in diagnosis of fractures. Their use should be limited to the minority of patients with persistent symptoms in whom plain film radiography including special views (e.g. scaphoid series at 10 days post-injury) fails to yield a result.

Suspected fracture is an appropriate indication for three-phase bone scintigraphy, with abnormal increased signal expected in all three phases of the scan [15]. Unlike other parts of the body, where fractures may produce linear abnormalities on the bone scan, fractures in the hand and carpal bones tend to have a more focal,

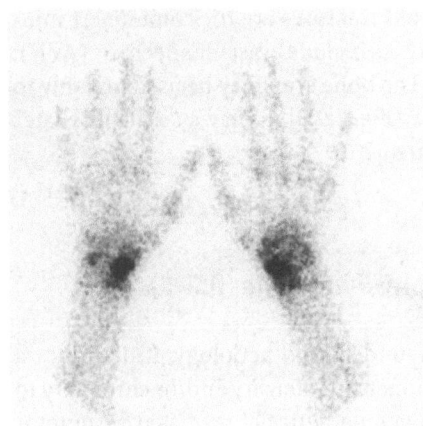

Fig. 7.7. Three-hour images from a ^{99m}Tc-MDP bone scan in a patient with bilateral scaphoid fractures which were confirmed on radiographs acquired 6 weeks after trauma

rounded appearance. Sometimes it is useful to manipulate image intensity to improve the definition of the lesion and assist in localisation of the abnormality. Previous studies have shown that bone scintigraphy in suspected scaphoid fracture has a sensitivity of 100% and a specificity of up to 75% with good inter-observer agreement [11, 15, 16]. More recently, MRI has been evaluated against bone scans in suspected scaphoid fracture and it compares favourably, producing a similar level of sensitivity but fewer false positive results [17]. False positive results on bone scans can be produced by poor anatomical localisation or the presence of alternative pathology. MRI has the added advantage of demonstrating soft tissue pathology, such as ligamentous injury, that may not be evident on scintigraphy [18].

Like scaphoid fractures, undisplaced fractures of the distal radius and ulna may also be difficult to diagnose on radiographs in the acute phase. This is especially true of some of the Salter-Harris type injuries to the growth plates in the immature skeleton. Bone scintigraphy can be extremely useful in this situation and positive findings should be evident in the acute stage (Fig. 7.8). It is particularly important in paediatric cases to image both limbs for comparison and to pay meticulous attention to radiographic positioning to appreciate subtle abnormalities in the growth plates.

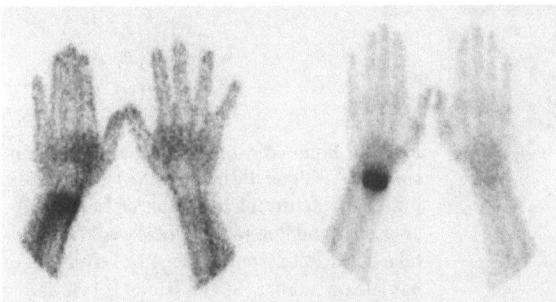

Fig. 7.8. Fracture of the distal radius. Early blood pool images (*left*) and 2-h ^{99m}Tc-MDP images of the wrists (*right*) show abnormal tracer localisation at the level of the distal right radius

Distal radial fractures and carpal scaphoid fractures are the commonest injuries to the wrist [19]. Complications of fractures include avascular necrosis (AVN), arthritis, infection and tendon injury [14]. The bone scan may be used not only to demonstrate the fracture in the acute stage (Fig. 7.9), but may also identify later complications such as AVN, infection and arthritis.

7.5   Reflex Sympathetic Dystrophy Syndrome (RSDS)

RSDS is a complicated disorder of poorly understood aetiology. It describes a syndrome of limb pain which is disproportionate in intensity and/or chronicity to the initiating insult, and is associated with sympathetically mediated vasomotor disturbances and characteristic soft tissue changes such as swelling (early stages) and loss of function (late stages).

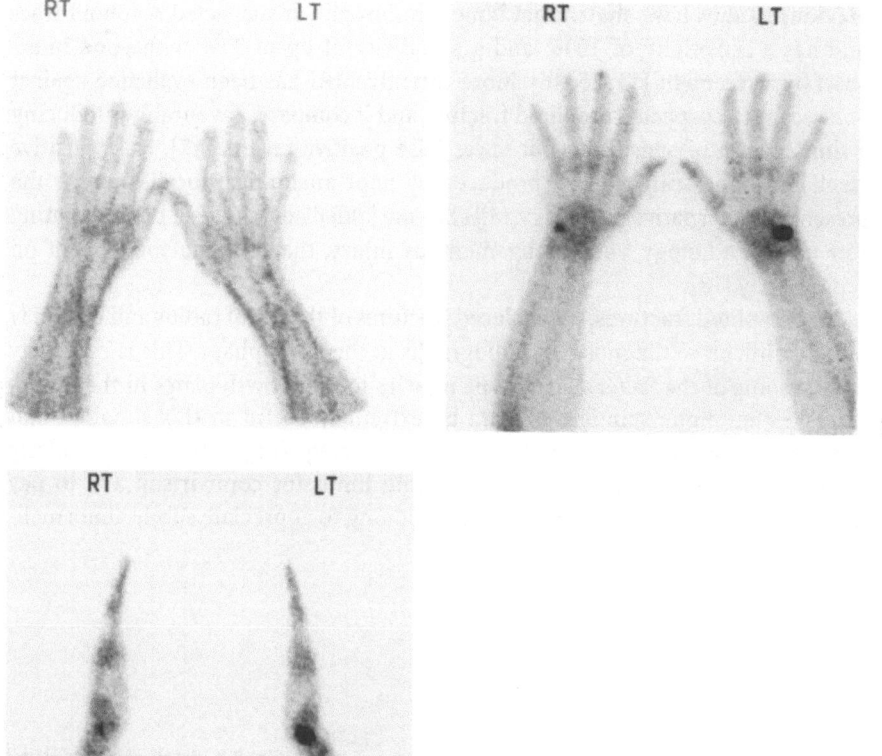

Fig. 7.9. Bone scan of the hands in a patient suffering a fall on the outstretched hand resulting in a fracture of the hook of hamate. Increased blood flow (a) and increased tracer uptake in the left carpus at the site of the hook of hamate on palmar (b) and lateral (c) views

In as many as a quarter of patients there is no history of a stimulus that triggered the onset of symptoms. Frequently however, a history of minor trauma or recent surgery may be obtained [20]. The diagnosis can be straightforward in florid cases but extremely difficult in patients with borderline symptoms and signs. This is not helped by the lack of consensus on pathophysiology, treatment and the lack of a specific objective diagnostic test. The controversy surrounding RSDS is even more overt in the literature, with the use of alternative names for this condition such as algodystrophy, Sudek's atrophy, shoulder-hand syndrome and sympathetically mediated pain syndrome amongst others.

In the absence of a sound diagnostic test for RSDS, the bone scan is an extremely useful adjunct to clinical findings. This is an appropriate indication for three-phase bone scintigraphy since vasomotor instability will cause abnormalities in all three phases of the scan [21]. As with other aspects of this disease there is marked variation in the pattern of bone scan abnormalities demonstrated and in different published series different criteria are used in scan interpretation which may explain why published studies have shown quite variable results for bone scan sensitivity and specificity in the diagnosis of RSDS [22–24]. One of the largest published series, in which 145 scintigrams were examined, showed a sensitivity of 96% and a specificity of 98% with a positive predictive value of 88% [24]. Each series, however, appears to have used the authors' own diagnostic criteria for RSDS and the patient populations differ in the duration of symptoms experienced. Despite this, the most commonly associated and reliable pattern on bone scintigraphy is diffuse increase in tracer uptake with juxta-articular accentuation in the affected limb in the third phase of the scan (Fig. 7.10). This is not specific for RSDS and may be seen in other pathologies such as arthritis, so it is important to interpret the scan in the appropriate clinical context.

Information from the first and second phases of the scan may be useful and Demangeat et al. [25] found that patterns of abnormalities on the three-phase bone scan corresponded to different time points after the onset of symptoms. In patients scanned between 0 and 60 weeks from the onset of symptoms, the majority showed increased activity in the third phase of the scan. Patients with less

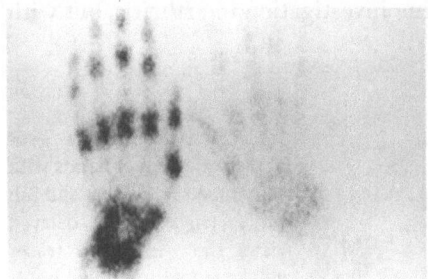

Fig. 7.10. Two-hour ^{99m}Tc-MDP bone scan image of the hands showing prominent juxta-articular tracer uptake and diffuse increase in tracer uptake in the right hand compared with the left

chronic symptoms (0–20 weeks after onset) had increased vascularity and blood pool in the affected limb. This work has been supported by other authors and it has been suggested that this may be a reliable indicator of the stage of the disease [26].

7.6   Arthritis

Polyarthritis or polyarthralgia is not a common indication for nuclear medicine imaging but hand and wrist scintigrams may be acquired as part of a full joint scan for arthritis. Sometimes the patterns of joint involvement can be helpful for initial diagnosis. On other occasions functional imaging may be used to assess disease activity, response to treatment or complications arising from medication such as avascular necrosis from prolonged steroid use.

The arthritides can be broadly divided into those associated with synovitis, such as rheumatoid arthritis, ankylosing spondylitis, gout and Reiter's disease, and those without an active inflammatory component, the commonest of which is osteoarthritis (Fig. 7.11). This is not a rigorous classification and there is some overlap between the two groups; for example aggressive osteoarthritis may exhibit inflammatory synovitis [27]. This division of the arthritides is useful in nuclear medicine image interpretation. Inflammatory arthritides may produce increased signal on all three phases of the bone scan with the pattern of abnormality mirroring the anatomical boundaries of the synovium and adjacent bone. Other radioactive tracers which are used as markers of inflammation will show abnormally increased activity at inflamed joints. This group of tracers includes labelled white cells [28] (Fig. 7.12), polyclonal human immunoglobulin [29], gallium-67 citrate [30] and, more recently, labelled anti-E-selectin monoclonal antibody [31] (Fig. 7.13).

The distribution of the involved joints may help to indicate the type of arthritis. In rheumatoid arthritis the typical pattern is that of symmetrical small joint involvement including the metacarpophalangeal and proximal interphalangeal joints of the hand (Fig. 7.14), whereas osteoarthritis typically is asymmetrical and has an affinity for the distal interphalangeal joints of the hands. Again, these patterns are not to be relied upon with great conviction and bone scans are by no means a routine investigation in arthritis, but with

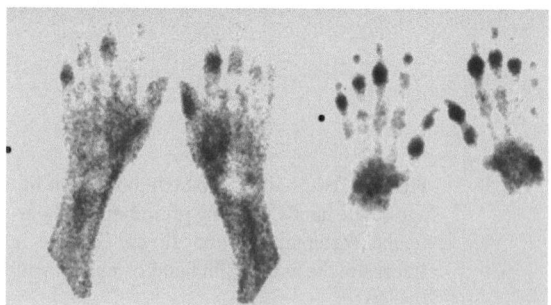

Fig. 7.11. Osteoarthritis. Two-phase bone scan of hands with early blood pool (*left*) and 3-h views (*right*). The delayed views show increased tracer uptake at multiple small joints in the hand. There is some increased blood pool at several of the joints consistent with an inflammatory component

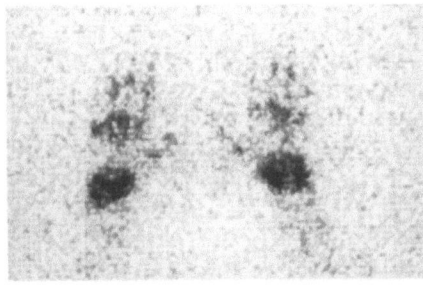

Fig. 7.12. Views of the hands 24 h after injection of indium-111-labelled leucocytes. There is white cell localisation at the wrists, most of the metacarpophalangeal joints and several of the proximal interphalangeal joints in a patient with active synovitis at these sites

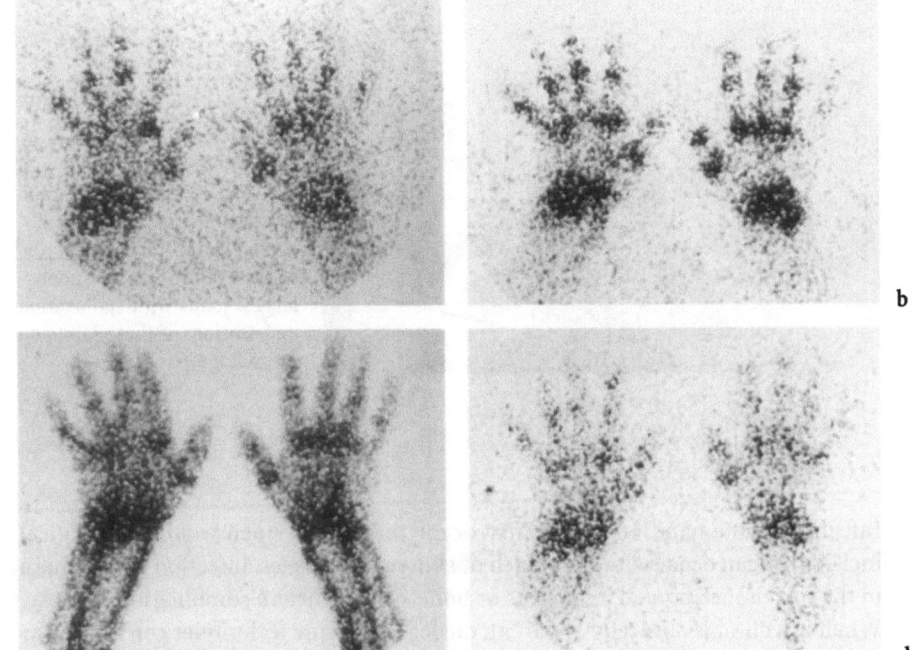

Fig. 7.13. Images of the hands in a patient with active rheumatoid arthritis using indium-111-labelled anti-E-selectin monoclonal antibody with 4-h (a) and 24-h imaging (b). The same patient was studied with ^{99m}Tc-labelled polyclonal human immunoglobulin with 4-h (c) and 24-h imaging (d)

an unusual presentation or equivocal radiographs, the bone scan may have some value in clinical management.

Some tracers have been shown to be more reliable than physical examination in assessing the degree of disease activity, and some tracers can identify sub-clinical disease [32]. It is difficult to see how this has a direct influence on patient management, but it could be beneficial in development of drugs to combat arthritis and in assessing disease response to treatment.

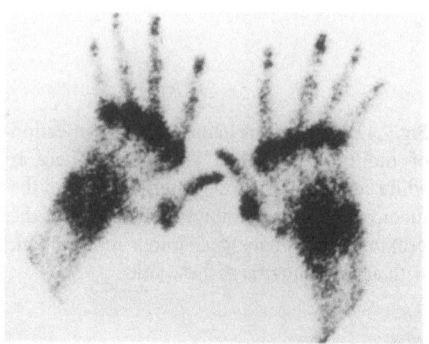

a

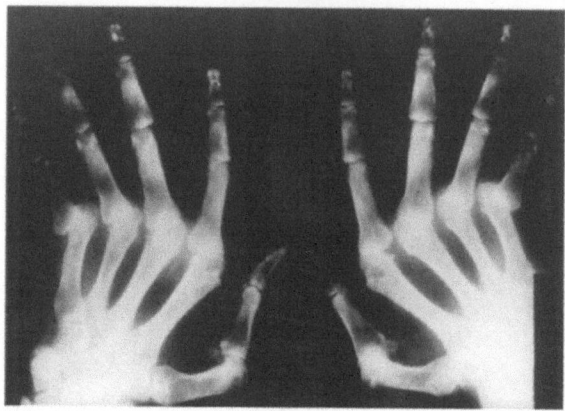

b

Fig. 7.14a, b. Rheumatoid arthritis. Images of the hands with ^{99m}Tc-MDP (a) and radiograph (b) demonstrating grossly abnormal bone turnover at the wrists and metacarpophalangeal joints with subluxation and erosions at these joints on the radiograph

7.7   Infection

Infection in the hand and wrist may occur through an open wound or surgical incision, or can occur without breach of skin or soft tissues. Infection may remain in the soft tissues, spread into joints or bone, or present as a combination of these. When infection is clinically apparent, nuclear medicine techniques can assess for the presence of spread to bone or joints. Different radioactive tracers are available including labelled white cells and gallium-67 citrate, but the most commonly used tracer is ^{99m}Tc-MDP, although a white cell scan may be performed subsequently. In the presence of infection ^{99m}Tc-MDP will demonstrate increased vascularity, blood pool and bone uptake of tracer [33]. This pattern of bone scan appearances is not specific to infection and can be seen in other conditions including the post-operative state. Sometimes the distribution of uptake allows the differentiation of osteomyelitis from septic arthritis. In septic arthritis, both sides of the joint are affected equally whereas in osteomyelitis the increased tracer uptake is accentuated in the affected epiphysis.

In the presence of bone scan abnormalities that could be explained by non-infective processes such as post-surgical/post-traumatic remodelling, specific infection-seeking agents may be helpful. White cells can be labelled with either ^{99m}Tc [7] or indium-111 [34]. ^{99m}Tc-labelled white cells give better image resolution than

[111]In-labelled white cells and the lower radiation dose (effective dose equivalent of ^{99m}Tc-labelled white cell scan is 3 mSv whereas the effective dose equivalent of ^{111}In-labelled white cell scan is 9 mSv) is beneficial in paediatric imaging. With its longer radioactive half-life (2.8 days for In-111 compared with 6 h for ^{99m}Tc), ^{111}In-labelled white cells can be imaged up to 48 or even 72 h after re-injection, which may be helpful in chronic or low-grade infection. Owing to the physical characteristics of indium-111 and gallium-67, gamma camera image resolution can be poor and a ^{99m}Tc-MDP bone scan may be performed as an adjunct to help delineate the bony structures of the hand and wrist to aid localisation of abnormal white cell or gallium uptake [35]. Gallium binds to circulating metal-binding proteins such as transferrin and also shows some localisation in granulocytes. It is not readily available and there is a significant delay of 48–72 h after injection before imaging takes place, but it avoids the hazards of white cell labelling and obviates the need for proficiency in this technique.

The situation is more complicated in patients with active synovitis, such as rheumatoid arthritis, who are suspected also of having septic arthritis. Unfortunately, all the infection-seeking tracers accumulate at sites of active synovitis and so the reliability of scintigraphic criteria to differentiate active synovitis from septic arthritis is poor [28, 30].

7.8 Other Focal Bone Scan Abnormalities

7.8.1 Avascular Necrosis

Avascular necrosis in the carpal bones is demonstrated well with MR scans but can also be diagnosed on bone scintigrams [36, 37]. In the scaphoid bone, an undiagnosed or non-healed fracture can lead to avascular necrosis of the proximal pole [14]. Because the blood supply begins distally in the scaphoid and runs proximally, a fracture through the middle of the bone disrupts the blood supply to the proximal pole causing it to die. In the chronic situation, radiographs are abnormal, with the dead bone becoming sclerotic and finally collapsing and fragmenting. In the early stages however, radiographs may be unremarkable, but bone scans can show decreased tracer uptake at the site of the affected bone reflecting bone ischaemia. As the pathological process continues, increased tracer uptake and vascularity can be demonstrated which represent an osteoblastic response in the surrounding bone [38] (Fig. 7.15). It may seem confusing to see increased vascularity at the site of a necrotic bone, but presentation of this condition is usually subacute and there is a profound hypervascular response in surrounding structures in an attempt to provide nutrients to the dying bone.

Avascular necrosis can occur in other carpal bones, most commonly the lunate, when it is known as Kienböck's malacia. The aetiology of this condition is not clear. In some cases it is believed to be idiopathic and in others it may be related to

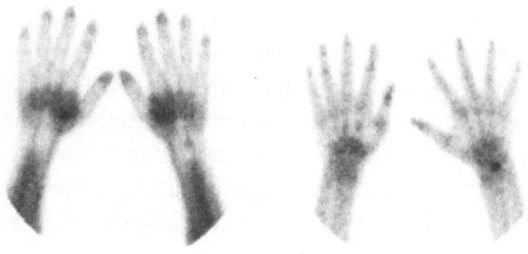

Fig. 7.15. Kienböck's malacia (avascular necrosis of the lunate). ^{99m}Tc-DP images demonstrate increased blood pool (*left*) and increased tracer uptake (*right*) in the left lunate bone

trauma. There is also an increased incidence in patients with negative ulnar variance (shortening of the ulna in relation to the radius). Once established, the necrotic lunate bone may require surgical bone grafting, removal or fusion of the proximal carpal row.

7.8.2 Paget's Disease

Although Paget's disease commonly involves the pelvis or long bones, it can occur in any bone in the body including the small bones of the hands and wrist (Fig. 7.16). Typically the involved bone is densely sclerotic, enlarged and may appear deformed on the radiograph, but early in the disease the radiographic findings may be quite subtle even when the bone scan is profoundly abnormal [39, 40]. In untreated Paget's disease there is uniform intensity of tracer uptake in the affected bone on the scintigram [41]. Paget's disease appears at the articular end of a bone and progresses along the shaft, so the bone scan shows increased uptake extending from the epiphysis along the diaphysis of affected metacarpals and phalanges.

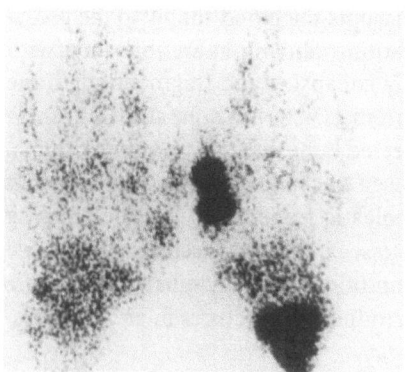
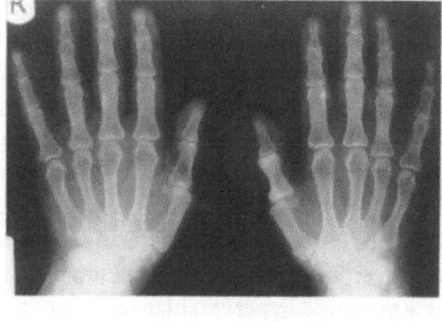

Fig. 7.16. Radiograph of the hands (**b**) of a patient with Paget's disease of the radius and right thumb proximal phalanx. The bone scan (**a**) shows grossly abnormally increased tracer uptake in the affected bones

7.8.3   Bone Tumours

Some malignant tumours can, rarely, produce solitary peripheral skeletal metastases. This group includes bronchogenic carcinoma, thyroid carcinoma, renal cell carcinoma and malignant melanoma. Therefore, when performing bone scans in these patients it is important to include images of the hands and feet, particularly if the patient is symptomatic, so as not to miss a solitary bone metastasis. Bone scans of the hands and wrists can also demonstrate hypertrophic pulmonary osteoarthropathy (HPOA) which is most commonly seen in the long bones of the forearm and legs (Fig. 7.17). The characteristic finding is the tramline sign which describes intense pericortical uptake of ^{99m}Tc-MDP. There may also be more focal uptake associated with the distal phalanges equating to the clinical presence of clubbing. The bone scan can return rapidly to normal after treatment of the underlying disease.

Primary bone or cartilage-based tumours may arise in the hands and wrists. Osteoid osteoma is a benign bone lesion that arises in one of the bones of the hand in as many as 8% of cases [42]. It occurs almost exclusively in patients under 30 years old and characteristically presents with night pain which is relieved by non-steroidal anti-inflammatory drugs. The diagnosis on radiographic appearances can be difficult although the lesion characteristically is sclerotic with a central lucent nidus. It is the nidus that causes pain, and if it is surgically removed then the pain disappears. Some surgeons have used nuclear medicine probes at operation to ensure that the nidus has been removed [43]. In osteoid osteoma, the bone scan typically shows a double density sign whereby the outer sclerotic area demonstrates increased tracer uptake and more intense tracer uptake is seen at the site of the nidus [44]. When a three-phase bone scan is performed, an osteoid osteoma shows increased signal in all three phases [45].

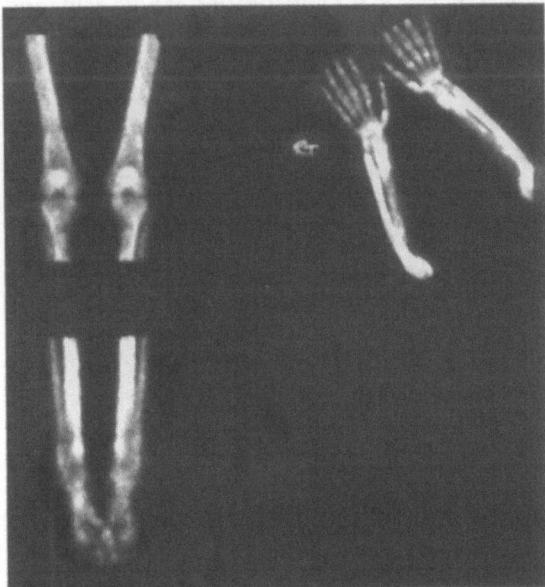

Fig. 7.17. Hypertrophic pulmonary osteoarthropathy. Bone scan images of the forearms, distal and proximal legs show the characteristic tramline sign of increased pericortical uptake of tracer

Other tumours do not produce such characteristic scintigraphic patterns but, in general, benign tumours such as enchondromas produce relatively low-grade uptake on bone scans [46], whereas those that are malignant or undergoing malignant transformation show increased intensity of uptake when compared with their benign counterparts. Bone scans, however, are not reliable at distinguishing benign from malignant lesions and probably their most useful application is in assessing the whole skeleton for distribution and multiplicity of lesions.

7.8.4   Miscellaneous Conditions

Bone scans of the hands and wrists may incidentally demonstrate soft tissue uptake of tracer at sites of heterotopic calcification regardless of the cause (Fig. 7.18), and in patients with hyperparathyroidism, brown tumours may sometimes be identified on the scintigram.

7.9   Conclusions

It is unusual for nuclear medicine to be the primary imaging modality undertaken for suspected pathologies in the hand and wrist; however, it remains an important adjunct to other imaging techniques, both when imaging the hand and wrist alone and also as part of an assessment of the entire skeleton. Although often lacking the specificity of conventional radiographs, bone scintigrams can be extremely sensitive and provide information regarding vascularity and blood pool in the hands and wrists, as well as identifying subtle abnormalities of bone metabolism. Scintigraphy continues to have an important role in the investigation of both acute and chronic hand and wrist conditions.

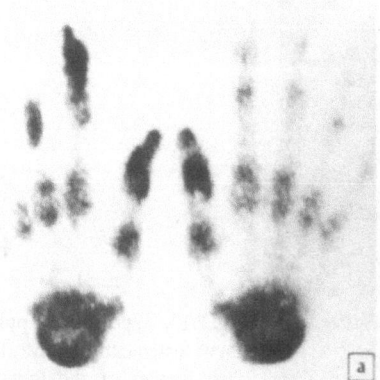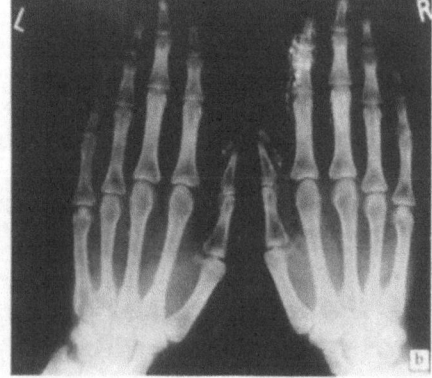

Fig. 7.18. Soft tissue calcification in a patient with systemic sclerosis. The calcification is visible on the radiograph (*right*) and corresponds to the sites of soft tissue uptake of ^{99m}Tc-MDP on the bone scan

Acknowledgements. We are grateful to Nick Bird for his valuable assistance and expertise in the preparation of the figures.

References

1. Administration of Radioactive Substances Advisory Committee (1998) Notes for guidance on the clinical administration of radiopharmaceuticals and use of sealed radioactive sources
2. RCR Working Party (1995) Making the best use of a Department of Clinical Radiology: guidelines for doctors, 3rd edn. Royal College of Radiologists, London
3. Subramanian G, McAfee JG, Blair RJ et al (1975) Technetium-99m-methylene diphosphonate – a superior agent for skeletal imaging: comparison with other technetium complexes. J Nucl Med 16:744–755
4. Paediatric Task Group of the European Association of Nuclear Medicine (1990) A radiopharmaceuticals schedule for imaging in paediatrics. Eur J Nucl Med 17:127–129
5. Mohamed A, Ryan PJ, Lewis M et al (1997) Registration bone scan in the evaluation of wrist pain. J Hand Surg [Br] 22:161–166
6. Bird NJ, Barber RW (1997) Co-registration of radionuclide images and plain film X-rays (abstract). Nucl Med Commun 18:291
7. Roddie ME, Peters AM, Osman S, et al (1988) Osteomyelitis. Nucl Med Commun 9:713–717
8. Jamar F, Manicourt D-H, Leners N et al (1995) Evaluation of disease activity in rheumatoid arthritis and other arthritides using ^{99m}technetium labeled nonspecific human immunoglobulin. J Rheumatol 22:850–854
9. Jamar F, Chapman PT, Manicourt D-H, et al (1997) A comparison between ^{111}In-anti-E-selectin mAb and ^{99}Tc^m-labelled human non-specific immunoglobulin in radionuclide imaging of rheumatoid arthritis. Br J Radiol 70:473–481
10. Arndt R (1987) Work, pace, stress, and cumulative trauma disorders. J Hand Surg 12:866–869
11. Rolfe EB, Garvie NW, Khan MA, et al (1981) Isotope bone imaging in suspected scaphoid trauma. Br J Radiol 54:762–767
12. Ganel A, Engel J, Oster Z, et al (1979) Bone scanning in the assessment of fractures of the scaphoid. J Hand Surg 4:540–543
13. Gilula LA, Destouet JM, Weeks PM, et al (1984) Roentgenographic diagnosis of the painful wrist. Clin Orthop 187:52–64
14. Leslie IJ, Dickson RA (1981) The fractured carpal scaphoid: natural history and factors influencing outcome. J Bone Joint Surg Br 63:225–230
15. Tiel-van Buul MMC, van Beek EJR, van Dongen A, et al (1992) The reliability of the 3-phase bone scan in suspected scaphoid fracture: an inter- and intraobserver variability analysis. Eur J Nucl Med 19:848–852
16. Brismar J (1988) Skeletal scintigraphy of the wrist in suggested scaphoid fracture. Acta Radiol 29:101–107
17. Thorpe AP, Murray AD, Smith FW, et al (1996) Clinically suspected scaphoid fracture: a comparison of magnetic resonance imaging and bone scintigraphy. Br J Radiol 69:109–113
18. Dalinka MK, Meyer S, Kricun ME, et al (1991) Magnetic resonance imaging of the wrist. Hand Clin 7:87–98
19. Taleisnik J (1988) Fractures of the carpal bone. In: Green DP (ed) Operative hand surgery, vol 2. Churchill Livingstone, New York, p 813
20. Veldman PJHM, Reynen HM, Arntz IE, et al (1993) Signs and symptoms of reflex sympathetic dystrophy: prospective study of 829 patients. Lancet 342:1012–1016
21. Mackinnon SE, Holder LE (1984) The use of three-phase radionuclide bone scanning in the diagnosis of reflex sympathetic dystrophy. J Hand Surg [Am] 9:556–563
22. Kozin F, Soin JS, Lawrence MR, et al (1981) Bone scintigraphy in the reflex sympathetic dystrophy syndrome. Radiology 138:437–443

23. Genant HK, Kozin F, Bekerman C, et al (1975) The reflex sympathetic dystrophy syndrome. A comprehensive analysis using fine-detail radiography, photon absorptiometry, and bone and joint scintigraphy. Radiology 117:21–32

24. Holder LE, Mackinnon SE (1984) Reflex sympathetic dystrophy in the hands: clinical and scintigraphic criteria. Radiology 152:517–522

25. Demangeat J-L, Constantinesco A, Brunot B, et al (1988) Three-phase bone scanning in reflex sympathetic dystrophy of the hand. J Nucl Med 29:26–32

26. Werner R, Davidoff G, Jackson D, et al (1989) Factors affecting the sensitivity and specificity of the three-phase technetium bone scan in the diagnosis of reflex sympathetic dystrophy syndrome in the upper extremity. J Hand Surg [Am]14:520–523

27. Goldenberg DL, Egan MS, Cohen AS, et al (1982) Inflammatory synovitis in degenerative joint disease. J Rheumatol 9:204–209

28. Al-Janabi MA, Jones AKP, Solanki K et al (1988) ^{99}Tc^m-labelled leucocyte imaging in active rheumatoid arthritis. Nucl Med Commun 9:987–991

29. Pons F, Moya F, Herranz R, et al (1993) Detection and quantitative analysis of joint activity inflammation with ^{99}Tc^m-polyclonal human immunoglobulin G. Nucl Med Commun 14:225–231

30. McCall IW, Sheppard H, Haddaway M, et al (1983) Gallium-67 scanning in rheumatoid arthritis. Br J Radiol 56:241–243

31. Chapman PT, Jamar F, Keelan ETM, et al (1996) Use of a radiolabeled monoclonal antibody against E-selectin for imaging of endothelial activation in rheumatoid arthritis. Arthritis Rheum 39:1371–1375

32. Soden M, Rooney M, Cullen A, et al (1989) Immunohistological features in the synovium obtained from clinically uninvolved knee joints of patients with rheumatoid arthritis. Br J Rheumatol 28:287–292

33. Maurer AH, Chen DCP, Camargo EE, et al (1981) Utility of three-phase skeletal scintigraphy in suspected osteomyelitis. J Nucl Med 22:941–949

34. Schauwecker DS (1989) Osteomyelitis: diagnosis with In-111-labeled leukocytes. Radiology 171:141–146

35. Schauwecker DS, Park HM, Burt RW, et al (1988) Combined bone scintigraphy and indium-111 leukocyte scans in neuropathic foot disease. J Nucl Med 29:1651–1655

36. Reinus WR, Conway WF, Totty WG, et al (1986) Carpal avascular necrosis: MR imaging. Radiology 160:689–693

37. Duong RB, Nishiyama H, Mantil JC, et al (1982) Kienböck's disease: scintigraphic demonstration in correlation with clinical, radiographic, and pathologic findings. Clin Nucl Med 7:418–420

38. Maurer AH, Holder LE, Espinola DA, et al (1983) Three phase radionuclide scintigraphy of the hand. Radiology 146:761–775

39. Fogelman I, Carr D (1980) A comparison of bone scanning and radiology in the assessment of patients with symptomatic Paget's disease. Eur J Nucl Med 5:417–421

40. Vellenga CJLR, Pauwels EKJ, Bijvoet OLM, et al (1984) Untreated Paget's disease of bone studied by scintigraphy. Radiology 153:799–805

41. Fogelman I, Ryan PJ (1996) Bone scanning in Paget's disease. In: Collier BD, Fogelman I, Rosenthall L (eds) Skeletal nuclear medicine. Mosby, St Louis, pp 171–181

42. Dahnert W (1993) Radiology review manual, 3rd edn. Williams and Wilkins, Baltimore, p 80

43. Ellison MJ, Issac L, Smith WI, et al (1984) Intraoperative scintigraphic localization of the nidus of osteoid osteoma. Clin Nucl Med 9:640–642

44. Helms CA (1987) Osteoid osteoma: the double density sign. Clin Orthop 222:167–173

45. Helms CA, Hattner RS, Vogler JB (1984) Osteoid osteoma: radionuclide diagnosis. Radiology 151:779–784

46. Vande Streek PR, Carretta RF, Weiland FL (1994) Nuclear medicine approaches to musculoskeletal disease: current status. Radiol Clin North Am 32:227–253

8 Normal Skeletal Development of the Hand

RICK R. VAN RIJN, CORNELIS VAN KUIJK

8.1 Introduction

The use of radiography to assess the skeletal development of the hand is almost as old as radiography itself. This may not be surprising as, in fact, the first radiograph of human tissue was that of the hand of Mrs. Röntgen [1]. In 1898, barely 3 years after the discovery of röntgen rays, the orthopaedist J. Poland published the first description of skeletal changes in the hand. In his book entitled *Skiagraphic Atlas Showing the Development of Bones of the Wrist and Hand*, he presented positive reprints (skiagraphs) of hand radiographs of 19 British children, aged 1–17 years, describing each radiograph in great detail (Fig. 8.1) [2]. He thus in fact preceded Pryor (1907) and Rotch (1909), who are generally credited as being the first to describe the changes in the radiological appearance of hand and wrist bones [3, 4]. In later years several scoring techniques were introduced [5–7]. These techniques are based on one of the following three methods.

The *numerical* technique constitutes the counting of the number of secondary ossification centres. In total seven regions of the body, amongst them the hand and wrist, are under consideration. It was introduced in 1946 by Elgenmark and later refined by Garn et al. [8–10]. This technique has several drawbacks. First, it uses an amount of radiation exposure which today would be totally unacceptable [11]. Secondly, the technique is not designed for use beyond the age of 5 years, as by the age of 6 years in boys 60 and in girls 65 of the 73 secondary ossification centres have already appeared [7]. The measurements are also very much influenced by the appearance of the phalangeal, metacarpal and metatarsal epiphysis. Due to this influence the range becomes extremely wide at approximately 20 months, and a 2-year-old infant may show 14 to 51 ossification centres. These drawbacks have led to this technique being abandoned.

Several authors have proposed the use of a *metrical* technique. Among the first were Baldwin et al., who used planimetric measurements to assess skeletal maturation. Later, simplification by only measuring the length and width of single bones was proposed by Schmidt and Moll [12]. As metrical techniques are tedious and time-consuming, implementation in a clinical setting cannot be advocated. These techniques are, however, by design suited to automated techniques and they have been used in recent publications in which automated skeletal age assessment techniques are presented [13].

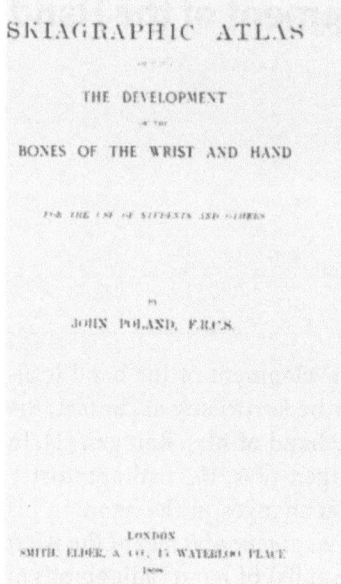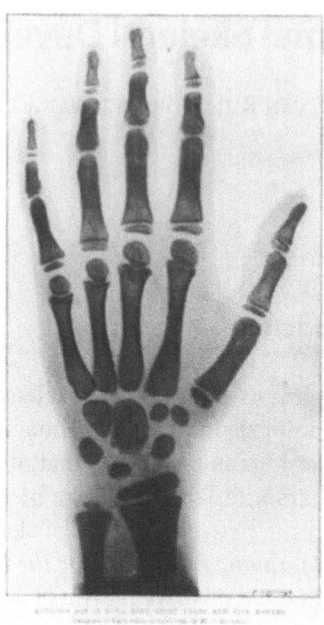

Fig. 8.1. *Left*: The title page of J. Poland's *Skiagraphic Atlas Showing the Development of Bones of the Wrist and Hand*. *Right*: A skiagraph of one of Poland's sons

The *morphological* technique is based on the assessment of the size and shape of the individual ossification centres. Todd introduced this technique in 1937 [14]. It was later refined by Walter Greulich and Idell Pyle with the introduction of their *Radiographic Atlas of Skeletal Development of the Hand and Wrist*, which has become the most widely used technique world-wide [15]. Years after the publication of Greulich and Pyle's standard work, two Dutch physicians, De-Roo and Schröder, published a similar atlas which, however, received little attention [16]. The technique proposed by Greulich and Pyle consists of comparing an individual's radiograph of the left hand with a set of "normal radiographs", thus obtaining a skeletal age. Later in this chapter we will discuss the Greulich and Pyle technique in depth. A different way of using normal radiographs was introduced by Acheson (1954), and later refined by Tanner, Whitehouse and Healy [17–19]. This technique is based on scoring separate bones in the wrist and hand and assigning a score to each. The total score is related to a table giving a Tanner score, which is not a skeletal age per se. As the Tanner-Whitehouse technique, as it currently is known, is the second most commonly used technique to assess skeletal maturation in the world today we will later discuss it in depth.

Before discussing the most commonly used skeletal age scoring techniques, i.e. Greulich and Pyle and Tanner-Whitehouse, the normal development of the hand skeleton is presented in the following section.

8.2   Pattern of Presentation of Ossification Centres

The development of the skeleton of the hand starts in an early embryonic state. Henke and Reyer described that in 18–20 mm embryos all skeletal elements, except for the distal phalanges and the os pisiforme, were present [20]. The elements of the hands have shapes, arrangements and relationships like those of the adult by 7 weeks of gestation (Fig. 8.2) [21]. With respect to the onset and sequence of joint formation of the hand there is less agreement. Leboucq stated that by 4 months all articular spaces are present [22]. Chondrification of the carpal elements occurs in a definite sequence, the capitate and hamate appearing first and the lunate and pisiform last [23]. Normally the digits chondrify in a proximodistal order, whereas the metacarpals appear slightly earlier than the carpals (Fig. 8.3).

After birth the bones of the hand begin to ossify and undergo specific changes in their shape in a regular order. In the majority of healthy children the sequence of ossification follows a set pattern. The only bone which cannot be placed in this sequence is the os naviculare (scaphoid). The pattern in which the bones appear is as follows: capitate, hamate, triquetral, lunate, trapezium (greater multangular), trapezoid (lesser multangular) and pisiform. In boys the scaphoid appears before the trapezium more often than in girls (Table 8.1).

In assessing the skeletal maturation of the hand one must bear in mind that although growth and development are concomitant in healthy children this may

Table 8.1. Mean age, in years-months, at which the onset of ossification is shown on radiographs [7]

Ossification centre	Boys	Girls
Capitate	0–3	0–2
Hamate	0–4	0–2
Triquetral	2–5	1–8
Lunate	4–1	2–7
Trapezium	5–10	4–1
Trapezoid	6–3	4–2

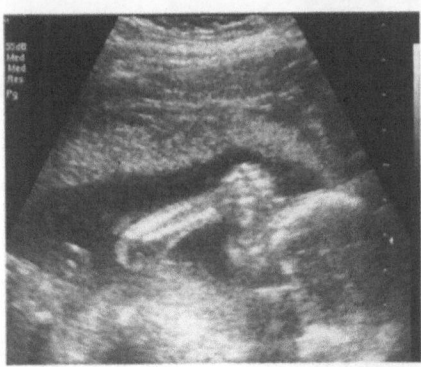

Fig. 8.2. Ultrasound examination of a 17-week-old fetus showing the phalanges and metacarpals of the developing hand (courtesy of Mrs. B.M. van Rijn)

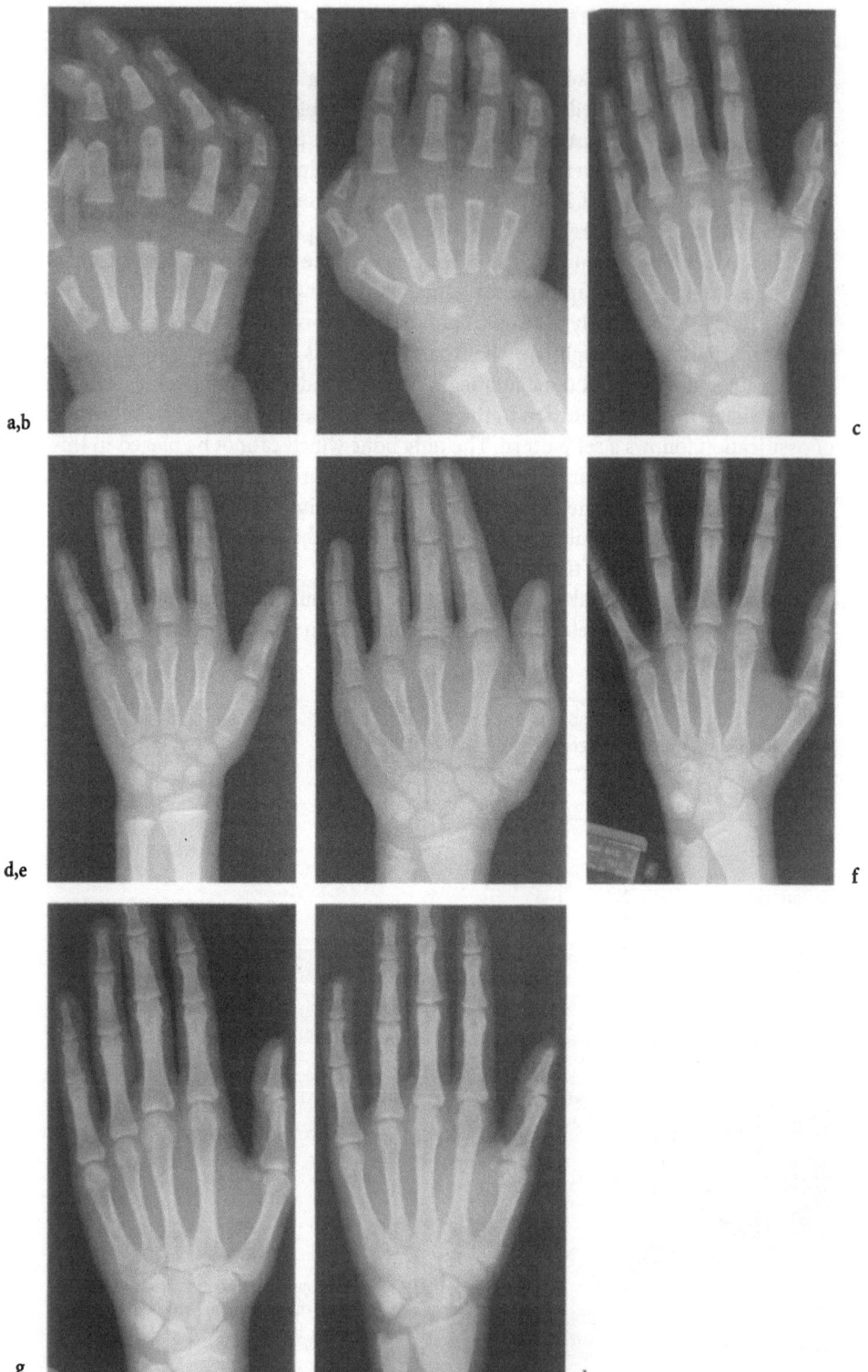

◊ **Fig. 8.3a–h.** Radiographs depicting the normal skeletal development of healthy Dutch girls (courtesy of the Department of Pediatric Radiology, University Children's Hospital "Sophia", Rotterdam, the Netherlands). By no means are these eight radiographs meant to give a full description of the maturation of the skeleton of the hand. Descriptions are adapted from the work of Greulich and Pyle [15]. **a** Newborn: the shafts of the second to fifth metacarpals are slightly tailored in the middle portion. The distal ends of the phalanges are slightly rounded whereas the proximal ends are widened and flattened. **b** 6 months: ossification of the hamate and capitate can be seen. **c** 3.6 years: the triquetrum, lunate and trapezium have now begun to ossify. The epiphyses of the second to fifth metacarpal have became visible since the previous stage. They have enlarged and their proximal margins are flattened. The proximal phalangeal epiphyses of the second to fifth fingers have thickened. **d** 6 years: ossification of the scaphoid, trapezium, trapezoideum, and the epiphysis of the ulna can now been seen. **e** 9 years: the ulnar epiphysis is flattened and the styloid process is seen. The radial epiphyses has widened and now is nearly as wide as the distal metaphyses. The carpals have begun to show articular surfaces. The proximal surfaces of the epiphyses of the second to fifth proximal phalanx are now almost as wide as the end of the shafts. They also have become convex. **f** 12 years: the styloid process has become more prominent and the radial epiphysis is by now overlapping the shaft. Articular surfaces of the capitate, hamate, trapezoid and trapezium are well defined. The sesamoid bone has begun ossification. The radiolucent spaces between the epiphyses and the shaft have significantly narrowed. **g** 15 years: the ulnar and radial epiphyses are beginning to fuse. Fusion is complete in all phalanges and the lines of fusion are almost obliterated. **h** 18 years: the skeleton of the hand is now fully grown, all epiphyses are closed and further growth is not possible. Although it is fully grown epiphyseal lines can persist throughout life; this especially true for the radius and the first metacarpal

---

not be true in diseased children. There are many diseases that can either accelerate or decelerate the development of the hand skeleton (Tables 8.2, 8.3). Besides an acceleration or deceleration, inborn errors of growth can influence the development of the hand [24]. For a discussion of these inborn errors we refer the reader to Chapter 9 in this book. Last but not least there are significant differences in skeletal maturation between the sexes and races, and this important factor should always be taken into account when assessing skeletal maturation [25].

8.3   Scoring Techniques

Currently there are two techniques in use for the assessment of skeletal maturation in routine clinical practice. The most widely adopted technique is that of Greulich and Pyle, it has been stated that 76% of all skeletal age assessments made by paediatricians were derived from this technique [5]. From our personal experience we feel that the same percentage or an even higher percentage applies to radiologists. The second most used technique is that of Tanner and Whitehouse, which is used by 20% of the paediatricians [5]. In this section we will discuss each technique in depth.

8.3.1   Greulich and Pyle

In 1959 Greulich and Pyle published their *Radiographic Atlas of Skeletal Development of the Hand and Wrist'* [15]. During the period between 1931 and 1942, 2,500 children from Cleveland, Ohio, were included in their research series. All these children came from social classes "somewhat above average in economic and

Table 8.2. Diseases decelerating skeletal development [24]

Endocrine disorders
    Hypothyroidism
    Cushing syndrome
    Hypogonadism
    Hypothalamic-hypophyseal disorders
        Panhypopituitarism
        Craniopharyngioma
    Constitutional growth retardation
    Laron dwarfism
Chromosomal disorders
    Down syndrome
    Trisomy 18
    Turner syndrome
    Other chromosomopathies
Other diseases
    Malnutrition
    Chronic disease
    Psycho-social deprivation
    Skeletal dysplasias
    Bone mineralisation anomalies (e.g. rachitis)
    Intra-uterine growth disorders (e.g. Silver-Russell syndrome)
    Idiopathic

Table 8.3. Diseases accelerating skeletal development [24]

Early sexual maturation
    True precocious puberty
    Pseudo-precocious puberty
        Androgenital syndrome
        Adrenal tumours
        Ovarian tumours
        Testicular tumours
        Gonadotropin-producing tumours (e.g. hepatoblastoma, germinoma)
        Iatrogenic (e.g. steroid use, anabolic steroid use)
    McCune-Albright syndrome
    Premature adrenarche
Other diseases
    Hyperthyroidism
    Cerebral gigantism
    Developmental syndromes
        Acrodysostosis
        Beckwith-Wiedemann syndrome
        Cockayne syndrome
        Marshall syndrome
        Weaver syndrome
        Pseudohypoparathyroidism
    Alimentary adipositas
    Idiopathic

educational status". The children were examined at 3-month intervals during the first post-natal year, at 6-month intervals from 1 to 5 years of age, and annually thereafter [15]. "The age of the children whose radiographs were used in the atlas differed not more than 2 percent from the calendar age at which the examinations were scheduled", i.e. the standard for a given age was selected using radiographs of children who at the time of their examination were exactly that age or no more than 2% older or younger [15]. Each standard was selected from 100 radiographs of children of the same age and sex, and in most cases the radiograph used in the atlas was, in the opinion of the authors, the most representative of this age. Wherever possible the radiographs of a single child were used over an interval of successive years or investigations.

The intervals between the standards are usually the same as the intervals between the examinations described above. However, in some instances the interval can be shorter or longer when the skeletal age does not correspond exactly to the calendar age of the child. After the chapters depicting the skeletal ages and their corresponding radiographs Greulich and Pyle presented maturity indicators for the separate bones of the hand and wrist. These maturity indicators are helpful in fine-tuning the skeletal age assessment. As stated by the authors "The modal chronological age at which a given maturity indicator first appears in the films of these children is the skeletal age that has been assigned to that maturity indicator in this atlas" [15].

One must bear in mind that the skeletal growth pattern shows a biological variation. Greulich and Pyle themselves stated in their atlas that: "it is probably safe to assume that one standard deviation above and below the skeletal age corresponding with the child's chronological age will include approximately one-third of the White children in this country who are adequately nourished and in good health; that two standard deviations will include about 90% of all such children, in addition to some whose skeletal development is retarded as a result of disease of nutritional inadequacy; and that a difference of more than two standard deviations above or below the mean would make it highly probable that the child is abnormally advanced or retarded"[15].

How should the atlas be used? Greulich and Pyle themselves described a procedure. They suggested that one should choose the standard of the same sex in approximately the same age group to begin with. However, later studies have shown that the accuracy of the Greulich and Pyle technique is greatly improved if the investigator is unaware of the biological age of the subject under investigation [26–28]. After the first step, one should compare the subject under investigation with the standards following and preceding the chosen Greulich and Pyle standard. The one that superficially resembles the radiograph of the subject most closely is selected. A more detailed comparison is then made on the individual bones. It is wise to use a standard approach by considering the bones in a regular order. A good order in which to assess the carpals is the sequence in which they appear; that way developmental disorders can be observed more readily [24].

A major advantage of the Greulich and Pyle atlas is the fact that the assessment is relatively easy to perform by a trained physician and can easily be incorporated in a day-to-day clinical practice.

8.3.2   Tanner and Whitehouse

Soon after the introduction of the Greulich and Pyle atlas the reliability of their technique was a matter of debate [26]. In particular the approach of comparing a standard radiograph with the radiograph in question was considered to be a weakness. In 1962 Tanner et al. introduced a new approach for the assessment of skeletal maturation, assessing each bone of the hand separately [18]. Later, in 1981, an update of this technique was published. In this chapter we will use the data published in the second edition originating from 1983 [29]. The normative data of their study were obtained from seven separate surveys, the data being collected between 1950 and 1972. In total approximately 2,200 radiographs (3–16 years) from cross-sectional surveys and 5,500 radiographs from 500 children (1–21 years) in mixed longitudinal studies were rated. According to the authors all subjects were drawn from an average socio-economic level in the British population in the 1950s.

In contrast to Greulich and Pyle the Tanner technique yields a maturity score instead of a skeletal age. Using standardised charts the maturity score can be expressed as a bone age. The rationale for the use of a maturity score lies in the fact that the use of an age scale has a significant drawback, as the relation between calendar age and maturity is not constant. In fact we know that it differs between the sexes and between populations [25].

Tanner et al. divided the continuous process of growth of each bone into discrete stages. "All stages could be described unambiguously by verbal criteria as well as illustrated in line drawings" [29]. Furthermore the stages had to be present in all subjects and absolute size was not taken into account. This approach yielded nine separate stages for the radius, metacarpals, phalanges, hamate and trapezium and eight separate stages for the rest of the carpal bones. The absence of a visible bone always relates to stage A. In this technique the bones of the second and fourth digits are ignored. Furthermore, the bones are given a biological weight in order to reduce the influence of the phalanges in the overall maturity score [30]. Tanner et al. also noted that the carpal bones often give worse information about maturity compared with the long bones. They therefore introduced a separate Tanner-Whitehouse RUS score consisting of the radius, ulna and finger bones (short bones).

How should the Tanner-Whitehouse technique be used? The radiograph of the hand is scored in a defined order: radius, ulna, metacarpals (1, 3, 5), proximal phalanges (1, 3, 5), middle phalanges (3, 5), distal phalanges (1, 3, 5), capitate, hamate, triquetral, lunate, scaphoid, trapezium and trapezoid. The bones are rated by comparing them with the descriptions and drawings. In case of doubt the description is conclusive. For each stage it is necessary that not only the criteria for that stage but also the criteria for the previous stage be met. Using tables the assigned stages are transcribed into a maturity stage.

The main advantage of the Tanner-Whitehouse technique is that it yields a scale ranging from 1 to 100 and therefore is a much finer scale than the rather crude Greulich and Pyle technique. A major disadvantage is the laborious character of this technique compared with the Greulich and Pyle atlas.

8.4   Automated Techniques

With the emergence of digital radiography renewed interest has been focused on automated techniques for scoring skeletal maturation. One might expect that a computer would outperform human operators in the field of skeletal maturation assessment. The implementation of automated techniques would definitely save a lot of time and human resources. Finally, the implementation of automated techniques would make it possible to compare studies performed at different institutes.

Most techniques are based on the implementation of the Tanner-Whitehouse (RUS) technique in an automated fashion [31–36]. The single match technique of Greulich and Pyle, which is easily applied in clinical practice, is difficult to incorporate in relatively simple software algorithms. The Tanner-Whitehouse technique, on the other hand, based on multiple comparison, is ideally suited to incorporation in automated techniques.

To extract data from a radiograph a two-step technique has been proposed. The first step consists of bone extraction and the second step is feature analysis. The bone extraction phase is technically difficult, as in radiography borders are often difficult to discern [35]. It is surprising to find that one technique uses a dark radiograph projected against a light background, a modern version of the original technique of "skiagraphy" [2, 33].

The variability in ossification of the hand that makes it suitable for bone age assessment, is at the same time a major obstacle in performing reliable segmentation of radiographs of the hand, i.e. extraction of bones from background and soft-tissue [35]. Segmentation can be performed according to two main protocols: edge-based and region-based. In edge-based segmentation edges of separate ossification centres are detected and grouped into boundaries. Region-based techniques work the other way round, i.e. boundaries are defined from the interiors of ossification centres [35]. After this procedure recognition of the individual bones followed by feature extraction is performed. Using the features of each individual bone classification is possible and a maturity score can be assigned to the radiograph in question.

With the advent of fast processors neural-network-based techniques are becoming available. These techniques are provided with knowledge about typical shapes during the various maturation stages. This in turn makes it possible to work without an extracted and explicitly described data set, and therefore the technically difficult process of bone segmentation can be avoided. However, operators are still needed to identify ossification centres using a mouse on the digitised radiograph [13]. Neural networks are by virtue of their design able to provide an optimal use of their acquired knowledge: for a given input stimulus, the output is generated by an efficient integration of data stored in the software with the actual input. Although most authors use the Tanner-Whitehouse technique, neural networks could also be used with the Greulich and Pyle atlas [13]. This neural network technique is fed with data based on measurements made on digitised images. It can therefore be considered to be a mix between a metric and a morphological technique. To date the automated techniques described in literature are mostly experimental and therefore cannot yet be implemented in a clinical setting.

8.5   Clinical Use and Problems

In this final section we will look at the clinical implementation of the Greulich and Pyle atlas and the Tanner-Whitehouse technique, as these are currently most widely used.

First the indications for skeletal age assessment should be discussed. In clinical practice the assessment of skeletal maturation is an important diagnostic tool. Several diseases and/or syndromes are characterised by an acceleration or deceleration of skeletal maturation [24]. Also the follow-up of therapeutic interventions as well as the side effects of treatment can be monitored. Furthermore, specific disharmonious ossification patterns are related to certain syndromes, i.e. the appearance of phalanges prior to carpals in children with trisomy 21 or cerebral gigantism. Skeletal maturation assessment can also be used for the prediction of a child's adult height. This application has implications in the treatment and counselling of "short" and "tall" children [37–41]. Besides physicians, lawyers might have an interest in skeletal age assessment. In the Netherlands, lawyers representing young refugees or delinquents regularly file requests for skeletal maturation assessment, raising the question whether the subject in question is older or younger than 18 years (i.e. adulthood). This has specific implications for the judicial technique: either juvenile or adult law, with the corresponding punishment. Furthermore the issue of age can be important in refugees seeking political asylum.

As discussed, the scoring techniques currently in use are based on radiographs of the hand. Therefore one might wonder whether the maturation of the hand is representative of total body maturation. In a study by Roche et al., in which the skeletal age as assessed using the Greulich and Pyle atlas was compared with knee bone ages, on average the age difference was zero [42]. Garn et al. showed an even distribution around zero for the fusion of the proximal tibial epiphysis and the small bone epiphysis of the hand [43]. These studies indicate that skeletal maturation of the hand is indeed representative of total body maturation.

It is shown that maturation of the hand is a reliable indicator of skeletal maturation. Therefore an important issue to address is the reliability of the different skeletal maturation assessment techniques [44–49]. Each technique has an inherent random error and systematic error. The random error can be assessed by intra-observer variance analysis. Acheson et al. compared the Greulich and Pyle and Tanner-Whitehouse techniques and found that the latter has a smaller 95% confidence limit, i.e. has a lower random error [17]. Proper training of the investigator can significantly reduce the random error. Simply reading the books by Greulich and Pyle or Tanner-Whitehouse is not enough. Roche et al. showed that discussion of inter-observer differences after reading a set of films significantly improved the replicability of the Greulich and Pyle technique [50]. Evaluating the inter-observer variance can assess the systematic error. Acheson et al. showed that there is a significant difference between the two techniques; in their study the Tanner-Whitehouse technique showed a greater systematic error [17]. Many publications state that the Tanner-Whitehouse technique is more accurate, most of them containing reference to the publication by Milner et al. to support this statement. However, in the above-mentioned article the authors state that "There is no doubt that these sophisticated methods (Tanner-Whitehouse) are essential for children with growth problems. For initial diagnosis a discrepancy with the chronological age of 2–3 years is the order of detection required. We feel that our results show that this is readily achievable routinely by the Greulich and Pyle method" [51]. The data presented in a study by Cole et al. implied that the "well-known" poor performance of the Greulich and Pyle method compared with Tanner-Whitehouse is based on differences between the reference populations [52].

As both the Tanner-Whitehouse and Greulich and Pyle techniques are claimed to be capable of assessing skeletal maturation the question can be raised whether the two techniques are equivalent, i.e. whether it matters which technique is used. One factor creating a difference between the techniques is the difference in the normal populations against which each technique was standardised [52]. Greulich and Pyle used a group of 2,500 North American children living in the region of Ohio, Cleveland, between 1931 and 1942 [15]. The population used by Tanner and Whitehouse, in contrast, consisted of a representative cross-section of British children [18]. Most authors agree that on average the skeletal age scored by the Greulich and Pyle technique yields a lower estimate than the Tanner-Whitehouse technique [17, 28, 51–55]. A second factor influencing compatibility of the two techniques is the obvious difference between them, i.e. the "mugshot"-like technique of Greulich and Pyle versus the bone by bone technique of Tanner and Whitehouse. Due to its laborious character of scoring each bone separately the Tanner-Whitehouse technique is more time-consuming. In a study amongst radiology registrars, who did not receive special training, it was found that on average a Greulich and Pyle study took 1.4 min and a Tanner-Whitehouse study 7.9 min [28]. We feel that the use of the Greulich and Pyle atlas is at least valid in day-to-day medical practice, as it is quick and more than accurate enough to find significant deviations from normal skeletal development [51, 56]. In the follow-up of medical intervention for growth acceleration or retardation, for centres specialised in paediatric endocrine diseases or for studies in physical anthropology, the use of the Tanner-Whitehouse technique is recommended as this offers a more finely calibrated scale [51, 57].

Since the two techniques originate from either the late 1930s or the 1950s one might wonder whether they still apply in a modern-day paediatric and adolescent population. First it should be stated that both techniques were designed for a Caucasian population and therefore will not necessarily apply to other ethnic groups [25, 27, 58–65]. The Tanner-Whitehouse technique was compared with a Belgian population in 1980 and French-Canadian population in 1970; both studies showed an advancement of skeletal maturity [66, 67]. We recently reassessed the applicability of the Greulich and Pyle technique in a Dutch Caucasian population at the Department of Pediatric Radiology, University Children's Hospital "Sophia", Rotterdam, the Netherlands. In a survey among 294 girls and 278 boys living in the Rotterdam area we found strong significant correlations between skeletal age (SA) as assessed with the Greulich and Pyle technique and the actual chronological age (CA) ($CA_{boys}=0.915 \times SA_{boys}+1.290$, $r=0.979$; and $CA_{girls}=0.996 \times SA_{girls}+0.195$, $r=0.974$; for both, $P<0.001$; Fig. 8.4). The chronological age was underestimated in girls by 1 month and in boys by 3 months; however, in neither group was this difference significant. However, if the children are divided into groups based on puberty stages according to Tanner, a significant trend is found in boys. At lower puberty stages calendar age preceded skeletal age whereas at higher puberty stages the reverse was seen. Analysis of the data showed that the Greulich and Pyle atlas is still applicable in a modern-day Dutch Caucasian population.

To conclude this chapter we wish to provide the reader with some helpful hints in assessing skeletal maturation:

· The first thing to consider is that most bone ages are normal; this does not apply in specialised clinical settings such as paediatric hospitals.
· The objectivity of the assessment is higher if the investigator is unaware of the patient's calendar age and clinical condition.
· It is mandatory to know the genetic gender of the patient in question.
· When using the Greulich and Pyle technique the finger epiphysis resemble "real life" more closely than the other regions.
· Each skeletal maturation assessment technique has a certain variable error. It is important to keep in mind that when, for example,. this variable error is 4 months the assessor must allow for a difference of 11.1 months to obtain confidence limits with 95% probability [68].
· Last but not least one must always bear in mind that skeletal maturation assessment is by *no means* a simple and unimportant radiological investigation. Unjust interpretation, i.e. under or overrating of skeletal maturation, of these films may have serious repercussions in the follow-up of young children.

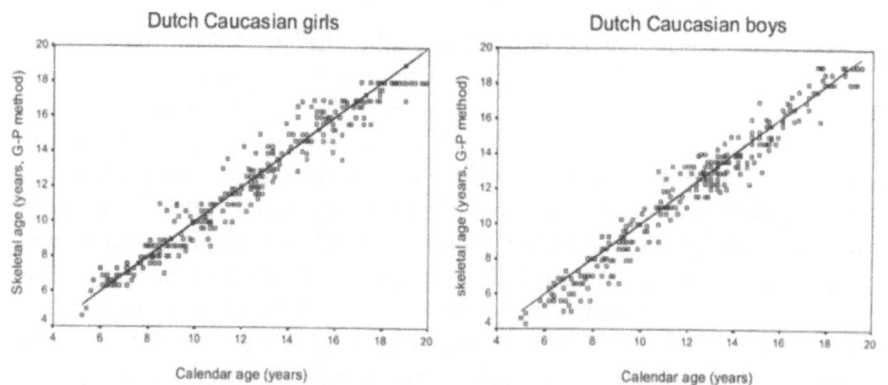

Fig. 8.4. Data obtained in 294 Dutch Caucasian girls (**a**) and 278 Dutch Caucasian boys (**b**) living in the Rotterdam area. The *dotted line* represents the line of unity. The *dots* represent calendar age plotted against the skeletal age as assessed using the Greulich and Pyle technique

References

1. Eisenberg RL (1992) Röntgen and the discovery of X-rays. Radiology: an illustrated history. Mosby Year Book, St Louis, pp 22–42
2. Poland J (1898) Skiagraphic atlas showing the development of bones of the wrist and hand. Smith Elder, London
3. Pryor JW (1907) The hereditary nature of variation in the ossification of bones. Anat Rec 1:84–88
4. Rotch TM (1909) A study of the development of bones in childhood by the roentgen method with the view of establishing a development index for the grading of and the protection of early life. Trans Am Assoc Physicians 24:603
5. Buckler JMH (1983) How to make most of bone ages. Arch Dis Child 58:761–763
6. Fendel H (1976) Methods of radiological bone age assessment (author's translation). Radiologe 16:370–380
7. Graham CB (1972) Assessment of bone maturation: methods and pitfalls. Radiol Clin North Am 10:185–202
8. Elgenmark O (1946) The normal development of the ossification centers during infancy and childhood: clinical, roentgenologic, and statistical study. Acta Paediatr 33 [Suppl 1]
9. Garn SM, Rohmann CG (1966) "Communalities" in the ossification timing of the growing foot. Am J Phys Anthropol 24:45–50
10. Yarbrough C, Habicht JP, Klein RE, Roche AF (1973) Determining the biological age of the preschool child from a hand-wrist radiograph. Invest Radiol 8:233–243
11. Freeman WL (1994) Research with radiation and healthy children: greater than minimal risk. IRB 16:1–5
12. Schmidt F, Moll H (1960) Atlas der normalen und pathologischen Handskeletentwicklung. Springer, Berlin Heidelberg New York
13. Gross GW, Boone JM, Bishop DM (1995) Pediatric skeletal age: determination with neural networks. Radiology 195:689–695
14. Todd TW (1937) Atlas of skeletal maturation (hand). Mosby, St Louis
15. Greulich WW, Pyle SI (1959) Radiographic atlas of skeletal development of the hand and wrist, 2nd edn. Stanford University Press, Stanford, Calif
16. DeRoo T, Schroder HJ (1976) Pocket atlas of skeletal age. Martinus Nijhoff, The Hague
17. Acheson RM, Vicinus JH, Fowler GB (1966) Studies in the reliability of assessing skeletal maturity from x-rays. 3. Greulich-Pyle atlas and Tanner-Whitehouse method contrasted. Hum Biol 38:204–218
18. Tanner JM, Whitehouse RH, Healy MJR (1962) A new system for estimating skeletal maturity from the hand and wrist with standards derived from a study of 2600 healthy British children. Centre International de L'enfance, Paris
19. Tanner JM (1971) The essential characteristics of a rating system. Am J Phys Anthropol 35:339–340
20. Henke W, Reyer C (1874) Studiën über die Entwicklung der Extremitäten des Menschen, insbesondere der Gelenkflächen. Sitzungsb k Akad Wiss Math Naturw Klasse 70:217–273
21. Hesser C (1926) Beitrag zur Kenntis der Gelenkentwicklung beim Menschen. Morphol Jahrb 55:489–567
22. Leboucq H (1884) Recherches sur la morphologie du carpe chez les mammifères. Arch Biol 5:35–102
23. Senior HD (1929) The chondrification of the human hand and foot skeleton. Anat Rec 42:35
24. Heinrich UE (1986) Die Bedeutung der radiologischen Skelettalterbestimmung für die Klinik. [Significance of radiologic skeletal age determination in clinical practice.] Radiologe 26:212–215
25. Ontell FK, Ivanovic M, Ablin DS, Barlow TW (1996) Bone age in children of diverse ethnicity. AJR 167:1395–1398

26. Acheson RM, Fowler G, Fry EI, Janes M, Koski K, Urbano P, et al. (1963) Studies in the reliability of assessing skeletal maturation from X-rays. I. Greulich-Pyle atlas. Hum Biol 37:317–349

27. Groell R, Lindbichler F, Riepl T, Gherra L, Roposch A, Fotter R (1999) The reliability of bone age determination in central European children using the Greulich and Pyle method. Br J Radiol 72:461–464

28. King DG, Steventon DM, O'Sullivan MP, Cook AM, Hornsby VPL, Jefferson IG et al (1994) Reproducibility of bone ages when performed by radiology registrars: an audit of Tanner and Whitehouse versus Greulich and Pyle methods. Br J Radiol 67:848–851

29. Tanner JM, Whitehouse RH, Cameron N, Marshall WA, Healy MJR, Goldstein H (1983) Assessment of skeletal maturity and prediction of adult height (TW2 method). Academic Press, London

30. Roche AF (1970) Associations between the rates of maturation of the bones of the hand-wrist. Am J Phys Anthropol 33:341–348

31. Tanner JM, Gibbons RD (1994) Automatic bone age measurement using computerized image analysis. J Pediatr Endocrinol 7:141–145

32. Rucci M, Coppini G, Nicoletti I, Cheli D, Valli G (1995) Automatic analysis of hand radiographs for the assessment of skeletal age: a subsymbolic approach. Comput Biomed Res 28:239–256

33. Hill K, Pynsent PB (1994) A fully automated bone-ageing system. Acta Paediatr Suppl 406:81–83

34. Cox LA (1994) Preliminary report on the validation of a grammar-based computer system for assessing skeletal maturity with the Tanner-Whitehouse 2 method. Acta Paediatr Suppl 406:84–85

35. Manos GK, Cairns AY, Rickets IW, Sinclair D (1994) Segmenting radiographs of the hand and wrist. Comput Methods Prog Biomed 43:227–237

36. Drayer NM, Cox LA (1994) Assessment of bone ages by the Tanner-Whitehouse method using a computer-aided system. Acta Paediatr 406 [Suppl]:77–80

37. Bayley N, Pinnea SB (1952) Tables for predicting skeletal height from skeletal ages revised for use with Greulich-Pyle hand standards. J Pediatr 40:423–441

38. Tanner JM, Whitehouse RH, Marshall WA, Carter BS (1975) Prediction of adult height from height, bone age, and occurrence of menarche at ages 4 to 16 with allowance for parent height. Arch Dis Childh 50:14–26

39. Roche AF, Wahner H, Thissen D (1975) The RWT method for the prediction of adult stature. Pediatrics 56:1026–1033

40. Sproul A, Peritz E (1971) Assessment of skeletal age in short and tall children. Am J Phys Anthropol 35:433–439

41. Harris EF, Weinstein S, Weinstein L, Poole AE (1980) Predicting adult stature: a comparison of methodologies. Ann Hum Biol 7:225–234

42. Roche AF, French NY (1970) Differences in skeletal maturity levels between the knee and hand. Am J Roentgenol Radium Ther Nucl Med 109:307–312

43. Garn SM, Rohmann CG, Blumenthal T (1966) Developmental communalities of homologous and non-homologous body joints. Am J Phys Antrop 25:147–151

44. Roche AF, Eyman SL, Davila GH (1971) Skeletal age prediction. J Pediatr 78:997–1003

45. Roche AF, Davila GH, Pasternack BA, Walton MJ (1970) Some factors influencing the replicability of assessments of skeletal maturity (Greulich-Pyle). Am J Roentgenol Radium Ther Nucl Med 109:299–306

46. Johnson GF, Dorst JP, Kuhn JP, Roche AF, Davila GH (1973) Reliability of skeletal age assessments. Am J Roentgenol Radium Ther Nucl Med 118:320–327

47. Cox LA (1996) Tanner-Whitehouse method of assessing skeletal maturity: problems and common errors. Horm Res 45 [Suppl 2]:53–55

48. Medicus H, Gron AM, Moorrees CF (1971) Reproducibility of rating stages of osseous development. (Tanner-Whitehouse system). Am J Phys Anthropol 35:359–372

49. Wenzel A, Melsen B (1982) Replicability of assessing radiographs by the Tanner and Whitehouse-2 method. Hum Biol 54:575–581

50. Roche AF, Rohmann CG, French NY, Davila GH (1970) Effect of training on replicability of assessments of skeletal maturity (Greulich-Pyle). Am J Roentgenol Radium Ther Nucl Med 108:511–515

51. Milner GR, Levick RK, Kay R (1986) Assessment of bone age: a comparison of the Greulich and Pyle, and the Tanner and Whitehouse methods. Clin Radiol 37:119–121

52. Cole AJ, Webb L, Cole TJ (1988) Bone age estimation: a comparison of methods. Br J Radiol 61:683–686

53. Andersen E (1971) Comparison of Tanner-Whitehouse and Greulich-Pyle methods in a large scale Danish survey. Am J Phys Anthrop 35:373–376

54. Fry EI (1968) Assessing skeletal maturity: comparison of the atlas and individual bone techniques. Nature 220:496–497

55. Vignolo M, Milani S, DiBattista E, Naselli A, Mostert M, Aicardi G (1990) Modified Greulich-Pyle, Tanner-Whitehouse, and Roche-Wainer-Thissen (knee) methods for skeletal age assessment in a group of Italian children and adolescents. Eur J Pediatr 149:314–317

56. Anderson M (1971) Use of the Greulich-Pyle "Atlas of Skeletal Development of the Hand and Wrist" in a clinical context. Am J Phys Anthropol 35:347–352

57. Malina RM (1971) A consideration of factors underlying the selection of methods in the assessment of skeletal maturity. Am J Phys Anthrop 35:341–346

58. Jimenez-Castellanos J, Carmona A, Catalina-Herrera CJ, Vinuales M (1996) Skeletal maturation of wrist and hand ossification centers in normal Spanish boys and girls: a study using the Greulich-Pyle method. Acta Anat (Basel) 155:206–211

59. Lejarraga H, Guimarey L, Orazi V (1997) Skeletal maturity of the hand and wrist of healthy Argentinian children aged 4–12 years, assessed by the TWII method. Ann Hum Biol 24:257–261

60. Loder RT, Estle DT, Morrison K, Eggleston D, Fish DN, Greenfield ML et al (1993) Applicability of the Greulich and Pyle skeletal age standards to black and white children of today. Am J Dis Child 147:1329–1333

61. Shakir A, Zaini S (1974) Skeletal maturation of the hand and wrist of young children in Baghdad. Ann Hum Biol 1:189–199

62. So LL (1997) Correlation of sexual maturation with skeletal age of southern Chinese girls. Aust Orthod J 14:215–217

63. Ye YY, Wang CX, Cao LZ (1992) Skeletal maturity of the hand and wrist in Chinese children in Changsha assessed by TW2 method. Ann Hum Biol 19:427–430

64. Yeon KM (1997) Standard bone-age of infants and children in Korea. J Korean Med Sci 12:9–16

65. Zhen OY, Baolin L (1986) Skeletal maturity of the hand and wrist in Chinese school children in Harbin assessed by the TW2 method. Ann Hum Biol 13:183–187

66. Baughan B, Demirjian A, Levesque GY (1979) Skeletal maturity standards for French-Canadian children of school-age with a discussion of the reliability and validity of such measures. Hum Biol 51:353–370

67. Beunen G, Lefevre J, Ostyn M, Renson R, Simons J, Van Gerven D (1990) Skeletal maturity in Belgian youths assessed by the Tanner-Whitehouse method (TW2). Ann Hum Biol 17:355–376

68. Mainland D (1954) Evaluation of the skeletal age of estimating children's development II. Variable errors in the assessment of roentgenograms. Pediatrics 13:165–173

9 Congenital Defects, Malformation Syndromes and Skeletal Dysplasias

ALESSANDRO CASTRIOTA SCANDERBEG, BRUNO DALLAPICCOLA

9.1 Introduction

The hand is involved to a significant extent in a number of malformation syndromes and skeletal dysplasias. Moreover, the hand is the anatomic site where isolated congenital defects of various types may occur. Isolated anomalies are often of no clinical significance, occurring in otherwise normal children.

As in many other fields of radiology, pathologic changes border on normal variations. Knowledge of the normal pattern of variation is therefore important in the recognition of relevant pathologic changes.

Some hand defects are not isolated but reflect a generalized bone disease, or they occur as part of a more complex malformation disorder. The radiographic interpretation of the defect, together with the family history and clinical examination, may provide insight into the recognition of the underlying disorder. Overall diagnostic specificity of these skeletal defects can be increased by careful evaluation of their location within the hand, their shape and size. It is known, for example, that a pseudo-epiphysis located at the base of the second metacarpal or at the distal end of the first metacarpal is a normal variant, while its location in other sites may suggest a pathologic condition, such as cleidocranial dysostosis, brachydactyly C, or spondyloepiphyseal dysplasia. Similarly, cone-shaped epiphyses in the first distal phalanx and in the fifth middle phalanx are normal findings in most cases, while their presence in the third or fourth middle phalanx, in the first proximal phalanx and in the fifth distal phalanx has been seen only in abnormal children. In some occasions, definition of the specific configuration of bone defects provides important clues to the diagnosis. For example, the presence of Giedion's type 24 cone-shaped epiphysis in the distal phalanx, and of types 19 and 20 in the middle phalanges, are distinct features of cleidocranial dysostosis. Similarly, drumstick-like appearance of the tufts of the distal phalanges strongly suggests the 45,X Turner syndrome.

Some acquired disorders can mimic congenital abnormalities. This is the case for erosions of the tufts which occur in idiopathic osteolysis (Cheney's syndrome), but can be seen in several acquired disorders, including infection and trauma. Another example is shortening of a digit, which can be genetically determined or due to acquired factors damaging the epiphysis, such as rheumatoid arthritis, infarcts, infections or trauma.

Since some terms used in this chapter can be confusing for readers who are not familiar with congenital abnormalities, a few general concepts and some basic definitions are provided below.

9.2   Terminology and Classifications

The term *congenital* refers to the presence of a given malformation since birth. Structural defects of prenatal onset can be divided into those representing a *single primary developmental defect* and those representing a *multiple malformation syndrome*. According to the nature of the event occurring during morphogenesis, single primary defects are classified as malformation, deformation or disruption defects. *Malformation* refers to a single primary defect arising from a localized error in morphogenesis. Most individuals with localized malformations are otherwise normal. In addition, once the malformation is surgically corrected, prognosis is excellent. A *deformation* is an alteration in shape and/or structure of a part which has differentiated normally. Most persons presenting with these anomalies are otherwise completely normal. Spontaneous correction usually occurs in 90% of cases, while the remainder simply benefit from early postural intervention. The term *disruption* is used to designate a structural defect resulting from destruction of a previously normally formed part. The prognosis is entirely determined by the extent and location of the tissue loss. Thus, a child with a limb amputation has an excellent prognosis, whereas a child with porencephalic lesions in the brain does not. On clinical grounds, malformations are divided into *major*, when associated with a gross structural change carrying serious medical, surgical or cosmetic consequences, and *minor* or *normal variation* when they do not have clinical consequences.

In contrast to the concept of single primary defect, the designation *multiple malformation syndrome* refers to several structural defects originating from the same known or presumed etiology. They usually include a number of anatomically unrelated errors in morphogenesis, often resulting from pleiotropy of a given gene mutation (e.g. TBX5 gene and hand and heart defects in Holt-Oram syndrome). *Association* is used to indicate a pattern of malformations for which no specific etiology has been recognized. The term *morphogenic complex* or *sequence* refers to a pattern of multiple anomalies deriving from a single primary defect in early morphogenesis. This single primary event results in multiple abnormalities through a cascading process of secondary and tertiary errors in morphogenesis [1]. The terminology for the various limb malformations is even more confusing. Terms such as phocomelia, hemimelia and ectromelia date back to 1837 [2]. Since then, several classifications have been proposed, among others the Frantz-O'Rahilly and the Temtamy-McKusick classifications [3, 4]. In the classification by Frantz-O'Rahilly, deficiencies were divided into terminal and intercalary. A modified version of the Frantz-O'Rahilly classification was adopted in 1969 [5], and terms such as amelia (absence of a limb) and meromelia (partial absence of a limb) were introduced. Meromelia was then distinguished according to its location, whether terminal or intercalary, and each of these categories was grouped as to whether it occurred along the transverse or the longitudinal axis [6]. In 1974, an international classification system was formulated [7]. Temtamy and McKusick have classified hand malformations into seven main groups, based on anatomic and genetic characteristics. These groups include: absence deformities, brachydactyly, syndactyly, polydactyly, contracture deformities, symphalangism and hand malformations with congenital ring constrictions. Each of these groups is divided into isolated forms and forms associated with other anomalies.

In the absence of a generalized agreement on terminology to describe hand abnormalities, radiographic description of the hand defect should include which parts are present, which are absent and which are deformed.

Also the classification of malformation syndromes involving the hand is quite confusing. A number of approaches have been proposed, including eponyms, anatomic sites of involvement, the patient's name, the author name, names of the city where they were originally discovered, the biochemical defect, and general clinical and pathologic findings. A standard nomenclature was established in 1970 by the European Society of Pediatric Radiology, chaired by Maroteaux [8].

9.3　　Embryology and Genetics

Each limb consists of four segments, including a root or zonoskeleton; a proximal segment or stylopodium, consisting of a single bone (humerus, femur); a medial segment or zeugopodium, consisting of two bones (radius and ulna, tibia and fibula); a distal part or autopodium, corresponding to hand and foot. Several complex processes are involved in the formation of these segments. Their action is coordinated, but so far only little understood.

The limb develops from an embryonic limb bud, in which a rapid cell proliferation of the apical ectodermal ridge (AER) occurs within the so-called progress zone. Closely linked to this growth is the limb bud polarization along anteroposterior and dorsoventral axes. The processes of cell proliferation and regeneration are in constant equilibrium with the process of cell death (apoptosis), which in human embryos is also responsible for the separation of the digits around days 51–53.

A major role in proximodistal axis patterning is played by the fibroblast growth factors (FGF) pathway. For example, FGF-10 triggers the synthesis of FGF-8 in the ectoderm overlying the limb bud and the expression of Sonic Hedgehog (SHH) in the mesoderm. In mice Fgf-2, Fgf-4 and Fgf-8 are produced in the apical ectodermal ridge and some of the Fgf genes maintain the expression of Shh in the zone of polarizing activity, controlling the anteroposterior axis. FGF receptor (FGFR) gene -1, -2, and -3 mutations, and mutations of the TWIST gene, which encodes for a helix-loop-helix transcription factor and acts upstream of the FGF genes, have been associated with distinct craniostenoses with limb anomalies. They include FGFR1 in Pfeiffer syndrome or acrocephalosyndactyly (ACS) type V; FGFR2 in Apert syndrome (ACS type 1), Saethre-Chotzen syndrome (ACS type III), Pfeiffer syndrome (ACS type V), Jackson-Weiss syndrome, Baere-Stevenson syndrome, and Antley-Bixler syndrome; FGFR3 in Saethre-Chotzen syndrome (ACS type III), Muenke syndrome and SADDAN dysplasia [11].

The SHH pathway plays a major role in anteroposterior axis patterning. The Hedgehog genes encode proteins involved in intracellular signaling. In particular,

SHH is an important morphogen with a key role in establishing anteroposterior polarity of the limbs. Although no SHH mutation has been demonstrated so far in human limb anomalies, some evidence supports this role. Notable examples include syndactyly of second and third toes in Smith-Lemli-Opitz syndrome, and shortening of fourth metacarpal, pre- or postaxial polydactyly or second-third toe syndactyly in Gorlin syndrome. In addition, the zinc-finger transcription factor GLI3, which is involved in SHH repression, is implicated in Greig syndrome. This disorder is associated with syndactyly of hands and feet, preaxial polydactyly of toes and, sometimes, of postminimus of the hands. A deletion of the same gene is also implicated in postaxial polydactyly type A. Heterozygous mutations in the gene for cAMP-response element (CREB)-binding protein, which is a coactivator of different transcription factors including the GLI family, cause Rubinstein-Taybi syndrome, in which limb anomalies consisting of broad deviated thumbs and great toes, eventually with preaxial polydactyly of feet, are found. Therefore, while in mice absence of SHH signaling results in limb amputations, in humans anomalies of SHH pathway cause syndactyly and polydactyly, preaxial in the case of upregulation, and postaxial in the case of downregulation.

The dorsoventral axis of the limb bud is determined by several transcription factors, but most of them are unknown. LMX1B mutations are involved in the autosomal dominant nail-patella syndrome.

The determination of limb identity and morphogenesis is defined by multiple other genes, most of which are unknown. At present four major groups of genes have been implicated in limb malformations: those encoding for T-box transcription factors (TBX), bone morphogenesis proteins (BMP), cartilage-derived morphogenetic protein (CDMP), and homeobox (HOX) genes.

TBX are probably relevant to the specification of limb identity. Mutations of TBX-5, mapping at 12q24, have been related to Holt-Oram syndrome, an autosomal dominant disorder with malformations of the radial ray, including absent, hypoplastic, or triphalangeal thumb. TBX-3 is mutated in the Schnizel ulnar-mammary syndrome, presenting with a wide range of ulnar ray abnormalities, including agenesis or duplication of the fifth finger.

BMPs are key regulators of the anteroposterior limb axis and HOX expression, playing a major role in initiation of chondrogenesis and cartilage differentiation. However, at present no mutation of BMP has been found in any of the human limb malformations. The Noggin (NOG) gene, which is an antagonist of the BMP signals, has been implicated in the autosomal dominant proximal symphalangism, presenting with ankylosis of the proximal interphalangeal joints, fusion of carpal and tarsal bones, and with multiple synostosis syndrome, characterized by brachydactyly. Mutations in the transcription factor SALL1, which functions in the BMP pathway, have been found in patients with the Townes-Brocks syndrome, an autosomal dominant disorder with preaxial polydactyly and triphalangeal thumb associated with imperforate anus and ear and urogenital tract anomalies.

CDMP or growth differential factor 5 is implicated in chondrogenesis and positioning of the joints. Homozygous mutations cause the autosomal recessive Hunter-Thompson acromesomelic dysplasia, in which anomalies are limited to the limbs. A similar and more severe disease, the autosomal recessive Grebe dysplasia, is also caused by CDMP1 mutations. Patients show impressively dysmorphic limbs, with a proximodistal gradient severity, consisting of carpal and tarsal fusions, agenesis of several carpal and tarsal bones and proximal and middle phalanges, sometimes with postaxial polydactyly. Heterozygous parents of Grebe dysplasia patients are affected by brachydactyly, sometimes with postaxial polydactyly. A distinct type of brachydactyly, with characteristics intermediate between A1 and C types, consisting of a short first metacarpal, and short second, third, and fifth middle finger phalanges, has been associated with CDMP1 mutations. The gene responsible for brachydactyly type B (absent or hypoplastic distal and middle phalanges; short, flattened, and bifid thumb) has been mapped to 9q22, while the gene for brachydactyly C (Haw-type) has been assigned to 12q24.

The homeodomain-containing transcription factors HOX, and in particular those of A and D complexes, are critical for limb development. For example, HOXD13 has been implicated in the formation of the autopodium and its mutations cause synpolydactyly. Heterozyotes have partial duplication and syndactyly of the third and fourth hand rays, and fourth and fifth foot rays, sometimes with pre- and postaxial polydactyly or isolated postaxial polydactyly. Severe limb anomalies are found in HOXD13 homozygotes, in which complete disorganization of the bone structure, syndactyly of all fingers, pre-, meso-, and postaxial polydactyly, abnormal carpus, tarsus, metacarpals and phalanges, and fusion of the metatarsals are found. Mutations of HOXA13 gene have been associated with hand-foot-genital syndrome, an autosomal dominant disorder with short first metacarpal, distal phalanx of the thumb and middle phalanx of the fifth finger, fusion or retarded maturation of the carpus.

In conclusion, recent molecular discoveries have detected a complex heterogeneity underlying limbs defects. While current classification, based on clinical features, remains useful, it is likely that a new classification, based on genetic defects, will replace previous groupings in the near future. This, in turn, will facilitate understanding of the mechanisms responsible for these defects [9–11].

9.4 Etiology

For most *single primary defects* the etiology is unknown. Most are explained on the basis of multifactorial inheritance, which implies an empiric recurrence risk figure in the range of 2–5% for the next child of healthy parents with an affected child. The fact that single primary defects are etiologically heterogeneous indicates that some have a non-genetic etiology (e.g., craniosynostosis due to in utero constraint), while others result from mendelian mutations (e.g., postaxial polydactyly). If neither dominant nor recessive inheritance is established for a given genetic *malformation*, multifactorial recurrence risk factors usually apply to unaffected parents. The majority of *deformations* are caused by intrauterine molding. Impaired ability of the fetus to kick results in decreased fetal movement. On the other hand, a *disruption* can be produced by amputation of a normally developed structure, usually a digit, an arm, or a leg (amniotic bands), or by interruption of blood supply to a developing part leading to infarction, necrosis, and/or resorption of the involved structures (e.g. Poland syndrome). Genetic factors play a minor role in the pathogenesis of disruptions. Thus, most are sporadic events in otherwise normal families.

Multiple malformation syndromes can be caused by chromosomal imbalances, teratogens, and single gene defects. Recurrence risk ranges from being unremarkable in cases arising from new mutations or caused by environmental factors, to 100% in the rare Down syndrome families where one parent is heterozygous for a balanced 21q/21q translocation. Single gene mutations, either dominant or recessive, or X-linked recessive in males, also cause a number of recognizable multiple malformation syndromes of prenatal onset. Diagnosis is based on clinical recognition of the disorder. A family history of a similarly affected individual is extremely useful. However, in many patients with multiple malformation syndromes of genetic etiology, the occurrence is sporadic, thus suggesting new mutations. In such cases, all family members are normal, and diagnosis depends entirely on the evaluation of the patient's phenotype. Examples include de Lange syndrome, Williams syndrome, Prader-Willi syndrome and Rubinstein-Taybi syndrome. *Associations* usually occur sporadically in otherwise normal families. Therefore, it is important to differentiate multiple malformation syndromes from morphogenic sequences, since in the latter recurrence risk counseling for the multiple anomalies is defined by the risk of the single localized malformation.

9.5   Diagnosis

The ultimate goal in evaluating a child with structural defects is making a specific overall diagnosis. When this is achieved, recurrence risk in future pregnancies, proper treatment and prognostication can be assessed. Recognition of a malformation syndrome is often difficult because of the wide range of expression of each entity (pleiotropism) and eventual overlap with similar but different entities (genetic heterogeneity). Due to pleiotropism, the definition of the relevant diagnostic signs or symptoms for a given condition can be extremely difficult. In general, no single signs should be considered essential to the diagnosis of a syndrome since in most cases no sign is present 100% of the time.

For this reason, hand radiographs cannot be diagnostic in every condition, and in most cases the diagnosis will depend upon a combined clinical, radiological, biochemical, genetic and molecular evaluation of the patient. However, skeletal hand evaluation can provide important clues to the diagnosis, especially when different hand anomalies are associated. As anticipated, even minor anomalies can be relevant if combined to other defects in the body.

Proper radiologic examination of the hand includes single bone evaluation, together with evaluation of their relation to each other. In some instances, bone length measurement is also required to assess size modifications which are not obvious on clinical grounds. A valuable approach to objective appraisal of brachydactyly is the *pattern profile analysis* of Poznanski et al. [12]. This method consists of plotting the relative length of the tubular bones, expressed in terms of standard deviations (Z-score) from the norms, against the specific location in the hand. Subtle bone shortening, which can be overlooked by direct observation, may be detected by this technique. In addition, since the profiles are plotted against appropriate standards for age and sex, they allow direct comparison between dissimilar individuals. Several patterns for specific disorders have been recognized, with a good agreement of the profile among different patients with the same disorder. An up-to-date bibliography covering the use of this method in bone dysplasias and malformation syndromes has been recently compiled by Poznanski and Garn [13].

9.6 Normal Variants and Congenital Anomalies, Including Minor Anomalies

In the following sections, a symptom-based approach is used to describe the most relevant radiologic changes of congenital abnormalities, malformation syndromes and skeletal dysplasias. In the absence of a satisfactory classification, we believe it is more useful for a radiologist to learn the basics of pattern recognition than memorizing a number of radiologic signs pertaining to single disorders. A more systematic description of the radiologic changes occurring in malformation syndromes and skeletal dysplasias is available in several excellent textbooks [14–20]. Here, the relevant radiologic changes affecting the hand will be discussed, providing a list of conditions with which the defect can be associated.

9.6.1 Epiphyseal Abnormalities

9.6.1.1 Cone-Shaped Epiphyses

Cone-shaped epiphyses are defined as a central projection of the epiphysis extending toward the corresponding metaphysis. This defect can be seen in normal individuals and in several pathologic conditions. Cones of the distal phalanx of the thumb and of the fifth middle phalanx are commonly seen in normal subjects. Shortening of the involved phalanx may be an additional feature. Cone-shaped epiphyses at the second and fifth middle phalanges may occur in both normal and affected children. Their location at the proximal phalanges, or at the third and fourth middle phalanges, suggests a malformation syndrome (Figs. 9.1, 9.2). Epiphyseal coning can occur in the hands and feet as well. Giedion identified 38 different types of this defect and described the association of chronic renal failure and phalangeal cone-shaped epiphyses of the hands (*cono-renal syndrome*) [21]. The most characteristic association is with the tricho-rhino-phalangeal syn-

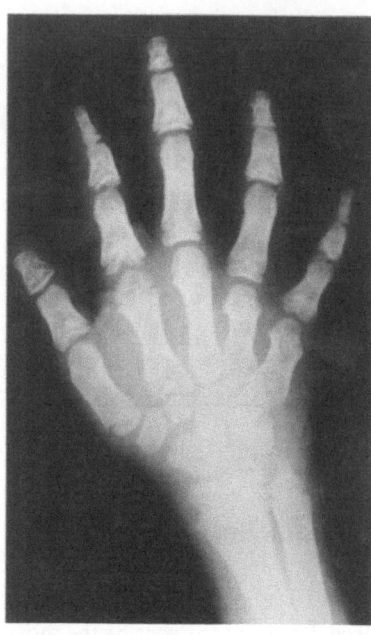

Fig. 9.1. Cone-shaped epiphyses. True cones of proximal and middle phalanges in a 10-year-old girl with tricho-rhino-phalangeal syndrome, type I. The epiphyses of second to fourth middle phalanges are sclerotic (ivory epiphyses). Shortening of tubular bones of the hand (mainly fourth and fifth metacarpals and first distal phalanges) and premature epiphyseal fusion are additional features

drome, type I and type II [22]. An association between cone epiphysis and ivory epiphyses has been established (Fig. 9.1). Epiphyseal changes similar to cones may be seen after any type of metaphyseal-epiphyseal insult, including fracture, osteomyelitis, bone infarction, radiation injury or drug administration [23].

On radiographs, variable central projection of the epiphysis into the corresponding metaphysis is found. In the most severe cases, this results in a U-shaped pattern. Possible associated features are shortening of the phalanx and ivory epiphysis.

Cone epiphyses may be found in acrodysostosis, tricho-rhino-phalangeal syndrome, asphyxiating thoracic dysplasia, chondroectodermal dysplasia, metaphyseal chondrodysplasia, chondrodysplasia punctata, cleidocranial dysplasia and peripheral dysostosis.

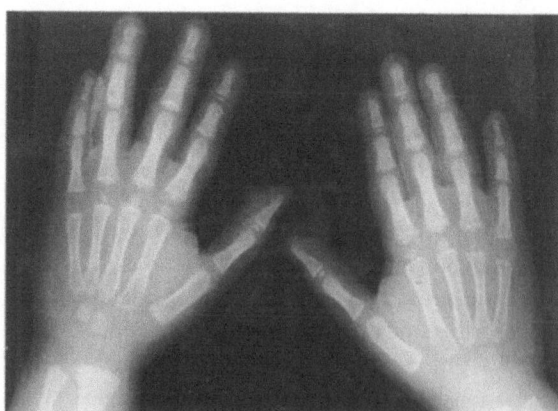

Fig. 9.2. Cone-shaped epiphyses of middle phalanges and ivory epiphyses of distal phalanges in a boy with tricho-rhino-phalangeal syndrome, type II (Giedion-Langer). Exostoses were present at other sites in the skeleton

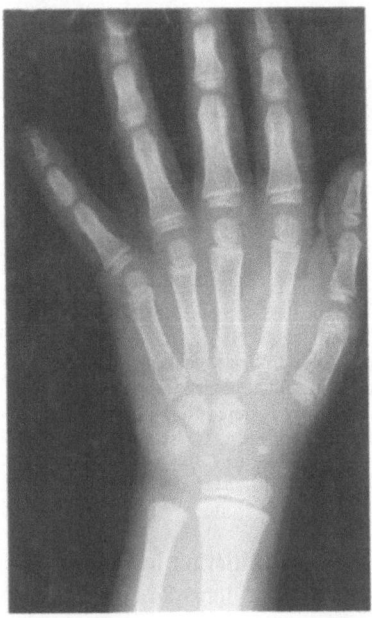

Fig. 9.3. Transverse notch in the distal end of the first metacarpal and true pseudo-epiphysis at the base of the second metacarpal in an otherwise normal child

9.6.1.2 Pseudo-epiphyses

The term pseudo-epiphysis refers to an epiphysis located at an abnormal site (Fig. 9.3). Indentation at the end of a bone which is normally not indented is also known as *transverse notch*. A transverse notch at the base of the second metacarpal and at the distal end of the first metacarpal is found, respectively, in about 60% and 80% of the general population. Transverse notching is also very common at the base of the fifth metacarpal. *True pseudoepiphyses* are less common, occurring in 1% of the general population [24]. Pseudoepiphyses, or even transverse notches, at different sites may be of diagnostic value, occurring in a selected group of skeletal dysplasias and malformation syndromes [16].

On radiographs, indentation (transverse notch) or fully developed extra epiphyses are found at sites where normally they are not present.

Pseudo-epiphyses can occur in brachydactyly C, cleidocranial dysplasia, chondroectodermal dysplasia, chromosomal abnormalities, Fanconi anemia, Kniest disease, Larsen syndrome, otopalatodigital syndrome and spondyloepiphyseal dysplasia.

9.6.1.3 Ivory Epiphyses

The term ivory epiphyses indicates increased density within the epiphysis

Sclerotic epiphyses may be found anywhere in the body in any condition in which the bones are abnormally dense (Fig. 9.4) [25]. Ivory epiphyses at the distal phalanges and at the fifth middle phalanx are commonly seen in normal children. Their location at the proximal phalanges strongly suggests a generalized bone disease (Figs. 9.1, 9.2) [26–28]. Individuals with ivory epiphyses are more likely to

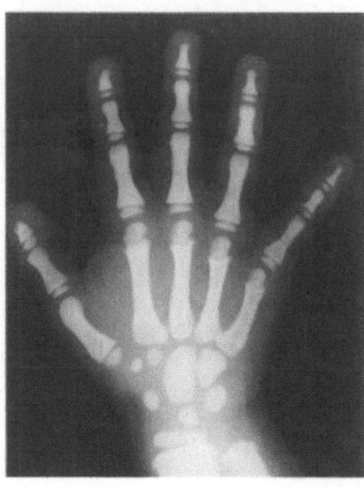

Fig. 9.4. Acro-osteolysis, phalangeal type. Small areas of tuft resorption of terminal phalanges are evident. The terminal phalanges are hypoplastic, with hypoplasia of the nails. Diffuse osteosclerosis is also evident in this 5-year-old girl with pyknodysostosis

have some retardation of skeletal maturation [29]. A distinction has been proposed between ivory epiphyses and epiphyses which appear dense as a result of an abnormal pattern of trabeculation.

Plain radiography shows sclerosis of the epiphyseal ossification centers (ivory epiphyses), or sclerosis of accessory ossification centers (ivory pseudoepiphyses).

Diseases associated with ivory epiphyses include tricho-rhino-phalangeal syndromes, Cockayne syndrome, Down syndrome, hypothyroidism, multiple epiphyseal dysplasia, spondylo-epiphyseal dysplasia, diastrophic dysplasia, hypopituitarism and mucopolysaccharidosis IV A (Morquio).

9.6.2   Normal Variation and Congenital Abnormalities of the Wrist

The shape and size of carpal bones, as well as their relative position often vary considerably among different individuals.

Small radiolucencies (cysts) are common variants in the carpus at any age, especially in adults. Gross alterations in structure, shape and configuration of the carpals may be seen in any condition affecting ossification, including mucopolysaccharidoses and epiphyseal dysplasia.

Carpal abnormalities can be isolated findings [30], or associated with other inborn defects. An association between a longitudinal defect in the forearm (radial, ulnar or central ray deficiency) and carpal abnormalities, including *aplasia, hypoplasia and fusion,* is well established (Fig. 9.5). In general, when the longitudinal defect involves the radial ray, the radially placed carpals are affected; when the defect is at the ulnar side, the medially placed carpals are involved. The congenital absence of the scaphoid alone, not associated with thumb or radial hypoplasia, has been reported. *Scalloping deformities* of the carpal bones most commonly are found in multiple epiphyseal dysplasia, but can be seen also in neurofibromatosis type 1 and soft tissue hemangiomas. *Irregular carpal bones* are observed in multi-

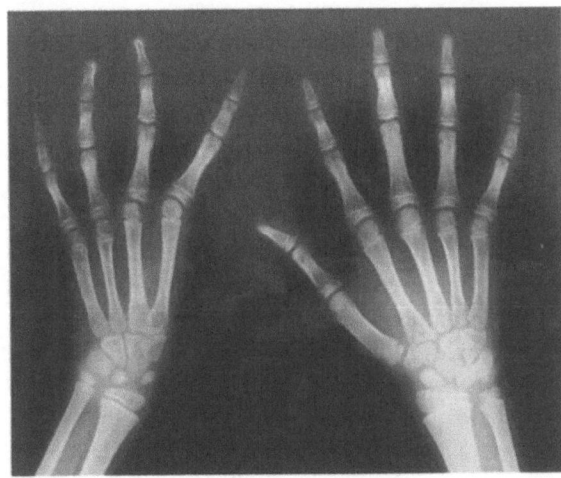

Fig. 9.5. Carpal abnormalities. Aplasia of trapezium and pisiform, hypoplasia of scaphoid and lunate (left hand) and fusion between lunate and triquetrum (right hand) in a 10-year-old boy. The left thumb is missing

ple epiphyseal dysplasia, punctate epiphyseal dysplasia, spondyloepiphyseal dysplasia, Morquio disease, rheumatoid arthritis, Winchester syndrome, or following trauma or infection. *Small carpal bones of bizarre shape* have been reported in Seckel syndrome, mostly as a consequence of disharmonic carpal maturation [31], and in diastrophic dysplasia (Fig. 9.6).

9.6.2.1 Carpal Angle Abnormalities

Changes in the normal relation between carpals and radius/ulna result in carpal angle abnormalities. The proximal row of carpal bones articulates with the distal radius and ulna. The distal row of the carpal bones articulates with the bases of the metacarpals (the trapezium with the first metacarpal, the trapezoid with the second, the capitate mainly with the third, and the hamate with the fourth and fifth).

The carpal angle is formed by the intersection of two lines, the first tangential to the proximal surfaces of the scaphoid and lunate, the second tangential to the

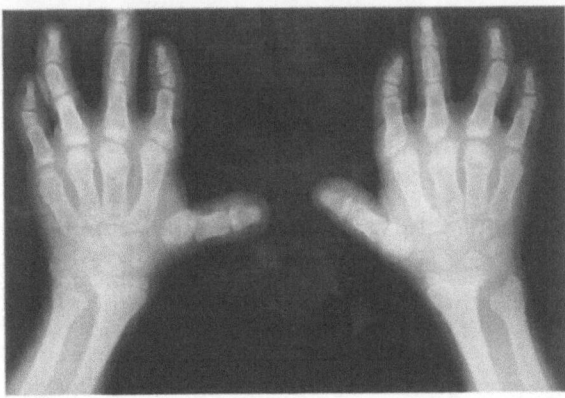

Fig. 9.6. Carpal abnormalities. Small, irregular carpal bones in a 5-year-old child with diastrophic dysplasia. Undermodeled tubular bones, ovoid first metacarpal with proximally located thumb (hitchhiker thumb), hypoplastic second and fifth middle phalanges, metaphyseal widening, severe epiphyseal abnormalities, finger clinodactyly and osteopenia are also present

proximal margins of the triquetrum and lunate (Fig. 9.7). Changes in the carpal angle may result from abnormalities of the end-portion of the radius or ulna [32]. In the Madelung deformity, a condition associated with decreased carpal angle, the primary deformity is a dorsal bowing of the distal end of the radius, with unequal growth of its epiphysis, resulting in wedging of the carpus between the deformed radius and protruding ulna, with the lunate at the apex of the wedge (Fig. 9.8). In mucopolysaccharidosis type 1 (Hurler) and mucopolysaccharidosis type IVA and IVB (Morquio disease), changes in the carpal angle are secondary to distal tapering of radius and ulna. An increased carpal angle can result from deformed or extra carpal bones. An example is diastrophic dysplasia.

The normal values for the carpal angle in children between 4 and 14 years of age have been established [32]. The normal values in adults are in the range of 130° to 137°.

On radiographs, a decreased (more acute) carpal angle appears as slanting of the radius; slanting or protrusion of the ulna; and overall triangulation of the carpus. Decreased carpal angle is associated with Turner syndrome [33, 34], dyschondrosteosis, multiple exostoses, Madelung deformity and mucopolysaccharidosis.

Increased carpal angle is depicted on radiographs as flattening of the proximal carpal row. Conditions associated with increased carpal angle include arthrogryposis, Down syndrome, diastrophic dysplasia, epiphyseal dysplasias, frontometaphyseal dysplasia, otopalatodigital syndrome, Pfeiffer syndrome and spondylometaphyseal dysplasia.

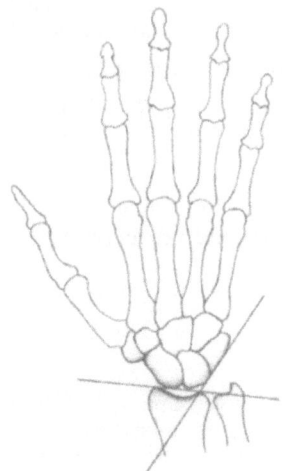

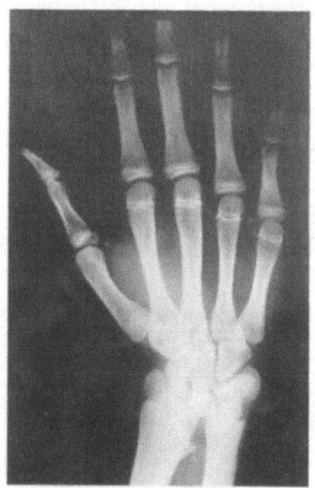

Fig. 9.7. The carpal angle. This angle is defined by two lines, one tangential to the proximal surfaces of the scaphoid and lunate and the second tangential to the proximal margins of the triquetrum and lunate

Fig. 9.8. Decreased carpal angle. Madelung deformity in a 17-year-old girl with chromosome X monosomy syndrome. The picture shows triangulation of distal radial epiphysis, widening of distance between radius and ulna, wedging of carpal bones between the deformed radius and protruding ulna, with the lunate at the apex of the wedge

9.6.2.2   Supernumerary Carpal Bones

Supernumerary carpal bones are extra ossicles scattered throughout the carpus, additional to the normal eight carpal bones. Up to 25 different carpal ossicles have been listed [35]. In general, extra carpal ossicles are asymptomatic and have no clinical relevance. However, they can be found in some distinct malformation syndromes. The so-called *os centrale*, an ossicle between capitate and scaphoid, can occur as an isolated finding but can also be found in hand-foot-uterus syndrome, Holt-Oram syndrome, otopalatodigital syndrome and Larsen syndrome. Extra ossicles of the *distal row* are seen in brachydactyly A-1, diastrophic dysplasia, Ellis-van Creveld syndrome, Larsen syndrome and otopalatodigital syndrome. In ulnar dimelia, a symmetric distribution of duplicated carpals is found, with a few unpaired bones at the center of the carpus. Accessory ossicles must be differentiated from *small fracture fragments*. In some subjects, a normal carpal bone is split into two or three small fragments on an idiopathic basis. In Larsen syndrome, a completely *bizarre rearrangement* of carpals occurs. On radiographs, the carpals can be deformed and hypoplastic, with squared-off borders.

9.6.2.3   Carpal Fusion

Carpal fusion consists in the fusion of two or more carpal bones into a single bone. It may occur as an isolated anomaly or as part of a generalized malformation complex. As a rule, fusions within the same row, either proximal (Figs. 9.5, 9.36, 9.43) or distal (Fig. 9.11), are likely to be an isolated anomaly, while fusions across the rows, massive fusion, or fusion between carpals and radius or ulna, usually occur in malformation syndromes [35–37].

Carpal fusion is secondary to failure in segmentation of primitive cartilaginous matrix, with lack of formation of the intervening joints. As an isolated anomaly, it occurs in about 1% of the general population, is bilateral in about 60% of cases, and has no clinical relevance. Pain is recorded as an uncommon complication, mainly in the presence of *partial fusion*. Isolated coalition most commonly affects the triquetrum and lunate [38]. Less common sites are capitate-hamate, trapezium-trapezoid and pisiform-hamate. Carpal synostosis and tarsal synostosis can be associated findings. Carpo-tarsal fusion associated with synostosis of the elbow joint, and progressive ankylosis of other joints, including the proximal interphalangeal, cervical vertebrae, hips and humeroradial joints, are features of *multiple synostosis syndrome 1*.

Carpal ankylosis can occur also after infections, inflammatory or traumatic processes, or surgery.

Plain radiography shows absence of the gap in trabecular pattern between two or more carpal bones; widening of the scapho-lunate interosseous space (fusion between lunate and triquetrum); and, less frequently, an intraosseous cyst adjacent to the area of coalition. Carpal fusion occurs in acrocephalosyndactyly (Apert type), acromegaly, arthrogryposis, chondroectodermal dysplasia, Turner syndrome, Crouzon craniofacial dysostosis [39], diastrophic dysplasia, dyschondrosteosis, fetal alcohol syndrome, frontometaphyseal dysplasia, hand-foot-genital syndrome, Holt-Oram syndrome, Kniest dysplasia, mesomelic dysplasia (Nievergelt type), multiple synostosis syndrome, oto-palato-digital syndrome (type 1), spondyloepimetaphyseal dysplasia (Irapa type), congenital synspondylism [40] and thalidomide embryopathy.

9.6.2.4   Multicentric Acro-osteolysis

Extensive osteolysis in the carpal and tarsal bones can occur either in idiopathic or in acquired conditions. The osteolytic process can be confined to the carpus/ tarsus, or involve other anatomic sites. Idiopathic osteolysis of the carpo-tarsal bones has been classified into two major forms: multicentric osteolysis with nephropathy, and hereditary multicentric osteolysis. Clinical manifestations in *multicentric osteolysis with nephropathy* [41–44], an autosomal dominant disorder, begin in early childhood with arthritis-like episodes involving ankles and wrists, extensive osteolysis of carpus and tarsus, and progressive renal failure. Nephropathy typically appears several years later. Symptom onset in adulthood can be associated with the involvement of other skeletal sites, including ribs, clavicles, sternum and mandible.

Hereditary multicentric osteolysis [45] is a distinct autosomal recessive disorder with characteristic features, including collapse, sclerosis and bone resorption of carpals, tarsals, elbows and shoulders; joint swelling, soft tissue thickening and flexion contractures of the knees, hip and elbows. There may be associated renal abnormalities. Other multicentric osteolyses do not fit with any of the disorders described above. Considerable overlap occurs between familial and nonfamilial cases, patients with and without nephropathy, and among different radiographic patterns. *Winchester syndrome* is characterized by short stature, severe joint contractures, peripheral corneal opacities, coarsened facies, dissolution of carpal and tarsal bones, and generalized osteoporosis [46].

Plain radiography shows progressive disappearance of the carpus and tarsus, with tapering of adjacent tubular bones in multicentric osteolysis with nephropathy; collapse and resorption of the carpal and tarsal bones, osteoporosis, cortical thinning and increased caliber of the tubular bones without tapering in hereditary multicentric osteolysis.

Other conditions associated with multicentric osteolysis include dermo-chondro-corneal dystrophy of François, diabetes mellitus, neuropathic osteoarthropathy, Farber disease, juvenile chronic arthritis, leprosy and neuropathic osteoarthropathy.

9.6.2.5   Acro-osteolysis, Phalangeal Type

In acro-osteolysis of the phalangeal type, bone resorption occurs at the distal phalanges. Bone destruction can be seen in several neoplastic, infectious, traumatic, vascular and congenital conditions. Ungual tuft resorption can also occur after frostbite, thermal and electrical burns.

The *acro-osteolysis syndrome of Hajdu-Cheney*, a dominantly inherited disorder, is characterized by resorption of the distal phalanges of hands and feet, osteoporosis, short stature, hypoplasia of the ramus of the mandible, and dolichocephalic skull with basilar impression. Changes in the phalanges, including tuft resorption and band-like areas of lucency, are similar to those encountered in vinyl chloride occupational exposure, renal osteodystrophy, pyknodysostosis and collagen vascular disorders. Although the pathogenesis is unknown, an abnormality of osteoblasts and a neurovascular dysfunction with local release of osteolytic mediators have been proposed as possible mechanisms [47–52].

An autosomal recessive disorder characterized by progressive phalangeal osteolysis, with skin ulceration and sensory neuropathy, so-called *neurogenic acroosteolysis*, is also known. Similar peripheral lesions affecting the phalanges and skin also occur in the *acro-osteolysis of Shinz*, an autosomal dominant disorder without neurologic compromise [53].

Plain films show tuft resorption and band-like areas of lucency across the waist of the terminal phalanges.

Other conditions associated with phalangeal osteolysis include cleidocranial dysplasia, dermatomyositis, diabetes mellitus, disseminated lipogranulomatosis, dysostosclerosis, ectodermal dysplasia, Ehlers-Danlos syndrome, epidermolysis bullosa, hyperparathyroidism, hypertrophic osteoarthropathy, malabsorption syndrome, mixed connective tissue disease, neurotropic disease, osteomalacia, osteopetrosis, osteopoikilosis, pityriasis rubra, polymyositis, porphyria, progeria, psoriasis, pyknodysostosis, rheumatoid arthritis, Raynaud disease, Reiter syndrome, sarcoidosis, scleroderma, Sjögren syndrome, Werner syndrome and Winchester syndrome.

9.6.3 Shortening or Absence of Components of the Hands

Deficiency of hand tubular bones ranges from minimal shortening of the fifth middle phalanx (Fig. 9.9) to complete absence of the hand *(acheiria)* (Fig. 9.10). These defect can be isolated or part of an extensive malformation complex and are commonly found in the feet. Short distal phalanges may be associated with cone-shaped epiphyses as a result of their premature fusion. Reduction deformities can occur in association with fusion or malsegmentation deformities.

Causative factors for tubular bone shortening are either congenital or acquired. At present, a number of genes responsible for split hand/split foot malformation and brachydactyly type C have been localized. Among the acquired conditions, any disorder causing closure of, or damage to, the epiphyses may result in shortening of the respective finger. Acquired forms are often differentiated from congenital ones because of their asymmetric and random involvement. Destroyed or eroded terminal phalanges on a acquired basis can mimic congenital shortening of the distal phalanges. Congenital shortening is often associated with hypoplastic fingernails.

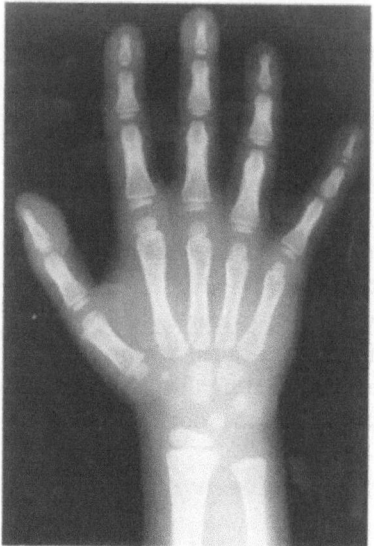

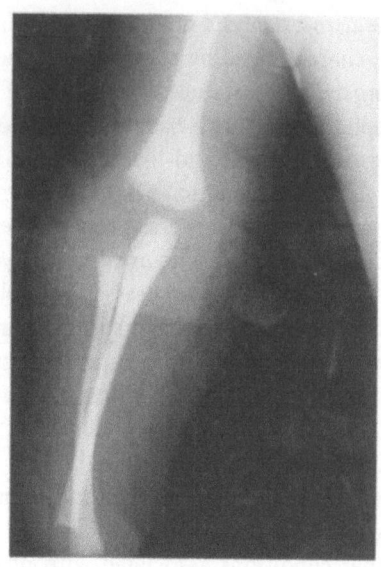

Fig. 9.9. Short middle fifth finger phalanx, associated with hypoplasia of the distal phalanx in a 4-year-old male with Coffin-Siris syndrome

Fig. 9.10. Acheiria. Isolated congenital defect in an otherwise normal newborn infant

According to Temtamy and McKusick, limb deficiencies are classified as transverse or longitudinal depending on whether they extend across the width of the hand or run parallel to its long axis [4, 7]. In a study based on 271 limb reduction defects, 35% were terminal transverse, 35% longitudinal (13% preaxial, 12% postaxial, 10% intercalary), 26% split limbs, and 4% multiple types. Overall, 75% of the defects involved upper limbs and 25% lower limbs. Associated anomalies, affecting the musculoskeletal (clubfoot, hip dislocation, congenital contractures), cardiovascular, gastrointestinal and genitourinary systems were present in about one-half of the patients [54].

Shortening of the distal phalanges (*brachytelephalangy*) (Fig. 9.11), middle phalanges (*brachymesophalangy*) (Fig. 9.12) or proximal phalanges, as well as shortening of the metacarpals (*brachymetacarpalia*), may contribute, individually or in variable association, to shortening of the fingers (*brachydactyly*) and, as a consequence, of the entire hand (*acromelia*).

In general, severe brachytelephalangy is clinically obvious, especially when associated with nail hypoplasia, while accurate radiographic measurements are required to identify milder cases.

Shortening of the middle phalanges can be generalized or localized to one or more fingers. Isolated shortening of the proximal phalanges is exceedingly rare.

9.6.3.1 Brachydactyly

The term brachydactyly literally means short digit. Eight major types of brachydactyly have been recognized [55]. However, several other forms of finger shorten-

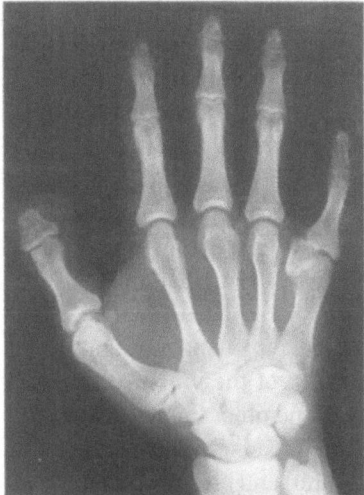

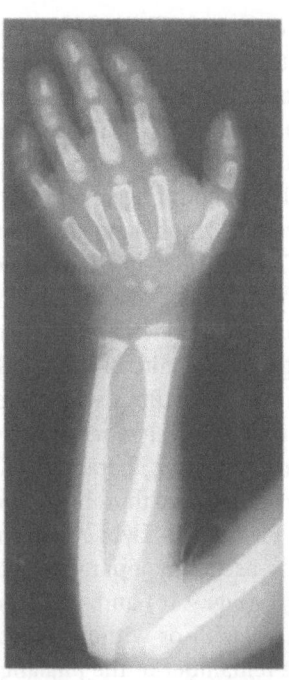

Fig. 9.11. Brachytelephalangy. All distal phalanges are abnormally short. Supernumerary carpal bones and carpal coalition (capitate and hamate) are also present. Note also distal symphalangism of the fifth digit and extreme hypoplasia of the proximal phalanx, which appears as a triangular remnant between the metacarpal and the middle phalanx. Fingernail hypoplasia was also a feature in this patient

Fig. 9.12. Brachymesophalangy, mainly of the second, fourth and fifth digits, in a 2-year-old child with Smith-Lemli-Opitz syndrome. Pseudoepiphyses are present at base of second and at end of first digit. Clinodactyly of the second and fifth fingers are also present

ing do not fit with these patterns described by Bell [56]. For example, acrodysostosis is associated with a generalized form of brachydactyly not included in the available classifications. Unusual patterns of phalangeal shortening are found in diastrophic dwarfism. Shortening of the middle phalanges occurring in Carpenter syndrome is indistinguishable from brachydactyly except for the presence of polydactyly. Shortening of the distal phalanges is not properly classified.

Type A brachydactyly is characterized by shortening of middle phalanges (brachymesophalangy) (Fig. 9.12). In *type A1*, middle phalanges of all digits are rudimentary, absent or fused with terminal phalanges. The proximal phalanges of the thumb and great toe are short. In the rare *A2 type*, shortening of the middle phalanges is confined to the index finger and second toe, all other digits being more or less normal. In *type A3*, shortening is limited to the middle phalanx of the fifth finger. This defect occurs in 0.5–24% in the general population. Because of the rhomboid or triangular shape of the rudimentary phalanx, radial curvature (clinodactyly) of the fifth finger is often an associated finding. This condition has distinct sex and racial distribution, being more common in females, in Mongoloids, and in American Indians than in males, Whites and Blacks. In the unusual *type A4*, brachymesophalangy affects mainly the second and fifth digits (Fig. 9.13).

When the fourth digit is affected, the abnormal middle phalanx leads to radial deviation of the distal phalanx. The feet show absence of middle phalanges in the lateral four toes. The disorder is inherited as an autosomal dominant trait.

Type B brachydactyly is the most severe form of brachydactyly. Similarly to type A brachydactylies, middle phalanges are short, while terminal phalanges are rudimentary or absent. Both fingers and toes are affected. The thumb and great toe are usually deformed. Symphalangism and mild syndactyly can also be present.

In *type C brachydactyly* digital anomalies are heterogeneous and include brachydactyly of the second and third middle phalanges, triangulation of the fifth middle phalanx, brachymetapody, hyperphalangy and symphalangism. A characteristic change is deformity of the middle and proximal phalanges of the second and third fingers, sometimes with hypersegmentation of the proximal phalanx. The fourth finger is grossly normal and projects beyond other fingers (Fig. 9.14).

Type D brachydactyly is characterized by short and broad terminal phalanges of the thumb (so-called stub thumb, or murderer's thumb) and great toe. This anomaly occurs in Rubinstein-Taybi syndrome (Fig. 9.15), pseudohypoparathyroidism (PHP), pseudo-pseudohypoparathyroidism (PPHP) and oto-palato-digital syndrome. In PHP (Fig. 9.16) and, less commonly, in PPHP, shortening also affects distal phalanges, with or without shortening of metacarpals, mainly the fourth and fifth. The remainder of the phalanges, with the exception of the fifth middle phalanx, is generally spared [57]. Distal phalangeal hypoplasia is a radiographic

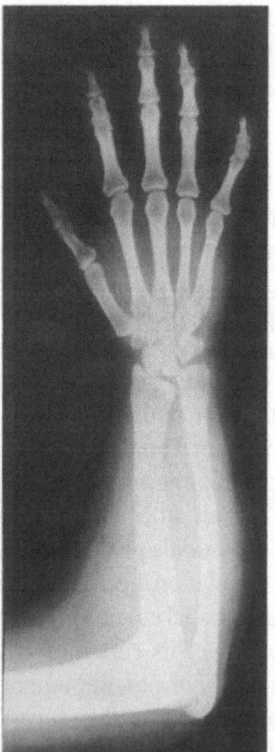

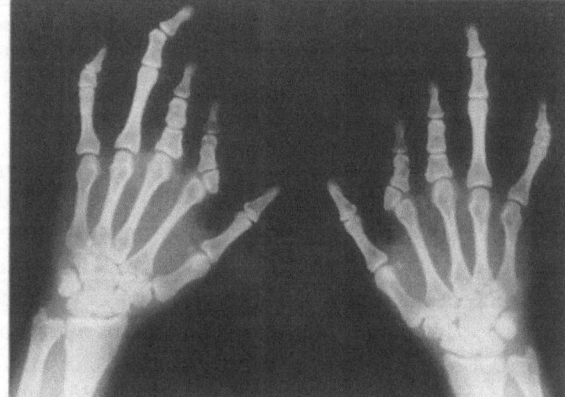

Fig. 9.14. Type C brachydactyly. Marked shortening of middle and proximal phalanges of the second and third digits, with hyperphalangy of the second. The fifth middle phalanx is also markedly short, while the fourth digit has a normal length and projects a clinodactylous distal phalanx beyond the other fingers

◊ **Fig. 9.13.** Type A4 brachydactyly. Shortening of the middle phalanges of the second and fifth digits

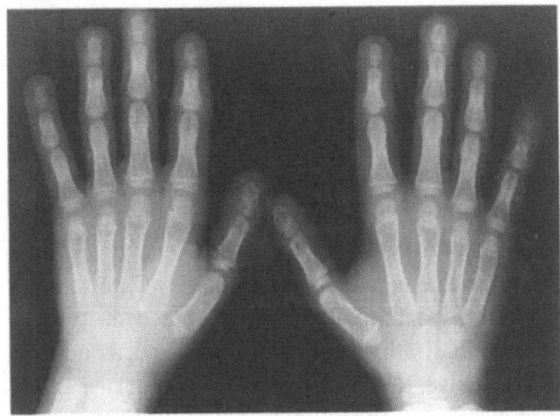

Fig. 9.15. Type D brachydactyly. Short and broad terminal phalanx of the thumbs in a 3-year-old boy with Rubinstein-Taybi syndrome. Note the irregularity of the external margin of the distal phalanges, probably suggesting an attempt at duplication. There is shortening and broadening of the distal phalanges of the fingers, involving both soft tissues and bones

feature in the X-linked recessive chondrodysplasia punctata. In this disorder, the distal phalanges have a characteristic triangular appearance, with the apex proximally placed. This is an important diagnostic finding in children over 3–4 years in whom puncta have normally disappeared [58].

In *type E brachydactyly* the metacarpals and metatarsals are abnormally short (*brachymetacarpalia* and *brachymetatarsalia*, respectively). A major involvement occurs in the fourth and fifth digits (Fig. 9.17), but also distal phalanges can be affected. The frequency of the association between short fourth-fifth metacarpal

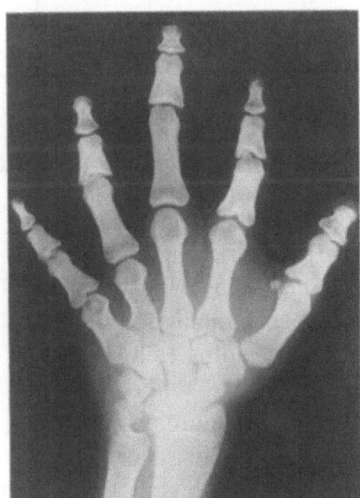

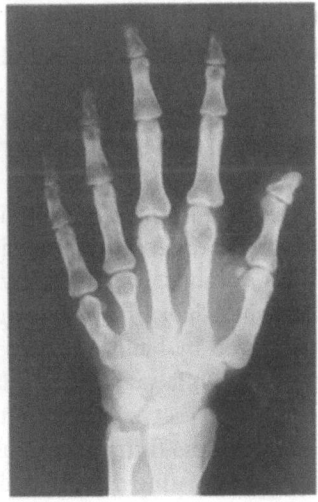

Fig. 9.16. Short distal phalanges and metacarpals in pseudohypoparathyroidism (PHP). Among the metacarpals the fourth and fifth are mostly involved, whereas phalangeal shortening is mainly in the distal phalanx of the thumb. Associated findings are fused cone-shaped epiphyses at the base of proximal and middle phalanges

Fig. 9.17. Type E brachydactyly. Shortening of the metacarpals affects mainly the fourth and fifth. The distal phalanx of the thumb is also short and radially deviated

and short distal phalanges progressively decreases in PHP-PPHP, brachydactyly E, brachydactyly D, Turner syndrome and acrodysostosis [59].

The radiographic study of brachydactylies is based on measurement of individual tubular bone lengths and comparison with the standard values for subjects matching for age and sex. The *pattern profile analysis* by Poznanski allows visualization of the specific defect in the hand [12, 13]. Plain radiography allows also recognition of associated features, including rhomboid middle phalanx in brachydactyly A2 and A3, symphalangism and syndactyly in brachydactyly B, brachymetapody, hyperphalangy and symphalangism in brachydactyly C, and fusion of the epiphyseal line at the base of the distal thumb phalanx in brachydactyly D.

The number of pathologic conditions, both congenital or acquired, associated with brachydactylous hands is impressive. Notable examples are maternal exposure to dilantin, hyperparathyroidism (secondary), hyperthyroidism, hypoparathyroidism, hypothyroidism, Aarskog syndrome, achondrogenesis, achondroplasia, acrodysostosis, acromesomelic dysplasia, asphyxiating thoracic dysplasia, atelosteogenesis, campomelic dysplasia, chondroectodermal dysplasia, chromosomal syndromes, cleidocranial dysplasia, Coffin-Siris syndrome, diastrophic dysplasia, Fanconi anemia, fetal alcohol syndrome, hand-foot-genital syndrome, Holt-Oram syndrome, Larsen syndrome, metaphyseal chondrodysplasia (McKusick), metatropic dysplasia, mucopolysaccharidoses, Noonan syndrome, oro-facio-digital syndrome 1 and 2, osteoglophonic dwarfism, osteosclerosis, oto-palato-digital syndrome types 1 and 2, peripheral dysostosis, Poland syndrome, progeria, pseudohypoparathyroidism (PHP), pseudo- pseudohypoparathyroidism (PPHP), pyknodysostosis, Rubinstein-Taybi syndrome, Silver-Russel syndrome, Smith-Lemli-Opitz syndrome, spondylo-epi-metaphyseal dysplasia (Irapa), TAR syndrome, thanatophoric dysplasia, tricho-rhino-phalangeal syndromes and Weill-Marchesani syndrome.

9.6.3.2 *Brachymetacarpalia*

Metacarpal shortening may be confined to one digit, or extend beyond more fingers and toes, in different combinations. Metacarpal shortening can be an isolated finding, or occur in association with other anomalies involving the hand or other skeletal sites. *Short first metacarpal* (Fig. 9.18) is commonly seen in conditions characterized by hand defect of the radial ray, including Holt-Oram syndrome, Fanconi anemia, acrocraniofacial dysostosis, de Lange syndrome, Juberg-Hayward syndrome, IVIC syndrome and radial hypoplasia syndrome. Shortening of the third, fourth, and fifth metacarpals (Fig. 9.19) is usually an isolated defect in late childhood, suggesting a cause-and-effect relationship with early epiphyseal closure. A mendelian dominant inheritance has been suggested for this defect. However, many other conditions, both acquired and congenital, are known in which shortening of the third, fourth and fifth metacarpals does occur. They include juvenile rheumatoid arthritis, infection, sickle cell disease, trauma, nevoid basal cell carcinoma syndrome (Gorlin syndrome), Beckwith-Wiedemann syndrome, multiple epiphyseal dysplasia, Ruvalcaba syndrome and tricho-rhino-pha-

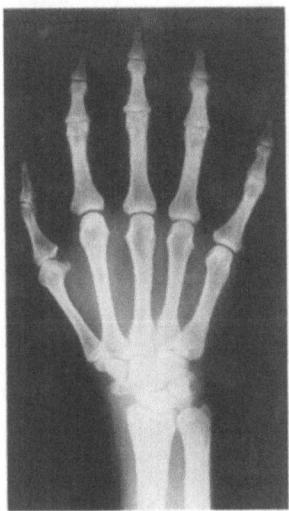

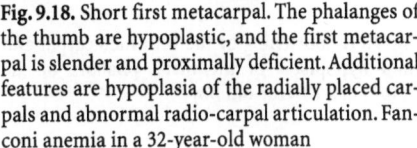

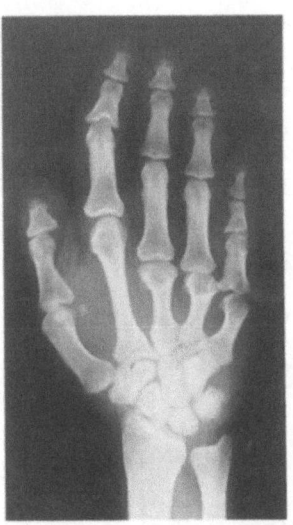

Fig. 9.18. Short first metacarpal. The phalanges of the thumb are hypoplastic, and the first metacarpal is slender and proximally deficient. Additional features are hypoplasia of the radially placed carpals and abnormal radio-carpal articulation. Fanconi anemia in a 32-year-old woman

Fig. 9.19. Shortening of the third, fourth and fifth metacarpal. Additional features include hypoplastic distal phalanges, mainly of the thumb, and cone-shaped epiphyses at the base of the middle second phalanx.

langeal syndrome. *Shortening of the fourth and fifth metacarpals* (Fig. 9.20, 9.21) occurs in pseudohypoparathyroidism (PHP), pseudo-pseudohypoparathyroidism (PPHP), brachydactyly E, Turner syndrome and acrodysostosis [59]. In 65% of PHP-PPHP, the fourth metacarpal is shortened, while the second metacarpal is less commonly involved. In these disorders, also distal phalanges, mainly of the thumb (75%), are affected. *Shortening of the fifth metacarpal* (Fig. 9.21) is also seen in the chromosome 5p syndrome (cri-du-chat) and Silver-Russel syndrome. *Shortening of all the metacarpals* is typically found in acrodysostosis, but it is also a feature of PHP-PPHP and brachydactyly E. Skeletal characteristics alone cannot distinguish between these conditions. Brachydactyly E has been lumped with PHP-PPHP, although a different pattern of inheritance was reported (X-linked dominant/autosomal recessive for PHP-PPHP, autosomal dominant for brachydactyly E). Patients with brachydactyly E are mildly short in stature and have round facies, but lack ectopic calcifications, mental retardation and cataract, unlike patients with PPHP.

The radiographic examination is used to assess and localize the bone defect. This can be achieved by either using crude measurements of the bone length or plotting their relative length against the specific location in the hand (pattern profile analysis).

The metacarpal sign (*Archibald sign*) is used to evaluate the relative shortening of the fourth metacarpal [60, 61]. A line is drawn tangential to the distal portion of the fourth and fifth metacarpals. In normal subjects, this line does not intersect the third metacarpal or just reaches its boundary. When simple intersection is used, the sign is positive in about 9.6% of normal individuals, but if more than 2 mm of intersection

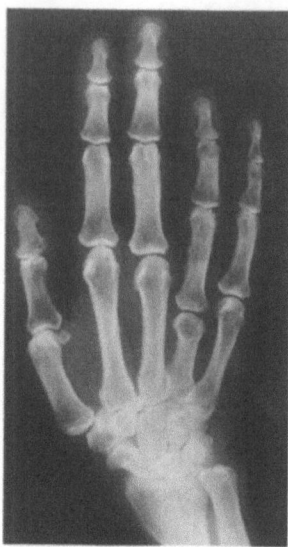
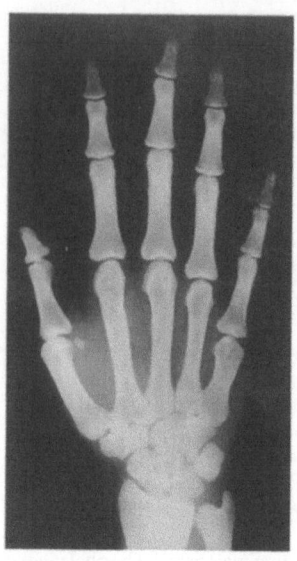

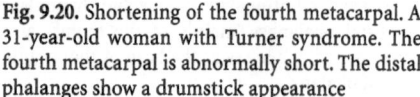

Fig. 9.20. Shortening of the fourth metacarpal. A 31-year-old woman with Turner syndrome. The fourth metacarpal is abnormally short. The distal phalanges show a drumstick appearance

Fig. 9.21. Shortening of the fifth metacarpal and mild hypoplasia of the distal phalanx of the thumb in a 18-year-old boy

is taken as the threshold, then the false positive results are less than 0.5% in the general population. The metacarpal sign may also provide false negative results when the third metacarpal is very short, or if the fifth is as short as the fourth. This sign is also unreliable when slight shortening affects several metacarpals.

Most of the conditions associated with brachymetacarpalia overlap those with brachydactyly, including acrodysostosis, acromesomelic dysplasia, atelosteogenesis, Beckwith-Wiedemann syndrome, brachydactyly A1, brachydactyly C, brachydactyly E, C syndrome, chondrodysplasia punctata, chromosomal disorders, Cockayne syndrome, Cohen syndrome, de Lange syndrome, diastrophic dysplasia, Dyggve-Melchior-Clausen syndrome, dyschondrosteosis, exostoses, Fanconi anemia, fetal alcohol syndrome, hand-foot-genital syndrome, Holt-Oram syndrome, hypoparathyroidism, hypothyroidism, Larsen syndrome, mucolipidosis, mucopolysaccharidosis, multiple epiphyseal dysplasia, nevoid basal cell carcinoma syndrome (Gorlin syndrome), oto-palato-digital syndrome type 2, Poland syndrome, PHP-PPHP, short rib polydactyly syndrome types 1-2-3, Silver-Russel syndrome, Sjögren-Larsson syndrome, tricho-rhino-phalangeal syndrome and Weill-Marchesani syndrome.

9.6.3.3 Radial Ray Deficiency

The term radial ray deficiency refers to a hand malformation consisting of hypoplasia/aplasia involving the radius, the radially placed carpals (scaphoid, trapezium and trapezoid) and the thumb.

Radial ray anomalies can occur as isolated defects or as a component of genetic syndromes. Syndrome identification is important for prognostic purposes, since every condition is associated with distinct complications. Radial ray deficiency varies from mild hypoplasia (Fig. 9.22) to total aplasia (Fig. 9.23). Absent radius is associated with curved ulna and short forearm. In the case of total aplasia, the hand is radially deviated and clubbed. The elbow may show fixed extension contracture, or deficit in active motion. Bilateral radial defects are common, since they occur in malformation syndromes more frequently than unilateral defects [62]. A number of hematologic syndromes are known in which the radial defect is a cardinal feature (e.g., Fanconi anemia, TAR association) [63]. Congenital heart disease (ventricular septal defect, atrial septal defect, pulmonary artery atresia, patent ductus arteriosus), spina bifida, cleft palate, renal anomalies and thrombocytopenia may be found in association with radial defects. The *VATER* sequence includes vertebral, anal, tracheoesophageal, renal and radial limb anomalies. In a series of 98 patients presenting with 160 hypoplastic thumbs, VATER association and Holt-Oram syndrome accounted for 44% of the cases [64]. Absence of the radius is associated with polydactyly and duplication of the ulna in the rare ulnar dimelia (mirror hand). This anomaly is likely to be secondary to differentiation failure of a part of the ray, rather than to its pure duplication [65].

Most cases of radial ray deficiency are sporadic. Some are consistent with an autosomal dominant or recessive pattern of inheritance. Still other cases result from a chromosome imbalance.

Plain radiography shows hypoplasia/aplasia of the radius, scaphoid, trapezium, trapezoid and thumb. The ulna and the whole forearm may be short and curved. The hand is radially deviated in patients with total radial aplasia.

Radial ray deficiency occurs in aminopterin embryopathy, trisomy 13 and 18 syndromes, craniosynostosis-radial defects, de la Chapelle syndrome, de Lange syndrome, dyschondrosteosis, Fanconi anemia, fetal varicella syndrome, Golden-

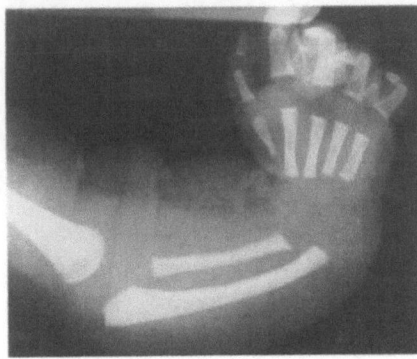

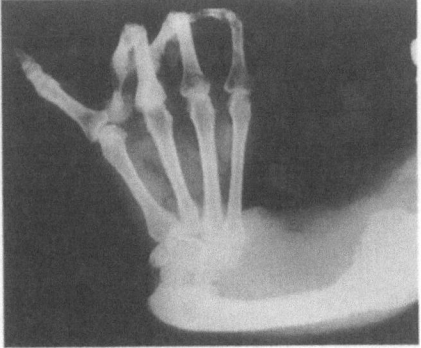

Fig. 9.22. Radial hypoplasia. Hypoplasia involves both proximal and distal radial portions. The thumb is also hypoplastic, and the hand radially curved. Newborn child with Fanconi anemia

Fig. 9.23. Absent radius. The radius, the radially placed carpals (scaphoid and trapezium) and the thumb are absent. The ulna is abnormally curved and short, and the hand is radially deviated and clubbed. Fanconi anemia in a 30-year-old woman

har syndrome, Holt-Oram syndrome, Klippel-Feil syndrome, mesomelic dysplasia, Nager syndrome, phocomelia, radial ray aplasia-renal anomalies, radial ray hypoplasia syndrome, radio-digito-facial dysplasia, Seckel syndrome, TAR syndrome, thalidomide embryopathy, thrombocytopenia-absent radius, Treacher Collins syndrome and VATER sequence.

9.6.3.4 Ulnar Ray Deficiency

Ulnar ray deficiency consists in the association between hypoplasia/aplasia affecting the ulna, the ulnar placed carpals (pisiform and hamate, rarely triquetrum and capitate) and the fourth and fifth fingers [66, 67]. Ulnar defects are much less common and less severe than radial defects. Three major abnormalities are known, i.e., *ulnar hypoplasia; partial ulnar aplasia*, consisting in the presence at birth of an ossified proximal segment of the ulna (Fig. 9.24); and *total ulnar aplasia*. In the partial aplasia, the distal ulna may consist of a fibrocartilaginous band extending from the proximal ossification center to the distal radial epiphysis, or to the ulnar side of the carpus, or both. A tethering effect of this band is supposed to cause ulnar deviation of the hand and wrist, as well as dislocation of the radial head in utero [68]. *Bilateral ulnar aplasia* is exceedingly rare and is associated with lower limb defects in half of the cases and with non-skeletal internal organ malformations in one-third. Total or partial ulnar defects with humeroradial synostosis can be associated with hypoplasia of the shoulder and proximal part of the humerus. In rare patients, combined central digit defects (syndactyly, delta phalanx, cleft hand) and ulnar ray defects are found.

A few ulnar ray defects have a mendelian pattern of inheritance, while most are sporadic.

This defect can occur in cardiomelic syndrome with ulnar agenesis, craniosynostosis-ulnar aplasia, de la Chapelle syndrome, de Lange syndrome, femurfibula-ulna syndrome, Klippel-Feil syndrome-absent ulna, mesomelic dysplasia

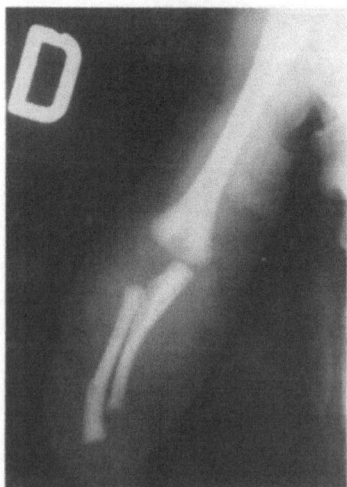

Fig. 9.24. Partial aplasia of the ulna. The proximal part of the ulna is normally developed, while the distal part is deficient. The radius is also deficient and abnormally curved. Isolated congenital acheiria in a newborn child

(Nievergelt type), Pallister syndrome, postaxial acrofacial dysostosis syndrome (Miller), Schinzel syndrome and symphalangism.

9.6.3.5 Central Ray Deficiency

The term central ray deficiency refers to the presence of hypoplasia/aplasia involving the central rays of the hand (and often the centrally placed carpals) [69]. Split-hand, cleft hand and lobster-claw deformity are often used as synonyms. Central ray deficiency (Fig. 9.25) can be either sporadic or part of genetic and non-genetic syndromes. In the isolated forms, one hand is generally involved while the feet are not affected. Genetically determined defects are usually bilateral and often associated with cleft feet (Figs. 9.26, 9.27). Tibial hemimelia can be an associated finding. The severity of this anomaly ranges from *simple clefts* (more or less complete absence of the third digit, Fig. 9.26) to *monodactyly* (deficiency of radial ray with no cleft, Fig. 9.28). In the monodactylous anatomic type, the fifth digit is invariably present. The anatomic classification has no genetic relevance because all types may occur in the same family or in different limbs of the same person. Mild cases of cleft hand resemble simple syndactyly on clinical grounds. Severe clefts can be associated with deformity of the carpal bones (fusion, aplasia) or with central polysyndactylies (Fig. 9.29).

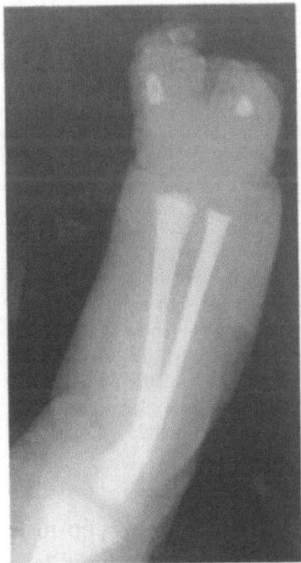 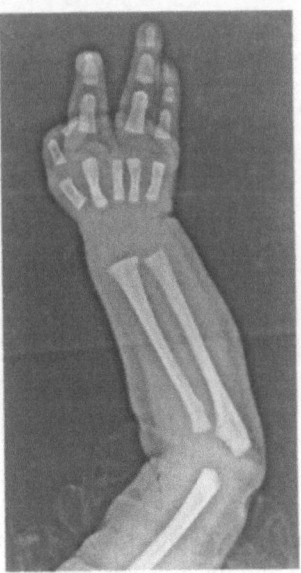

Fig. 9.25. Split-hand. Severe split hand, with absent digits 2 to 4, and remnants of digit 1 and 5. The contralateral hand and feet were normal. Isolated (sporadic) anomaly in a newborn girl

Fig. 9.26. Split-hand. The third digit is missing, while the others are more or less normal. Hypoplastic middle fifth phalanx is also evident. Isolated split-hand and split-foot deformity in a 10-day-old child

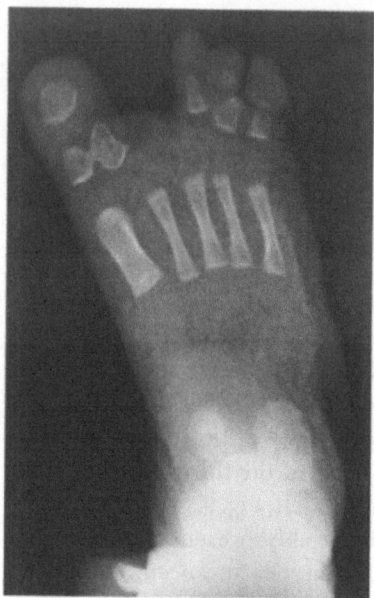

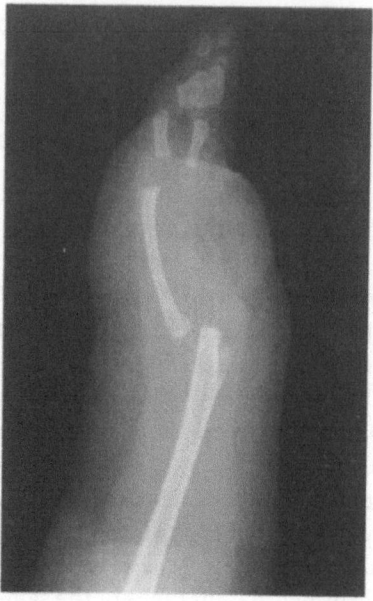

Fig. 9.27. Split-foot in the same patient as in Fig. 9.26. The second digit is missing. The second proximal phalanx is medially dislocated and fused with the first proximal (partial syndactyly)

Fig. 9.28. Monodactyly. Severe hand and forearm abnormality, with radial aplasia, ulnar shortening, elbow dislocation and monodactylous hand. Two digits are fused into one

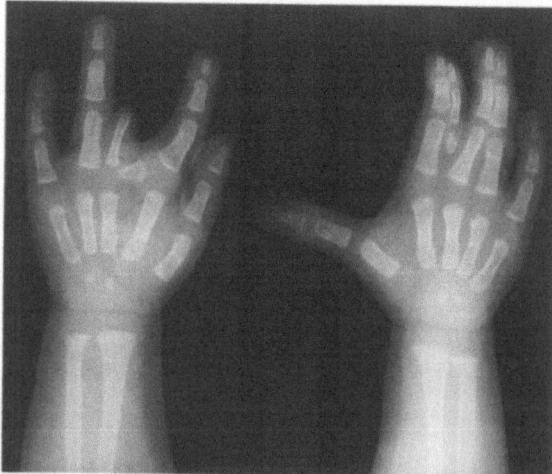

Fig. 9.29. Split-hand. Left hand splitting is associated with right polysyndactyly. The extra-digit is in the web of the second digit. Split-foot was also a feature in this 5-month-child

Clefting may result either from bone and soft tissue aplasia, or from synostosis of phalanges and metacarpals. This suggests that syndactyly and cleft hand take place at around the same week of gestation.

On the basis of its distribution, a mediolateral and a medial form of cleft hand have been recognized. Cleft hands with osseous aplasia often show a mediolateral form, while those with synostosis are mostly located at the medial side.

Congenital heart defects and cleft lip and palate have been described in association with cleft hand. In families with split hand, hypoplasia of the ulnar rays may also be present.

This anomaly is genetically highly heterogeneous, having been assigned to loci 2q3, 5q3, 6q21, 7q22 SHFM1, 10q25 SHFM3 and Xq26 SHFM2.

On radiographs, simple clefts are depicted as absence of the third digit, while more severe clefting implies the absence of more than one digit up to monodactyly. Phalangeal/metacarpal fusion with splitting of digits (without aplasia), central polysyndactyly, carpal fusion or carpal aplasia are found in cases of complex clefts.

Central ray defects occur in absent ulna-split hand and foot deformity, acrorenal syndrome, autosomal dominant split hand-split foot malformation, ectrodactyly-absence of long bones deformity, ectrodactyly-ectodermal dysplasia-cleft palate (EEC) syndrome, familial split hand-split foot anomaly, hypoglossia-hypodactylia syndrome, Möbius syndrome, Robinow syndrome [70], Treacher Collins syndrome and ulnar aplasia-lobster claw deformity [71].

9.6.3.6   Terminal Transverse Defect

The term terminal transverse defect refers to absence of the distal portions of extremities extending across the width of the hand. The defect may involve the phalanges (*aphalangia*) (Fig. 9.30), entire fingers (*adactylia*) (Fig. 9.31), or even the full hand (*acheiria*) (Fig. 9.10). In general, only one limb is affected [72], but cases with bilateral and symmetric defects have also been reported [73].

The association between terminal transverse defects and scalp-skull defects (*aplasia cutis congenita*) is found in Adam-Oliver syndrome, a heterogeneous group of disorders with various clinical features and a distinct pattern of inheritance (autosomal dominant, autosomal recessive, sporadic). Maternal smoking during pregnancy has been considered a possible cause for terminal transverse limb deficiencies [74].

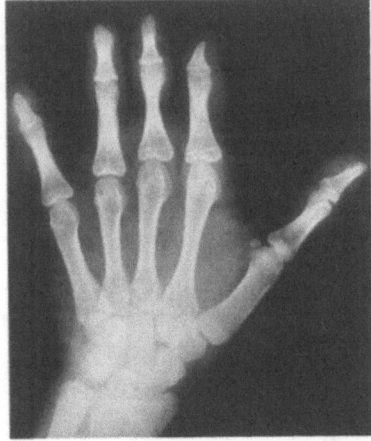

Fig. 9.30. Terminal transverse defects. Aplasia of second to fifth distal phalanges. The middle phalanges are hypoplastic (especially the second) and deformed. Fingernail hypoplasia was also present in this 13-year-old girl

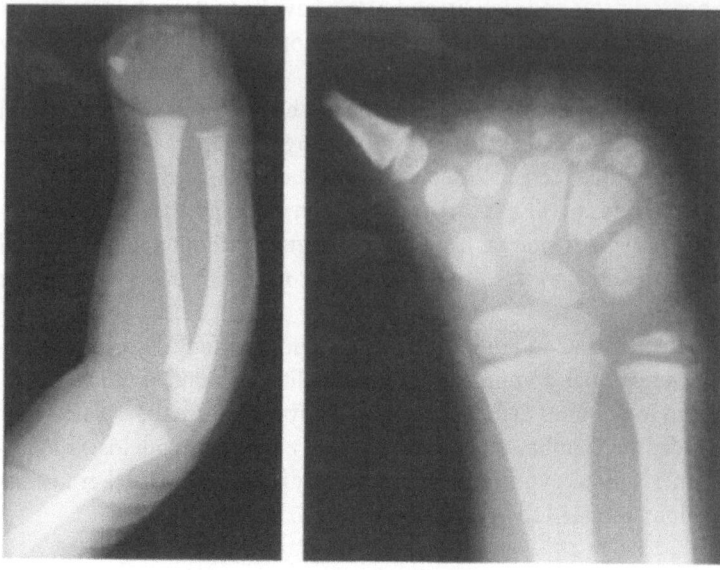

a   b

Fig. 9.31a, b. Terminal transverse defects. **a** Adactyly of all digits. The only visible bone within the hand is a small first metacarpal. The forearm is normally developed. Bilateral clubfoot was an additional finding in this 10-day-old boy. **b** The same boy at 8 years. The carpal bones are normally ossified. The second to fifth metacarpals are extremely hypoplastic, while a larger remnant of the first metacarpal is present

A non-mendelian condition causing different terminal transverse defects is known as *amniotic band sequence* [75]. In this disorder ring-like constriction bands are usually seen in the soft tissues. In utero vascular insults can cause ring constrictions similar to those encountered in the amniotic band disruption sequence. A number of these cases have been observed in babies born to mothers undergoing *early first trimester chorionic villi sampling* (<9 weeks of gestation).

In general, these defects are sporadic. In a few cases a mendelian pattern of inheritance is recognized.

On radiographs, there is absence of one or several tubular bones across the width of the hand without evidence of ring-like constrictions in the soft tissues.

Terminal transverse defects can be associated with aplasia cutis congenita, atelosteogenesis, Coffin-Siris syndrome, Goltz syndrome, hand-foot-genital syndrome, Holt-Oram syndrome, hypoglossia-hypodactylia syndrome, Poland syndrome and pyknodysostosis.

9.6.4   Other Anomalies, Including Configuration Anomalies, Malsegmentation, Fusion and Axial Deviation

This heterogeneous group of congenital hand defects originates from *differentiation failure* (syndactyly, symphalangism), from *duplication* (polydactyly), or from *overgrowth* (macrodactyly) of hand portions. A miscellaneous group of defects (camptodactyly, clinodactyly, arachnodactyly, angel-shaped phalanx) resulting in abnormal configuration of the involved segment is also included. In some instances, different defects are present together (polysyndactyly, polydactyly of a triphalangeal thumb, brachysyndactyly, etc.).

Polydactyly may occur in the hands and feet of the same person [76]. Very often, when polydactyly is postaxial in the hands, i.e., the extra digit is located at the ulnar side, it is postaxial also in the feet. More rarely, there is a discrepancy between hands and feet, a condition referred to as *crossed polydactyly* [77]. Unilateral polydactyly is more common in preaxial than in postaxial polydactyly.

The *delta phalanx* anomaly (longitudinally bracketed diaphysis) is a distinct fusion anomaly, characterized by a trapezoid-shaped diaphyseal-metaphyseal unit, with rhomboid appearance of the phalanx [78, 79]. A possible mechanism is the presence of a cartilaginous bracket along one side of the diaphysis, which subsequently ossifies, causing the malformed phalanx to be tipped 90° from the axes of the proximal and distal phalanges. The first proximal phalanx and the fifth middle phalanx in the hands and feet are most commonly involved. The delta phalanx can occur as an isolated anomaly, associated with other defects such as polydactyly, hyperphalangism, symphalangism, clinodactyly and brachydactyly type A2, or as part of malformation syndromes, such as Down syndrome, acrocephalosyndactyly and Rubinstein-Taybi syndrome.

The *angel-shaped phalanx*, a rather complex anomaly of the phalanx and corresponding epiphysis, is potentially a specific marker for genetic disease.

9.6.4.1 Preaxial Polydactyly

The term preaxial polydactyly is used to describe the presence of supernumerary digits located at the radial (preaxial) side of the hand. Four types have been recognized: *thumb polydactyly* (Figs. 9.46, 9.47); *polydactyly of triphalangeal thumb*; *polydactyly of index finger*; and *polysyndactyly* (Fig. 9.29) [80, 81]. Polysyndactyly refers to the presence of both polydactyly (with the thumb normally showing the mildest degree of duplication) and syndactyly, usually in the third and fourth digit. It has been suggested that type IV polydactyly and *type I crossed polydactyly* are the same disorder. Type I crossed polydactyly consists of postaxial polydactyly in the hands and preaxial polydactyly in the feet. In *type II crossed polydactyly* the extra digit is preaxial in the hands and postaxial in the feet. Preaxial polydactyly is generally unilateral, while postaxial polydactyly is often bilateral. Although some evidence suggests that preaxial polydactyly is genetically determined, the pattern of inheritance has not been established, most cases being sporadic.

Hand radiographs show complete or partial duplication of first or second fingers. In the case of polysyndactyly, fusion usually occurs between the third and fourth digits.

Diseases associated with preaxial polydactyly include acro-renal-ocular syndrome, Down syndrome, cranio-fronto-nasal dysplasia, Diamond-Blackfan syndrome, DiGeorge syndrome, Dubowitz syndrome, Fanconi anemia, Holt-Oram syndrome, Levy-Hollister syndrome, Nager syndrome, Poland syndrome, short rib-polysyndactyly type 2 (Majewski type), VATER association and velo-cardiofacial syndrome.

9.6.4.2   Postaxial Polydactyly

When the supernumerary digit is located on the ulnar side of the hand, the term postaxial polydactyly is used. Two distinct phenotypes are known. In *type A polydactyly*, the supernumerary digit is fully developed and articulates with the fifth digit (Fig. 9.32), or with an extra metacarpal (Fig. 9.33). In *type B polydactyly*, the extra digit is rudimentary and often appears as a skin tag (Fig. 9.34). When metacarpals are duplicated, carpals are often fused. Among the chromosomal disorders, postaxial polydactyly occurs almost exclusively in trisomy 13 syndrome [82]. In a large study of 2,271 cases of postaxial polydactyly ascertained from 1,582,289 births, it was found that hand postaxial polydactyly is a distinct genetic disorder with respect to postaxial polydactyly in the feet [83]. Hand postaxial polydactyly was the most frequent type (76%), followed by foot postaxial polydactyly (15%) and hand/foot postaxial polydactyly (9%). Hand polydactyly occurred more frequently at the left side (77%), and was associated with African Black ethnicity,

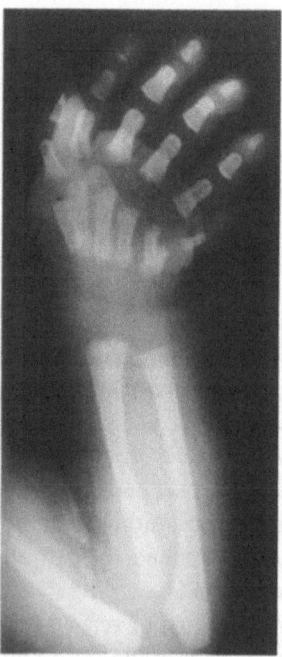
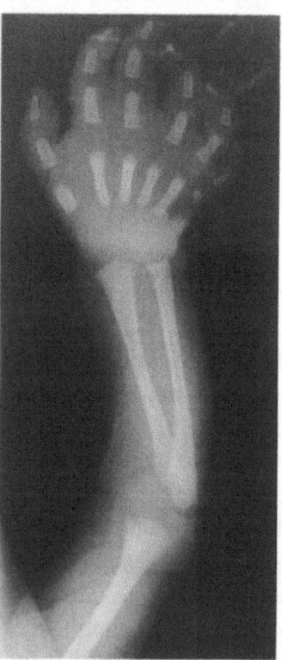

Fig. 9.32. Type A postaxial polydactyly. A bifid fifth metacarpal is harboring the extra digit. One-month-old infant with chromosome 13 trisomy syndrome

Fig. 9.33. Type A postaxial polydactyly. A fully developed supernumerary digit on the ulnar side articulates with an extra rudimentary metacarpal. Newborn infant with chromosome 13 trisomy syndrome

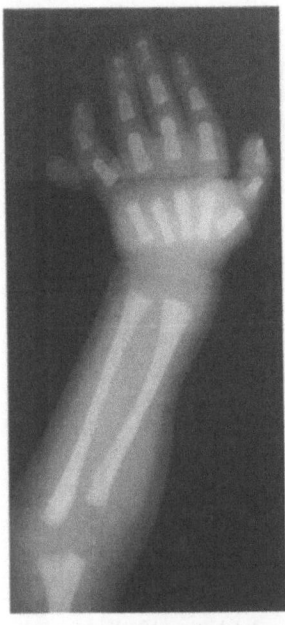

Fig. 9.34. Type B postaxial polydactyly. The extra digit is rudimentary (skin tag) and is connected with the mid-portion of the fifth digit. Newborn infant with chromosome 13 trisomy syndrome

male sex, twinning and parental consanguinity. In the majority of cases, hand/foot polydactyly was associated with other defects.

The inheritance is autosomal dominant, with high penetrance. GLI3 mutations have been found in a number of patients with type A polydactyly [84]. The pattern of inheritance of isolated polydactyly type B is unclear. However, an autosomal recessive model has been suggested based on the association of this defect with some recessive disorders, including Ellis-van Creveld and Bardet-Biedl syndrome.

Plain radiography shows a fully developed extra digit on the ulnar side in type A polydactyly, with inconstant carpal fusion; and a rudimentary extra digit in the form of a skin tag in type B polydactyly.

Disorders in which this defect occurs include acro-renal association, acrocallosal syndrome, acrocephalopolysyndactyly (Carpenter type), asphyxiating thoracic dysplasia, C syndrome, Goltz syndrome, Kaufman-McKusick syndrome, Meckel syndrome, Pallister-Hall syndrome, Rubinstein-Taybi syndrome, short rib-polydactyly syndromes and Smith-Lemli-Opitz syndrome.

9.6.4.3 Syndactyly

Syndactyly literally means "fingers-together" and refers to the fusion of two or more digits, due to lack of differentiation. Fusion can be confined to the soft tissues (*simple*) (Fig. 9.35), or involve the soft tissues and the bones (*complex*) (Fig. 9.36). In the latter, the neurovascular structures are also involved. Syndactyly is *partial* when it is located at the proximal segments of the digits, and *complete* when it extends towards their tips. Fusion involving only the distal portions of the digits is termed *acrosyndactyly*.

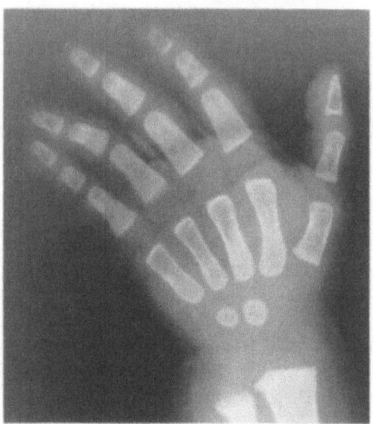

Fig. 9.35. Simple syndactyly. Fusion between digits 4 and 5 is limited to the soft tissues. Isolated finding in a 1-year-old child

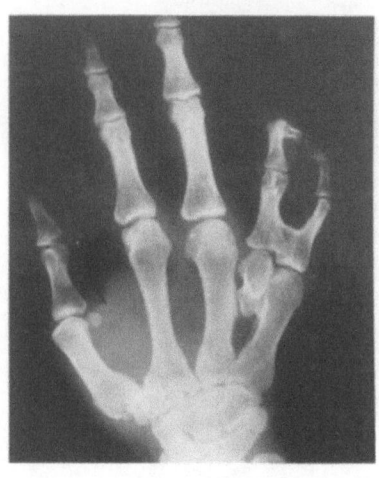

Fig. 9.36. Complex syndactyly. Fusion between digits 4 and 5 involves both soft tissues and bones. Syndactyly in this case is termed "partial" since it involves only the proximal portions of the digits (proximal phalanges). Additional findings include proximal deficiency of the fourth metacarpal and carpal coalition (lunate-triquetrum)

Five phenotypes of syndactyly have been recognized [4]. *Type I syndactyly* is complete or partial webbing between the third and fourth fingers (Fig. 9.37), occasionally associated with fusion of distal phalanges (*zygodactyly*). Other locations are less common. Complete or partial webbing in the feet occurs between the second and third toes. The overall prevalence of type I syndactyly is about 3 per 10,000 newborns, with the most common type being isolated syndactyly of toes 2 and 3, followed by syndactyly of fingers 3 and 4 and syndactyly of toes 4 and 5 [85]. *Type II syndactyly* consists of syndactyly of the third and fourth fingers, with duplication of fingers 3 and 4 in the web (*polysyndactyly*) (Fig. 9.38) [86]. Feet show syndactyly of toes 4 and 5 with polydactyly of the fifth toe in the web. Males are affected more commonly than females. Associated aplasia/hypoplasia of the middle phalanges of the toes can also occur. *Type III syndactyly* refers to complete and bilateral syndactyly of the ring and little fingers. The fifth finger is short, with a rudimentary or absent middle phalanx. Feet are not involved. Since this type of syndactyly was found in a family whose individuals were affected by oculo-dento-digital dysplasia, it has been suggested that the two conditions are encoded by the same gene (6q22–q24) [87]. In *Type IV syndactyly*, there is complete soft tissue syndactyly of all the fingers in the hand with *hexadactyly* (the extra digit can be either preaxial or postaxial). Cutaneous syndactyly in the feet with hexadactyly is a possible associated finding. Syndactyly type IV with hexadactyly of the feet is probably a complex entity which can include a variety of lower limb malformations [88]. In *type V syndactyly*, there is soft tissue fusion of fingers 3 and 4 (and toes 2 and 3) as well as bone metacarpal (and metatarsal) fusion (mainly fourth and fifth, or third and fourth) [89].

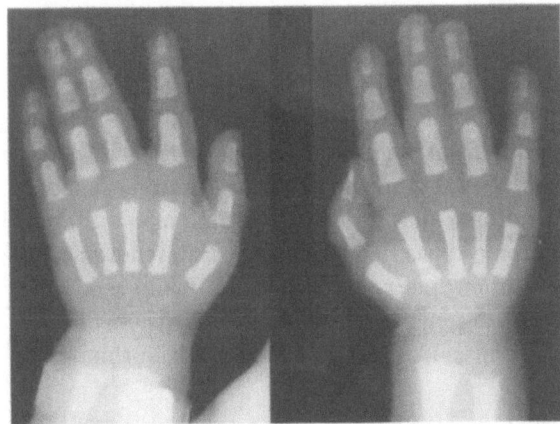

Fig. 9.37. Type I syndactyly. Complete (left hand) and partial (right hand) webbing between fingers 3 and 4

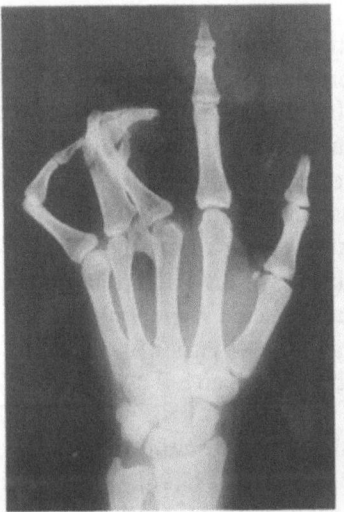
a

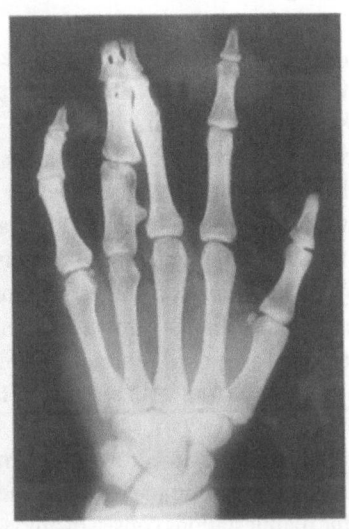
b

Fig. 9.38a, b. Type II syndactyly. **a** Soft tissue fusion between the third and fourth fingers is associated with duplication of the fourth digit in the web. The extra digit is partially formed and fused with the fourth. **b** Distal syndactyly between fingers 3 and 4 and attempt at duplication of digit 4

The overall prevalence of syndactyly is 1 in 2,500 births [85]. These defects are twice as frequent in males as in females, and 10 times more common in whites than in blacks. In about 10% of subjects with syndactyly, Poland syndrome is also present [90].

The inheritance is autosomal dominant; however, sporadic cases have also been reported.

Radiography permits the differentiation of simple from complex syndactylies, and the classification of different types on the basis of their specific features.

Syndactyly can be found in Aarskog syndrome, acrocephalopolysyndactyly (Carpenter, Goodman), acrocephalosyndactyly (Apert), acrocephalosyndactyly (Pfeiffer, Saethre-Chotzen), acro-renal syndrome, aminopterin fetopathy, amniotic band sequence, aplasia cutis congenita, arthrogryposis, Bardet-Biedl syndrome, brachydactyly (A2, B), C syndrome, chondrodysplasia punctata, chromosomal abnormalities (13, 18, 21), Cohen syndrome, de Lange syndrome, Dubowitz syndrome, Ehlers-Danlos syndrome, Fanconi anemia, fetal hydantoin syndrome, fibrodysplasia ossificans progressiva, frontodigital syndrome, Hallermann-Streiff syndrome, Holt-Oram syndrome, Meckel syndrome, Möbius syndrome, multiple synostosis syndrome, Nager syndrome, nevoid basal cell carcinoma syndrome (Gorlin), oto-palato-digital syndrome, types 1 and 2, Pallister-Hall syndrome, Poland syndrome, Prader-Willi syndrome, pterygium syndrome, Robin syndrome, Rubinstein-Taybi syndrome, short rib-polydactyly syndromes, Silver-Russel syndrome, Smith-Lemli-Opitz syndrome, TAR syndrome and tricho-rhino-phalangeal dysplasia types 1 and 2.

9.6.4.4   Symphalangism

The term symphalangism refers to the fusion between two phalanges within the same digit. Symphalangism occurring at the proximal interphalangeal joints (*proximal symphalangism*) was first described by Cushing in 1916 [91]. Both hands and feet can be involved (the thumb is usually spared). Carpal and tarsal fusions frequently are also present. Deafness is a common associated defect [92], suggesting pleiotropy of the same gene. Other associations include absent first metacarpal, clubfoot and humero-ulna synostosis [93]. Metacarpals are generally short or flat. *Distal symphalangism* consists of ankylosis of distal interphalangeal joints (Fig. 9.11). The index finger is most frequently affected. Hypoplasia/aplasia of fingernails or toenails are possible associated features [94]. Fusion involving the interphalangeal joints of the toes with sparing of the hands is an isolated inherited anatomic variant.

Proximal symphalangism is an autosomal dominant trait resulting from mutation of the noggin gene, mapping to chromosome 17q21–q22 [95, 96].

The radiographic manifestations consist of ankylosis between two contiguous phalanges, eventually in association with carpal fusion. In infants, symphalangism can be detected with difficulty because of the radiographically occult cartilaginous tissues.

The defect occurs in brachydactyly (B, C), diastrophic dysplasia, facio-audiosymphalangism syndrome, familial distal symphalangism, multiple synostosis syndrome, pterygium syndrome and short rib-polydactyly syndrome.

9.6.4.5   Clinodactyly

The term clinodactyly applies to radial curvature of a given finger, usually the fifth (Fig. 9.39). The defect can be an incidental finding in otherwise normal persons, or part of a number of malformation syndromes [97]. Clinodactyly results from hypoplasia or asymmetric configuration of the phalanx, which is shorter along one side than the other. Both acquired and genetically determined conditions account for this deformity. Among the acquired conditions, infectious or traumatic injuries can cause clinodactyly via a damage to the phalangeal epiphysis [98]. In

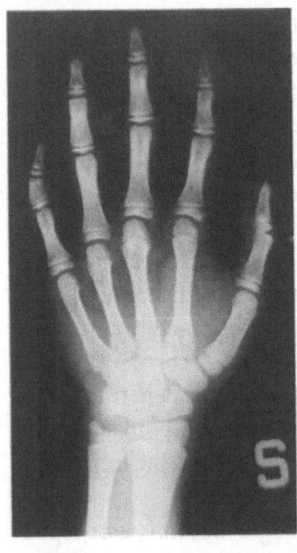

Fig. 9.39. Clinodactyly of the fifth digit. The middle fifth phalanx is hypoplastic so that radial deviation of the finger occurs. Isolated finding in a 12-month-old child

type A3 brachydactyly, the presence of a rudimentary fifth middle phalanx is responsible for the radial deviation of the digit. A similar mechanism is involved in the clinodactyly associated with delta phalanx [78]. In macrodystrophia lipomatosa, the affected (enlarged) digit is almost invariably clinodactylous, as a result of the side-to-side variation in growth rate acceleration.

This defect can be inherited as autosomal dominant trait in most cases, but it occurs also sporadically.

The radiographic examination depicts radial deviation and possible associated changes in the middle phalanx, including asymmetry, hypoplasia or delta phalanx.

Conditions associated with clinodactyly include Aarskog syndrome, acrocephalopolysyndactyly (Carpenter, Goodman), acrocephalosyndactyly (Saethre-Chotzen), aminopterin embryopathy, Bardet-Biedl syndrome, brachydactyly (A1, A2, A3, C), camptomelic dysplasia, cerebro-costo-mandibular syndrome, chromosomal trisomy syndromes (13, 18, 21), Cohen syndrome, de Lange syndrome, Dubowitz syndrome, Ehlers-Danlos syndrome, Fanconi anemia, fetal alcohol syndrome, fibrodysplasia ossificans progressiva, hand-foot-genital syndrome, Holt-Oram syndrome, Kabuki make-up syndrome, Marfan syndrome, Meckel syndrome, mesomelic dysplasia (Nievergelt), nail-patella syndrome, Noonan syndrome, oto-palato-digital syndrome type 1, Poland syndrome, Prader-Willi syndrome, pterygium syndrome, Robinow syndrome, Rubinstein-Taybi syndrome, Seckel syndrome, Silver-Russel syndrome, Treacher-Collins syndrome, tricho-rhino-phalangeal syndromes, Williams syndrome and Zellweger syndrome.

9.6.4.6 Camptodactyly

The defect in camptodactyly consists of a contracture deformity of the proximal interphalangeal joints. Camptodactyly is most often an isolated anomaly, but can be a feature in a number of genetic diseases. The fifth digit is most commonly affected (Fig. 9.40), but any finger may be involved. The defect is bilateral in about 50% of cases. Although its pathogenesis is not definitely understood, a possible mechanism is the imbalance between the flexor and extensor forces at the interphalangeal joint, related to anomalies of the lumbrical muscle [99]. Flexion contractures at the interphalangeal joints may also be secondary to genetic or nongenetic arthropathy [100, 101]. Acquired causes of flexion deformities include burning and infectious or traumatic injuries to the digits. The diagnosis is primarily clinical, based on demonstration of a fixed contracture of the flexor digitorum muscle. The rare *Kirner deformity* is a combination of camptodactyly and clinodactyly of the fifth distal phalanx.

The inheritance is usually autosomal dominant with reduced penetrance. Radiographs, which may be unable to distinguish between true camptodactyly and faulty positioning, are important for disclosing associated findings, including joint damage and osteoporosis.

Disorders associated with this defect include Aarskog syndrome, acrocephalopolysyndactyly (Goodman), Antley-Bixler syndrome, arthropathy-camptodactyly, camptobrachydactyly, chromosomal trisomy syndromes (8, 13, 18, 21), contractural arachnodactyly, craniofrontal dysplasia, fetal alcohol syndrome, Freeman-Sheldon syndrome, Goltz syndrome, Holt-Oram syndrome, Marfan syndrome, Meckel syndrome, nail-patella syndrome, Pena-Shokeir syndrome types I and II, Poland syndrome, pterygium syndrome, Roberts syndrome, Williams syndrome and Zellweger syndrome.

9.6.4.7 Angel-Shaped Phalanges

Giedion et al. defined the angel-shaped phalanx as an abnormal appearance of middle phalanges resembling that of the little angels used in the decoration of Christmas trees [102]. This appearance is due to a diaphyseal cuff (the wings of the

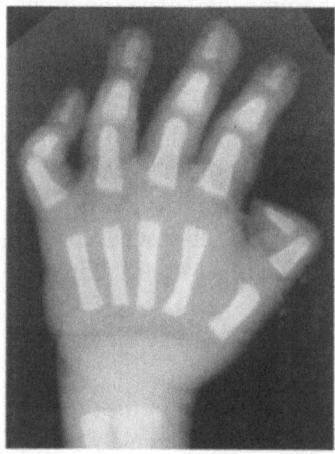

Fig. 9.40. Camptodactyly. The contracture deformity involves the proximal interphalangeal joint of the fifth digit. A flexion deformity of the first digit is also appreciable. Newborn child with isolated anomaly

angel), surrounding a meta-diaphyseal core (the body of the angel), plus a cone-shaped epiphysis at the bottom (the skirt) and a distal pseudoepiphysis at the top (the head). Eight angel-shaped epiphyses types have been identified, differing from each other in the "body" appearance (empty or structured), in the configuration of the "wings" (completely separated or joined to the body), in the configuration of the "skirt" (metaphyseal stalk with normal physis, true cone epiphysis, metaphyseal irregularities) and in the shape of the "head" (true pseudoepiphysis, indentation of the phalangeal tip). This unique appearance tends to normalize over time, giving rise to a short middle phalanx. This anomaly is part of the condition known as *angel-shaped phalango-epiphyseal dysplasia (ASPED)* [102], which is likely due to an auto-somal dominant mutation associated with epiphyseal dysplasia, delayed bone age, coxarthrosis and hyperextensibility of the interphalangeal joints.

This anomaly can occur also in brachyphalangy type C and spondylo-megaep-iphyseal-metaphyseal dysplasia.

9.6.4.8 Macrodactyly

Macrodactyly is a grotesque enlargement of a finger. The existence of isolated macrodactyly is questioned. In most cases this anomaly is associated with other regional or generalized overgrowth of the body. Fingers and toes can be affected, especially on the preaxial side [103, 104]. Phalanges, metacarpals and metatarsals are enlarged, with enlargement involving all the anatomic components of the digit, i.e., bones, tendons, nerves, vessels, subcutaneous fat and skin (Fig. 9.41). Clino-dactyly, either medial or lateral, can be an additional feature. Sometimes, a dorsal angulation of the finger is also present. In *macrodystrophia lipomatosa* [105], the localized, progressive overgrowth of the mesenchymal components of a digit leads to gigantism of one or two digits. Macrodactyly in *neurofibromatosis* [106] is uncommon and results from plexiform neurofibromas, combined with mesoder-mal dysplasia. *Arteriovenous malformation* of the digits can occur as an isolated

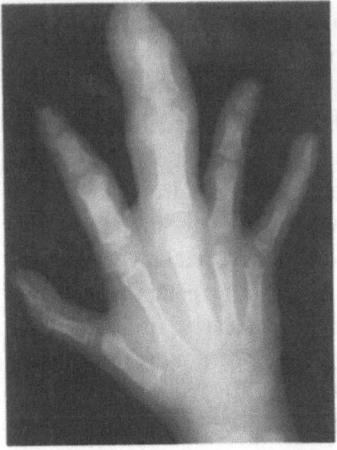

Fig. 9.41. Macrodactyly. Osseous and soft tissue enlargement affecting the third digit. The other digits are more or less normal with the exception of finger 2, which shows subtle abnormalities of both osseous and soft-tissue components. Macrodystrophia lipomatosa

anomaly, or in the context of *Klippel-Trenaunay-Weber syndrome* [107]. Acquired causes of localized finger gigantism include infectious dactylitis, trauma, infarction, Still disease and osteoid osteoma.

Most of the isolated macrodactylies are sporadic. When the defect is part of a malformation complex, the inheritance pattern pertains to the one of the primary disorder.

Plain films depict soft-tissue and bone overgrowth within the digit and can improve diagnostic specificity. For example, in macrodystrophia lipomatosa overgrowth is most marked at the distal end of the digit and along its volar surface, with a possible involvement of adjacent digits, while the trabecular pattern is normal. By contrast, in neurofibromatosis type 1 distal phalanges are less severely affected, distribution is bilateral, growth plates are prematurely fused and cortices are dense and wavy. In hemangiomas and lymphangiomas soft tissues are hypertrophic and bone overgrowth is symmetric.

Disorders with macrodactyly also include enchondromatosis (Ollier disease), fibrous dysplasia, Maffucci syndrome, melorheostosis, plexiform neuroma, proteus syndrome and tuberous sclerosis.

9.6.4.9   *Arachnodactyly*

Arachnodactyly is an abnormal elongation of the hand tubular bones. Elongation of metacarpals and phalanges is a cardinal feature in a group of inherited disorders of the connective tissue, in which skin, ligaments, tendons, skeleton and cardiovascular system are variably involved. These disorders include Marfan syndrome, congenital contractural arachnodactyly or Beals syndrome, homocystinuria, and Ehlers-Danlos syndrome [108]. Since "marfanoid" skeletal changes, including arachnodactyly, are seen in other heterogeneous disorders, their diagnostic value is limited. The metacarpophalangeal pattern profile can distinguish Marfan from marfanoid syndromes with 86% sensitivity and 81% specificity [109]. However, clinical history, histologic and genetic studies remain the mainstream of diagnosis. The metacarpal index, a radiographic measure of metacarpal slenderness, has been used to support the clinical diagnosis of Marfan syndrome [110]. However, application of this analysis may provide false-positive and false-negative results. Racial and ethnic variability may account for this low accuracy.

Marfan syndrome is due to an autosomal dominant mutation within the fibrillin-1 (FBN1) gene, mapping to 15q21.1. Congenital contractural arachnodactyly is due to mutations of the fibrillin-2 (FBN2) gene, mapping to 5q23–q31. Homocystinuria is an autosomal recessive disorder, while Ehlers-Danlos syndrome includes a group of diseases resulting from autosomal dominant or recessive mutations.

The radiographic examination discloses metacarpal and phalangeal elongation, an abnormality which can be more precisely assessed by using the metacarpophalangeal pattern profile. Another parameter is the metacarpal index, which is defined by dividing the lengths of second through fifth metacarpals by their width, and averaging the ratios obtained. The metacarpal index is increased in arachnodactyly. The normal range for the metacarpal index in children has been established [111]. The metacarpal index is less than 8.8 in normal adult males, and less than 9.4 in normal adult females [112]. Depending on the primary disorder, other possible radiographic features include: a 90° flexion deformity of the fifth digit, and marked soft tissue reduction, in Marfan syndrome; carpal deformities, meta-physeal flaring, stippled growth plates of the distal radius and ulna, osteoporosis, and multiple contractures, in homocystinuria; dislocations and subluxations and capitate-scaphoid malalignment, in Ehlers-Danlos syndrome.

Arachnodactyly can be also a feature of Antley-Bixler syndrome, chromosome XYY syndrome, frontometaphyseal dysplasia, ichthyosis syndromes, multiple endocrine neoplasia type 2b, myotonic dystrophy, nevoid basal cell carcinoma syndrome (Gorlin), Rieger syndrome and Sotos syndrome.

9.6.5   Thumb Abnormalities

Although thumb abnormalities are randomly associated with other abnormalities, they often represent a key sign for diagnosing some rare disorders. In general, each patient has a distinct anomaly, but multiple different defects can occur within the same digit. For example, *broad thumbs* are commonly also short, and vice versa. Likewise, an *extra digit* on the radial side can also be *triphalangeal, or hypoplastic* (e.g. acro-renal-ocular syndrome) [113, 114]. *Short, broad and abducted thumbs* can be associated with similar defects in the halluces [115]. Congenital *hypoplasia* of the thumb is often seen in association with longitudinal failure of radial formation. Other thumb anomalies include *abnormally placed thumb, bifid thumb* and *hyperextensible thumb.*

9.6.5.1   Short, Hypoplastic or Absent Thumb

The group of defects encompassing short, hypoplastic or absent thumb includes anomalies ranging from poorly formed to unformed thumb. Short thumb can result from shortening of either all its components or individual bones. *Hypoplasia of the distal phalanx* is found in about 3% in the general population. Short and broad terminal phalanges of the thumb and big toe are referred to as brachydactyly type D. *Shortening of the proximal phalanx* is a common non-specific variant, but can be seen also in type A1 brachydactyly. Hypoplasia/aplasia of the thumb is seen in association with longitudinal radial ray deficiency [116, 117]. In general, the severity of thumb dysplasia correlates with the severity of radial dysplasia. A short thumb is often malpositioned (Fig. 9.42). Deficiency of the intrinsic and extrinsic muscles goes often along with thumb hypoplasia. A *floating thumb* is rudimentary and distally placed, with very hypoplastic surrounding muscles (Fig. 9.43). In a series of 98 patients with 160 hypoplastic thumbs, the defect was more common in males than females (6 to 4), was bilateral in about two-thirds cases, and associated with radial dysplasia in more than of half cases; additional defects occurred in 85% of the patients. Distinct disorders, including Holt-Oram and VATER association, occurred in 44% of the sample [118]. *Total absence of the*

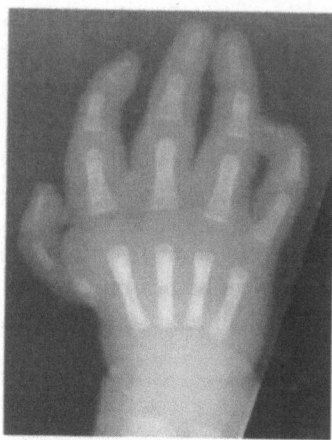 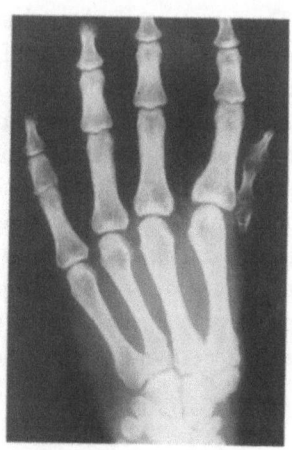

Fig. 9.42. Thumb hypoplasia. The thumb, in addition of being hypoplastic, is also malpositioned. Clinodactyly of the fifth finger is also evident

Fig. 9.43. Thumb hypoplasia. A rudimentary, distally placed thumb, with severely deficient first metacarpal (floating thumb) is present in a male with Holt-Oram syndrome. Carpal abnormalities, including aplasia of trapezium, hypoplasia of scaphoid, and fusion between lunate and triquetrum, are also evident

thumb may be an isolated anomaly, but is often associated with other congenital malformations (Fig. 9.44). Thumb aplasia in one hand and thumb hypoplasia in the other hand can occur in the same patient.

Distal brachyphalangy results from an autosomal dominant mutation, while absent thumb is genetically heterogeneous.

Radiographs show hypoplasia/aplasia of one or more tubular bones, while the pattern profile analysis of Poznanski allows graphic visualization of the specific defect. Associated thumb deformities, including malpositioning of variable degree, can also be easily detected. In general, radiography allows an accurate assessment of the longitudinal radial ray defects.

These anomalies occur also in acrocephalopolysyndactyly/acrocephalosyndactyly syndromes, aminopterin fetopathy, Baller-Gerold syndrome, cephaloskeletal dysplasia (Taybi-Linder), chromosomal aneuploidy syndromes (9, 13, 18, and others), de Lange syndrome, diastrophic dysplasia, DOOR syndrome, Dyggve-Melchior-Clausen syndrome, dyssegmental dysplasia, ectodermal dysplasia, Fanconi anemia, fibrodysplasia ossificans progressiva, hand-foot-genital syndrome, Holt-Oram syndrome, Nager syndrome, oto-palato-digital syndrome types 1 and 2, PHP-PPHP, pterygium syndrome, radial hypoplasia syndromes, Rubinstein-Taybi syndrome, TAR syndrome, Smith-Lemli-Opitz syndrome and thalidomide embryopathy.

9.6.5.2 Broad Thumb

The term broad thumb refers to a thumb wider than normal. A broad thumb, with *broad short terminal phalanges*, is a cardinal sign in Rubinstein-Taybi syndrome

a

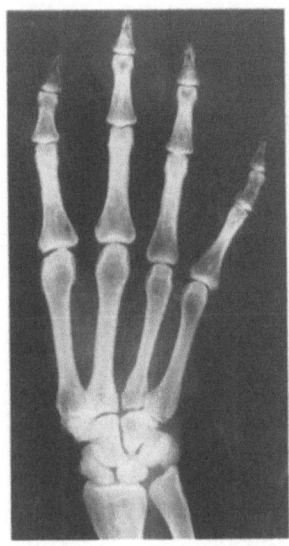

b

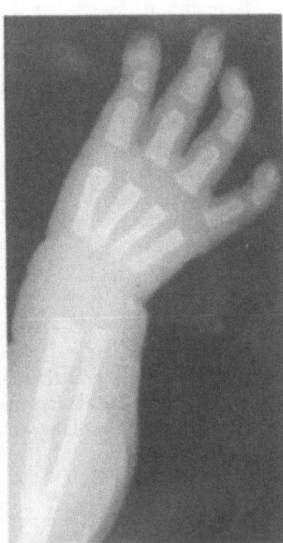

Fig. 9.44a, b. Thumb aplasia. **a** Total absence of the thumb and trapezium in a 18-year-old boy with Holt-Oram syndrome. **b** Thumb aplasia in a newborn child with Nager syndrome

[119, 120]. *Widening of the tubular bones of the digits,* including the thumbs, most marked in the proximal and middle phalanges, occurs in acromesomelic dysplasia. The *proximal thumb phalanx* is broad and short in acrocephalosyndactyly syndromes. Broadening of individual thumb bones is associated with distal duplication in thumb polydactylies.

Plain radiographs disclose widening (and shortening) of one or more tubular bones in the thumb.

A broad thumb can occur in acrocephalopolysyndactyly (Carpenter syndrome), acrocephalosyndactyly (Apert and Pfeiffer syndromes), trisomy 13 syndrome, diastrophic dysplasia, fibrodysplasia ossificans progressiva, frontodigital syndrome, hand-foot-genital syndrome, Larsen syndrome, Meckel syndrome, oto-palato-digital syndrome types 1 and 2, Robinow syndrome and Rubinstein-Taybi syndrome.

9.6.5.3 Triphalangeal Thumb

This anomaly of triphalangeal thumb (TPT) consists of a long, fingerlike thumb, presenting with three rather than two phalanges. TPT (Fig. 9.45) is rare, occurring either alone or in association with other hand and foot abnormalities (polydactyly, brachydactyly, cleft hand, etc.) [121, 122]. It can also be part of a syndrome, becoming a distinct feature of its classification. By contrast, TPT is of little help in the recognition of skeletal dysplasias. Distinct phenotypic variations of this defect are known.

The association TPT-polydactyly syndrome is referred to as *TPT type I*. In this disorder, thumb anomalies are highly variable, ranging from an opposable thumb with a delta phalanx to an extreme form of preaxial polydactyly with a triphalangeal index finger replacing the thumb. The inheritance is autosomal dominant, and the disease-gene mapped to chromosome 7q [123]. Sporadic cases of TPT have also been reported.

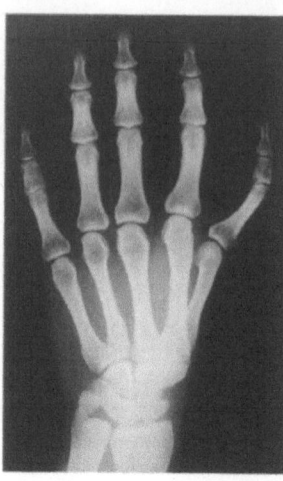

Fig. 9.45. Triphalangeal thumb. Finger-like thumb consisting of three well-formed phalanges in a male with Holt-Oram syndrome. Carpal abnormalities of the same type of those seen in Fig. 9.43 are present

On radiographic examination, the accessory phalanx can appear as a well-formed phalanx, or a small, triangular ossicle. In addition, extra phalanges and large pseudoepiphyses can be easily differentiated. A typical metacarpophalangeal pattern profile has been reported [124].

The most common disorders associated with TPT include some aneuploidy syndromes (mainly trisomy 13) Diamond-Blackfan syndrome, DOOR syndrome, Fanconi anemia, fetal hydantoin syndrome, Goodman syndrome, Holt-Oram syndrome, Levy-Hollister syndrome, Poland syndrome, thalidomide embryopathy, TPT-brachydactyly-ectrodactyly, TPT-polydactyly syndrome, TPT-polydactyly-syndactyly, tricho-rhino-phalangeal dysplasia and VATER association.

9.6.5.4   Thumb Polydactyly

The term thumb polydactyly designates the duplication of one or more of the skeletal components in the thumb. *Thumb polydactyly* corresponds to type 1 preaxial polydactyly, and consists of duplication of one or more of the skeletal components of a biphalangeal thumb. Thumb polydactyly has been further classified into six types, depending on whether the distal or proximal phalanx, or the metacarpal are bifid or duplicated (Fig. 9.46). The most common type is a duplicated proximal phalanx resting on a broad metacarpal (Fig. 9.47). Preaxial polydactyly type 2 designates the association of *polydactyly and triphalangeal thumb.*

Thumb duplication can occur as an isolated anomaly or in association with other defects. When isolated, it is usually unilateral and sporadic. Thumb polydactyly is the most common form of polydactyly, and is 3–4 times more frequent in American Indians than in Caucasians, with a higher prevalence in females compared with males. Aplasia or hypoplasia of the thumb musculature (*Fromont anomaly*), inherited as an autosomal dominant trait, has been regarded as a minor expression of thumb polydactyly [125, 126].

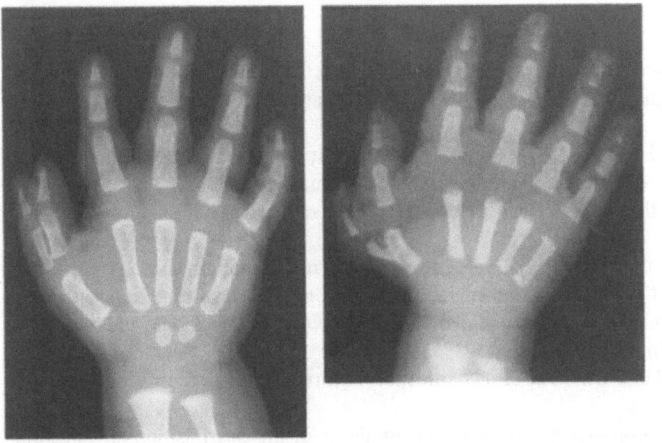

a

b

Fig. 9.46a, b. Thumb polydactyly. **a** Duplication of both proximal and distal phalanges (type 4 thumb polydactyly). Isolated anomaly in a 10-month-old girl. **b** Bifid metacarpal and duplicated proximal and distal phalanges (type 5 thumb polydactyly) in a newborn child with VATER association

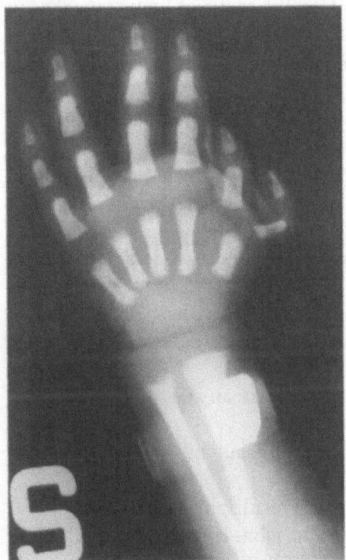

Fig. 9.47. Thumb polydactyly. Duplication of proximal phalanx resting on a broad first metacarpal. Sporadic defect in a newborn child

On radiographs duplication of one or more thumb tubular bones is found, together with a broad (or bifid) tubular bone proximal to the duplication, on which the duplicated bone rests.

This anomaly can be found also in acro-renal-ocular syndrome, Bloom syndrome, Down syndrome, cranio-fronto-nasal dysplasia, Diamond-Blackfan syndrome, Dubowitz syndrome, Fanconi anemia, Holt-Oram syndrome, Levy-Hollister syndrome, Nager syndrome, Poland syndrome, short rib-polysyndactyly type 2 (Majewski), and VATER association.

References

1. Jones KL (1987) Dysmorphology. The approach to structural defects of prenatal onset. In: Behrman RE, Vaughan VC (eds) Nelson textbook of pediatrics, 13th edn. Saunders, Philadelphia, pp 273–276
2. Geoffrey Saint-Hilaire I. (1837) Histoire générale et particulière des anomalies de l'organisation chez d'homme et les animaux. Baillière, Paris, pp 1832–1837
3. Frantz CH, O'Rahilly R (1961) Congenital skeletal limb deficiencies. J Bone Joint Surg Am 43:1202
4. Temtamy SA, McKusick VA (1978) The genetics of hand malformation. Liss, New York
5. Burtch RL (1969) Classification nomenclature of congenital skeletal limb deficiencies. In Swinyard CA (ed) Limb development and deformity: problems of evaluation and rehabilitation. Thomas, Springfield, Illinois, pp 505–524
6. Mital MA (1976) Limb deficiencies: classification and treatment. Orthop Clin North Am 7:457
7. Kay HW (1974) A proposed international terminology for the classification of congenital limb deficiencies. Orthot Prosth 28:33–44
8. Maroteaux P (1970) Nomenclature internationale des maladies osseuses constitutionneles. Ann Radiol 13:455–464
9. Winter RM, Tickle C (1993) Syndactylies and polydactylies: embryological overview and suggested classification. Eur J Hum Genet 1:96–104
10. Manouvrier-Hanu S, Holder-Espinasse M, Lyonnet S (1999) Genetic of limb anomalies in humans. Trends Genet 15:409–417
11. Jabs EW (1998) Toward understand the pathogenesis of craniosynostosis though clinical and molecular correlates. Clin Genet 53:79–86
12. Poznanski AK, Garn SM, Nagy JM, Stern AM (1972) Metacarpophalangeal patterns profiles in the evaluation of skeletal malformation. Radiology 104:1–11
13. Poznanski AK, Garn S (1997) A bibliography covering the use of metacarpophalangeal pattern profile analysis in bone dysplasias, congenital malformation syndromes, and other disorders. Pediatr Radiol 27:358–365
14. Taybi H, Lachman RS (1995) Radiology of syndromes, metabolic disorders and skeletal dysplasias, 4th edn. Year Book, Chicago
15. Poznanski AK (1984) The hand in radiologic diagnosis, 2nd edn. Saunders, Philadelphia
16. Kozlowski K, Beighton P (1995) Gamut index of skeletal dysplasias: an aid to radiodiagnosis, 2nd edn. Springer, Berlin Heidelberg New York
17. Spranger JW, Langer LO, Wiedemann HR (1974) Bone dysplasias: an atlas of constitutional disorders of skeletal development. Saunders, Philadelphia
18. Beighton P (1988) Inherited disorders of the skeleton, 2nd edn. Churchill Livingstone, Edinburgh
19. Maroteaux P (1979) Bone diseases of children. Lippincott, Philadelphia
20. McKusick VA (1994) Mendelian inheritance in man, 11th edn. Johns Hopkins Press, Baltimore
21. Giedion A (1979) Phalangeal cone-shaped epiphyses of the hands (PhCSEH) and chronic renal disease: the conorenal syndromes. Pediatr Radiol 8:32–38
22. Giedion A (1967) Cone-shaped epiphyses of the hands and their diagnostic value: the tricho-rhino-phalangeal syndrome. Ann Radiol 10:322–329
23. Nishimura G, Mugishima H, Hirao J, Yamato M (1997) Generalized metaphyseal modification with cone-shaped epiphyses following long-term administration of 13-cis-retinoic acid. Eur J Pediatr 156:432–435
24. de Iturriza JR, Tanner JM (1969) Cone-shaped epiphyses and other minor anomalies in the hands of normal British children. J Pediatr 75:265–272
25. Swischuk LE, John SD (1995) Differential diagnosis in pediatric radiology, 2nd edn. Williams and Wilkins, Baltimore
26. Allison A, Blumberg BS (1958) Familial osteoarthropathy of the fingers. J Bone Joint Surg Br 40:538–545

27. Gewanter H, Baum J (1985) Thiemann's disease. J Rheumatol 12:150–153
28. Giedion A (1976) Acrodysplasias: peripheral dysostosis, acrodysostosis and Thiemann's disease. Clin Orthop 114:107–115
29. Kuhns LR, Poznanski AK, Harper HA, Garn SM (1973) Ivory epiphyses of the hands. Radiology 109:643–648
30. Kuz JE, Smith JM (1997) Congenital absence of the scaphoid without other congenital abnormality: a case report. J Hand Surg Am 22:489–491
31. Poznanski AK, Iannaccone G, Pasquino AM, Boscherini B (1983) Radiological findings in the hand in Seckel syndrome (bird-headed dwarfism). Pediatr Radiol 13:19–24
32. Poznanski AK, Garn SM, Shaw HA (1976) The carpal angle in congenital malformation syndromes. Ann Radiol 19:141–150
33. Kosowicz J (1962) Carpal sign in gonadal dysgenesis. J Clin Endocrinol Metab 22:949–952
34. Kosowicz J (1965) The roentgen appearance of hand and wrist in gonadal dysgenesis. AJR 93:354–357
35. O'Rahilly R (1953) Survey of carpal and tarsal anomalies. J Bone Joint Surg Am 35:626–642
36. Cockshott WP (1963) Carpal fusions. AJR 89:1260–1264
37. Cope JR (1974) Carpal coalition. Clin Radiol 25:261–266
38. Garn SM, Frisancho AR, Poznanski AK, et al (1971) Analysis of triquetral-lunate fusion. Am J Phys Anthropol 34:431–433
39. Anderson PJ, Hall CM, Evans RD, Jones BM, Hayward RD (1997) Hand anomalies in Crouzon syndrome. Skeletal Radiol 26:113–115
40. Wiles CR, Taylor TFK, Sillence DO (1992) Congenital synspondylism. Am J Med Genet 42:288–295
41. Tyler T, Rosenbaum HD (1976) Idiopathic multicentric osteolysis. AJR 126:23–31
42. Whyte MP, Murphy WA, Kleerekoper M, Teitelbaum SL, Avioli LV (1978) Idiopathic multicentric osteolysis: report of an affected father and son. Arthritis Rheum 21:367–376
43. Renie WA, Pyeritz RE (1981) Idiopathic multicentric osteolysis in a 78-year-old woman. Johns Hopkins Med J 148:165–171
44. Carnevale A, Canun S, Mendoza L, del Castillo V (1987) Idiopathic multicentric osteolysis with facial anomalies and nephropathy. Am J Med Genet 26:877–886
45. Torg JS, DiGeorge AM, Kirkpatrick JA, Trujillo MM (1969) Hereditary multicentric osteolysis with recessive transmission: a new syndrome. J Pediatr 75:243–252
46. Winter RM (1989) Winchester's syndrome. J Med Genet 26:772–775
47. Hajdu N, Kauntze R (1948) Cranioskeletal dysplasia. Br J Radiol 21:42–48
48. Cheney WD (1965) Acro-osteolysis. AJR 94:595–607
49. Giaccai L (1952) Familial and sporadic neurogenic acro-osteolysis. Acta Radiol 38:17–29
50. Lamy M, Maroteaux P (1961) Acro-osteolyse dominante. Arch Franc Pediatr 18:693–702
51. Elias AN, Pinals RS, Anderson HC, Gould LV, Streeten DHP (1978) Hereditary osteodysplasia with acro-osteolysis (the Hajdu-Cheney syndrome). Am J Med 65:627–636
52. O'Reilly MAR, Shaw DG (1994) Hajdu-Cheney syndrome. Ann Rheum Dis 53:276–279
53. Schinz HR, Baensch WE, Friedl E, Uehlinger E (1951) Roentgen-diagnostics. Grune and Stratton, New York
54. Lin S, Marshall EG, Davidson GK, Roth GB, Druschel CM (1993) Evaluation of congenital limb reduction defects in upstate New York. Teratology 47:127–135
55. Bell J (1951) On brachydactyly and symphalangism: I. In: Penrose LS (ed) The treasury of human inheritance. Cambridge University Press, Cambridge
56. Fitch N (1979) Classification and identification of inherited brachydactylies. J Med Genet 16:36–44
57. Steinbach HL, Young DA (1966) The roentgen appearance of pseudohypoparathyroidism (PH) and pseudo-pseudohypoparathyroidism (PPH). Differentiation from other syndromes associated with short metacarpals, metatarsals, and phalanges. AJR 97:49--66
58. Lawrence JJ, Schlesinger AE, Kozlowski K, Poznanski AK, Bacha L, Dreyer GL, Barylak A, Sillence DO, Rager K (1989) Unusual radiographic manifestations of chondrodysplasia punctata. Skeletal Radiol 18:15–19

59. Poznanski AK, Werder EA, Giedion A (1977) The pattern of shortening of the bones of the hand in PHP and PPHP. A comparison with brachydactyly E, Turner syndrome, and acrodysostosis. Pediatr Radiol 123:707–718

60. Archibald RM, Finby N, De Vito F (1959) Endocrine significance of short metacarpals. J Clin Endocrinol Metab 19:1312–1322

61. Slater S (1970) An evaluation of the metacarpal sign (short fourth metacarpal). Pediatrics 46:468–471

62. Spranger S, Weber M, Troger J, Tariverdian G, Opitz JM (1996) Bilateral radial deficiency with lower limb involvement. Am J Med Genet 63:193–197

63. Semmekrot BA, Haraldsson A, Weemaes CM, Smeets DF, Geven WB, Brunner HG (1992) Absent thumb, immune disorder, and congenital anemia presenting with hydrops fetalis. Am J Med Genet 42:736–740

64. James MA, McCarrol HR Jr, Manske PR (1996) Characteristics of patients with hypoplastic thumbs. J Hand Surg [Am] 21:104–113

65. Chinegwundoh JO, Gupta M, Scott WA (1997) Ulnar dimelia. Is it a true duplication of the ulna? J Hand Surg [Br] 22:77–79

66. Ogden JA, Watson HK, Bohne W (1976) Ulnar dysmelia. J Bone Joint Surg Am 58:467–475

67. Swanson AB, Tada K, Yonenobu K (1984) Ulnar ray deficiency: its various manifestations. J Hand Surg [Am] 9:658–664

68. Resnick D (1995) Additional congenital or heritable anomalies and syndromes. In: Resnick D (ed) Diagnosis of bone and joint disorders, 3rd edn. Saunders, Philadelphia, p 4282

69. Blauth W, Falliner A (1986) Morphology and classification of cleft hands. Handchir Mikrochir Plast Chir 18:161–195

70. Balci S, Ercal MD, Atasu M (1993) Robinow syndrome: with special emphasis on dermatoglyphics and hand malformations (split hand). Clin Dysmorphol 2:199–207

71. Franceschini P, Vardeu MP, Dalforno L, Signorile F, Franceschini D, Lala R, Matarazzo P (1992) Possible relationship between ulnar-mammary syndrome and split hand with aplasia of the ulna syndrome. Am J Med Genet 44:807–812

72. Graham JM, Brown FE, Struckmeyer CL, Hallowell C (1986) Dominantly inherited unilateral terminal transverse defects of the hand (adactylia) in twin sisters and one daughter. Pediatrics 78:103–106

73. Harmon JV, Osathanondh R, Holmes LB (1995) Symmetrical terminal transverse limb defects: report of a twenty-week fetus. Teratology 51:237–242

74. Czeizel AE, Kodaj I, Lenz W (1994) Smoking during pregnancy and congenital limb deficiency. BMJ 308:1473–1476

75. Van Allen MI, Siegel-Bartelt J, Dixon J, Zuker RM, Clarke HM, Toi A (1992) Constriction bands and limb reduction defects in two newborns with fetal ultrasound evidence for vascular disruption. Am J Med Genet 44:598–604

76. Miura T, Nakamura R, Imamura T (1987) Polydactyly of the hands and feet. J Hand Surg 12:474–476

77. Goldstein DJ, Kambouris M, Ward RE (1994) Familial crossed polysyndactyly. Am J Med Genet 50:215–223

78. Jones GB (1964) Delta phalanx. J Bone Joint Surg Br 46:226–228

79. Ogden JA, Light TR, Conlogue GJ (1981) Correlative roentgenography and morphology of the longitudinal epiphyseal bracket. Skeletal Radiol 6:109–117

80. Bingle GJ, Niswander JD (1975) Polydactyly in the American Indian. Am J Hum Genet 27:91–99

81. Handforth JR (1950) Polydactylism of hand in southern Chinese. Anat Rec 106:119–125

82. Lewandowski RC, Yunis JJ (1977) Phenotypic mapping in man. In: Yunis JJ (ed) New chromosomal syndromes. Academic Press, New York

83. Castilla EE, Dutra MG, da Fonseca RL, Paz JE (1997; Hand and foot postaxial polydactyly: two different traits. Am J Med Genet 73:48–54

84. Radhakrishna U, Blouin JL, Mehenni H, Patel UC, Patel MN, Solanki JV, Antonarakis SE (1997) Mapping one form of autosomal dominant postaxial polydactyly type A to chromosome 7p15–q11.23 by linkage analysis. Am J Hum Genet 60:597–604

85. Castilla EE, Paz JE, Orioli-Parreiras IM (1980) Syndactyly: frequency of specific types. Am J Med Genet 5:357–364

86. Camera G, Camera A, Pozzolo S, Costa M, Mantero R (1995) Synpolydactyly (type II syndactyly) with aplasia/hypoplasia of the middle phalanges of the toes: report on a family with eight affected members in four generations. Am J Med Genet 55:244–246

87. Brueton LA, Huson SM, Farren B, Winter RM (1990) Oculodentodigital dysplasia and type III syndactyly: separate genetic entities or disease spectrum? J Med Genet 27:169–175

88. Rambaud-Cousson A, Dudin AA, Zuaiter AS, Thalji A (1991) Syndactyly type IV/hexadactyly of feet associated with unilateral absence of the tibia. Am J Med Genet 40:144–145

89. Robinow M, Johnson GF, Broock GJ (1982) Syndactyly type V. Am J Med Genet 11:475–482

90. Lord MJ, Laurenzano KR, Hartmann RW Jr (1990) Poland's syndrome. Clin Pediatr 29:606–609

91. Cushing H (1916) Hereditary ankylosis of proximal phalangeal joints (symphalangism). Genetics 1:90–106

92. Gorlin RJ, Kietzer G, Wolfson J (1970) Stapes fixation and proximal symphalangism. Z Kinderheilkd 108:12–16

93. Learman Y, Katznelson MB, Bonne-Tamir B, Engel J, Hertz M, Goodman RM (1981) Symphalangism with multiple anomalies of the hands and feet: a new genetic trait. Am J Med Genet 10:245–255

94. Poush JR (1991) Distal symphalangism: a report of two families. J Hered 82:233–238

95. Polymeropoulos MH, Poush J, Rubenstein JR, Francomano CA (1995) Localization of the gene (SYM1) for proximal symphalangism to human chromosome 17q21-q22. Genomics 27:225–229

96. Krakow D, Reinker K, Powell B, Cantor R, Priore MA, Garber A, Lachman RS, Rimoin DL, Cohn DH (1998) Localization of a multiple synostoses-syndrome disease gene to chromosome 17q21-22. Am J Hum Genet 63:120–124

97. Martinot-Duquenoy V, Ducos S, Herbaux B, Pellerin P, Debeugny P (1990) Clinodactyly in children. Apropos of 34 cases. Therapeutic choices. Chir Pediatr 31:337–340

98. Fingerhut A, Brocard M, Ronat R (1982) Clinodactylie par brulure electrique. Quelques reflexions à propos de deux cas. Ann Chir Main 1:347–350

99. Frank U, Krimmer H, Hahn P, Lanz U (1997) Surgical therapy of camptodactyly. Handchir Mikrochir Plast Chir 29:284–290

100. Athreya BH, Schumacher HR (1978) Pathologic features of a familial arthropathy associated with congenital flexion contractures of fingers. Arthritis Rheum 21:429–437

101. Hamza M, Bardin T (1989) Camptodactyly, polyepiphyseal dysplasia and mixed crystal deposition disease. J Rheumatol 16:1153–1158

102. Giedion A, Prader A, Fliegel C, Krasikov N, Langer L, Poznanski A (1993) Angel-shaped phalango-epiphyseal dysplasia (ASPED): identification of a new genetic bone marker. Am J Med Genet 47:765–771

103. Chen SH, Huang SC, Wang JH, Wu CT (1997) Macrodactyly of the feet and hands. J Formos Med Assoc 96:901–907

104. Kalen V, Burwell DS, Omer GE (1988) Macrodactyly of the hands and feet. J Pediatr Orthop 8:311–315

105. Goldman AB, Kaye JJ (1977) Macrodystrophia lipomatosa: radiographic diagnosis. AJR 128:101–105

106. Meszaros WT, Guzzo F, Schorsch H (1966) Neurofibromatosis. Am J Roentgenol Radium Ther Nucl Med 98:557–569

107. You CK, Rees J, Gillis DA, Steeves J (1983) Klippel-Trenaunay syndrome: a review. Can J Surg 26:399–403

108. Parrish JD (1960) Heritable disorders of connective tissue. Proc R Soc Med 53:515–521

109. De Oliveira SRP, Moretti-Ferreira D, Contini A, Norato DY (1997) Metacarpophalangeal pattern profile in Marfan and Marfan-like patients. Am J Med Genet 72:159–163

110. Nelle M, Troger J, Rupprath G, Bettendorf M (1994) Metacarpal index in Marfan's syndrome and in constitutional tall stature. Arch Dis Child 70:149–150

111. Rand TC, Edwards DK, Bay CA, Jones KL (1980) The metacarpal index in normal children. Pediatr Radiol 9:31–32

112. Walker TM (1979) The normal metacarpal index. Br J Radiol 52:787–791

113. Miura T, Nakamura R, Horii E, Sano H (1990) Three cases of syndactyly, polydactyly, and hypoplastic triphalangeal thumb (Haas's malformation). J Hand Surg [Am] 15:445–449

114. Halal F, Homsy M, Perreault G (1984) Acro-renal-ocular syndrome: autosomal dominant thumb hypoplasia, renal ectopia, and eye defect. Am J Med Genet 17:753–762

115. Sharma AK, Haldar A, Phadkee SR, Agarwal SS (1994) Preaxial brachydactyly with abduction of thumbs and hallux varus: a distinct entity. Am J Med Genet 49:274–277

116. Tsuyuguchi Y, Yukioka M, Kawabata H, Kawai H, Ono K (1987) Radial ray deficiency. J Pediatr Orthop 7:699–704

117. Giampietro PF, Auerbach AD, Elias ER, Gutman A, Zellers NJ, Davis JG (1998) New recessive syndrome characterized by increased chromosomal breakage and several findings which overlap with Fanconi anemia. Am J Med Genet 78:70–75

118. James MA, McCarrol HR Jr, Manske PR (1996) Characteristics of patients with hypoplastic thumbs. J Hand Surg [Am] 21:104–113

119. Rubinstein JH, Taybi H (1963) Broad thumbs and toes and facial abnormalities. Am J Dis Child 105:588–608

120. Rubinstein JH (1990) Broad thumb-hallux (Rubinstein-Taybi) syndrome 1957–1988. Am J Med Genet Suppl 6:3–16

121. Poznanski AK, Garn SM, Holt JF (1971) The thumb in the congenital malformation syndromes. Radiology 100:115–129

122. Wood VE (1985) Congenital thumb deformities. Clin Orthop 195:7–11

123. Heutink P, Zguricas J, van Oosterhout L, Breedveld GJ, Testers L, Sandkuijl LA, Snijders PJ, Weissenbach J, Lindhout D, Hovius SER, Oostra BA (1994) The gene for triphalangeal thumb maps to the subtelomeric region of chromosome 7q. Nature Genet 6:287–292

124. Zguricas J, Dijkstra PF, Gelsema ES, Snijders PJ, Wustefeld HP, Venema HW, Hoius SE, Lindhout D (1997) Metacarpophalangeal pattern (MCPP) profile analysis in a family with triphalangeal thumb. J Med Genet 34:55–62

125. Fromont NI (1895) Anomalies musculaires multiples de la main, absence du fléchisseur propre du ponce; absence des muscles de l'eminence thénar; lombricaux supplementaire. Bull Soc Anat Paris 70:395–401

126. Graham JM, Brown FE, Hall BD (1987) Thumb polydactyly as a part of the range of genetic expression for thenar hypoplasia. Clin Pediatr 26:142–148

10 The Hand in Endocrine Disorders

Daphne J. Theodorou, Stavroula J. Theodorou, Donald Resnick

Introduction

The hand is well recognized as a mirror of disease for various endocrine disorders. The bones of the hands and wrists comprise more than 25% of the total bones of the skeleton. In and about the hand and wrist, adjacent bones of different shapes and sizes form several joints, and with the surrounding soft tissues they provide the upper extremity with unique, functional capabilities of highly sophisticated and precise mobility. Because of the relative paucity of overlying soft tissue, the hand is accessible to radiographic studies using film without intensifying screens, the latter allowing high resolution imaging of the fine trabecular architecture in the hand. Given that endocrine disorders may be manifested by certain osseous, articular, and soft tissue abnormalities, radiologic evaluation of the hand may provide the clinician with invaluable aid in diagnosing a systemic disorder, particularly in the setting of nonspecific or inconclusive clinical, pathologic, and biochemical findings.

Pituitary, thyroid, and parathyroid disease may severely derange skeletal growth, development, and maturation with musculoskeletal manifestations depending upon the age of onset and duration of the disease. With radiographic examination of the hand and wrist, skeletal growth and maturation may be assessed efficiently. Evaluation of the relative length and width of tubular bones and comparison of measurements between tubular bones, or between digits and the carpal region, may be helpful in the identification of congenital growth disturbances. Thorough radiographic evaluation of the musculoskeletal manifestations of endocrine disorders in the hand, includes assessment of various anatomic structures and interpretation of different pathologic signs. Assessment of the thickness of articular cartilage and synovium, joint effusion, osseous deformity, osteopenia, marginal erosion, and periarticular and subcutaneous calcification or ossification are among the parameters of diagnostic importance in endocrine disease involving the hand. This chapter focuses on the imaging features of endocrine disorders affecting bones, joints, soft tissues, and blood vessels in the hand and wrist, and reviews the differential diagnosis associated with these clinical syndromes.

10.1   Pituitary Disorders

10.1.1   Acromegaly and Gigantism

Hypersecretion of growth hormone (GH, somatotropin) usually secondary to acidophilic adenomas of the anterior lobe of the pituitary gland, or less frequently,
GH hypersecretion associated with diffuse hyperplasia of the acidophilic cells,
leads to different skeletal manifestations depending on the age of the patient. In
the immature skeleton in which growth plates are open, excess production of GH
leads to proportional overgrowth of bone. The resulting clinical syndrome is
termed *pituitary gigantism* and is associated with extreme height and a large
skeleton with normal bone age. In the mature skeleton, after physeal closure, excessive GH production leads to an increase in width of bone and soft tissue enlargement manifested particularly in the acral parts of the skeleton. The resulting
clinical term for this syndrome is *acromegaly* (literally large extremities).

Radiographic manifestations of the hand in patients with acromegaly include
soft tissue thickening of the digits, osseous enlargement and increased width by
means of thickening and squaring of the phalanges and metacarpal bones, over-
constriction or overtubulation of the shafts of the phalanges with normal or increased cortical thickness, widening of the articular spaces due to thickening of
articular cartilage, bone proliferation at tendon and ligament attachment sites
(enthesopathy) simulating peripheral manifestations of diffuse idiopathic skeletal
hyperostosis (DISH), and enlargement of the ungual tufts, which characteristically
may appear spade-like (occasionally with pseudoforamina) (Fig. 10.1). Radiographic changes about the wrist, however, resemble those in the hand [1].

In diagnosing early acromegalic changes in the hand, Kleinberg et al. [2]
introduced the sesamoid index. According to this particular method, the size of
the medial sesamoid at the first metacarpophalangeal joint is measured. The

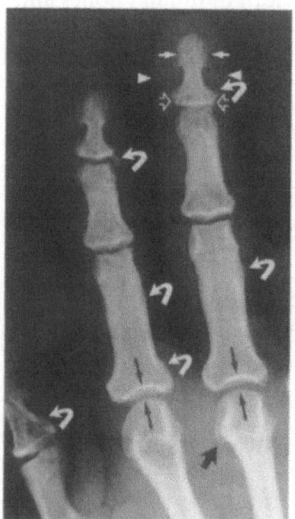

Fig. 10.1. Acromegaly: radiographic features of the hand. Observe
the soft tissue thickening of the digits (*arrowheads*). Enlargement
of the ungual tufts (*small arrows*) and bases of terminal phalanges
(*open arrows*), as well as the broad caliber of all phalanges, can be
appreciated. Small diaphyseal exostoses of the phalanges can be
seen (*curved arrows*). Widening of the metacarpophalangeal joints
(*arrows*) and a beak-like osseous outgrowth on the radial aspect of
the third metacarpal head is noted (*thick arrow*). (Courtesy of P.
Kline, M.D., Denver, Col.)

sesamoid index is the product of the height and length of the sesamoid bone of the first digit. In controls, the sesamoid index was 20 (range 12–29), while in acromegalic patients, the sesamoid index in men was 40 (range 30–63) and in women it was 33 (range 31–35). This study recorded a direct correlation between age and sesamoid index in patients with acromegaly. As indicated by other investigators [3, 4], however, reliability of the sesamoid index in diagnosing acromegaly is limited because of the significant overlap in measurements in acromegalic patients and controls.

Anton [3] used radiographic measurements of the tuftal width of the third finger although he noted highly significant sex differences. He found that a tuft width of 12 mm or more in men, and 10 mm or more in women, was highly diagnostic of acromegaly. In addition, Anton [3] reported that radiographic measurements of the second metacarpophalangeal joint thickness were helpful in evaluating acromegaly. In acromegalic patients, the width of the second metacarpophalangeal joint was 2.4 mm (range 2–3 mm) and in the control group was 1.6 mm (range 1–2.5 mm).

In their investigative study Lin and Lee [5] calculated different measurements of the hand including interstyloid distance, width of the phalanges, width of the fingers, width of the metacarpophalangeal joints, and sesamoid index. These investigators noted considerable variations between the sexes, and significant differences between the acromegalic and control groups. They concluded that although there is no measurement universally specific for acromegaly, the constellation of findings including thickening of the soft tissues of the fingers, widening of the metacarpophalangeal joints with beak-like marginal bone outgrowths, widening of the phalanges, an increased sesamoid index, and an increased interstyloid index, usually allows accurate diagnosis of acromegaly.

As bone resorption accompanies bone proliferation in acromegaly [1], bone density tends to be decreased, particularly in the late stages of disease [6]. However, the most important complication of the disease is secondary osteoarthritis owing to premature degeneration of the excessively stimulated cartilage by the elevated serum GH. As a result, initial joint space widening is followed by joint space narrowing, bone sclerosis, cyst formation, and osteophytosis [1].

Differential diagnosis of acromegaly must include pachydermoperiostosis. In this latter disorder, however, there is mild prominence of the phalangeal tufts without enlargement of the articular space as opposed to the severe enlargement of the phalangeal tufts and articular space seen in acromegaly. However, tuftal enlargement can be a normal finding occurring more commonly in men than in women, and in persons who perform heavy manual labor. Furthermore, irregular excrescences occur in the tufts of senile persons. With regard to the soft tissue thickening seen in acromegaly, similar thickening also can be observed in other diseases, related to edema, hemorrhage, or fatty tissue infiltration. Differential diagnosis of the initial phase of acromegaly from other disease processes is usually straightforward. The later stages of acromegalic joint disease include findings similar to those of primary degenerative joint disease. Involvement of non-weight-bearing joints, prominent osteophytes, and beak-like excrescences of articular bone surfaces are characteristic of acromegaly. Finally, the distribution of degenerative changes in acromegaly may be similar to that in calcium pyrophosphate dihydrate (CPPD) crystal deposition disease. Although acromegaly and CPPD may coexist in the same person, the presence of articular and periarticular calcification, and more severe and progressive joint destruction, are features consistent with CPPD crystal deposition disease [1].

10.1.2 Hypopituitarism

Hypopituitarism is associated with various causative factors including neoplasms, surgery, irradiation, injury, vascular insult, infection, and granulomas of the pituitary gland or the hypothalamus. Familial pituitary deficiency, however, is reported in 10% of cases. Isolated GH deficiency during the period of skeletal growth leads to abnormality of osseous development. The effect on the growing skeleton is a delay in appearance and growth of ossification centers and a similar delay in their fusion and disappearance [7].

Growth failure usually is not apparent at birth but is recognized when the child is 1–3 years of age. Growth in children with hypopituitarism is markedly slow, at the rate of 50–60% of normal, but it is constant. The effect of GH deficiency is greater on length of bones than it is on skeletal maturation [8]. Radiographic manifestations in the hand of patients with hypopituitarism include shortening and broadening of the metacarpal bones and distal phalanges or, less commonly, a hypoplastic appearance of the distal phalanges, metaphyseal irregularity, flattening and absence of closure of the physes, and severe osteoporosis. Open epiphyses may be observed in the distal portions of the radius and ulna as well, but articular abnormalities rarely are seen [7].

In their study of male patients with isolated GH deficiency, Hernandez and coworkers [9] observed that the length of the second metacarpal bone was the most significantly decreased measurement as compared with the chronologic age. In addition, retardation of skeletal maturation, with the carpal bones showing more significant retardation than the tubular bones, was found. Depression in the carpal age was similar to depression in the height age, indicating that the carpal age may correlate closely with height.

Treatment with human GH results in an increase in skeletal maturation paralleling the increase in chronological age, and an increase in cortical thickness [7]. Carpal bones respond more dramatically to treatment than the tubular bones [10], as does the second metacarpal bone [9]. Occasionally, widening of the growth plates may be seen. In addition, treatment with GH may result in metaphyseal sclerosis, although sclerotic "ivory" epiphyses may be seen also in untreated GH deficiency [10].

The differential diagnosis of hypopituitarism includes hypothyroidism, gonadal dysgenesis (Turner's syndrome), malnutrition, diabetes mellitus, chronic renal disease, achondroplasia, rickets, pseudohypoparathyroidism, and neurofibromatosis [7]. Most of these conditions are differentiated easily from hypopituitarism owing to additional and distinctive radiologic findings.

10.2   Thyroid Disorders

10.2.1   Hyperthyroidism

Abnormality in thyroid function can be associated with various factors including alteration in autoimmune mechanisms. Thyroid hormone increases bone remodeling [11] and although both osteoblastic and osteoclastic activities are increased by excessive thyroid hormone, osteoclastic activity predominates, with resultant bone resorption.

Radiographic changes of the skeleton in patients with hyperthyroidism are well known and vary in frequency from 3.5% to 50% [12]. In the hand, *hyperthyroid osteopathy* leads to bone loss which is manifested as a lattice-like appearance in the phalanges, and "flaky" cortices due to radiolucent intracortical striations [12]. Meema and Schatz [13], using magnification techniques, noted cortical striations in the second metacarpal bone in more than 50% of patients with hyperthyroidism. Using radiodensitometry techniques in examining the third metacarpal bone, Fraser and coworkers [14] observed osseous rarefaction in women with hyperthyroidism but not in the control group. Meunier and coworkers [15] also investigated bone resorption in hyperthyroidism and confirmed the presence of linear striations predominantly in cortical bone. Although osteoid seams representing new bone formation by activated osteoblasts have been reported in hyperthyroidism [16], significantly increased cortical bone porosity [11] and an overall decrease in bone density place patients at a higher risk for pathologic fractures [12, 17] and deformity. Decreased bone density in thyrotoxic patients, however, is partially reversible after effective treatment and remains constantly depressed compared with normal levels. A minor radiographic sign in hyperthyroidism is the visualization of Plummer's nails (onycholysis), characterized by material collecting in the undersurface of the nail [18].

In children, hyperthyroidism is associated with abnormalities affecting skeletal maturation. Acceleration of skeletal maturation may be associated with premature physeal fusion and a more advanced skeletal age than expected for the patient's chronological age, the former remaining retarded compared with that of normal children. Riggs and associates [19] published a case of a child 5 weeks old whose skeletal maturation was about 2.5 years; at 3 months, it was 4 years. In their series of neonates with hyperthyroidism, these investigators observed cone epiphyses and early physeal fusion resulting in brachydactyly of the metacarpal bones, and the middle and distal phalanges. In neonates with hyperthyroidism, widening of the middle and distal phalanges of the fingers also may be seen. Bonakdarpour and associates [20] described a case where three carpal ossification centers, as well as some degree of phalangeal ossification, were already present at birth.

Although osteoporosis also may be found in children with hyperthyroidism, severe generalized osteoporosis remains the most important radiographic finding in adult patients. Finally, when hyperthyroidism occurs in association with other autoimmune diseases (e.g., scleroderma, rheumatoid arthritis, systemic lupus erythematosus), the radiographic findings of these diseases also may be manifested in the hand [12].

10.2.2   Thyroid Acropachy

Thyroid acropachy is an unusual manifestation of thyroid disease affecting 0.5–1% of patients with thyrotoxicosis [21]. This disorder usually follows treatment of hyperthyroidism, when the patient is euthyroid or hypothyroid, or it may also occur when patient is in the hyperthyroid state. Thyroid acropachy, also indicated by its Greek name, is the clinical term used to designate thickening of the extremities.

The primary musculoskeletal effect of thyroid acropachy is active periosteal reaction involving most commonly the diaphyses of the metacarpal bones, proximal and middle phalanges, and occasionally the long bones. Terminal tufts usually are spared. From a radiographic standpoint, periostitis is usually asymmetric in distribution and shows a predilection for the radial aspect of the bone. In thyroid acropachy, periostitis is dense and solid in appearance, with a feathery or spiculated contour (Fig. 10.2). Thick, shaggy periosteal new bone formation may produce irregular enlargement of the bone [22].

Soft tissue manifestations of thyroid acropachy include localized swelling and digital clubbing [23]. Osseous abnormalities in thyroid acropachy are not progressive; however, resolution of the condition is poorly correlated with correction of thyroid function [22].

Differential diagnosis in thyroid acropachy should include other diseases associated with periosteal bone formation. Hypertrophic osteoarthropathy is characterized by bony proliferation but the distribution, location and pattern of periostitis are different. In pachydermoperiostosis periosteal reaction is not limited to bone diaphyses, whereas in hypervitaminosis A, venous stasis, vascular insufficiency, infectious and traumatic disorders, and additional clinical and radiographic features, permit accurate diagnosis [22].

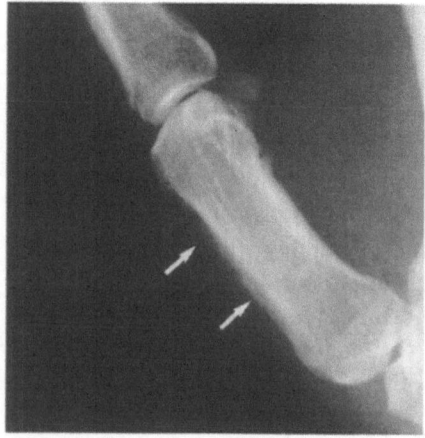

Fig. 10.2. Thyroid acropachy: radiographic features of the hand. Note the extensive, spiculated periosteal new bone formation predominating along the radial aspect of the diaphysis of the first metacarpal bone (*arrows*). (Courtesy of G. Greenway, M.D., Dallas, Tex.)

10.2.3 Hypothyroidism

Hypothyroidism and *myxedema* are general terms indicating physiologic and bio-chemical abnormalities that result from deficiency of the thyroid hormones. In the primary form of hypothyroidism, hormonal deficiency is attributed to dysfunction of the thyroid gland itself, whereas in the secondary form of hypothyroidism there is deficiency in thyroid stimulating hormone. The causes of hypothyroidism are variable and include thyroiditis (Hashimoto's disease), damage to the thyroid gland after surgery or radioactive iodine therapy, deficiency in iodine, thyroid atrophy, neoplastic and infiltrative disorders (lymphoma, metastasis, amyloidosis), and pituitary disorders.

Musculoskeletal effects of hypothyroidism depend upon the age of onset and duration of the disorder. Congenital thyroid deficiency (cretinism) and hypothyroidism in children (juvenile myxedema) are associated with severe developmental abnormalities. In adult-onset hypothyroidism, bone abnormalities are mild [24]. In neonates, children, and young adults, the primary skeletal manifestation of hypothyroidism is retardation of skeletal maturation resulting in retardation in growth.

From a radiographic standpoint, delayed appearance and growth of epiphyseal ossification centers are most characteristic, and abnormality of physeal development is accompanied by delayed physeal closure. Despite persistence of the physeal growth plate, longitudinal growth of bones is diminished as the plate itself is "closed off" by osseous tissue of the metaphysis, which is apposed to the cartilage growth zone [24]. In the hand, arrest in growth is manifested as shortening and widening of the metacarpal bones, which present endosteal cortical thickening [25]. The ratio of the second metacarpal bone length to skeletal age is greater than 1 [26]. Hypoplastic phalanges of fifth finger may be seen [27]. A distinctive osseous projection in the mid-portion of the metaphyses of the distal phalanges also has been described in 79% of patients with untreated hypothyroidism [28]; this finding however, resolves with therapy.

In affected epiphyses, ossification proceeds from multiple centers rather than from a single site (pseudoepiphyses). Abnormal epiphyseal ossification results in a characteristic irregular and fragmented epiphyseal appearance recognized as epiphyseal dysgenesis [29, 30]. In hypothyroidism, epiphyses tend to be stippled during infancy, fragmented during childhood, and cone-shaped during adolescence [27]. In the hand, fragmented ossification of carpal centers or phalangeal epiphyses may be an occasional radiographic finding [31]. With appropriate treatment, epiphyseal dysgenesis may resolve. Delayed or inadequate therapy, however, may lead to secondary articular degeneration, intra-articular osseous and cartilaginous bodies, and deformity [24]. Despite effective thyroid replacement therapy, the carpal scaphoid often remains deformed after other carpal centers have gradually re-formed [25]. An additional helpful diagnostic sign of hypothyroidism is the rapid improvement in ossification that results during therapy [24]. Lusted and Pickering [31] showed that serial radiographs of the hand and wrist obtained during therapy with thyroid hormone are the most sensitive indicators for assessing advancing skeletal maturation. Increased radiopacity of epiphyses and metaphyses, particularly about the radius and ulna, also has been noted in hypothyroid patients [32]. Increased bone sclerosis, however, may be seen in association with soft tissue calcific deposits [33].

Finally, a wide spectrum of additional disorders may be seen in hypothyroid patients. Included among them are carpal tunnel syndrome, synovial thickening and effusion in the metacarpophalangeal joints and wrists, calcium pyrophosphate dihydrate (CPPD) crystal deposition with joint space narrowing, ligament laxity and intra-articular osseous bodies, osteoporosis, and bilateral destructive arthropathy with predilection for the proximal interphalangeal joints [24]. Connective tissue diseases including rheumatoid arthritis, systemic lupus erythematosus, and seronegative polyarthritis, also have been described in patients with Hashimoto's disease, probably relating to an autoimmune reaction [24].

10.3   Parathyroid Disorders and Renal Osteodystrophy

10.3.1   Hyperparathyroidism

Hyperparathyroidism is the term describing a clinical state of elevation of serum parathyroid hormone concentration. The condition may be primary, secondary, or tertiary. In primary hyperparathyroidism, hypersecretion of parathyroid hormone is due to abnormality in the parathyroid glands. Hyperparathyroidism may have many causes, including single or multiple adenomas, diffuse hyperplasia, and carcinoma. Secondary hyperparathyroidism usually is secondary to chronic renal disease (in the latter case rickets or osteomalacia coexist) or, occasionally, malabsorption states including pancreatic insufficiency and nontropical sprue. Tertiary hyperparathyroidism occurs in patients with chronic renal disease and secondary hyperparathyroidism who develop autonomous parathyroid function.

In hyperparathyroidism, initial osseous involvement may be mild and inconspicuous on radiographic evaluation, although histopathologic examination of bone reveals exaggerated osteoclastic activity on the surface of trabeculae within the cancellous bone and on the walls of the haversian canals within the cortical bone [34]. The hand is almost always involved in hyperparathyroidism, and radiographs may provide considerable aid in establishing the diagnosis when clinical findings are not specific. The sensitivity of bone resorption in the hands in the early stages of the disease has been documented repeatedly, indicating that high-quality radiography (with macroradiography or digitized radiography) of this region is adequate in detecting and monitoring the course of skeletal changes in primary and secondary hyperparathyroidism [35].

Subperiosteal bone resorption is most frequently observed along the radial aspect of the phalanges of the hand, particularly in the middle phalanges of the index and middle fingers, whereas the ulnar aspect is usually spared [35] (Fig. 10.3). There is a lace-like appearance of the phalangeal bone, which may progress

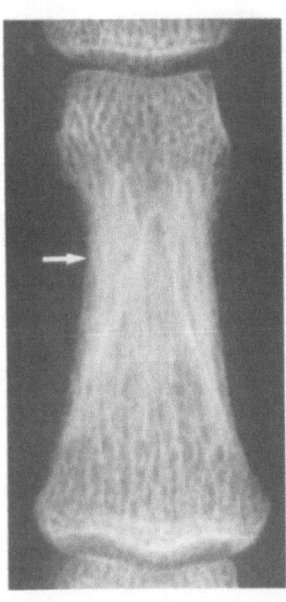

Fig. 10.3. Hyperparathyroidism: radiographic features of the hand. Observe the subperiosteal bone resorption, most evident on the radial aspect of the middle phalanx (*arrow*)

to a spiculated contour and ,eventually, to complete resorption of the entire cortex with loss of definition between cortex and spongiosa. Subperiosteal bone resorption involves the phalangeal tufts as well, where loss of the cortical "white line" represents the earliest sign of disease [36] (Fig. 10.4). It should be differentiated carefully from the normal contour irregularity of the tufts. Furthermore, a distinctive pattern of acro-osteolysis in the terminal phalanges of the hands consists of band-like radiolucent areas that may separate the tuft and the base of the phalanx completely [35] (Fig. 10.5). With osseous healing, brachydactyly or soft tissue clubbing may be seen.

Subperiosteal bone resorption also may be evident at the margins of joints in the hand and wrist, simulating changes of rheumatoid arthritis, although in some places the erosions are intra-articular (Fig. 10.4). They also may be juxta-articular, located slightly farther from the joint margin, and usually they are associated with resorption of the adjacent phalangeal shafts. Furthermore, this pattern of subperiosteal resorption of bone predominates on the ulnar aspect of the metacarpal heads (compared with a radial predilection in rheumatoid arthritis), involves the distal interphalangeal joints sparing proximal interphalangeal joints (compared with the opposite situation in rheumatoid arthritis), is associated with a normal-appearing joint space (compared with early joint space narrowing in rheumatoid arthritis), and is characterized by a shaggy, irregular osseous contour with bony "whiskering" (compared with the mild or absent bone proliferation in rheumatoid arthritis) [35].

In hyperparathyroidism, subperiosteal resorption of bone almost always is associated with intracortical resorption [35]. Superficial intracortical bone loss produces pseudoperiostitis [35]. Because of rapid or severe bone loss, multiple intracortical, radiolucent areas may be observed in the metacarpal cortex (Fig. 10.6).

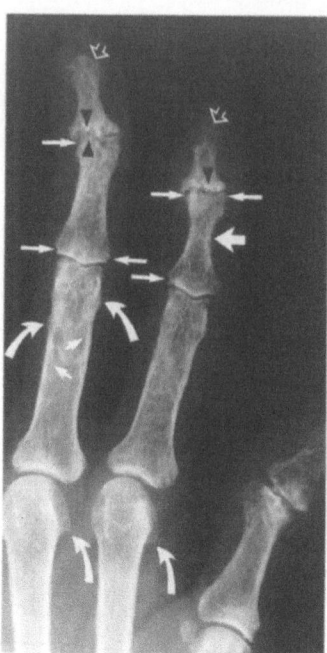

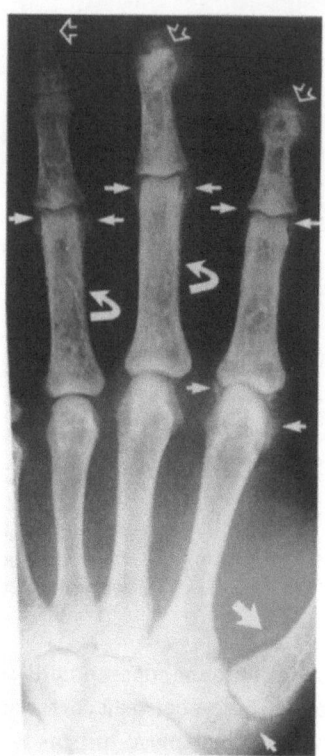

Fig. 10.4. Hyperparathyroidism: radiographic features of the hand. Subperiosteal bone resorption involving the phalangeal tufts with loss of definition of the cortical "white line" of the tufts is observed (*open arrows*). At the distal interphalangeal joints, severe subchondral bone resorption (*arrowheads*) can be seen. Associated subperiosteal resorption at the corners of the joints (*arrows*) results in a squared appearance of the phalanges. Note the severe subperiosteal bone resorption prominent on the radial aspect of the second middle phalanx (*thick arrow*). Hook-like erosions occur on the phalanges and metacarpal heads (*curved arrows*). The phalanges appear diffusely abnormal. Endosteal bone resorption and scalloping of the endosteal margin of the cortex of the proximal phalanges (*small arrows*) can be appreciated. (Courtesy of A. Brower, M.D., Norfolk, Va.)

Fig. 10.5. Hyperparathyroidism: radiographic features of the hand. Severe acro-osteolysis with complete destruction of the phalangeal tufts is evident (*open arrows*). Observe the extensive periarticular soft tissue calcification (*arrows*), subperiosteal bone resorption (*curved arrows*), and vascular calcification (*thick arrow*)

These intracortical linear striations or tunneling are best visualized in the cortex of the second metacarpal bone [37].

In the hand, osteoclastic resorption occurs along the endosteal surface of bone. Radiographic findings include localized scalloped or pocket-like defects along the endosteal margin of the cortex (Fig. 10.4), which can simulate abnormalities occurring in multiple myeloma, and more generalized cortical thinning, which can simulate abnormalities of osteoporosis [35].

Subchondral resorption of bone occasionally can be seen in the hands and wrists of patients with hyperparathyroidism. Given that subperiosteal resorption,

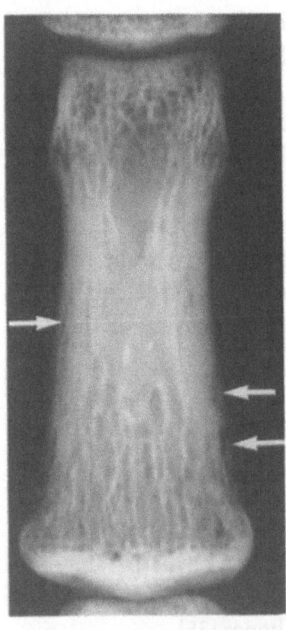

Fig. 10.6. Hyperparathyroidism: radiographic features of the hand. Observe the intracortical bone resorption manifested as multiple radiolucencies of the phalangeal cortices (*arrows*). (Courtesy of C. Gundry, M.D., Minneapolis, Minn.)

"osteogenic" synovitis, and crystal-induced arthritis also may occur in hyperparathyroidism, it often is hard to ascertain the exact contribution of subchondral resorption to the radiographic appearance of joint abnormalities in the hand and wrist. Furthermore, in the clinical setting of chronic renal disease and dialysis, factors such as renal osteodystrophy, dialysis bone disease, amyloidosis, and CPPD, urate, calcium hydroxyapatite, and oxalate crystal deposition contribute essentially in the production of intra- and periarticular erosive alterations [35].

In children with primary or secondary hyperparathyroidism, irregular radiolucent areas may be apparent in the metaphysis adjacent to the growth plate of tubular bones of the hand [35]. In the absence of osteomalacia, these metaphyseal alterations are attributable to hyperparathyroidism. Using sequential radiographic examinations in patients with chronic renal failure, Young and coworkers [38] observed progressive metaphyseal sclerosis, which in some cases persisted even after fusion of the adjacent physis. Growth plate fracture involving the bones of the hands may occasionally occur in secondary hyperparathyroidism and renal osteodystrophy [39].

In the hyperparathyroid state, osseous resorption may occur at sites of tendon and ligament attachment to bone [35] and this also may apply to the hand and wrist. Trabecular resorption within medullary bone, particularly in the advanced stages of the disease, may involve the tubular bones of the hand. Bone assumes a characteristic granular appearance, with loss of distinct trabecular detail, and subsequent osseous deformities may simulate the changes of osteomalacia [35].

Brown tumors, or osteoclastomas, are included among the radiographic manifestations of hyperparathyroidism. Although they were described initially in primary hyperparathyroidism, brown tumors occur with greater frequency in secondary hyperparathyroidism. Brown tumors represent localized accumulations of osteoclasts, fibrous tissue, and giant cells, which can replace bone and occasionally produce osseous expansion. They appear as single or multiple well or poorly demarcated osteolytic lesions with an eccentric or cortical location [35]. Following removal of the parathyroid adenoma, brown tumors may present healing with increased radiodensity.

A prominent radiographic feature of hyperparathyroidism is generalized osteopenia. Fine-detail, magnification radiography and quantitative bone mineral analysis may be of substantial help in detecting not only the degree and rate of bone loss in the early stages of disease, but also a partial recovery of this loss following therapeutic parathyroidectomy.

As hyperparathyroidism may induce either bone resorption or formation, increased radiodensity of bones may become a prominent radiographic feature. Osteosclerosis is observed more frequently in patients with renal osteodystrophy and secondary hyperparathyroidism, although it also may be evident in primary hyperparathyroidism. Diffuse increase of bone density may be seen in patients with secondary hyperparathyroidism and, rarely, in the primary form of disease. In primary hyperparathyroidism, bone sclerosis may be localized or patchy, with close-meshed thickened spongy trabeculae, evident in the metaphyseal regions of the long bones [35].

There is a meaningful association between primary hyperparathyroidism and CPPD crystal deposition that may lead to the pseudogout syndrome. Less frequently, CPPD crystal deposition may occur in chronic renal disease. Radiographic features of such crystal deposition usually are related to the presence of cartilage calcification (chondrocalcinosis), although deposits in intra-articular and periarticular structures also may be observed (Fig. 10.7). However, patients with hyperparathyroidism and CPPD crystal deposition also may develop structural

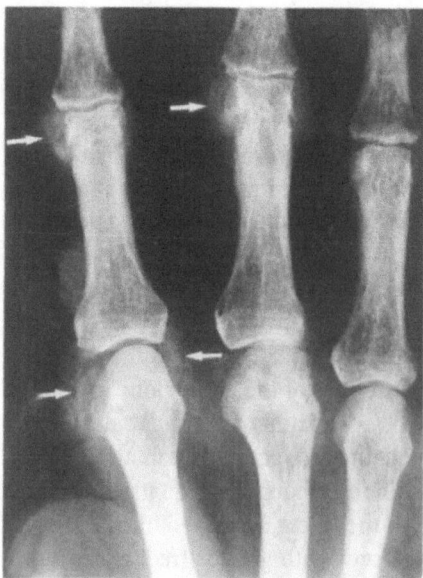

Fig. 10.7. Hyperparathyroidism and calcium pyrophosphate dihydrate (CPPD) crystal deposition disease: radiographic features of the hand. In this patient with primary hyperparathyroidism and CPPD crystal deposition, extensive periarticular calcification can be seen in the metacarpophalangeal and proximal interphalangeal joints (*arrows*). (Courtesy of M. Recht, M.D., Cleveland, Ohio)

joint damage (pyrophosphate arthropathy) characterized by osteosclerosis, osteophytosis, and joint space narrowing [35] (Fig. 10.8).

In addition to these clinical and radiographic features of hyperparathyroidism, other rheumatic manifestations also may be encountered. In particular, findings may relate to subperiosteal bone resorption at the margins of the joint, subchondral resorption leading to cartilage and bone disintegration and fragmentation (Fig. 10.9), subligamentous and subtendinous resorption, intra-articular crystal deposition in cartilage, synovium and capsule, periarticular crystal deposition in soft tissues, and tendinous and ligamentous injury and rupture [35]. Because parathyroid hormone may affect ligaments and tendons themselves, resultant capsular and ligamentous laxity, as well as rupture, may be contributory to joint instability, cartilaginous and osseous destruction, and traumatic synovitis [35]. In the hand, spontaneous tendon avulsion and tendinous rupture in either primary or secondary hyperparathyroidism can involve the flexor and extensor tendons of the fingers. Ligamentous laxity however, may result in subluxation at the metacarpophalangeal and phalangophalangeal joints (Fig. 10.10). Finally, an association between rheuma-

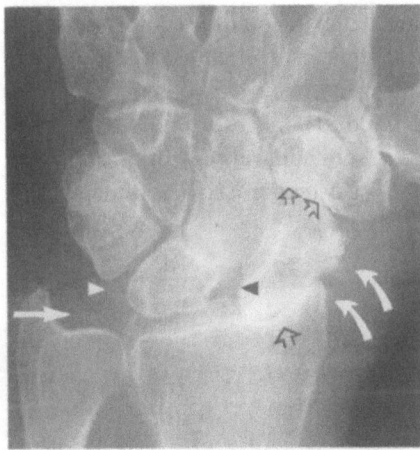

Fig. 10.8. Hyperparathyroidism and calcium pyrophosphate dihydrate (CPPD) crystal deposition disease: radiographic features of the wrist. In a different patient with primary hyperparathyroidism and CPPD crystal deposition, observe the intra-articular calcification (*arrowheads*), chondrocalcinosis in the triangular fibrocartilage complex (*arrow*), and severe structural joint deformity (pyrophosphate arthropathy) most prominent in the radiocarpal, scaphotrapezium, and scaphotrapezoid joints (*open arrows*). Note the osteophyte formation in the distal radius and scaphoid bone (*curved arrows*) (Courtesy of M. Austin, M.D., Newport Beach, Calif.)

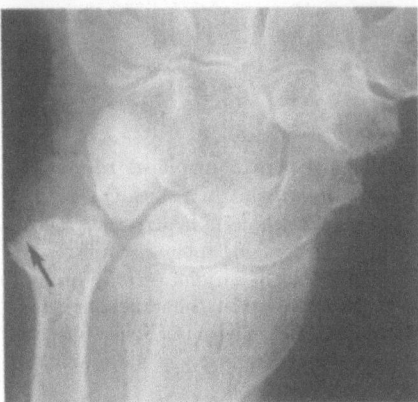

Fig. 10.9. Hyperparathyroidism: radiographic features of the distal ulna. Observe the considerable bone resorption (*arrow*) in the distal ulna. (Courtesy of A. Brower, M.D., Norfolk, Va.)

toid arthritis or rheumatoid arthritis-like syndromes, gouty arthritis, and hyperparathyroidism has been suggested [40].

Primary hyperparathyroidism in infants and children may have its counterpart in radiographic changes. Severe osseous involvement with subperiosteal resorption in both metaphyses and epiphyses, extensive erosions of tubular bones, osteopenia, marked periostitis, and pathologic fractures are findings frequently encountered in hyperparathyroid children. A second, self-limited disorder, transient hyperparathyroidism of the neonate, occurring secondary to hypoparathyroidism in the mother, presents radiographic changes similar to congenital primary hyperparathyroidism. Radiographic changes of the skeleton in older children with hyperparathyroidism include clubbing of the fingers, osteopenia, cystic lesions of bone, metaphyseal irregularity, and fractures [35] (Fig. 10.11).

The combination of radiographic findings in hyperparathyroidism is adequately characteristic that precise diagnosis is not difficult, although individual radiographic signs, which are evident in this disease, may be encountered also in other disorders.

Extensive subperiosteal resorption of bone is a typical sign of hyperparathyroidism, whereas focal areas of subperiosteal bone resorption may be seen in different processes including tumor, infection, gout, and xanthomatosis. In the latter disorders, contour defects in bone are better defined in comparison with defects in hyperparathyroidism. Intracortical bone resorption may be observed in hyperthyroidism and acromegaly, while endosteal bone resorption may be noted in osteoporosis and multiple myeloma. Subchondral bone resorption may be associated with osteoporosis, although widespread subchondral resorption and articular collapse are rarely encountered features of osteoporosis. Severe depression

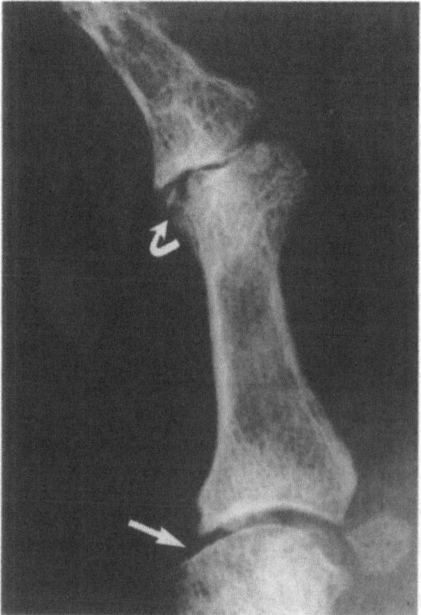

Fig. 10.10. Hyperparathyroidism: radiographic features of the hand. In a patient with the osseous manifestations of hyperparathyroidism, observe the minimal subluxation at the first metacarpophalangeal joint (*arrow*), owing to ligamentous laxity. Subchondral bone resorption at the interphalangeal joint, is evident (*curved arrow*). (Courtesy of A. Brower, M.D., Norfolk, Va.)

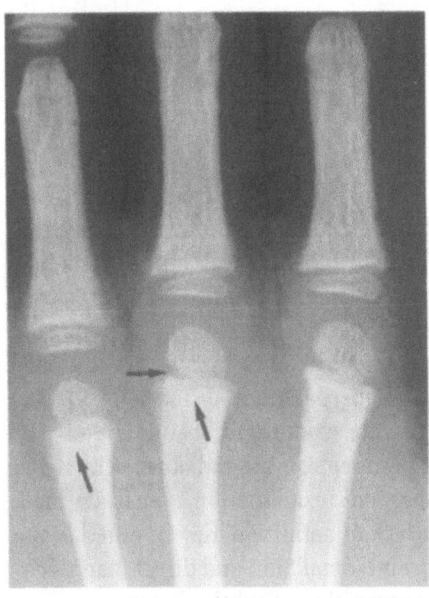

Fig. 10.11. Secondary hyperparathyroidism: radiographic features of the hand. Observe the irregular and widened physes in the metacarpal bones (*arrows*) related to hyperparathyroidism

and fragmentation of subchondral bone in hyperparathyroidism may resemble the findings of osteonecrosis, septic arthritis, or crystal-induced arthropathy. In the interphalangeal joints of the hand, changes may simulate inflammatory osteoarthritis, psoriasis, or rheumatoid arthritis.

In hyperparathyroidism, brown tumors resemble various neoplastic or neoplastic-like diseases, including giant cell tumor and fibrous dysplasia. Diffuse bone sclerosis also is common in fluorosis, hypoparathyroidism, irradiation, sickle cell anemia, metastatic neoplasm, sarcoidosis, mastocytosis, Paget's disease, and myelofibrosis. CPPD crystal deposition associated with primary and, less commonly, secondary hyperparathyroidism is identical to that occurring in idiopathic CPPD crystal deposition disease and hemochromatosis. Monosodium urate crystal deposition (secondary gout) in hyperparathyroidism resembles primary gout, although involvement of unusual articular sites is more common in secondary gout. Finally, severe periostitis and extensive bone resorption in hyperparathyroid children may resemble the findings of syphilis or leukemia [35].

10.3.2   Renal Osteodystrophy

Renal osteodystrophy is the clinical term indicating bone disease in patients with chronic renal failure. The cause of chronic renal insufficiency is variable and includes inflammatory disorders, congenital abnormalities of the urinary tract, and obstructive uropathy. The radiographic manifestations of renal osteodystrophy reflect hyperparathyroidism and deficiency of 1,25-dihydroxyvitamin D [$1,25(OH)_2D$], rickets and osteomalacia, osteoporosis, soft tissue and vascular calcification, and miscellaneous changes. Skeletal involvement in renal osteodystrophy has been well documented.

Musculoskeletal abnormalities include osteitis fibrosa cystica, rickets or osteomalacia (or both), osteoporosis, osteosclerosis, soft tissue and vascular calcification, and miscellaneous changes.

10.3.2.1 Hyperparathyroidism

As with primary hyperparathyroidism, radiographic features in renal osteodystrophy with *secondary hyperparathyroidism* include subperiosteal, intracortical, endosteal, trabecular, subchondral, subligamentous and subcutaneous bone resorption, brown tumors, bone sclerosis, and chondrocalcinosis, although the frequency of some of these findings may be different in renal osteodystrophy with secondary hyperparathyroidism compared with primary hyperparathyroidism [41].

In adults, the earliest radiographic changes most commonly are observed in the hands. Subperiosteal resorption of bone prominent on the radial aspects of the index and long fingers is visualized on radiographic examination as an ill-defined, blunt "lacy" outline of the cortex. A similar lack of definition may be noted in the cortex of the terminal phalangeal tufts [41]. Fine-detail film and direct magnification may be of invaluable help in the early recognition of subtle changes.

In patients with renal osteodystrophy and secondary hyperparathyroidism, brown tumors are reported with increasing frequency, although they occur less frequently than they do in primary hyperparathyroidism. In renal osteodystrophy, brown tumors generally are single and may be the presenting feature of the disease. In brown tumors, progressive osteolysis and cortical expansion (Fig. 10.12) may result in pathologic fracture [41].

Osteosclerosis (increased bone density) is a well-known feature of renal osteodystrophy involving most commonly the axial skeleton, although the appendicular

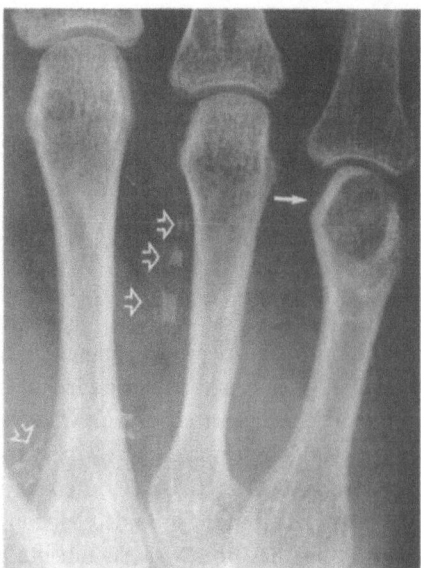

Fig. 10.12. Renal osteodystrophy: radiographic features of the hand. In this patient with chronic renal disease and secondary hyperparathyroidism, a brown tumor of the fifth metacarpal bone manifested as a well-defined osteolytic area with cortical expansion can be observed (*arrow*). Note the extensive vascular calcification (*open arrows*)

skeleton also may be involved, particularly the metaphyseal regions of long bones.

Periosteal neostosis represents periosteal bone formation in patients with renal osteodystrophy and is most commonly seen in those patients with severe hyperparathyroid bone disease. In the hand, periosteal neostosis occurs in the metacarpal bones and phalanges and tends to assume an asymmetric distribution. Monostotic involvement is rarely encountered. On radiographic examination, periosteal neostosis is manifested as laminated periosteal new bone formation and usually a radiolucent zone is visualized between the periosteal and host bone; fusion of the two areas finally may occur [41] (Fig. 10.13).

Following renal transplantation, further osteopenia resulting from the combined effects of steroid therapy and continued secondary hyperparathyroidism may occur.

In uremia, soft tissue calcifications may occur in skeletal muscle (amorphous calcium deposition), periarticular areas in the capsule and tendons of large and small joints (hydroxyapatite deposition, or amorphous calcium deposition), and arteries (Fig. 10.12). Chondrocalcinosis due to CPPD crystal deposition is not as common as it is in primary hyperparathyroidism. Localized cartilage calcification in the triangular fibrocartilage complex (TFCC) of the wrist has been observed [42], although widespread chondrocalcinosis and pyrophosphate arthropathy are rare manifestations of this disorder.

10.3.2.2 Rickets and Osteomalacia

Rickets and osteomalacia are general terms indicating pathologic, histologic, biochemical, and radiologic abnormalities that result from inadequate or delayed mineralization of osteoid in mature cortical and spongy bone (osteomalacia) and an interruption in orderly development and mineralization of the growth plate

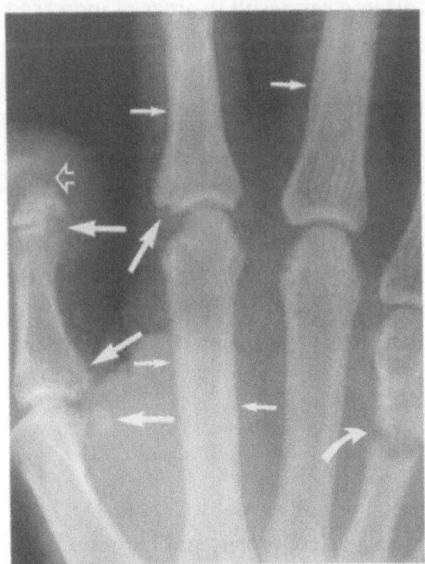

Fig. 10.13. Renal osteodystrophy: radiographic features of the hand. In this patient with renal osteodystrophy, periosteal neostosis is manifest as thick, laminated periosteal new bone formation (*arrows*). Observe the pathologic fracture in the mid-diaphysis of the fourth metacarpal bone (*curved arrow*). Acro-osteolysis (*open arrow*), subperiosteal and subchondral bone resorption (*long arrows*) are additional features of secondary hyperparathyroidism. (Courtesy of A. Brower, M.D., Norfolk, Va.)

(rickets) [43]. Osteomalacia occurs in association with chronic renal disease, and although factors such as absence of 1,25-dihydroxycholecalciferol, deficiency or resistance to vitamin D, and malabsorption of calcium contribute to bone disease, the precise cause of osteomalacia is not well defined. Rachitic abnormalities of bone are common in children with chronic renal disease. Rickets-like changes also may be seen in children with primary hyperparathyroidism.

Regardless of their causes, the osteomalacic and rachitic syndromes display remarkably similar histologic and radiographic features [43]. Because rachitic changes are more evident in regions of the most active bone growth, in the hand target sites of rickets include the distal ends of ulna and radius [44]. General radiographic features of rickets include retardation in bone growth and osteopenia. Alterations appearing at the growth plate are characteristic of the disease, as slight axial widening at the physis represents the earliest specific radiographic finding [45]. This is followed by a decrease in bone density on the metaphyseal side of the growth plate. Progressive widening and irregularity of the growth plate may be observed. Disorganization and "fraying" of the spongy bone occur in the metaphyseal region, which eventually demonstrates widening and cupping [43]. In the hand of rachitic children, irregularities and widening of the physes seen in the metacarpals and phalanges also may be associated with changes in bone resorption. Slipped epiphyses in the distal portion of the radius and ulna and, on rare occasions, in the small bones of the hand, also may be seen [46]. Swelling about joints is an additional feature of rickets.

Radiographic diagnosis of osteomalacia may be challenging, as changes such as osteopenia are nonspecific for the disease. Medullary bone shows a decrease in the total number of trabeculae, owing to a loss of secondary trabeculae (Fig. 10.14). The remaining bone trabeculae are prominent and present a "coarsened" pattern with unsharp margins reflecting deposition of inadequately mineralized osteoid. Deposition of immature osteoid in the cortical bone is manifested as lucent sites [43]. Nevertheless, excessive deposition of osteoid can result in areas of increased radiodensity. Looser's zones, or pseudofractures, are a feature of osteomalacia. They appear as broad radiolucent bands, perpendicular to the cortex, with defined, mild to moderately sclerotic margins, and absence of callus formation.

10.3.2.3 Osteoporosis

In renal osteodystrophy, osteopenia is an additional feature. Decreased bone density, however, results not only from osteoporosis, but also from osteitis fibrosa cystica and osteomalacia. Cortical thinning observed in renal osteodystrophy is due to osteoporosis and endosteal and subperiosteal resorption of hyperparathyroidism.

10.3.2.4 Fractures

Pathologic fractures are a complication of renal osteodystrophy (Fig. 10.13). They result from hyperparathyroidism, osteomalacia, osteoporosis, and aluminum in-

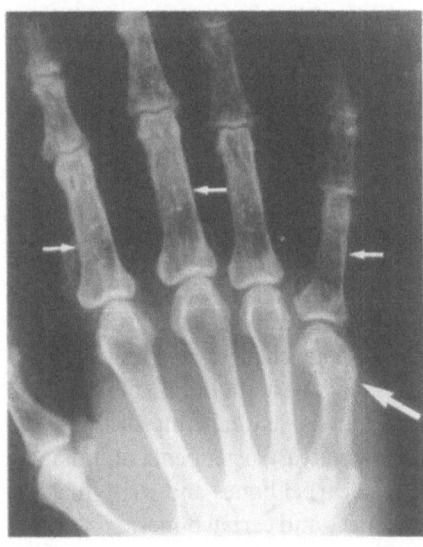

Fig. 10.14. Renal osteodystrophy and osteomalacia: radiographic features of the hand. In this patient with renal osteodystrophy, note the typical findings of osteomalacia, which include thin cortex of the tubular bones of the hand (*arrows*), and sparse or absent bone trabeculae. Deformity of the fifth metacarpal bone owing to a healed fracture, can be seen (*long arrow*)

toxication [43]. Fractures also may be seen in areas of brown tumors. Insufficiency fractures may be observed in the short tubular bones of the hand of uremic patients.

10.3.2.5 Soft Tissue and Vascular Calcification

Soft tissue calcification in renal osteodystrophy can be prominent and can lead to symptoms and signs that simulate the findings of articular disease [43]. Soft tissue deposits in the musculoskeletal system can occur in viscera, vasculature (Fig. 10.12), and subcutaneous and periarticular tissue. Calcium hydroxyapatite material tends to accumulate in subcutaneous tissues, vessels, and periarticular regions, whereas magnesium whitlockite-like material accumulates in muscles. In chronic renal disease, calcific deposition in periarticular regions may induce an acute aseptic inflammatory reaction of soft tissues, including tendon sheaths. In the wrists, periarticular calcific deposits may be of significant size and may produce patchy or tumoral radiodense areas [43]. Bilateral symmetric deposits about multiple joints are common and, in some instances, may be associated with radiodense lesions in the joint capsule. In uremic disease, ligamentous calcification may also be seen. Bone erosions beneath periarticular calcific accumulations associated with intra-articular hydroxyapatite crystal deposition can be noted.

10.3.2.6 Miscellaneous Abnormalities

Because patients with chronic renal failure have hyperuricemia, they may develop gouty arthritis. Radiographic findings of secondary gout simulate those of primary gout, with eccentric bone erosions and asymmetric soft tissue swelling [43]. Long-standing gouty arthritis may lead to destruction of the involved metacarpophalangeal or interphalangeal joint. Oxalosis of bone may be an additional secondary manifestation of chronic renal insufficiency.

10.3.3   Hemodialysis and Renal Transplantation

Most of the musculoskeletal manifestations in patients undergoing hemodialysis, peritoneal dialysis, or renal transplantation are secondary to renal osteodystrophy. During treatment, these manifestations are modified to some extent, and additional manifestations related to the type of therapy become evident as well.

With sufficient hemodialysis, many of the osseous changes of renal osteodystrophy may resolve. The effect of hemodialysis on hyperparathyroid bone disease and osteomalacia, however, may vary, as hemodialysis may halt, improve, or worsen bone disease. Inadequate hemodialysis may increase osteopenia and may be associated with pathologic fractures in the metacarpal bones and wrist. In addition, dialysis cysts tend to develop in the phalanges and carpal bones.

10.3.3.1   Aluminum Toxicity

Patients with chronic renal disease may develop aluminum toxicity, resulting in a low-turnover osteomalacia, termed *dialysis osteomalacia* or *aluminum osteomalacia.* The source of the aluminum is related to the contents of phosphate binding gels or the ambient water or dialysate, or to the orally administered aluminum-containing phosphate-binding medications prescribed for uremic patients. In children, aluminum contamination may contribute to rachitic bone disease.

Aluminum accumulation at the interface between bone and unmineralized osteoid inhibits mineralization. Aluminum "contamination" blocks skeletal uptake of bone, resulting in hypercalcemia and development of secondary hypoparathyroidism. Radiographic manifestations of aluminum-associated osteopathy include osteopenia, rachitic alterations at the physeal zones, and pathologic fractures [47]. In the musculoskeletal system, high aluminum levels are found not only in bone, but also in the synovial membrane, cartilage, and joint fluid.

10.3.3.2   Soft Tissue and Vascular Calcification

Soft tissue and vascular calcification are common findings in patients treated with hemodialysis, and large tumoral deposits occur with highest frequency in this condition. During dialysis, reversal of periarticular and, less frequently, vascular calcification may be observed.

10.3.3.3   Musculoskeletal Infection

Included among the potential complications of hemodialysis and renal transplantation are septicemia, osteomyelitis, and septic arthritis [48]. Arteriovenous fistulae are an ideal site of entry for infectious organisms. Staphylococci, streptococci,

Pseudomonas spp., *Mycobacterium* spp., and fungi are the pathogens most commonly involved in osteomyelitis and septic arthritis.

10.3.3.4   Carpal Tunnel Syndrome

Carpal tunnel syndrome is a well-recognized complication of renal hemodialysis that usually is attributed to alterations in vascular hemodynamics at the access site, resulting in edema, venous distention, and compression of the medial nerve within the carpal canal. Deposition of amyloid occurs in the synovium and adjacent tendons, as well as in the accompanying small cystic lesions in the carpal bones [48].

10.3.3.5   Amyloid Deposition

The association of amyloid deposition with renal hemodialysis is well recognized. In patients receiving hemodialysis, deposition of beta-2-microglobulin occurs in the wrist, which may result in carpal tunnel syndrome. Musculoskeletal manifestations of beta-2-microglobulin-associated amyloidosis include periarticular soft tissue masses, cystic lesions in long and short tubular bones, pathologic fractures, joint subluxations and dislocations, and digital contractures. Amyloid deposition may lead to arthropathy in the wrist; amyloidomas in periarticular bone may produce radiolucent lesions that may fracture; and amyloid accumulation in soft tissues may lead to neurovascular compromise, particularly about the wrist [48].

Deposition of amyloid in soft tissue, ligaments, joint capsule, and synovium results in bulky periarticular masses about the wrist. Accumulation of amyloid in the synovial membrane may account for joint effusions in hemodialyzed patients. Synovial collections of amyloid may invade marginal regions of intra-articular bone directly. Amyloid deposition in the carpal bones is associated with well defined osteolytic lesions. Most commonly, these lesions are multiple, and may be bilateral, and they produce a geographic pattern of bone destruction. Radiolucent lesions are found in both central and marginal regions of periarticular bone, and progressive enlargement of cystic lesions may lead to collapse of the articular surface and pathologic fractures [48]. Amyloid deposition in cartilage may be a causative factor in joint arthropathy and destruction. Although accumulation of amyloid in articular cartilage occurs in asymptomatic senile persons, in patients with dialysis-related arthropathy, amyloid accumulates in capsulosynovial insertions and may spread from these insertional sites along the superficial layers of cartilage, leading to surface fibrillation, irregularity, and deep fissuring [49]. Additional musculoskeletal manifestations of amyloidosis in patients treated with hemodialysis include flexor tendon contracture, trigger finger, and tendon rupture. Tendinous and ligamentous laxity resulting in reducible deformities of small joints in the hand may be seen. Digital clubbing confined to one or more fingers may be induced by anoxia distal to the site of the fistula, and hemarthrosis also may be an additional complication of hemodialysis.

10.3.3.6 Abnormalities of the Hand and Wrist Occurring after Peritoneal Dialysis and Renal Transplantation

Musculoskeletal abnormalities in patients with chronic renal disease undergoing peritoneal dialysis are well known. Tumoral soft tissue calcific deposits in the hand and wrist of these patients may lead to tendon rupture. Rarely, osseous erosions associated with soft tissue calcific collections may occur. Amyloid and CPPD crystal deposition, destructive arthropathy about the interphalangeal joints and intraosseous lytic lesions, and carpal tunnel syndrome are additional abnormalities occurring in association with chronic peritoneal dialysis.

Bone and soft tissue abnormalities also have been observed in patients treated with renal transplantation. In the post-transplantation period, radiologic features of hyperparathyroidism may be noted in some patients, whereas in others, these features may either disappear or become exaggerated. After renal transplantation, osteopenia may remain unchanged or worsen; a few patients may present an increase in bone mineral density. Osteomalacia and periarticular calcifications may resolve completely after renal transplantation. Osteonecrosis represents a well-known complication occurring in the post-transplant period due to various factors including steroid administration, osteopenia, hyperparathyroidism, hypophosphatemia, and immune response to the renal graft. In the hand, osteonecrosis most commonly involves the carpal bones and destruction of the articular surface and cartilage induces synovial effusions. Spontaneous fractures also may occur after renal transplantation. Additional abnormalities occurring in patients who have had renal transplants include bone and joint infection, tendinitis and tendon disruption, and the severe complication of development of an osseous malignancy.

10.3.3.7 Differential Diagnosis

Radiographic features of hyperparathyroidism occurring in renal osteodystrophy should be distinguished from those of primary hyperparathyroidism. In this regard, radiographic features of secondary hyperparathyroidism include an increased frequency of soft tissue and vascular calcification, more common and extensive osteosclerosis, and a decreased frequency of chondrocalcinosis. In renal osteodystrophy, diffuse bone sclerosis must be differentiated from the increased radiodensity associated with other endocrine, metabolic, and neoplastic diseases. In addition, periosteal neostosis in renal osteodystrophy must be distinguished from the periosteal bone formation occurring in hypertrophic osteoarthropathy, neoplasms, and infections.

Osteomalacia and rickets accompanying chronic renal disease present radiographic features identical to those accompanying other types of osteomalacia and rickets related to dietary deficiencies. Slipped epiphyses, however, tend to be more common in rickets of renal osteodystrophy.

Periarticular calcification occurring in renal osteodystrophy is found in idiopathic tumoral calcinosis, collagen vascular diseases, idiopathic calcium hydroxyapatite crystal deposition disease, hypervitaminosis D, and milk-alkali syndrome. In renal osteodystrophy, periarticular, soft tissue, and vascular calcifications also accompany other manifestations of the disorder.

10.3.4 Hypoparathyroidism

Hypoparathyroidism is a general term describing a clinical state of parathyroid hormone deficiency, which results in hypocalcemia and neuromuscular dysfunction. Hypoparathyroidism may have many causes, including excision of or trauma to the parathyroid glands during thyroid surgery; congenital absence or atrophy of the parathyroid glands; and parathyroid gland destruction after radiation. Rarely, the disease occurs in infants as a response to hyperparathyroidism in the mother owing to transplacental transport of calcium with suppression of fetal parathyroid activity. End-organ resistance to the action of parathyroid hormone, however, is seen in pseudohypoparathyroidism and pseudopseudohypoparathyroidism.

The major radiographic manifestations of hypoparathyroidism are osteosclerosis, which may be generalized or localized, and soft tissue calcification. In the hand, the radiographic findings of hypoparathyroidism are usually subtle. Subcutaneous, ligamentous and tendinous calcification, premature fusion of the physes, enthesopathy, and osteoporosis are among the radiographic features of hypoparathyroidism which are less commonly encountered [50].

The differential diagnosis of osteosclerosis seen in hypoparathyroidism includes osteoblastic metastasis, Paget's disease, renal osteodystrophy, fluorosis, myelofibrosis, sickle cell anemia, and mastocytosis. Most of these conditions are differentiated easily from hypoparathyroidism because of other radiographic features that are not characteristic of hypoparathyroidism. Subcutaneous calcification observed in hypoparathyroidism also may be observed in collagen vascular disease, renal osteodystrophy, hypervitaminosis D, and milk-alkali syndrome [50].

10.3.5 Pseudohypoparathyroidism and Pseudopseudohypoparathyroidism

Pseudohypoparathyroidism (PHP) or Albright's hereditary osteodystrophy, is a congenital disorder that is characterized by hypocalcemia and hyperphosphatemia similar to that seen in idiopathic hypoparathyroidism. Although the disease shares many features with hypoparathyroidism, it also differs in many aspects; it involves an end-organ resistance to parathyroid hormone, and it manifests a characteristic somatotype that includes short stature, obesity, and brachydactyly. *Pseudopseudohypoparathyroidism (PPHP)* is the normocalcemic form of PHP and is also caused by failure of end-organ response to parathyroid hormone.

The clinical and radiographic manifestations of PPHP are identical to those of PHP. In the hand, radiographic findings of PHP and PPHP include shortening of the metacarpal bones and phalanges secondary to premature physeal closure, widening and shortening of the phalanges with presence of cone-shaped and pseudo-epiphyses, soft tissue calcification, and small diaphyseal exostoses that extend perpendicularly from the surface of the bone (Figs. 10.15, 10.16). In most cases of PHP and PPHP, metacarpal shortening shows predilection for the first, fourth, and fifth rays. The first metacarpal bone may present excessive width and curvature. Shortening of metacarpal bones may lead to a positive metacarpal sign. Normally, a line drawn tangential to the heads of the fourth and fifth metacarpal

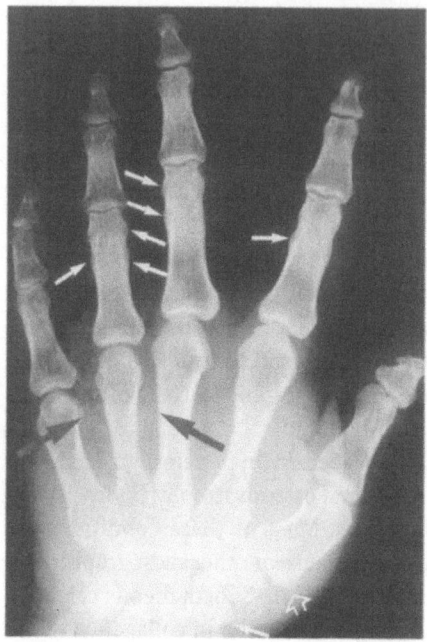

Fig. 10.15. Pseudohypoparathyroidism (Albright's hereditary osteodystrophy): radiographic features of the hand and wrist. In this patient with pseudohypoparathyroidism, observe the shortening and widening of the bones of the first digit, and broad-based bone excrescences (exostoses) on the phalanges of the long fingers and the scaphoid bone (*arrows*). A single bone excrescence can be seen on the base of the first metacarpal bone, as well (*open arrow*). Stippled soft tissue calcification of the third and fourth intermetacarpal space is observed (*long arrows*)

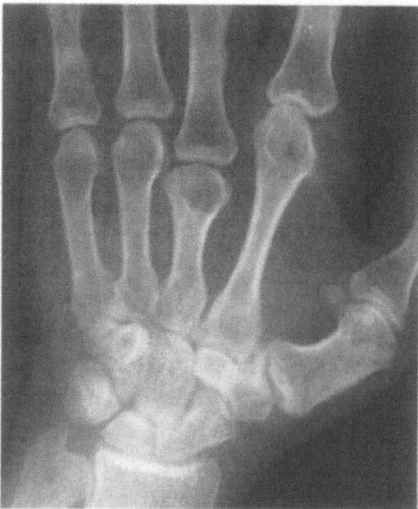

Fig. 10.16. Pseudohypoparathyroidism (Albright's hereditary osteodystrophy): radiographic features of the hand. In this patient with pseudohypoparathyroidism and brachydactyly, shortening of several metacarpal bones, particularly the third, is present

bones does not intersect the end of the third metacarpal bone or just contacts its articular surface. In patients with PHP or PPHP such a line may intersect the third metacarpal bone, indicating disproportionate shortening of the fourth and fifth metacarpal bones. This sign is not specific, as it is positive in other congenital conditions such as the basal cell nevus syndrome, Beckwith-Wiedemann syndrome, isolated developmental variation, multiple epiphyseal dysplasia, Turner's syndrome, and Noonan syndrome, as well as in acquired conditions including juvenile chronic arthritis, sickle cell anemia with infarction, growth plate injury, and neonatal hyperthyroidism. In addition, this sign sometimes is unreliable in diagnosing PHP and PPHP because the third metacarpal bone also may be short in these conditions [51]. Soft tissue calcification in PHP and PPHP is characterized as plaque-like in appearance, is subcutaneous, and is asymmetrically distributed. Soft tissue ossification also may be seen, and usually it is limited and periarticular in distribution and not associated with soft tissue swelling or tenderness. Bone density may be increased, normal, or decreased in PHP and PPHP. The carpal angle may be reduced [52].

Radiographic findings of hyperparathyroidism may be seen in some patients with PHP and PPHP. Radiographic abnormalities common to these disorders include typical subperiosteal resorption in the phalanges in association with cortical erosion of the distal portions of the radius and ulna, osteosclerosis, soft tissue calcification, brown tumors, and periosteal neostosis [51].

In the hand, although radiographic manifestations of PHP and PPHP are identical, shortening of the distal phalanges occurs at a relatively higher rate in PHP, whereas relative shortening of the metacarpal bones occurs more frequently in PPHP. These hand abnormalities should be differentiated from findings in acrodysostosis (with a significantly smaller size of the bones in this latter condition), and Turner's syndrome (mild changes in comparison with both PHP and PPHP). Additionally, thin bones and drumstick phalanges may be evident in Turner's syndrome and brachydactyly E and D. Some radiographic features of PHP and PPHP, however, resemble those of myositis ossificans progressiva and multiple hereditary exostoses [51].

Acknowledgements. This work was supported by VA grant SA-360 and the A.S. Onassis Public Benefit Foundation Educational Stipend U-033.

References

1. Resnick D (1995) Acromegaly and gigantism. In: Resnick D (ed) Diagnosis of bone and joint disorders. Saunders, Philadelphia, pp 1971–1992
2. Kleinberg D, Young I, Kupperman H (1966) The sesamoid index. An aid in the diagnosis of acromegaly. Ann Intern Med 64:1075–1078
3. Anton H (1972) Hand measurements in acromegaly. Clin Radiol 23:445–450
4. Duncan T (1975) Validity of the sesamoid index in the diagnosis of acromegaly. Radiology 115:617–619

5. Lin S, Lee K (1971) Relative value of some radiographic measurements of the hand in the diagnosis of acromegaly. Invest Radiol 6:426–431

6. Sartoris D (1996) Acromegaly. In: Sartoris D (ed) Musculoskeletal imaging. Mosby-Year Book, St Louis, pp 302–303

7. Resnick D (1995) Hypopituitarism. In: Resnick D (ed) Diagnosis of bone and joint disorders. Saunders, Philadelphia, pp 1992–1993

8. Hernandez R, Poznanski A, Hopwood N (1979) Size and skeletal maturation of the hand in children with hypothyroidism and hypopituitarism. AJR 133:405–408

9. Hernandez R, Poznanski A, Kelch R, et al (1977) Hand radiographic measurements in growth hormone deficiency before and after treatment. AJR 129:487–492

10. Poznanski A (1984) Hypopituitarism. In: Poznanski A (ed) The hand in radiologic diagnosis: with gamuts and pattern profiles. Saunders, Philadelphia, pp 778–780

11. Mosekilde L, Eriksen E, Charles P (1990) Effects of thyroid hormone on bone and mineral metabolism. Endocrinol Metab Clin North Am 19:35–63

12. Resnick D (1995) Hyperthyroidism. In: Resnick D (ed) Diagnosis of bone and joint disorders. Saunders, Philadelphia, pp 1995–1999

13. Meema H, Schatz D (1970) Simple radiologic demonstration of cortical bone loss in thyrotoxicosis. Radiology 97:9–15

14. Fraser S, Smith D, Wilson G (1967) Effet des troubles thyroidiens sur le metabolisme et la densité osseuse actualités endocrinologiques 11° serie. Expansion Scientifique Française, Paris, p 3

15. Meunier P, S-Bianchi G, Edouard C, et al (1972) Bony manifestations of thyrotoxicosis. Orthop Clin North Am 3:745–774

16. Follis R (1953) Skeletal changes associated with hyperthyroidism. Bull Johns Hopkins Hosp 92:405–421

17. Cummings S, Nevitt M, Browner W, et al (1995) Risk factors for hip fracture in white women. Study of osteoporotic fractures research group. N Engl J Med 332:767–773

18. Lentino W, Poppel M (1960) The roentgen manifestations of Plummer's nails (onycholysis) in hyperthyroidism. AJR 84:941–944

19. Riggs W, Wilroy R, Etteldorf J (1972) Neonatal hyperthyroidism with accelerated skeletal maturation, craniosynostosis, and brachydactyly. Radiology 105:621–625

20. Bonakdarpour A, Kirkpatrick J, Renzi A, et al (1972) Skeletal changes in neonatal thyrotoxicosis. Radiology 102:149–150

21. Gimlette T (1960) Thyroid acropachy. Lancet I:22–24

22. Resnick D (1995) Thyroid acropachy. In: Resnick D (ed) Diagnosis of bone and joint disorders. Saunders, Philadelphia, pp 1999–2001

23. Sartoris D (1996) Thyroid acropachy: important features. In: Sartoris D (ed) Musculoskeletal imaging. Mosby-Year Book, St Louis, pp 300–301

24. Resnick D (1995) Hypothyroidism. In: Resnick D (ed) Diagnosis of bone and joint disorders. Saunders, Philadelphia, pp 2001–2009

25. Steinbach H, Gold R, Preger L (1975) Congenital hypothyroidism (cretinoid epiphyseal dysplasia). In: Steinbach H, Gold R, Preger L (eds) Roentgen appearance of the hand in diffuse disease. Year Book Medical Publishers, Chicago, pp 239–241

26. Thijn C (1986) Hypothyroidism. In: Thijn C (ed) Radiology of the hand. Springer, Berlin Heidelberg New York, pp 201–205

27. Sartoris D (1996) Hypothyroidism. In: Sartoris D (ed) Musculoskeletal imaging. Mosby-Year Book, St Louis, pp 301–302

28. Hernandez R, Poznanski A, Hopwood N (1979) Distinctive appearance of the distal phalanges in children with primary hypothyroidism. Radiology 132:83–84

29. Borg S, Fitzer P, Young L (1975) Roentgenologic aspects of adult cretinism. Two case reports and review of the literature. AJR 123:820–828

30. Parker B (1981) Hypothyroidism with epiphyseal dysgenesis. Pediatric case of the day. AJR 136:1030–1031

31. Lusted L, Pickering D (1956) Hypothyroid infant and child; role of roentgen evaluation in therapy. Radiology 66:708–717
32. Poznanski A (1984) Hypothyroidism. In: Poznanski A (ed) The hand in radiologic diagnosis: with gamuts and pattern profiles. Saunders, Philadelphia, pp 751–758
33. Bateson E, Chandler S (1965) Nephrocalcinosis in cretinism. Br J Radiol 38:581–584
34. Jaffe H (1972) Primary and secondary hyperparathyroidism. In: Jaffe (ed) Metabolic, degenerative, and inflammatory diseases of bones and joints. Lea and Febiger, Philadelphia, pp 301–331
35. Resnick D (1995) Hyperparathyroidism. In: Resnick D (ed) Diagnosis of bone and joint disorders. Saunders, Philadelphia, pp 2012–2036
36. Sundaram M, Joyce P, Shields J, et al (1979) Terminal phalangeal tufts: Earliest site of renal osteodystrophy findings in hemodialysis patients. AJR 133:25–29
37. Meema H, Meema S (1972) Microradioscopic and morphometric findings in the hand bones with densitometric findings in the proximal radius in thyrotoxicosis and in renal osteodystrophy. Invest Radiol 7:88–96
38. Young W, Sevcik M, Tallroth K (1991) Metaphyseal sclerosis in patients with chronic renal failure. Skeletal Radiol 20:197–200
39. Kirkwood J, Ozonoff M, Steinbach H (1972) Epiphyseal displacement after metaphyseal fracture in renal osteodystrophy. AJR 115:547–554
40. Scott J, Dixon A, Bywaters E (1964) Association of hyperuricemia and gout hyperparathyroidism. BM J I:1070–1073
41. Resnick D (1995) Renal osteodystrophy. In: Resnick D (ed) Diagnosis of bone and joint disorders. Saunders, Philadelphia, pp 2036–2043
42. Braunstein E, Menerey K, Martel W, et al (1987) Radiologic features of a pyrophosphate-like arthropathy associated with long-term dialysis. Skeletal Radiol 16:437–441
43. Resnick D (1995) Rickets and osteomalacia. In: Resnick D (ed) Diagnosis of bone and joint disorders. Saunders, Philadelphia, pp 1885–1922
44. Park E (1932) Blackader lecture on some aspects of rickets. Can Med Assoc J 26:3–15
45. Steinbach H, Noetzli M (1964) Roentgen appearance of the skeleton in osteomalacia and rickets. AJR 91:955–972
46. Arvin M, White S, Braunstein E (1990) Growth plate injury of the hand and wrist in renal osteodystrophy. Skeletal Radiol 19:515–517
47. Resnick D (1995) Aluminum toxicity. In: Resnick D (ed) Diagnosis of bone and joint disorders. Saunders, Philadelphia, pp 1905–1906
48. Resnick D (1995) Musculoskeletal abnormalities occurring after hemodialysis. In: Resnick D (ed) Diagnosis of bone and joint disorders. Saunders, Philadelphia, pp 2047–2061
49. Solé M, Muñoz-Gomez J, Campistol J (1990) Role of amyloid in dialysis-related arthropathies. A morphological analysis of 23 cases. Virchows Archiv A Pathol Anat Histopathol 417:523–528
50. Resnick D (1995) Hypoparathyroidism. In: Resnick D (ed) Diagnosis of bone and joint disorders. Saunders, Philadelphia, pp 2061–2064
51. Resnick D (1995) Pseudohypoparathyroidism and pseudopseudohypoparathyroidism. In: Resnick D (ed) Diagnosis of bone and joint disorders. Saunders, Philadelphia, pp 2064–2069
52. Steinbach H, Young D (1966) The roentgen appearance of pseudohypoparathyroidism (PH) and pseudopseudohypoparathyroidism (PPHP). Differentiation from other syndromes associated with short metacarpals, metatarsals and phalanges. AJR 97:49–66

11 Bone Densitometry and Osteoporosis at the Hand and Wrist

GIUSEPPE GUGLIELMI, MARIO CAMMISA, ANTONIO DE SERIO

11.1 Introduction

Osteoporosis is one of the most devastating disorders associated with aging. The disease is characterized by decreased bone mineral density (BMD) and microarchitectural deterioration in bone tissue, resulting in an increased risk of atraumatic fracture. In the preclinical state the disease is characterized simply by low bone mass without fractures. This totally asymptomatic state is often termed "osteopenia" [1]. Osteoporosis and osteopenia are the most common metabolic bone diseases in the developed countries [2]. In order to be able to evaluate more completely the prevalence and incidence of osteoporosis, the World Health Organization (WHO) convened an expert panel to define osteoporosis on the basis of bone mass measurement [3]. The diagnostic categories for women that were established by that panel are as follows:
- Normal: bone mineral density (BMD) or bone mineral content (BMC) less than 1 standard deviation (SD) of the young adult reference mean (T-score)
- Low bone mass (osteopenia): BMD or BMC between −1.0 and −2.5 SD lower than the young adult reference mean
- Osteoporosis: BMD or more than −2.5 SD below the young adult reference mean
- Severe (established) osteoporosis: with one or more osteoporotic fragility fractures.

Osteoporotic fractures may affect any part of the skeleton except the skull. Most commonly, fractures occur in the distal forearm (Colles' fracture), thoracic and lumbar vertebrae, and proximal femur (hip fracture).

11.1.1 Classification of Osteoporosis

In addition to describing osteoporosis as being of the high- or low-turnover type, there are several other classification systems [4]. The first is the classification into "primary" and "secondary", the latter being osteoporosis for which a clearly identifiable etiological mechanism is recognized. Primary osteoporosis is further characterized into "postmenopausal" and "senile". In "postmenopausal" osteoporosis there is an apparent excess loss of cancellous bone with relative sparing of cortical bone, and the clinical syndromes involve Colles' fracture and vertebral fracture. In "senile" osteoporosis there is a more simultaneous loss of both cortical and cancellous bone. The pathogenesis of senile osteoporosis is uncertain, but it is postulated to result from an age-related decline in renal production of 1,25-dihydroxyvitamin D and calcium malabsorption, with subsequent secondary hyperparathyroidism. Fracture syndrome often seen in the patient with senile osteoporosis characteristically involves the hip and pelvis [5].

Most risk factors are in five major categories: age, or age-related; genetic; environmental; endogenous hormones and chronic diseases; and physical characteristic of bone tissue [6] (Table 11.1).

11.1.2   Detection of Osteoporosis

There is a growing demand from patients, general medical practitioners and specialists (obstetricians, orthopedists, surgeons, rheumatologists and endocrinologists) for clinical services that provide for the detection, assessment and management of osteoporosis [7,8]. Whether a fracture is sustained depends on a variety of factors; however, BMD is the single most important determinant as to whether or not a fracture occurs [9]. Reduced bone mass is therefore a useful predictor of increased fracture risk. Studies have shown large (5–20%) annual losses in trabecular BMD in women undergoing surgical or natural menopause [10, 11]. Osteoporosis-related fractures result in significant morbidity and mortality [12]. As

Table 11.1. Risk factors for osteoporosis

Age, or age-related
    Each decade associated with 1.4 to 1.8 fold increased risk
Genetic
    Ethnicity: Caucasian and Oriental > Blacks and Polynesians
    Gender: female > male
    Family history
Environmental
    Nutrition; calcium deficiency
    Physical activity and mechanical loading
    Drugs, e.g., corticosteroids, anticoagulants, anticonvulsants
    Smoking
    Alcohol
    Falls (trauma)
Endogenous hormones and chronic diseases
    Estrogen deficiency
    Androgen deficiency
    Chronic diseases, e.g., gastrectomy, cirrhosis, hyperthyroidism, hypercortisolism
Physical characteristic of bone tissue
    Density
    Size and geometry
    Microarchitecture
    Composition

BMD assessment techniques have progressed from simple radiography to more sensitive methods, the quality of BMD measurements has improved substantially. With advances in noninvasive detection techniques, osteoporosis can now be detected early and a course of treatment established. The availability of reliable BMD assessment techniques also makes it possible to monitor response to therapy. Furthermore, the capability now exists to evaluate any part of the skeleton with a high degree of precision and accuracy, thereby making it possible to assess bone strength reliably and predict fracture risk [13].

This chapter addresses the current role and application of peripheral measurement techniques for the assessment of osteoporosis at the hand and wrist site. Besides traditional approaches such as radiological diagnosis of osteoporosis, radiographic absorptiometry (RA) and radiogrammetry, new peripheral approaches have been developed that offer powerful ways to assess skeletal status in osteoporosis. These include single X-ray absorptiometry (SXA), peripheral dual X-ray absorptiometry (pDXA), peripheral quantitative computed tomography (pQCT), quantitative ultrasound (QUS) techniques and magnetic resonance imaging (MRI) approaches.

11.2   Radiological Diagnosis of Osteoporosis

Indications of bone loss on radiographs are generally a reduction in density and changes in morphology. Radiographic findings suggestive of osteopenia and osteoporosis are frequently encountered in daily medical practice and can result from a wide spectrum of diseases ranging from highly prevalent causes such as postmenopausal and involutional osteoporosis to very rare endocrinological and hereditary disorders [14, 15]. It has been estimated that in most cases early osteoporosis (osteopenia) becomes detectable on conventional radiographs only after a loss of at least 20–40% of the skeletal bone mass [16, 17]. The visual estimation of bone quality and skeletal status may not be adequate for the assessment and quantification of osteopenia, but is an important part in the standard routine of a radiologist reading a radiograph. Nevertheless, conventional radiography is widely available, and it remains useful for the detection of specific alterations in certain instances (e.g., subperiosteal resorption in hyperparathyroidism). Alone, and in conjunction with modern, computer-aided, imaging techniques, conventional radiography is widely used for the detection of fractures, for the differential diagnosis of osteopenia, or for follow-up examinations in specific clinical settings (i.e., secondary hyperparathyroidism and renal osteodystrophy) [18, 19].

Several different approaches have been established to quantify the information available from a radiograph. Semiquantitative grading techniques have not proven to be precise or sensitive enough to diagnose osteopenia at an early stage, but were employed successfully in epidemiological studies in the assessment of osteoporosis [20–22].

11.2.1   Principal Radiographic Findings in Osteopenia and Osteoporosis

In osteoporosis, the amount of calcium per unit mineralized bone volume remains constant at about 35% [23]. Therefore, a decrease in the mineralized bone volume results in a decrease of the total bone calcium and a decreased absorption of the X-ray beam. This phenomenon is then referred to as increased radiolucency. As bone mass is lost, changes in the bone structure occur. Bone is composed of two compartments: cortical bone and trabecular bone. The structural changes seen in cortical bone represent bone resorption at different sites (e.g., the inner and outer surfaces of the cortex, or within the cortex in the Haversian and Volkmann channels). These three sites (endosteal, intracortical and periosteal) may react differently to distinct metabolic stimuli.

Cortical bone remodeling typically occurs in the endosteal "envelope", and the interpretation of subtle changes in this layer may be difficult. With increasing age there is a widening of the marrow canal due to an imbalance of endosteal bone formation and resorption that leads to a "trabeculization" of the inner surface of the cortex (Fig. 11.1). Endosteal scalloping due to resorption of the inner bone surface can be seen in high-bone turnover states such as reflex sympathetic dystrophy.

Intracortical bone resorption may cause longitudinal striation or tunneling. These changes are seen in various high-turnover metabolic diseases affecting the bone such as hyperparathyroidism, osteomalacia, renal osteodystrophy, and acute osteoporoses from disuse or reflex sympathetic dystrophy syndrome, but also rapidly evolving postmenopausal osteoporosis. Intracortical tunneling is a hallmark of rapid bone turnover. It is usually not apparent in disease states with relatively low turnover such as senile osteoporosis.

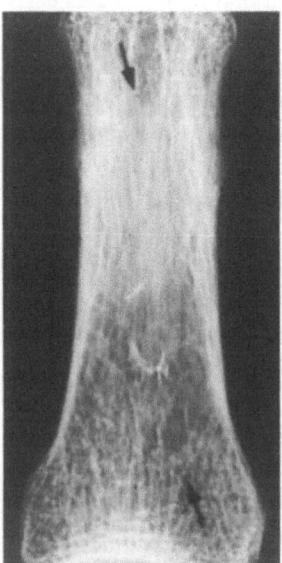

Fig. 11.1. High-resolution radiographic technique of the phalanx with magnification depicts the widening of the marrow canal due to an imbalance of endosteal bone formation and resorption that leads to a "trabeculization" of the inner surface of the cortex

Accelerated endosteal and intracortical resorption, with intracortical tunneling and indistinct border of the inner cortical surface, is best depicted with high-resolution radiographic techniques with optical magnification (Fig. 11.2).

Subperiosteal bone resorption is associated with an irregular definition of the outer bone surface. This finding is pronounced in diseases with a high bone turnover, principally primary and secondary hyperparathyroidism. However, rarely it may also be present in other diseases.

11.3 Radiogrammetry

One of the first descriptions of these measurements assessing aging bone was the paper published by Barnett and Nordin in 1960 [20]. They introduced a hand score (measured at the shaft of the second metacarpal), a femoral score and a spine score. Several dimensions can be measured, such as total bone width, cortical thickness, the ratio of cortical width to total bone width, and the cortical area. These measurements are usually performed on radiographs depicting tubular bones [24–26]. More recently Meema and coworkers [27, 28] have published several papers discussing radiogrammetry of the radius and the second metacarpal, maintaining that the technique is suitable for screening in osteoporosis. Rico et al. [29, 30] have also published several papers using radiogrammetry in a variety of studies including those on the treatment of osteoporosis. The number of recent papers on radiogrammetry of the metacarpal, phalangeal and forearm bones, however, is limited, and these publications come primarily from a few dedicated research groups.

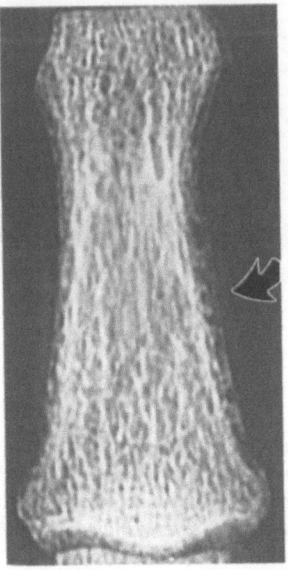

Fig. 11.2. High-resolution radiographic technique of the phalanx with magnification well demonstrates intracortical tunneling and indistinct border of the inner cortical surface, as a hallmark of rapid bone turnover

Radiogrammetry now has two major applications in osteoporosis research. The first is in measurement of the phalangeal and metacarpal indices. This is based on the fact that when osteopenia develops, the cortical thickness of these small tubular bones decreases while the medullary cavity enlarges due to endosteal resorption of bone. The second application is in measurement of geometric dimensions of the hip (especially the hip axis length).

The oldest application is the measurement of dimensions on images of tubular bones, the basic idea of which is simple: one measures the outer diameter of the tubular bone (D) and its inner diameter (d) (Fig. 11.3). The ratio $(D-d)/D$ is called the cortical index, $D-d$ being the combined cortical thickness. When endosteal resorption occurs, the cortical shell becomes thinner while the medullary cavity enlarges; in this case the cortical index and the combined cortical thickness decrease.

These measurements are usually performed on the metacarpal bones and, rarely, the radius. The precision errors with these techniques are generally in the order of 3%. One of the major deficiencies of the technique is that it does not measure intracortical porosity or the resorption of trabecular structures, both well-known features of bone loss.

Radiogrammetry has been used in a variety of studies. Van Hemert et al. [31] showed in a large epidemiological study that the relative cortical area decreases an average of 1% in women aged 45-64 years. In another study the same authors reported that the metacarpal cortical area when used as a risk factor for osteoporotic fractures shows a clear trend toward more fractures when the cortical area is decreased [32]. Comparing a group of healthy peri- and postmenopausal women with a group of women with osteoporotic vertebral deformities, Meema and Meindoket [28] showed that the measurement of combined cortical thickness at the metacarpal bones can be useful in identifying osteoporotic women when a "fracture threshold" is used. Rico et al. [30] used radiogrammetry in a prospective study evaluating the effect of salmon calcitonin on bone mass and they showed that the combined corti-

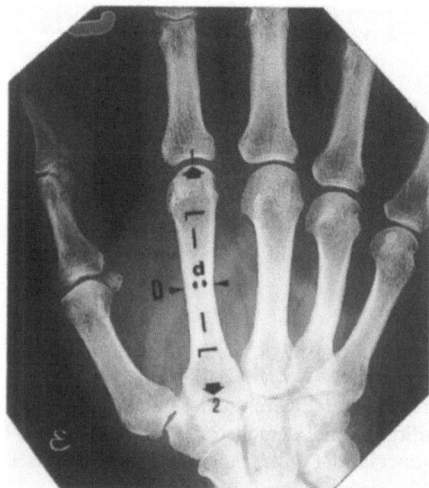

Fig. 11.3. Radiogrammetry of the second metacarpal bone. The inner (medullary cavity: d) and outer diameter (total bone width: D) of the bone are measured. Several indices can be calculated from these simple measurements

cal thickness increased significantly in the treated group. Another study comparing DXA with QUS and radiogrammetry showed that all measurements were correlated significantly [33]. Wishart et al. [34] compared metacarpal radiogrammetry with SPA and spinal QCT and concluded that radiogrammetry yields cross-sectional information about bone density and fracture risk comparable to that obtained by the other methods. Derisquebourg et al. [35] used digitized images to measure the appropriate dimension on standardized hand radiographs and found that radiogrammetry can be of value in mass screening for osteoporosis. Adami et al. [36] recently showed that the metacarpal index is very moderately correlated with spinal, femoral and forearm DXA measurements. One major limitation leading to the potential insensitivity of radiogrammetry is related to the failure to measure intracortical resorption or porosity and irregular endosteal scalloping or erosion. Because intracortical resorption and trabecular bone resorption are indicators of high-bone-turnover states, the fact that they are not measured by this technique is significant. Despite its shortcomings when applied to individual patients, radiogrammetry remains an important research tool to study changes in cortical bone.

11.4 Radiographic Absorptiometry

Radiographic absorptiometry is one of the first quantitative techniques developed to estimate BMD [37–40]. Standardized radiographs of bones are obtained simultaneously with an aluminum step-wedge phantom. However, an X-ray beam, which passes through an absorbing tissue is scattered according to the composition and physical thickness of this tissue. Variations in the amount of soft tissue overlying the bone are not accounted for. Therefore, reasonable accuracy can only be assured at appendicular bones, which are surrounded by a relatively negligible amount of soft tissue (e.g., metacarpals or phalanges). The optical density of appendicular bone on the exposed film is determined by comparison with the defined density of the aluminum step-wedge using an optical densitometer. The results are given in aluminum equivalent values. Radiographic absorptiometry is a low cost technique, which measures integral bone (trabecular and cortical). Numerous physical factors that influence the radiographic image such as inconsistencies in beam quality, instability of the X-ray source, film response and beam hardening effects, also have an adverse effect on precision and accuracy of the method [40]. Error sources include the impact of inhomogeneity of the X-ray beam and overlying soft tissue mass, the film developing process, the calibration procedure and the delineation of the region of interest. Some of these are minimized if central evaluation is performed. Several methods are currently in use. One of these is the method developed by CompuMed (Osteogram; Calif., USA). This technique makes two posteroanterior radiographs of the hand, one at 50 kVp and the other at 60 kVp, using nonscreen film. An aluminum reference wedge is placed parallel to the middle phalanx of the index finger (Fig. 11.4). The radiographs are analyzed at a central

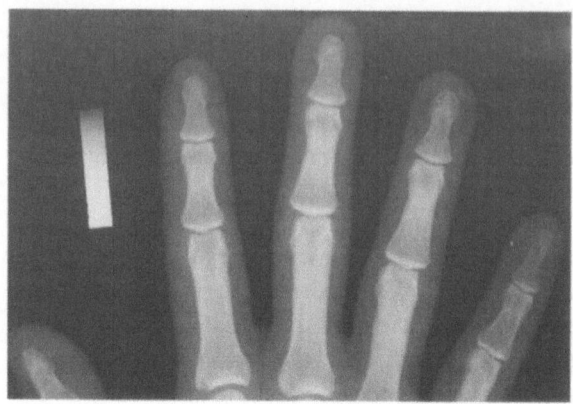

Fig. 11.4. Radiograph of a hand made for the CompuMed radiographic absorptiometry technique. An aluminum wedge is placed alongside the second finger for calibration purposes. Results are given in arbitrary units.

laboratory. The short-term precision error is reported to be 1.5% (coefficient of variation) in vivo [41] and 1% in vitro [42]. Other systems are those provided by NIM (Osteoradiometer; Verona, Italy) for metacarpal bone and radius measurements [36, 43], by Teijin (Bonalyzer; Tokyo, Japan) for radius measurements [44] and by Chugai (Tokyo, Japan) for metacarpal measurements [45]. The performance of RA has been evaluated in a number of studies. Precision errors down to 1% to 3.5% and accuracy errors of 3% to 6% have been achieved. However, newer computer-aided calibration and analysis techniques have enhanced the suitability of the method [46].

11.5 Peripheral X-Ray Absorptiometry

As the technological successors of previous photon source absorptiometry techniques, two approaches are now used for the assessment of the peripheral skeleton: single X-ray absorptiometry (SXA) and peripheral dual X-ray absorptiometry (pDXA). Both techniques use an X-ray tube instead of a radioactive source. The physical principle of the SXA is based on an X-ray system (55 kV, 300 A with K-edge filtration and solid state detectors). If a single-energy X-ray beam is used, then the arm is placed in a water bath to allow correction for soft tissue overlying bone. If a dual-energy X-ray beam is used the water bath is not necessary. The equipment is relatively compact and mobile; scanning takes about 5 min. The position of the forearm is standardized by the patient gripping a vertical rod. Both techniques allow evaluation of weight-bearing and non-weight-bearing bones. It is also possible to select predominantly cortical or trabecular measurements sites. The scan is performed in a rectilinear fashion at a distal (87% cortical bone) and ultradistal (predominantly 65% trabecular bone) site. Accuracy is 3%, precision is better than 1% and radiation dose is 0.1 μSv.

Advantages of SXA include the small footprint of the device, its relatively low price, and ease of operation. Recently special-purpose peripheral DXA devices have been introduced commercially. pDXA devices offer the same advantages as SXA devices plus an even simpler positioning procedure. Some manufacturers are discontinuing their SXA devices, moving to pDXA. There are only a few studies that address the question of whether performance of pDXA is more precise or more accurate than that of SXA. The accuracy error sources of varying soft tissue composition and thickness were previously considered to be of lesser importance for forearm measurements, and it remains to be seen whether pDXA will indeed perform better than SXA at equivalent measurement sites [47, 48].

11.6 Peripheral Quantitative Computed Tomography

Bone mineral measurement of the radius has been used for many years in the evaluation of osteoporosis [49, 50]. In the forearm, typically 70% trabecular and 30% compact bone is found at the ultradistal radius [51]. Peripheral quantitative computed tomography (pQCT) was introduced some 20 years ago and has been proposed as a relatively inexpensive method to assess trabecular BMD in single-slice mode [52, 53]. pQCT measures the apparent volumetric BMD (mg/cm^3), in contrast to projection techniques such as DXA or SXA of the radius, and allows separate assessments of trabecular and cortical bone [54, 55] (Fig. 11.5). Since 1976, pQCT has been used on a research basis [52], and it has recently become commercially available for measuring the radius and tibia [56, 57]. Spinal QCT

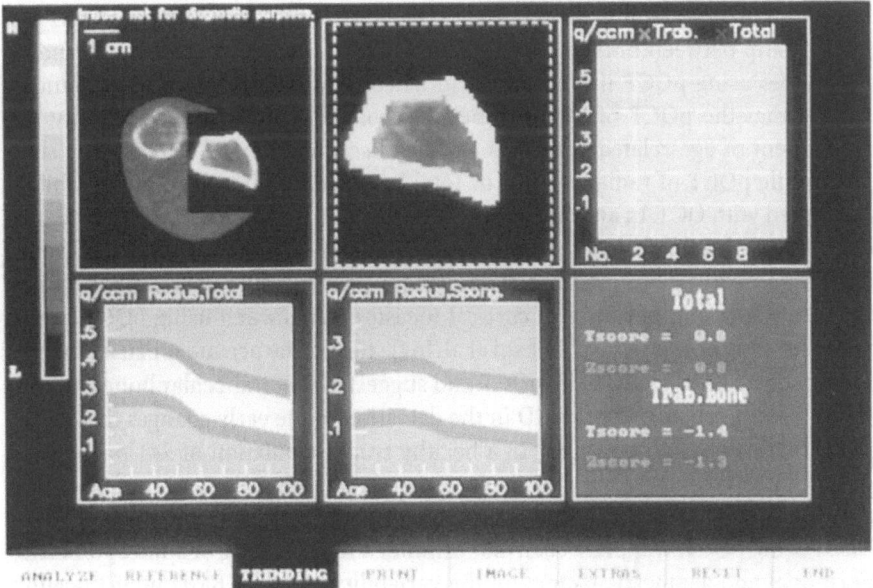

Fig. 11.5. The XCT-960 (Stratec, Germany) pQCT scanner allows the analysis of total and trabecular bone mineral density

demonstrates the apparent volumetric BMD, selecting vertebral trabecular bone. Advantages of pQCT over axial QCT are that pQCT generates a lower radiation dose (1–2 µSv in pQCT compared with 50 µSv in spinal QCT), and that it provides substantially higher reproducibility [58]. Advantages of pQCT over DXA are high accuracy, separate measurement of cortical and trabecular bone, and cross-sectional bone imaging to offer additional information [59].

Two different pQCT systems are commercially available: the XCT-960 (Stratec, Germany) and the Densiscan 1000 (ScancoMedical, Switzerland). On a coronal scout view of the distal portion of the non-dominant forearm, the operator manually places a reference line at the medial end of the radial endplate. Using this line, the standard scan position is found automatically; a single-slice scan position is obtained proximal to the distal medial end of the radius at 4% of the distance from the ulnar styloid to the olecranon process.

11.6.1 Assessment of BMD

Numerous clinical studies have employed peripheral QCT at the forearm to assess skeletal changes with aging. Recent studies calculated the precision in vivo of pQCT for the trabecular and cortical measurements using healthy subjects. Butz et al. [60] in a German reference population observed peak values of trabecular and total BMD at the ages 40–50 years in women and 30–40 years in men. In this study, beyond these ages, both trabecular and total BMD showed a linear decline with age. Schneider et al. [61] reported in a multicenter German reference database study an annual decrease of 1% in trabecular bone density and 1.5% decrease in total bone density in postmenopausal women. Grampp et al. [62] evaluated the relationship between BMD measurements of the lumbar spine using QCT and of the radius using pQCT in a healthy and osteoporotic population. They demonstrated that the pQCT of radial trabecular bone showed a weak capability for assessment of age-related bone loss and for discrimination of osteoporotic subjects while pQCT of radial cortical or total bone showed intermediate capability compared with QCT. In another study, Grampp et al. [63] assessed the age-related bone loss with aging in healthy pre- and postmenopausal, and osteoporotic women using forearm pQCT and radial and spinal DXA measurements. In this paper they showed the importance of cortical measurements when using pQCT of the radius to assess osteoporosis. Takagi et al. [64] studied the perimenopausal change in trabecular BMD assessed by pQCT and suggested that trabecular bone connectivity is more sensitive than BMD in the detection of the early changes that occur in osteoporosis. Gatti et al. [65] in a healthy study population of 241 postmenopausal and 29 premenopausal women, reported that trabecular and compact bone densities in combination with their cross-sectional areas, can be accurately measured using pQCT. Wapniarz et al. [66] examined the influence of anthropometric, hormonal and geometric factors on the variability of radial BMD in 583 healthy pre- and postmenopausal Caucasian women. In this study they evaluated the radial total and trabecular BMD measured by pQCT and showed that radial BMD is influenced strongly by geometric variables such as cross-sectional bone area, and that years since menopause and body mass index are predictors of postmenopausal BMD [66]. Hasegawa et al. [67],using pQCT in 617 healthy Japanese women and 75 subjects with osteoporosis with at least one vertebral fracture, showed a significant correlation with spinal DXA measurement (r=0.8) and a linear postmenopausal decline averaging 1.1% per year. In this study, the diagnostic sensitivity of osteoporosis expressed as a T-score was –3.0 for integral BMD, –2.4 for trabecular BMD, and –2.9 for cortical and subcortical BMD [67]. Guglielmi et al. [68] described the normal cross-sectional pattern of radial bone loss in healthy women and generated a normative database for an Italian population.

11.6.2 Assessment Beyond BMD

pQCT offers additional possibilities that have only recently been recognized. Using the high-resolution pQCT device, osteoporotic changes are apparent on images of both the radius and the tibia. The radiation dose is small, and structural parameters such as trabecular separation and number can be measured with precision errors of less than 0.5% [69]. Provided that bone structure contributes to fracture risk independently of BMD, high-resolution pQCT may allow improvement in fracture risk prediction. Moreover, pQCT provides complete information about the distribution of bone mineral within the CT slice imaged. Therefore, it is possible to calculate biomechanically relevant parameters describing bone strength, including the cross-sectional moment of inertia and the bone strength index, which, compared with BMD alone, allow a more accurate assessment of bending strength [70–72].

In conclusion, there are various indications for the appropriate use of pQCT in the diagnosis of osteoporosis. To investigate the mechanism of bone metabolism, it is helpful to evaluate the trabecular and cortical bone separately. The analysis of cortical BMD and cortical cross-sectional geometry are important in the assessment of age-related changes and bone fragility. The measurement of trabecular BMD can be useful for assessing the effect of therapy, and repeated measurements are possible because of the low-radiation dose.

11.7 Quantitative Ultrasound

Fracture occurrence in osteoporosis does not depend on bone density alone, other factors that appear to be relevant being bone microarchitecture or the elasticity of the bone. Several studies have shown that these factors are related to fracture independently of BMD [73–75]. During the past few years numerous approaches for the assessment of skeletal status by means of quantitative ultrasound (QUS) have been developed [76–78]. The attractiveness of QUS as an alternative or complementary technique to BMD measurements lies in its low cost, portability, ease of use and the lack of exposure to ionizing radiation. These benefits combined with clinical results showing good diagnostic sensitivity for fracture discrimination have encouraged further basic investigation and commercial development. Current available systems measure US parameters primarily in trabecular bone (calcaneus, patella) [79, 80], cortical bone (tibia) [81] or integral bone (phalanges) [82]. The QUS measurement methods take into account either US velocity or speed of sound (SOS) or broadband US attenuation (BUA), or both. Ultrasound velocity is considered to be related mainly to bone density and trabecular structure [83–85].

Several studies have shown that the phalanges of elderly women have relatively high decrements in QUS parameters from peak adult bone mass compared with other techniques such as BMD of the spine, femoral neck and forearm [75, 82, 83, 86]. Finally, the computer-assisted re-evaluation of hand radiographs by radiographic absorptiometry taken over the past 20 years has shown that phalangeal analysis is able to predict the risk of fracture [39, 87]. The hand phalanges are short tubular bones and are a trabecular-rich site that, with aging or osteoporosis, undergo early important morphological changes, particularly at the level of metaphysis, within the medullary canal [88, 89]. It has been demonstrated that medullary canal width changes strongly interfere with US transmission velocity, both in vitro and in vivo [90, 91].

One system is commercially available for measurement of QUS parameters at the finger phalanges (DBM Sonic, Igea, Italy) (Fig. 11.6). The device uses two US

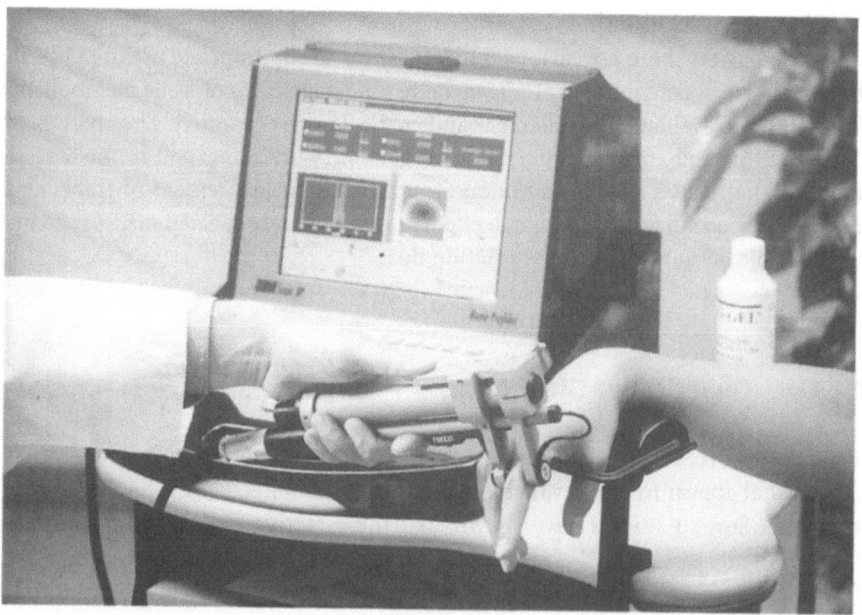

Fig. 11.6. The site of measurement of the new DBM Sonic Bone Profiler device (Igea, Italy)

probes mounted on a precision caliper. One probe, positioned on the medial surface of the distal metaphysis of the proximal phalanx, generates the US signal and the other one, positioned on the opposite surface, receives the US energy after it has crossed the phalanx. The device automatically calculates the velocity taking into consideration the distance between the probes and the time required by the US signal to cross the phalanx. The reproducibility of the measurements with phalangeal QUS ranges from a minimum of 0.4% to a maximum of 0.8% [33,82,92,93]. US transmission at the phalanx for the study of osteoporosis was successfully utilized for many years. Jergas et al. [94] and Fredfeldt [95], using US techniques, discriminated between normal and osteoporotic subjects. In an in vitro study Amo et al. [96] demonstrated that measurements of bone mass made with US velocity are well correlated with DXA measurements in rat bone specimens. Cadossi and Cané [90], using pig phalanges, showed that the US velocity measured is strictly dependent on the characteristics of the medullary canal. Several clinical investigations have demonstrated that US velocity at the phalanges is sensitive to age-related bone mass changes and showed that the parameter amplitude-dependent speed of sound (AD-SoS) was able to discriminate women in pre-, peri-, and post-menopause [82, 92, 93, 97]. A good correlation of QUS parameters at the phalanges and ultradistal radial BMD measurement has been reported [98]. Alenfeld et al. [99] and Sili-Scavalli et al. [100] using the same phalangeal US device reported good discrimination between osteoporotic patients and age- and gender-matched controls. Recent data from a prospective 3-year longitudinal study have shown that US velocity measured at the phalanx is associated with an increased risk of fracture, although the number of incident fractures was small in that study [97]. Guglielmi et al. [101] reported that phalangeal US velocity has a good correlation with spinal BMD measurement and can be used to discriminate between normal and subjects with vertebral fracture.

11.8   Magnetic Resonance Imaging

Magnetic resonance imaging (MRI) offers alternative ways of assessing skeletal properties beyond BMD. In the context of osteoporosis, MRI cannot be used to image trabecular bone directly because bone lacks water/fat content and thus appears as a signal void like the image background [102–104]. However, two different techniques have been developed to circumvent this problem: high-resolution MRI and quantitative MRI. High-resolution MRI (HRMRI) generates "inverse" images of trabecular microstructure by depicting the marrow structure. To achieve this, spatial resolution has to be optimized, a challenge that can only be achieved at peripheral measurement sites. Quantitative magnetic resonance imaging (QMRI), however, exploits the phenomenon that the presence of bony structure modifies the local magnetic field, causing changes in the measured relaxation times [105–108]. Current use of HRMRI has been targeted to peripheral skeletal sites (calcaneus, radius or finger phalanges), in order to achieve a reasonable signal-to-noise ratio [109–111] (Fig. 11.7). HRMRI in clinical applications can depict trabecular bone structure using a 1.5 T scanner and can be used to quantify stereology measures with high accuracy [112–114]. In QMRI, the differences in the magnetic susceptibility of bone and bone marrow cause local field inhomogeneities. The resultant dephasing of magnetization of bone marrow cause a shortening of transverse relaxation times T2*, which can be imaged using gradient echo sequences. Trabecular bone consequently shows variable gray-level patterns at different anatomical locations. Early investigations confirmed the associations between 1/T2* and BMD and also observed aging patterns typical for standard densitometry parameters [106–108]. Experimental and theoretical studies indicate that bone structure should have an impact on 1/T2* that is independent of BMD [113, 115–117].

11.9   Conclusions

Most peripheral measurement techniques are attractive for practical and safety reasons. Compared with more sophisticated techniques such as DXA and QCT, equipment cost is substantially lower, the devices require less space, and sometimes they are even portable. Because of the measurement site, which is far away from radiation-sensitive organs, radiation exposure is small, with effective dose equivalents of less than 10 µSv. Peripheral measurements performed by means of QUS techniques appear to match the performance of the X-ray-based peripheral approaches, and they have additional advantages and potentials beyond bone densitometry. Finally, operation is usually easier and, therefore, less error prone. An exception is MRI techniques, but these approaches offer unique capabilities for radiation-free imaging of trabecular structure and, therefore, are particularly interesting for cutting edge research investigations.

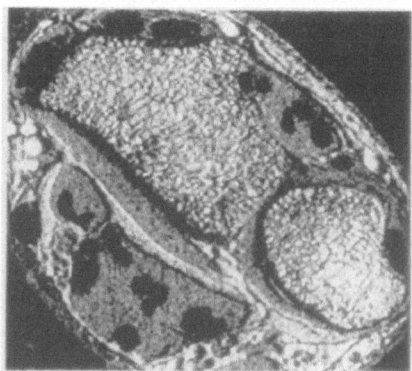

Fig. 11.7. Axial high-resolution MR images of the distal radius of a young normal subject. Note the differences in trabecular structure in vivo obtained with a spatial resolution of 98×98×500 µm

References

1. Avioli LV, Kleerekoper M (1998) Osteoporosis: the clinical problem. In: Genant HK, Guglielmi G, Jergas M (eds) Bone densitometry and osteoporosis. Springer, Berlin Heidelberg New York, pp 1–19
2. Avioli LV (1991) Significance of osteoporosis: a growing international health care problem. Calcif Tissue Int 49:S5–S7
3. World Health Organization (1994) Assessment of fracture risk and its application to screening for postmenopausal osteoporosis. Report of a WHO study group. World Health Organ Tech Rep Ser 843:1–129
4. Pacifici R (1998) The physiology of bone turnover. In: Genant HK, Guglielmi G, Jergas M (eds) Bone densitometry and osteoporosis. Springer, Berlin Heidelberg New York, pp 43–60
5. Ross PD (1998) Epidemiology of osteoporosis. In: Genant HK, Guglielmi G, Jergas M (eds) Bone densitometry and osteoporosis. Springer, Berlin Heidelberg New York, pp 21–42
6. Wasnich RD (1999) Epidemiology of osteoporosis. In: Favus MJ (ed) Primer on the metabolic bone diseases and disorders of mineral metabolism. Lippincott / Williams and Wilkins, Philadelphia, pp 257–259
7. Adams JE (1998) Single and dual energy X-ray absorptiometry. In: Genant HK, Guglielmi G, Jergas M (eds) Bone densitometry and osteoporosis. Springer, Berlin Heidelberg New York, pp 305–334
8. Genant HK (1998) Current state of bone densitometry for osteoporosis. Radiographics 18:913–918
9. Baran DT, Faulkner KG, Genant HK, Miller PD, Pacifici R (1997) Diagnosis and management of osteoporosis: guidelines for the utilization of bone densitometry. Calcif Tissue Int 61:433–440
10. Riggs BL, Melton LJ III (1986) Involutional osteoporosis. N Engl J Med 314:1676–1686
11. Lane JM, Riley EH, Wirganowicz PZ (1996) Osteoporosis: diagnosis and treatment. J Bone Joint Surg Am 78:618–632
12. Ray NF, Chan JK, Thamer M, Melton LJ III (1997) Medical expenditures for the treatment of osteoporotic fractures in the United States in 1995: report from the National Osteoporosis Foundation. J Bone Miner Res 12:24–35
13. Link TM, Majumdar S, Lin J, Newitt D, Augat P, Ouyang X, Mathur A, Genant HK (1998) A comparative study of trabecular bone properties in the spine and femur using high resolution MRI and CT. J Bone Miner Res 13:122–132
14. Steiner E, Jergas M, Genant HK (1996) Radiology of osteoporosis. In: Marcus E (ed) Osteoporosis. Academic, San Diego, pp 1019–1054
15. Grampp S, Steiner E, Imhof H (1997) Radiological diagnosis of osteoporosis. Eur Radiol 7 [Suppl 2]:S11–S19
16. Virtama P (1960) Uneven distribution of bone mineral and covering effect of non-mineralized tissue as reasons for impaired detectability of bone density from roentgenograms. Ann Med Int Fenn 49:57–65
17. Grampp S, Jergas M, Glüer CC, Lang P, Brastow P, Genant HK (1993) Radiological diagnosis of osteoporosis: current methods and perspectives. Radiol Clin North Am 31:1133–1145
18. Jergas M, Genant HK (1999) Radiology of osteoporosis. In: Favus MJ (ed) Primer on the metabolic bone diseases and disorders of mineral metabolism. Lippincott / Williams and Wilkins, Philadelphia, pp 160–168
19. Genant HK, Engelke K, Fuerst T, Glüer CC, Grampp S, Harris ST, Jergas M, Lang T, Lu Y, Majumdar S, Mathur A, Takada M (1996) Noninvasive assessment of bone mineral and structure: state of the art. J Bone Miner Res 11:707–730
20. Barnett E, Nordin BEC (1960) The radiological diagnosis of osteoporosis: a new approach. Clin Radiol 11:166–174
21. Singh M, Nagrath AR, Maini PS (1970) Changes in trabecular pattern of the upper end of the femur as an index of osteoporosis. J Bone Joint Surg Am 52:457–467
22. Herrs Nielsen VA, Pødenphant J, Martens S, Gotfredsen A, Juel Riis B (1991) Precision in assessment of osteoporosis from the spine radiographs. Eur J Radiol 13:11–14

23. LeGeros RZ (1994) Biological and synthetic apatites. In: Brown PW, Constantz B (eds) Hydroxyapatite and related materials. CRC Press, Boca Raton, pp 3-28

24. Horsman A, Simpson M (1973) The measurement of frequential changes in cortical bone geometry. Br J Radiol 48:471-476

25. Bloom RA, Pogrund H, Libson E (1983) Radiogrammetry of the metacarpal: a critical reappraisal. Skeletal Radiol 10:5-9

26. Kalla AA, Meyers OL, Parkyn ND, Kotze TJvW (1989) Osteoporosis screening -radiogrammetry revisited. Br J Rheumatol 28:511-517

27. Meema HE (1991) Improved fracture threshold in postmenopausal osteoporosis by radiogrammetric measurements: its usefulness in selection for preventive therapy. J Bone Miner Res 6:9-14

28. Meema HE, Meindok H (1992) Advantages of peripheral radiogrammetry over dual-photon absorptiometry of the spine in the assessment of prevalence of osteoporotic vertebral fractures in women. J Bone Miner Res 7:897-903

29. Rico H, Aguada F, Revilla M, Villa LF, Martin J (1994) Ultrasound bone velocity and metacarpal radiogrammetry in hemodialyzed patients. Miner Electrolyte Metab 20:103-106

30. Rico H, Revilla M, Hernandez ER, Villa LF, Alvarez de Buergo M (1995) Total and regional bone mineral content and fracture rate in postmenopausal osteoporosis treated with salmon calcitonin: a prospective study. Calcif Tissue Int 56:181-185

31. Van Hemert AM, Vandenbroucke JP, Hofman A, Valkenburg HA (1990) Metacarpal bone loss in middle-aged women: "horse racing" in a 9-year population based follow-up study. J Clin Epidemiol 43:579-588

32. Van Hemert AM, Vandenbroucke JP, Birkenhäger, Valkenburg HA (1990) Prediction of osteoporotic fractures in the general population by a fracture risk score. Am J Epidemiol 132:123-135

33. Aguado F, Revilla M, Hernandez ER, Villa LF, Rico H (1996) Dual-energy X-ray absorptiometry total body bone mineral content, ultrasound bone velocity, and computed metacarpal radiogrammetry, with age, gonadal status, and weight in healthy women. Invest Radiol 31:218-222

34. Wishart JM, Horowitz M, Bochner M, Need AG, Nordin BEC (1993) Relationship between metacarpal morphometry, forearm and vertebral bone density and fractures in postmenopausal women. Br J Radiol 66:435-440

35. Derisquebourg T, Dubois P, Devogelaer JP, Meys E, Duquesnoy B, Nagant de Deuxchaisnes C, Delcambre B, Marchandise X (1994) Automated computerized radiogrammetry of the second metacarpal and its correlation with absorptiometry of the forearm and spine. Calcif Tissue Int 54:461-465

36. Adami S, Zamberlan N, Gatti D, Zanfisi C, Braga V, Broggini M, Rossini M (1996) Computed radiographic absorptiometry and morphometry in the assessment of postmenopausal bone loss. Osteoporos Int 6:8-13

37. Cosman F, Herrington B, Himmelstein S, Linsday R (1991) Radiographic absorptiometry: a simple method for determination of bone mass. Osteoporos Int 2:34-38

38. Matsumoto C, Kushida K, Inoue T, Yamazaki K, Imose K, Inoue T (1994) Metacarpal bone mass in normal and osteoporotic Japanese women using computed X-ray densitometry. Calcif Tissue Int 55:324-329

39. Yates AJ, Ross PD, Lydick E, Epstein RS (1995) Radiographic absorptiometry in the diagnosis of osteoporosis. Am J Med 98 [Suppl 2A]:S41-S47

40. Ross PD (1997) Radiographic absorptiometry for measuring bone mass. Osteoporos Int 7 [Suppl 3]:S103-S107

41. Ravn P, Overgaard K, Huang C, Ross PD, Green D, McClung M, for the EPIC study group (1996) Comparison of bone densitometry of the phalanges, distal forearm and axial skeleton in early postmenopausal women participating in the EPIC study. Osteoporos Int 6:308-313

42. Yang SO, Hagiwara S, Engelke K, Dhillon MS, Guglielmi G, Bendavid EJ, Soejima O, Nelson DL, Genant HK (1994) Radiographic absorptiometry for bone mineral measurement of the phalanges: precision and accuracy study. Radiology 192:857-859

43. Maggio D, Pacifici R, Cherubini A, Aisa MC, Santucci C, Cucinotta M, Senin U (1995) Appendicular cortical bone loss after the age 65: sex-dependent event? Calcif Tissue Int 56:410–414

44. Seo GS, Shraky M, Aoki C, Chen JT, Aoky J, Imose K, Togawa Y, Inoue T (1994) Assessment of bone density in the distal radius with computer assisted X-ray densitometry (CXD). Bone Miner 27:173–182

45. Hayashi Y, Yamamoto K, Fukunage M, Ishibashi T, Takahashi T, Nishii Y (1990) Assessment of bone mass by image analysis of metacarpal bone roentgenograms: a quantitative digital image processing (DIP) method. Radiat Med 8:173–178

46. van Kuijk C, Genant HK (1998) Radiogrammetry and Radiographic Absorptiometry. In: Genant HK, Guglielmi G, Jergas M (eds) Bone densitometry and osteoporosis. Springer, Berlin Heidelberg New York, pp 291–304

47. Rossini M, Adami S (1997) The appendicular bone measurements. Ital J Mineral Electrolyte Metab 11:97–102

48. Glüer CC, Jergas M, Hans D (1997) Peripheral measurement techniques for the assessment of osteoporosis. Semin Nucl Med 3:229–247

49. Ruegsegger P, Durand E, Dambacher MA (1991) Differential effects of aging and disease on trabecular and compact bone density of the radius. Bone 12:99–105

50. Ruegsegger P, Durand E, Dambacher MA (1991) Localization of regional forearm bone loss from high resolution computed tomographic images. Osteoporos Int 1:76–80

51. Schlenker RA, Von Seggen WW (1976) The distribution of cortical and trabecular bone mass along the lengths of the radius and ulna and the implications for in vivo bone mass measurements. Calcif Tissue Int 20:41–52

52. Ruegsegger P, Elsasser U, Anliker M, Gnehm H, Kind HP, Prader A (1976) Quantification of bone mineral mineralization using computed tomography. Radiology 121:93–97

53. Schneider P, Borner W (1991) Periphere quantitative Computertomographie QCT-Scanner. · Fortschr Roentgenstr 154:178–182

54. Ito M, Tsurusaki K, Hayashi K (1997) Peripheral QCT for the diagnosis of osteoporosis. Osteoporos Int 7 [Suppl 3]:S120–S127

55. Schneider P, Reiners C (1998) Peripheral quantitative computed tomography. In: Genant HK, Guglielmi G, Jergas M (eds) Bone densitometry and osteoporosis. Springer, Berlin Heidelberg New York, pp 349–363

56. Muller A, Ruegsegger E, Ruegsegger P (1989) Peripheral QCT: a low-risk procedure to identify women predisposed to osteoporosis. Phys Med Biol 34:741–749

57. Schneider P, Borner W (1991) Peripheral quantitative Computed tomography for bone mineral measurement with a new special purpose QCT-Scanner: method, normal references, comparison to osteoporotic patients. Fortschr Roentgenstr 154:292–299

58. Guglielmi G, Cammisa M, De Serio A, Giannatempo GM, Bagni B, Orlandi G, Russo CR (1997) Long term in vitro precision of single slice peripheral Quantitative Computed Tomography (pQCT): multi center comparison. Technol Health Care 5:375–381

59. Ruegsegger P (1996) Bone density measurement. Rheumatology 18:103–116

60. Butz S, Wüster C, Scheidt-Nave C, Gotz M, Ziegler R (1994) Forearm BMD as measured by peripheral Quantitative Computed Tomography (pQCT) in a German reference population. Osteoporos Int 4:179–184

61. Schneider P, Butz S, Allolio B, Borner W, Klein K, Lehmann R (1995) Multicenter German reference data base for peripheral quantitative computer tomography. Technol Health Care 3:69–75

62. Grampp S, Jergas M, Lang P, Steiner E, Fuerst T, Glüer CC, Genant HK (1996) Quantitative CT assessment of the lumbar spine and radius in patients with osteoporosis. AJR 167:133–140

63. Grampp S, Lang P, Jergas M, Glüer CC, Mathur A, Engelke K, Genant HK (1995) Assessment of the skeletal status by peripheral Quantitative Computed Tomography of the forearm: short-term precision in vivo and comparison to Dual X-ray Absorptiometry. J Bone Miner Res 10:1566–1576

64. Takagi Y, Fujii Y, Miyauchi A, Goto B, Takahashi K, Fujta T (1995) Transmenopausal change of trabecular bone density and structural pattern assessed by peripheral Quantitative Computed Tomography in Japanese women. J Bone Miner Res 10:1830–1834

65. Gatti D, Rossini M, Zamberlan N, Braga V, Fracassi E, Adami S (1996) Effect of aging on trabecular and compact bone components of proximal and ultradistal radius. Osteoporos Int 6:355–360

66. Wapniarz M, Lehmann R, Reincke M, Schonau E, Klein.K, Allolio B (1997) Determinants of radial bone density as measured by pQCT in pre- and postmenopausal women: the role of bone size. J Bone Miner Res 12:248–254

67. Hasegawa Y, Kushida K, Yamazaki K, Inoue T (1997) Volumetric bone mineral density using peripheral Quantitative Computed Tomography in Japanese women. Osteoporos Int 7:195–199

68. Guglielmi G, De Serio A, Fusilli S, Scillitani A, Chiodini I, Torlontano M, Cammisa M (2000) Age-related changes assessed by peripheral QCT in healthy Italian women. Eur Radiol (in press)

69. Müller R, Hildebrand T, Häuselmann HJ (1996) In vivo reproducibility of three-dimensional structural properties of noninvasive bone biopsies using 3D-pQCT. J Bone Miner Res 11:1745–1750

70. Müller R, Hahn M, Vogel M (1996) Morphometric analysis of noninvasively assessed bone biopsies: comparison of high-resolution computed tomography and histologic sections. Bone 18:215–220

71. Augat P, Reeb H, Claes LE (1996) Prediction of fracture load at different skeletal sites by geometric properties of the cortical shell. J Bone Miner Res 11:1356–1363

72. Ferretti JL, Capozza RF, Zanchetta JR (1996) Mechanical validation of a tomographic (pQCT) index for noninvasive estimation of rat femur bending strength. Bone 18:97–102

73. Hans D, Dargent-Molina P, Schott AM, Sebert JL, Cormier C, Kotski PO, Delmas PD, Pouilles JM, Breart G, Meunier PJ (1996) Ultrasonographic heel measurements to predict hip fracture in elderly women: the EPIDOS prospective study. Lancet 348:511–514

74. Bauer DC, Glüer CC, Cauley JA, Vogt TM, Ensrud KE, Genant HK, Black DM (1997) Bone ultrasound predicts fractures strongly and independently of densitometry in older women: a prospective study. Arch Intern Med 157:629–634

75. Glüer CC, Cummings SR, Bauer DC (1996) Osteoporosis: association of recent fractures with quantitative US findings. Radiology 199:725–732

76. Glüer CC, Wu CY, Jergas M, Goldestein SA, Genant HK (1994) Three quantitative ultrasound parameters reflect bone structure. Calcif Tissue Int 55:46–52

77. van Daele PLA, Burger H, De Laet CEDH, Pols HAP (1996) Ultrasound measurement of bone. Clin Endocrinol 44:363–369

78. Hans D, Fuerst H, Guglielmi G, Genant HK (1998) Quantitative Ultrasound for assessing bone properties. In: Genant HK, Guglielmi G, Jergas M (eds) Bone densitometry and osteoporosis. Springer, Berlin Heidelberg New York, pp 379–405

79. Langton CM, Palmer SB, Porter RW (1994) The measurement of broadband ultrasound attenuation in cancellous bone. Eng Med 13:89–91

80. Heaney RP, Avioli LV, Chesnut CH III, Lappe J, Recker RR, Brandenburger GH (1995) Ultrasound velocity through bone predicts incident vertebral deformity. J Bone Miner Res 10:341–345

81. Orgee JM, Foster H, McCloskey EV, Khan S, Coombes G, Kanis JA (1996) A precise method for the assessment of tibial ultrasound velocity. Osteoporos Int 6:1–7

82. Sili-Scavalli A, Marini M, Spadaro A, Riccieri V, Cremona A, Zoppini A (1996) Comparison of ultrasound transmission velocity with computed metacarpal radiogrammetry and dual photon absorptiometry. Eur Radiol 6:192–195

83. Hans D, Fuerst T, Uffmann M (1996) Bone density and quality measurement using ultrasound. Curr Opin Rheumatol 8:370–375

84. Glüer CC, Wu CY, Genant HK (1993) Broad-band ultrasound attenuation signals depend on trabecular orientation: an in vitro study. Osteoporos Int 3:185–191

85. Glüer CC for the International Quantitative Ultrasound Consensus Group (1997) Quantitative ultrasound techniques for the assessment of osteoporosis: expert agreement on current status. J Bone Miner Res 12:1280–1288

86. Kleerekoper M, Nelson DA, Flynn MJ, Pawluska AS, Jacobsen G, Peterson EL (1994) Comparison of radiographic absorptiometry with dual energy X-ray absorptiometry and quantitative computed tomography in normal older white and black women. J Bone Miner Res 9:1745–1749

87. Trouerbach WT, Vecht-Hart CM, Collette HJA, Slooter GD, Zwamborn AW, Schmitz PIM (1993) Cross-sectional and longitudinal study of age-related phalangeal bone loss in adult females. J Bone Miner Res 8:685–691

88. Buckwalter JA, Glimcher MJ, Cooper RR, Recker R (1995) Bone biology. J Bone Joint Surg (Am) 77:1256–1289

89. Parfitt AM (1984) Age-related structural changes in trabecular and cortical bone. Calcif Tissue Int 36:123–128

90. Cadossi R, Cané V (1996) Pathways of transmission of ultrasound energy through the distal metaphysis of the second phalanx of pigs: an in vitro study. Osteoporos Int 36:123–128

91. Guglielmi G, Giannatempo GM, Scillitani A, Chiodini I, Liuzzi A, Cammisa M (1996) Phalangeal QUS and computed X-ray images of hand radiographs. Osteoporos Int 6 [Suppl 1]:S493

92. Ventura V, Mauloni M, Mura M, Patrinieri F, de Aloysio D (1996) Ultrasound velocity changes at the proximal phalanges of the hand in pre-, peri-, and postmenopausal women. Osteoporos Int 6:368–375

93. Duboeuf F, Hans D, Schott AM, Giraud S, Delmas PD, Meunier PJ (1996) Ultrasound velocity measured at the proximal phalanges: precision and age-related changes in normal females. Rev Rhum 63:427–434

94. Jergas M, Uffmann M, Muller P, Koster O (1993) Ultraschallgeschwindigkeitsmessungen zur diagnose der postmenopausalen Osteoporose. Fortschr Roentgenstr 158:207–213

95. Fredfeldt KE (1986) Sound velocity in the middle phalanges of the human hand. Acta Radiol Diagn 27:95–96

96. Amo C, Revilla M, Hernandez ER, Rico H (1996) Correlation of ultrasound bone velocity with dual energy X-ray bone absorptiometry in rat bone specimens. Invest Radiol 31:114–117

97. Mele R, Masci G, Ventura V, de Aloysio D, Bicocchi M, Cadossi R (1997) Three-year longitudinal study with quantitative ultrasound at the hand phalanx in female population. Osteoporos Int 7:550–557

98. Lusenti T, Cadossi R, Franco V, Soliani F, Rustichelli R, Borgatti PP (1994) Evaluation with ultrasound of bone quality at the proximal phalanges of the hand in patients suspected for type I osteoporosis. Minerva Ginecol 46:423–429

99. Alenfeld FE, Wüster C, Beck C, Meeder PJ, Ziegler R (1995) Quantitative ultrasound at the phalanges: separation of osteoporotic and non-osteoporotic fractures. J Bone Miner Res 10:S273

100. Sili-Scavalli A, Marini M, Spadaro A, Messineo D, Cremona A, Sensi F, Riccieri D, Taccari E (1997) Ultrasound transmission velocity of the proximal phalanxes of the non dominant hand in the study of osteoporosis. Clin Rheumatol 16:396–403

101. Guglielmi G, Cammisa M, De Serio A, Scillitani A, Chiodini I, Carnevale V, Fusilli S (1999) Phalangeal US velocity discriminates between normal and vertebrally fractured subjects. Eur Radiol 9:1632–1637

102. Sebag GH, Moore SG (1990) Effect of trabecular bone on the appearance of marrow in gradient echo imaging of the appendicular skeleton. Radiology 174:855–859

103. Majumdar S, Thomasson D, Shimakawa A, Genant HK (1991) Quantification of the susceptibility difference between trabecular bone and bone marrow: experimental studies. Magn Reson Med 22:111–127

104. Majumdar S, Genant HK (1992) In vivo relationship between marrow T2* and trabecular bone density determined with a chemical shift-selective asymmetric spin-echo sequence. J Magn Reson Imag 2:209–219

105. Wehrli FW, Ford JC, Haddad JG (1995) Osteoporosis: clinical assessment with quantitative MR imaging in diagnosis. Radiology 196:631–641

106. Grampp S, Majumdar S, Jergas M, Newitt DC, Lang P, Genant HK (1995) In vivo assessment of the distal radius by quantitative magnetic resonance imaging, peripheral computed tomography, and dual X-ray absorptiometry. Radiology 198:213–218

107. Majumdar S, Newitt DC, Jergas M, Gies A, Chiu E, Osman D, Keltner J, Keyak J, Genant HK (1995) Evaluation of technical factors affecting the quantification of trabecular bone structure using magnetic resonance imaging. Bone 17:417–430

108. Guglielmi G, Selby K, Blunt BA, Jergas M, Newitt DC, Genant HK, Majumdar S (1996) Magnetic resonance imaging of the calcaneus: preliminary assessment of trabecular bone-dependent regional variations in marrow relaxation time compared with dual X-ray absorptiometry. Acad Radiol 3:336–343

109. Chung HW, Wehrli FW, Williams JL, Wehrli SL (1995) Three dimensional nuclear magnetic resonance micro-imaging of trabecular bone. J Bone Miner Res 10:1452–1461

110. Hipp J, Jansujwicz A, Simmons C, Snyder B (1996) Trabecular bone morphology from micro-magnetic resonance imaging. J Bone Miner Res 11:286–292

111. Majumdar S, Newitt DC, Mathur A, Osman D, Gies A, Chiu E, Lotz J, Kinney J, Genant HK (1996) Magnetic resonance imaging of trabecular bone structure in the distal radius: relationship with X-ray tomographic microscopy and biomechanics. Osteoporos Int 6:376–385

112. Genant HK, Majumdar S (1997) High-resolution magnetic resonance imaging of trabecular bone structure. Osteoporos Int 7 [Suppl 3]:S135–S139

113. Hwang S, Wehrli FW, Williams J (1997) Probability-based structural parameters from three-dimensional nuclear magnetic resonance images as predictors of trabecular bone strength. Med Phys 24:1255–1261

114. Wehrli FW, Hwang S, Ma J, Song H, Ford J, Haddad J (1998) Cancellous bone volume and structure in the forearm: noninvasive assessment with MR microimaging and image processing. Radiology 206:347–357

115. Link TM, Majumdar S, Lin J Newitt DC, Augat P, Ouyang X, Mathur A, Genant HK (1998) A comparative study of trabecular bone properties in the spine and femur using high-resolution MRI and CT. J Bone Miner Res 13:122–132

116. Link TM, Majumdar S, Augat P, Lin J, Newitt DC, Lu Y, Lane N, Genant HK (1998) In vivo high resolution MRI of the calcaneus: differences in trabecular structure is osteoporosis patients. J Bone Miner Res 13:1175–1182

117. Link TM, Majumdar S, Grampp S, Guglielmi G, van Kuijk C, Imhof H, Glüeer CC, Adams JE (1999) Imaging of trabecular bone structure in osteoporosis. Eur Radiol 9:1781–1788

12 Degenerative Disease of the Hand and Wrist

J. M. ELLIOTT, A. J. GRAINGER, H. K. GENANT

12.1 Pathological Concepts: Overview

Since the early descriptions of osteoarthritis (OA), conventional radiography has been the primary imaging modality used in the confirmation and monitoring of the disease. In general, the radiographic abnormalities reflect different phases of the disease process which can be considered to have a destructive (regressive) component and a productive phase (progressive remodeling) [1]. The destructive phase is characterized by joint space narrowing, cyst formation, flattening and deformity (Fig. 12.1), whereas osteophyte formation and sclerosis are evident in the productive phase (Fig. 12.2). The two phases coexist in time although different segments of the joint may be affected. Conventional radiographs demonstrate primarily the subchondral effects of osteoarthritis, and any damage to cartilaginous surfaces must therefore be inferred from joint space narrowing. Despite this limitation, conventional radiography remains the most important imaging tool in the study of this disease, being readily available, inexpensive and reproducible.

Other imaging modalities such as radioisotope studies, computed tomography and magnetic resonance imaging have been used in the investigation of OA. Their role will be reviewed in this chapter but the discussion will concentrate on conventional radiography.

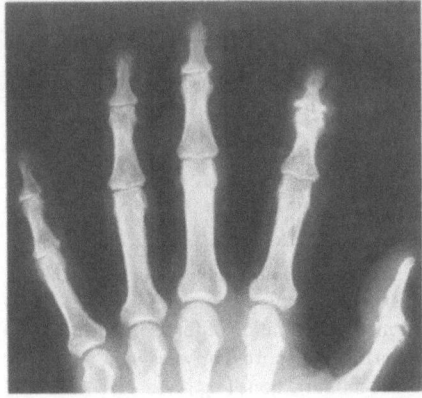

Fig. 12.1. Destructive phase of OA. In this hand of a 67-year-old woman, there is joint space narrowing and flattening of the distal interphalangeal (DIP) joints. Osteophytosis is also noted, particularly at the DIP joint of the index finger, where overlying soft tissue swelling can be seen

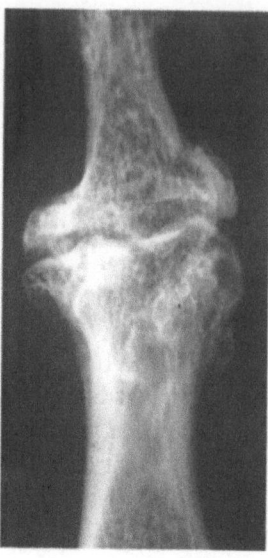

Fig. 12.2. Productive phase of OA. This DIP joint of the thumb demonstrates severe osteophyte formation at the joint margins. Note the continuity of the cortex. Sclerosis and joint space narrowing are also present, indicating the overlap between the destructive and productive phases of the process

12.2 Risk Factors and Pathogenesis

Degenerative joint disease in the form of OA is a ubiquitous disease affecting the majority of the population at some point. The disease is seen in other vertebrates and is not a modern disease, having been observed in ancient skeletons including those of Egyptian mummies and dinosaurs.

Traditionally OA has been classified as either primary – developing in the absence of any underlying condition; or secondary – resulting from a pre-existing condition which predisposes to OA. However, it has been suggested that this classification is inappropriate, since it is probable that all cases of OA arise as a result of some pre-existing abnormality in biomechanics which we are currently unable to detect in many cases. Mitchell and Crues [2] proposed an alternative classification of the disease involving four major categories (Table 12.1).

This classification emphasizes the fact that an underlying cause for the development of OA exists which may be the result either of abnormal force across a normal joint or of normal forces acting on a joint with one or more abnormal components. Nevertheless, despite a predisposing factor being identified in some cases of OA, in the majority of cases no such cause is found and the terms primary and secondary OA have become widely accepted.

Table 12.1. Major categories of the Mitchell & Crues classification [2]

Abnormal concentration of force on normal articular cartilage matrix	Normal concentration of force on abnormal articular cartilage matrix
Normal concentration of force on normal cartilage supported by stiffened subchondral bone (e.g., Paget's disease or osteopetrosis)	Normal concentration of force on normal cartilage supported by weakened subchondral bone (e.g., avascular necrosis)

Primary generalized OA or Kellgren's arthritis is a specific form of OA involving the hands. Genetic factors are thought to play an important part in the etiology of this variant. It has characteristic clinical and radiological findings as will be discussed later.

The prevalence of OA increases with age, being as high as 85% in the population over 70 years of age. The disease affects both men and women. However, there is a higher incidence of more severe disease in women. Before the age of 50 years, men have a higher prevalence of OA than women, but in later life women have a higher prevalence and incidence of the disease. Evidence suggests that these differences may arise because estrogen has a protective role against the development of OA. It is postulated that the increased risk that older women have of developing OA relates to the fall in estrogen associated with the menopause [3]. Another difference between the sexes is the pattern of disease involvement. Women are more likely than men to develop generalized OA which, in particular, involves multiple joints in the hands.

In addition to age and sex several other risk factors have been identified for the development of OA in the larger joints including excessive exercise, obesity and congenital and developmental disorders [4, 5]. However these are not thought to be so important in the development of OA of the hand and wrist. In these locations more significant risk factors include trauma, occupation and genetic factors. OA associated with trauma and occupation may be of importance in explaining some of the differences in the disease pattern seen between men and women. Genetic influences appear to be particularly relevant in the development of primary generalized OA, associated with Bouchard and Heberdon's nodes [6].

Degenerative joint disease changes may also develop secondary to another pre-existing joint disease (Fig. 12.3). Such conditions include the crystal-induced arthropathies, bleeding disorders and osteonecrosis. Congenital disorders or joint malalignment may predispose to the development of OA. This is seen with epiphyseal dysplasias in many joints. In the wrist OA may be associated with a disproportionally long ulna relative to the radius (positive ulnar variance).

12.3   Pathogenesis

In contrast to the inflammatory arthropathies such as rheumatoid arthritis, where the synovium is the target organ, in OA the target tissue is traditionally considered to be the articular cartilage. However, changes in subchondral bone are important and in idiopathic OA authors have suggested that the initial abnormality occurs in the subchondral bone [7, 8].

The structure of cartilage, comprising chondrocytes surrounded by a matrix of collagen and proteoglycans, confers on the tissue unique properties essential to the normal function of the joint. First it is able to act as an absorber of stress, and secondly it provides a smooth surface allowing low friction movement of the joint. In healthy individuals there is a constant, balanced process of synthesis and degra-

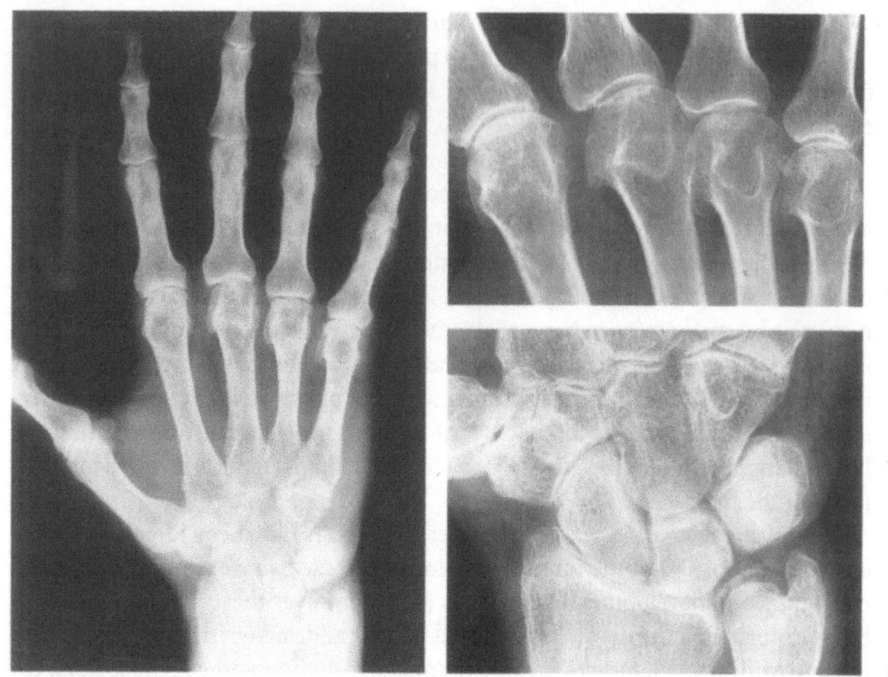

Fig. 12.3a–c. Secondary OA. **a** In this patient with hemochromatosis, joint space narrowing, flattening and sclerosis are present, particularly at the metacarpophalangeal (MCP) joints. **b** The changes at the MCP joints are better displayed and the beak-like osteophytes typical of this condition are well seen. **c** The calcification within the triangular fibrocartilage complex is illustrated

dation of the cartilage matrix. A widely accepted theory is that in the osteoarthritic joint this dynamic process becomes unbalanced, with changes in the matrix composition occurring as a result of increased degradation and possibly also decreased synthesis of collagen and the proteoglycans [9, 10]. Support for this theory comes from the increased presence of matrix metalloproteinases, produced by the chondrocytes, which degrade both proteoglycans and collagen in osteoarthritic cartilage [11, 12]. While these destructive processes are progressing there are efforts at repair. Despite their limited capacity for proliferation newly formed cells are found in osteoarthritic cartilage and synthesis of proteoglycans along with other matrix components increases. Nevertheless these repair mechanisms are inadequate and there is degradation of the cartilage matrix resulting in an alteration of the functional properties of the cartilage. The changes are also thought to allow increased water uptake by the cartilage which contributes to its inability to function normally. The end result is failure of the cartilage, initially in load-bearing areas, with fibrillation, softening and ulceration which may eventually lead to exposure of the underlying bone [4, 13, 14].

The reduced protection afforded the subchondral bone may initiate the osseous changes seen in OA. However, this is an area of some controversy and as indicated above an alternative view is that subchondral bone change is the initial event. It is argued that the subchondral sclerosis commonly seen in OA is not a response to failure of the cartilage but the result of microfracture repair. It is postulated that these microfractures occur as a result of abnormal loading across the joint. The subsequent reduced compliance of the underlying bone leads to an increase in the stresses to be absorbed by the overlying cartilage, which eventually fails [7, 8, 14].

12.4   Radiological-Pathological Correlation

The changes seen in the osteoarthritic synovial joint on radiological examination reflect the pathological changes occurring. These fall into three main groups:
  - Degradation and thinning of articular cartilage
  - Subchondral bone changes
  - Osteophyte formation

12.4.1   Cartilaginous Changes

The degradation of cartilage seen in OA is a progressive process. Initially the cartilage develops areas of fibrillation on its surface. In the large joints such as the hip and knee these changes occur primarily in the weight-bearing portions of the joint. However, in the joints of the hand and wrist, weight-bearing is not a factor, and cartilage degradation in these synovial joints is typically a diffuse although irregular process.

As the process of cartilage degradation continues, ulcers and fissures start to develop within the cartilage. In places these may extend through the full thickness of the cartilage exposing the underlying subchondral bone. As discussed above the cartilage undergoes attempts at repair and areas of denuded subchondral bone may become covered with regenerated cartilage [15]. Nevertheless, the process of cartilage fragmentation progresses with gradual thinning of the articular cartilage.

This process accounts for the reduction in joint space seen on radiographs, which is one of the fundamental radiological features of OA. Narrowing of the articular space occurs prior to changes indicative of eburnation.

12.4.2   Subchondral Bone Changes

The subchondral bone changes occurring in OA comprise sclerosis and cyst formation.

Subchondral sclerosis is a characteristic feature of OA and provides a useful distinguishing feature from those arthritic processes, such as rheumatoid arthritis, which are characterized by periarticular osteoporosis (Fig. 12.4). Subchondral sclerosis represents reparative processes which occur in the trabecular bone fol-

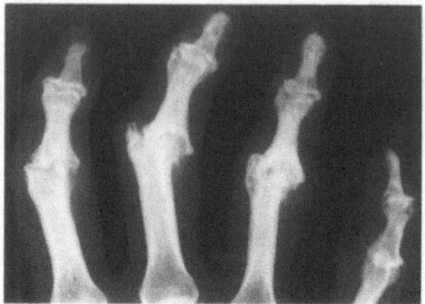

Fig. 12.4. Erosive OA. Despite the marked erosive change at the proximal interphalangeal (PIP) joints with loss of joint space and deformity, there is sclerosis in the adjacent bone. This is a useful distinguishing feature from rheumatoid arthritis, in which periarticular osteoporosis is characteristic. Osteophyte formation is prominent and there is involvement of the DIP joints

lowing microtrauma. This occurs as the protection normally afforded by the overlying cartilage is lost. Following cartilage loss, the opposing bone surfaces become closely applied leading to eburnation and eventual collapse. Areas of sclerosis which predominate on the pressure segments of the joints develop, and extend vertically into the subchondral bone. In addition there is horizontal extension over a larger proportion of the adjacent bone. Eventually, radiolucencies appear within the dense zones representative of cysts.

12.4.3   Cysts

The term "cyst" when used in connection with joint disease is not entirely accurate as such a cyst does not always represent a cavity with an epithelial lining. Various terms have been used including synovial cysts [16], subchondral cysts [17], subarticular pseudocysts [18], necrotic pseudocysts [19] and geodes [20]. The cystic spaces are visible in the sclerotic portion of the bone and it is sometimes possible to identify communication with the joint surface. The location of the cysts is helpful in allowing the differentiation of degenerative disease from other inflammatory arthropathies. In OA they are typically situated at the pressure segment of a joint, unlike in rheumatoid arthritis whereas cyst formation predominates at the junction of the cartilage and the bone following erosion by pannus. Although the cysts seen in calcium pyrophosphate dihydrate (CPPD) deposition resemble those of OA, they are larger and tend to be associated with more collapse and fragmentation of the subchondral plate. Another cystic entity is the intraosseous ganglion, although it is rare and often difficult to distinguish from a degenerative cyst [21]. An intraosseous ganglion occurs in nonpressure areas of a joint, is large and is associated with an otherwise normal joint – features which may allow differentiation from a subchondral cyst. While the pathogenesis of intraosseous ganglia is unclear, it is generally accepted that they do not arise as a result of an articular disorder.

It has been proposed that the subchondral cysts of OA arise as a result of intrusion of the synovial fluid into the subchondral bone leading to secondary resorption of the trabeculae [22, 23]. Clearly the fact that the cysts may communicate with the joint surface is compatible with this theory. In addition Landells [23] also supports this theory by noting that cartilage fragments may be seen within the cysts, and that the cyst contents are compatible with a derivation from synovial fluid.

An alternative model of cyst formation has been proposed by which cysts represent foci of osteonecrosis arising from the increased stresses occurring in the subchondral bone of osteoarthritic joints following cartilage degradation [24, 25]. Although these two separate theories of cyst pathogenesis have been proposed it has been suggested that the actual process may well involve simultaneous occurrence of both mechanisms [20].

Differentiation from bone neoplasms, such as giant cell tumors, chondroblastomas and metastases, is usually aided by other features associated with degenerative disease.

12.4.4   Osteophyte Formation

The tendency to form osteophytes is a distinctive feature of OA and represents part of the reparative process seen with this disease. Osteophytes may be classified according to their location as marginal, central, periosteal or capsular. Central osteophytes are most usually seen in the hip and knee, while periosteal osteophytosis, also termed buttressing, is most typically seen in the femoral neck of the osteoarthritic hip. Both marginal and capsular osteophytes are seen in the hand. Marginal osteophytes are thought to result from a process involving vascularization of the subchondral bone marrow (Fig. 12.5). This vascularization leads to calcification of the adjacent cartilage and stimulates endochondral ossification.

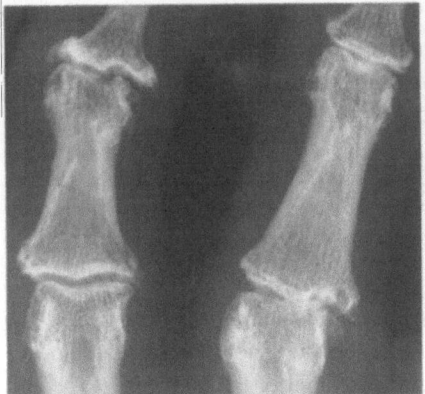
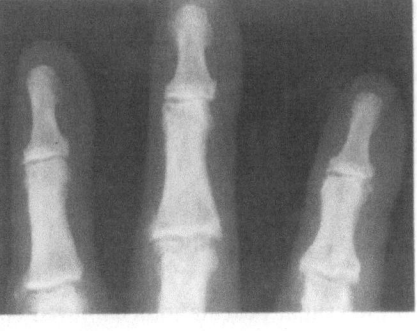

a

b

Fig. 12.5a, b. Osteophyte formation. **a** Marginal osteophytes are present at the DIP joint and PIP joints. Trabeculae can be seen within the bony protuberances and a "ghost" outline of the original calcified cartilage is noted deep to the new cortex. **b** the osteophytes at the PIP joints are larger, perhaps as a result of capsular pull

The resultant bony protuberances contain bone trabeculae and bone marrow and are usually covered with cartilage. In the case of capsular osteophytes the bony spurs develop in reaction to capsular traction forces. They develop along the direction of capsular pull at the site of capsular insertion [26]. Size is variable and initially the joint space is normal. Radiographically, it is possible to determine the edge of the original calcified cartilage, which remains as a "ghost" outline deep to the new region of endochondral ossification.

12.5 Other Articular Structures

Degenerative joint disease produces alterations in structures other than the articular surface and subchondral bone of the joint. In the wrist, as in the knee, there is a fibrocartilaginous disc which shows evidence of degeneration both in the older patient and as a result of trauma. Such degeneration is associated with tears which may progress to fragmentation.

There may also be inflammatory changes in the synovium. Evidence indicates that unlike the inflammatory arthropathies, where synovitis is the primary joint abnormality, the synovitis of OA is a reactive phenomenon which is considered to be secondary to the underlying degenerative process. Proliferative changes in the synovium may also result from the presence of articular debris within the joint. The synovial membrane alterations may be of significance in contributing to the pain and joint stiffness seen in some cases. This is particularly the case in those patients with erosive OA (see later discussion) [27].

12.5.1 Osteonecrosis

Osteonecrosis is associated with degenerative joint disease but radiographically its presence cannot be readily determined. However, primary osteonecrosis may eventually lead to destructive, degenerative changes which can obscure the underlying problem. This differentiation is important in the wrist, where the lunate is susceptible to necrosis.

12.5.2 Malalignment

In the weight-bearing joints, uneven stress leads to asymmetry in the loss of the articular surface and further abnormal stresses result in various degrees of deformity. This process also applies to the distal and proximal interphalangeal (DIP, PIP) joints, giving rise to "tilt" deformities. A similar problem in the wrist, perhaps related to altered stress from ligamentous and capsular supporting structures, is seen at the base of the first metacarpal on the trapezium, where severe subluxation and malalignment lead to a characteristic clinical and radiographic appearance (Fig. 12.6).

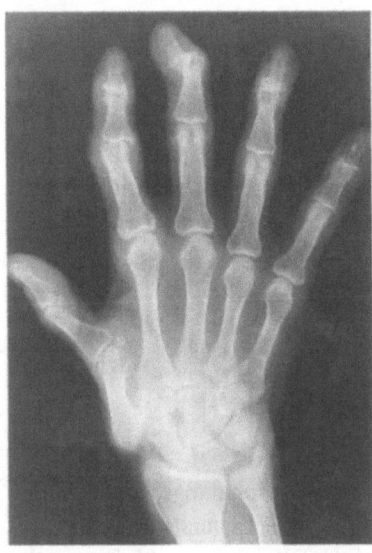

Fig. 12.6. Malalignment. As a result of irregular joint space narrowing, tilt deformities are seen, especially at the DIP joint of the middle finger and the PIP joint of the index finger. Subluxation and malalignment has also occurred at base of the first metacarpal

12.6   Classification and Assessment

Although the common features seen in OA are agreed upon, it has been more difficult to establish reliable criteria for classification, diagnosis and evaluation of disease progress. A system for clinical evaluation was developed by the American College of Rheumatology using a combination of symptoms, signs and radiographic findings [28]. This study found that clinical assessment was of more value than radiographic assessment and the criteria were most sensitive and specific when hard tissue enlargement of the DIP and PIP joints was present with no metacarpophalangeal (MCP) swelling. Conventional radiography was unable to detect osteophyte formation despite the presence of hard bony enlargement on physical examination. Detection of osteophytes radiographically has been an important part of the assessment of OA since the description of a system by Kellgren and Lawrence which considers osteophytes as pathognomonic [29], but on a single posteroanterior projection of the hand, dorsal or palmar osteophytes may not be visible. Subsequently, Altman et al. [28] found that a combined score of narrowing, osteophytes and erosions had the best overall diagnostic characteristics and that an evaluation limited to the second and third DIP joints, PIP joints and the trapezometacarpal joints was as useful as one involving all joints of the hand and wrist. Kallman et al. [30] developed a system utilizing the five DIP joints, four PIP joints, the first MCP joint, and the trapezoscaphoid joint of both hands which produced similar results to those of Altman. Kallman et al. applied their system in the follow-up of a male population in which joint space narrowing and doubtful osteophytes appeared to be the earliest signs of disease [30]. A modified version of this system was adopted by Lane et al. [31] and their study confirmed Kallman's findings with regard to narrowing and osteophyte formation.

These various systems have provided means of staging OA, and by giving equal weight to other features of the disease process the reliance upon osteophyte formation has been removed. Conventional radiography remains the most important technique for evaluation of OA due to its availability, low cost and detection of major change if scoring systems are used. However, detection of early abnormalities is not possible and an increasing role for other modalities such as scintigraphy, ultrasound and in particular magnetic resonance imaging is likely.

12.7   Radiological Features

12.7.1   Joints of the Hand

The most frequently affected joints in the hand are the interphalangeal joints of the fingers and thumb. While both the PIP and DIP joints of the fingers may be affected simultaneously (Fig. 12.7), isolated involvement of the DIP joint is not infrequently seen. In contrast it is relatively unusual to see PIP joint involvement in the absence of disease involving the DIP joints. MCP joint involvement is uncommon and virtually always associated with more distal disease of the interphalangeal joints.

This pattern of joint involvement is in contrast to the pattern seen in rheumatoid arthritis where the MCP and PIP joints are preferentially affected over the DIP joints.

12.7.2   Interphalangeal Joints

In common with other joints, the characteristic features of interphalangeal joint involvement in OA are joint space narrowing, subchondral sclerosis and peripheral

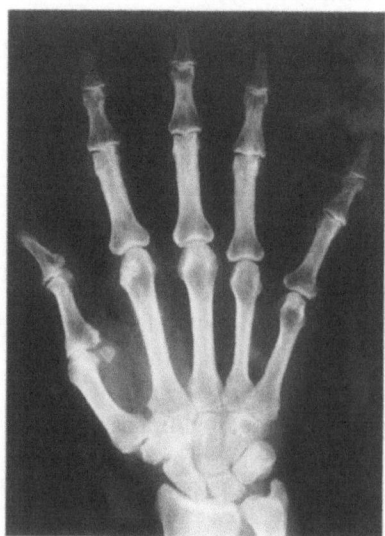

Fig. 12.7. DIP and PIP involvement. There is mild joint space narrowing, osteophyte formation and sclerosis affecting the DIP and PIP joints – a typical appearance in OA

osteophyte formation. Subchondral cyst formation may be prominent. As the process progresses the irregular cartilage loss results in characteristic tilt deformities. Further cartilage loss may lead to complete loss of joint space. The consequent mechanical erosion of bone on bone leads to a peculiar zig-zag appearance of the articular surfaces. Periarticular osteoporosis is not a feature of the disease. While erosive arthritis is described (see later discussion) erosions are not a typical finding in OA and their absence provides another means of distinction from the inflammatory arthropathies. However, if there is excessive crumbling and fragmentation of the subchondral bone the appearances may simulate a true erosive process.

Heberdon first described OA at the DIP joints in 1802. He drew attention to the nodal bony enlargements about these joints which are now termed Heberdon's nodes. Similar nodes can also be identified at the PIP joints and these are termed Bouchard's nodes. These nodes result from overgrowth of the phalangeal condyles, reflecting reparative processes in the pathophysiology of the disease. Such nodes are particularly characteristic of a form of OA, best thought of as a separate entity to "degenerative joint disease", that is most frequently seen in postmenopausal women and has been termed primary generalized or Kellgren's OA (Fig. 12.8). This variation is thought to occur in people with a genetic predisposition [6] and usually results in bilateral hand involvement, although sparing of the ipsilateral side in hemiparesis has been reported [32]. Although this form of OA runs its course over several years it usually leaves the patient with only moderate deformity and disability.

Soft tissue swelling is also seen about involved interphalangeal joints in OA. However, in contrast to the fusiform swelling seen in the inflammatory arthropathies, such as rheumatoid arthritis, that seen in OA is more focal and may have a lumpy appearance. Occasionally small mucoid cysts may develop adjacent to the interphalangeal joint, appearing as a particularly prominent focal soft tissue mass. These cysts are similar in nature to the ganglion cysts arising from joint capsules

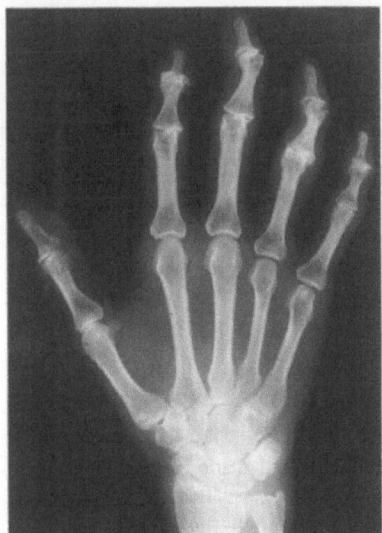

Fig. 12.8. Heberdon's and Bouchard's nodes. Osteoarthritic changes involve the DIP and PIP joints. Soft tissue swelling can be identified at both, consistent with Heberdon's and Bouchard's nodes respectively

or tendon sheaths, having gelatinous contents [33]. They may communicate with the articular capsule from which they arise.

12.7.3 Metacarpophalangeal Joints

At least some loss of joint space is seen in one or more of the MCP joints in the majority of patients with evidence of OA involving the interphalangeal joints [34]. In contrast to the diffuse but irregular joint space loss at the DIP and PIP joints, the joint space loss at the MCP joints tends to be uniform. However, in contrast to the interphalangeal joints and the joints of the wrist, other radiological features of OA such as subchondral sclerosis and osteophytosis are often not seen. When present, subchondral cysts are more frequently seen in the metacarpal heads than the phalangeal bases. If present, osteophytes are usually small.

12.7.4 Erosive Osteoarthritis

Erosive osteoarthritis or inflammatory arthritis are terms used in connection with a variant of primary generalized OA (described above) where the inflammatory component of the disease becomes particularly significant [35]. The disease has the same symmetrical joint distribution as non-inflammatory OA, classically involving the interphalangeal joints, and commonly the MCP and first carpometacarpal joints. Although the condition classically affects the joints of the hand, the wrist may occasionally be involved (Fig. 12.9).

Along with the expected findings in OA of joint space narrowing and proliferative changes (including osteophytosis) this form of the disease is characterized by

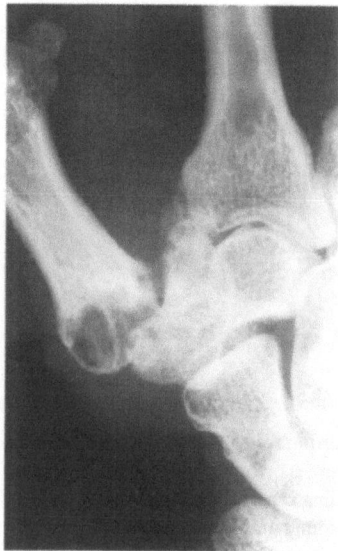

Fig. 12.9. Erosive OA. The articulation between the trapezium and first metacarpal is affected. Erosions are present on both sides of the joint space

the presence of bony erosions. Controversy exists as to the cause of the erosions, which may be the result of true synovial inflammation, although it is possible they may be related to collapse or pressure atrophy of the subchondral bone [26]. This latter theory would be in accordance with the observation that the erosions typically occur at sites of cartilage loss and therefore begin centrally within the joint. In contrast erosions of the inflammatory arthropathies are more marginally placed [36]. The pattern of central subchondral erosion seen in erosive OA gives the joint an appearance that resembles a seagull's wings. Adjacent periosteal new bone formation may be seen and bony ankylosis is a frequent occurrence in patients with erosive OA (Fig. 12.10) [36].

Erosive OA must be distinguished from the inflammatory arthropathies which result in erosions, such as rheumatoid arthritis and the seronegative arthropathies. In contrast to rheumatoid arthritis erosive OA has a more distal joint distribution in the hand, primarily involving the DIP joints. Rheumatoid arthritis lacks the proliferative features of OA such as subchondral sclerosis and osteophyte formation, typically showing instead juxta-articular osteoporosis. Furthermore, the pattern of bone destruction is different, with erosive OA showing the characteristic pattern of subchondral bone erosion discussed above.

Psoriatic arthritis typically has a more distal distribution similar to that seen in erosive OA. However, again the pattern of erosion is different and while periosteal bone apposition may be a feature of both diseases, that seen in psoriatic arthritis tends to be more irregular and exuberant in contrast to the mild linear periosteal new bone of erosive OA. The possibility of seronegative rheumatoid arthritis supervening on pre-existing OA must be considered, and may account for some cases diagnosed as erosive OA.

12.8 Joints of the Wrist

Approximately 95% of degenerative arthritis in the wrist relates to the scaphoid [37]. Three specific patterns have been described in periscaphoid degenerative disease of the wrist. The most common is that of SLAC wrist (scapholunate ad-

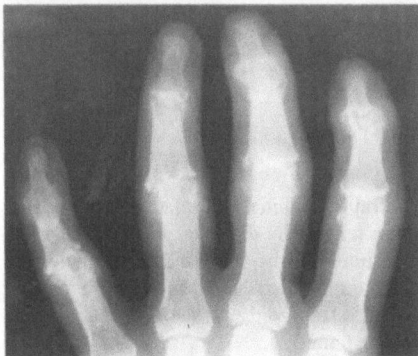

Fig. 12.10. Ankylosis. There is ankylosis of the DIP joint of the middle finger – a frequent occurrence in erosive OA

vanced collapse), which represents almost 55% of degenerative disease in the wrist. The second pattern is triscaphe arthritis affecting the trapezium, trapezoid and distal scaphoid, which is seen in 26% of wrist OA. A combination of these two patterns gives rise to the third, which involves the radioscaphoid, capitolunate and distal scaphoid-trapezium-trapezoid joints. This accounts for 14% of wrist arthritis, with the remaining 5% occurring between the distal ulna and lunate or lunate and triquetrum.

12.8.1   Pantrapezial Joints

The carpometacarpal joint between the trapezium and the thumb is frequently involved in OA, although the radiographic changes and clinical symptoms may not correlate [38]. In view of the four articulations of the trapezium with the thumb metacarpal, the index metacarpal, the trapezoid and the scaphoid, it has been helpful to consider this area as a single unit termed the pantrapezial or trapezio-centric joints (Fig. 12.11). A study comparing the accuracy of radiographic evaluation of the pantrapezial joints with anatomical dissection found that multifacet arthrosis was present in 73% of cases radiographically but in only 46% at anatomical dissection [39]. In none were all four facets involved. This overprediction radiographically appeared to relate to poor visualization of the trapezial articulation with the index metacarpal, trapezoid and scaphoid on standard radiographic views. The stress view of Eaton and Littler provides a clear view of all trapezial facets [40]. Other authors have also suggested additional views to improve the visualization of trapezial articulation [41–43].

The contours of the trapezium-thumb metacarpal joint have been studied in degenerative joints and normals, revealing that the saddle-shaped articulation is flatter in women than men and that as degenerative change progresses, a more

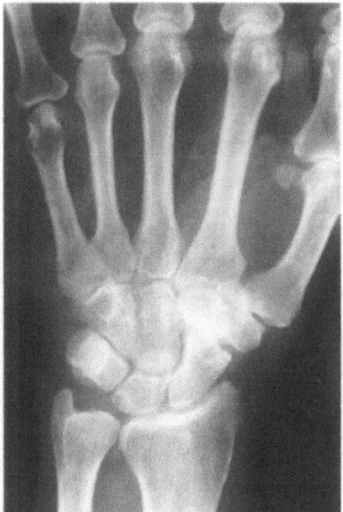

Fig. 12.11. Pantrapezial joints. Joint space narrowing and sclerosis are present at the distal scaphoid articulation with the trapezium and the trapezoid. Osteophyte formation is noted on the distal trapezium. In this projection, the trapezium-trapezoid articulation is obscured by the overlap of the bones

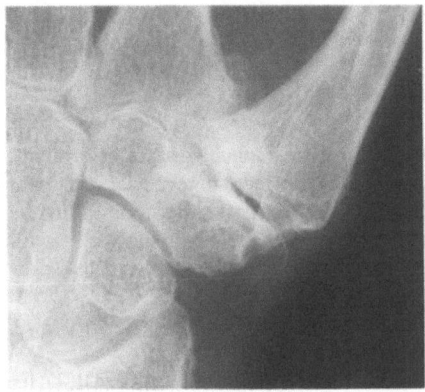

Fig. 12.12. Osteophytosis at the trapezium. Large osteophytes are present on the trapezium. The metacarpal demonstrates osteophytes but these are smaller. Accompanying sclerosis is also noted at this articulation

semi-cylindrical configuration develops [44]. Osteophytes were found earlier and were larger on the trapezium than on the metacarpal. When present, they tended to occur on the concave surfaces of the articulation (Fig. 12.12).

Eaton and Littler [40] described four stages of arthrosis visible radiographically. Slight widening of the joint space due to effusion occurs in stage I and mild subluxation can also be present. The joint space is narrow in stage II and at least one third subluxation is seen. Stage III is denoted by osteophytes and fragments greater than 2 mm in association with marked subluxation. By stage IV there is major subluxation, compensatory hyperextension at the interphalangeal joint and advanced cystic and sclerotic subchondral bone changes.

12.8.2   Periscaphoid Joints

The SLAC wrist results from disturbed alignment between the articular surfaces of the scaphoid and radius. The radial articular surface is composed of an ovoid fossa for the scaphoid and a spheroidal one for the lunate. The relationship of the scaphoid with this fossa has been described like two nesting boat hulls or two spoons, which, if congruous allow an even distribution of pressure [37]. Rotation, however, leads to contact between the proximal surface of the scaphoid and the edges rather than the concavity of the radial elliptical fossa. This in turn causes an uneven distribution of load and destructive change at these surfaces (Fig. 12.13).

The subsequent changes in the scaphoid, which collapses and rotates, alter the load distribution at the capitolunate joint. The ligamentous laxity allows separation of the scaphoid and lunate. Rotatory subluxation occurring at the scaphoid then permits the capitate to displace from the lunate in a shearing type of action. Cartilage destruction at the articular surfaces of the capitate and lunate is the end result. Interestingly, the sequence of events remains constant, with the process beginning in the radial portion of the radioscaphoid joint, extending to the remainder of this joint before affecting the capitolunate joint. The articulation of the proximal lunate with the radius is preserved. Despite large displacement of the lunate with volar interca-

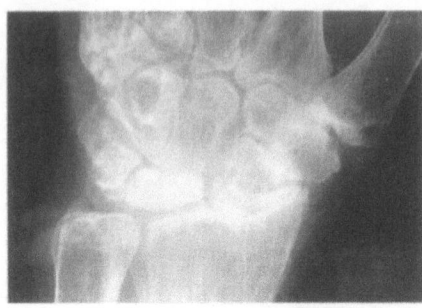

Fig. 12.13. Periscaphoid disease. Destructive change has occurred at the articular surfaces of the scaphoid and distal radius resulting in loss of joint space and sclerosis in this patient with calcium pyrophosphate dihydrate (CPPD) deposition

lated segment instability (VISI) or dorsal intercalated segment instability (DISI), its position within the spherical fossa of the distal radius remains perpendicular at the cartilage surfaces even in the advanced stages of the SLAC wrist.

Triscaphe arthritis between the scaphotrapezium and scaphotrapezoid joints occurs when the trapezium and trapezoid abut the dorsum of the distal scaphoid, particularly when the normal load distribution present on the radial aspect of the wrist is destroyed in SLAC wrist.

The SLAC wrist has also been described in CPPD but calcification was common in the triangular fibrocartilage complex (TFCC) and there was involvement of the radiolunate joint which allowed distinction from OA [45].

12.8.3 Ulno-carpal Disease

Ulnar-sided wrist disease will be considered, particularly as it relates to TFCC disorders and the ulnar impaction syndrome.

The TFCC is a cartilaginous, ligamentous structure arising from the radius and inserting into the ulna and adjacent carpus; it lies between the distal ulna and ulnar aspect of the proximal carpal row. The triangular fibrocartilage (TFC) proper is bordered anteriorly and posteriorly by the palmar and dorsal radioulnar ligaments. These attachments are further reinforced by some of the fibers inserting into the ulnar styloid base, lunate as the ulnolunate ligament, the triquetrum as the ulnotriquetral ligament, and the hamate and base of the fifth metacarpal as the ulnocollateral ligament. In this location, the TFCC functions as a cushion, stabilizing the distal radioulnar joint and the ulnar carpus. In the neutral position, the amount of load borne by the TFCC is constant irrespective of the presence of ulnar variance due to the relative thickness of the TFC in positive and negative variance [46–48]. Ulnar variance refers to the length of the ulna relative to the radius. Various methods of measurement have been used, although a study by Steyers and Blair [49] found compatibility between three of the most common methods. The three techniques compared were as follows: (1) Project a line. A line is drawn from the ulnar side of the articular surface of the distal radius toward the ulna. Variance is measured from this line to the carpal surface of the ulna [50, 51]. (2) The concentric circle technique of Palmer et al. [52]. The distal sclerotic line of the radius is marked and then a template of concentric circles placed over the radiograph. The distance from the line which most closely matches the concavity of the distal radial sclerotic line to the cortical rim of the ulnar head is measured. (3) The method of perpendiculars. The longitudinal axis of the radius is determined and then a line drawn perpendicular to it. The distance from this line to the distal cortical rim of the ulna is then measured [53]. Variation in the load transmitted on the ulnar aspect of the forearm occurs during supination and pronation, with supination resulting in a relative negative ulnar variance, and pronation in a more positive ulnar variance. Repetitive pronation and supination leads to loading of the ulnar aspect of the wrist, being variants of the ulnar impaction syndrome and causing damage to the proximal and distal aspects of the TFC. Cartilage loss of the lunate and ulnar head occurs and possibly perforation of the TFCC. Eventually, the lunotriquetral ligament ruptures leading to instability and degeneration of the ulnocarpal and distal radioulnar joints.

A classification was described based on clinical examination, conventional radiographs, arthrograms, arthroscopy and arthrotomy findings [54]. The major classification differentiates traumatic (based on lesion location) and degenerative lesions which depend on lesion location, degenerative change of TFCC, ulnar head, ulnocarpal bones and lunotriquetral ligament. As mentioned, the classification was based upon the imaging studies available at that time but similar findings have since been described at magnetic resonance imaging (MRI). Degenerative lesions are classified as class 2, traumatic lesions being class 1. In all the class 2 lesions, the posteroanterior radiograph in neutral position reveals a neutral or positive ulnar variant. Class 2A represents wear of the TFCC without perforation. Class 2B is similar but with chondromalacia of the ulnar aspect of the lunate or radial aspect of the ulnar head, or both. Subchondral erosion in these locations may also occur. Class 2C demonstrates an ovoid perforation of the TFCC in its ulnar avascular portion in addition to the findings in class 2B. Further progression seen in class 2D is characterized by degenerative change of the lunate and ulnar head, perforation of the horizontal portion of the TFCC and disruption of the lunotriquetral ligament. The end stages are seen in class 2E, in which the TFC is usually absent, the ulnocarpal and distal radioulnar joints show degenerative changes and the lunotriquetral ligament is completely disrupted.

MRI and bone scintigraphy have since demonstrated earlier detection of abnormalities in the carpal bones [55, 56]. Scintigraphy is sensitive but not specific and fails to demonstrate precise anatomical location. MRI depicts not only the signal abnormalities but also the anatomical distribution. Low signal on T1-weighted and corresponding high signal on T2-weighted sequences have been noted in the triquetrum, lunate and distal ulna, and the limited extent of the lunate signal changes allows differentiation from Kienböck disease. Fat suppression techniques enhance the detectibility of subtle lesions. Cartilage abnormalities have not been consistently identified in the wrist, but with improved techniques being employed elsewhere to evaluate cartilage, this may change in the future. MRI has also demonstrated perforations of the TFCC and, in combination with intra-articular gadolinium DTPA, it is now possible to visualize deficiencies in the other intrinsic ligaments such as the lunotriquetral ligament. Although this may allow more precise classification of the disease prior to surgery, various operative procedures are currently in use and the therapeutic implications for such detailed findings are not yet clear [55].

References

1. Trueta J (1968)Studies of the development and decay of the human frame. Saunders, Philadelphia
2. Mitchell NS, Cruess RL (1977) Classification of degenerative arthritis. Can Med Assoc J 117:763–765
3. Felson DT, Nevitt MC (1998) The effects of estrogen on osteoarthritis. Curr Opin Rheumatol 10:269–272
4. Creamer P, Hochberg MC (1997) Osteoarthritis. Lancet 350:503–508
5. Oddis CV (1996) New perspectives on osteoarthritis. Am J Med 100:10S–15S
6. Brooks PM, March LM (1995) New insights into osteoarthritis. Med J Aust 163:367–369
7. Burr DB (1998) The importance of subchondral bone in osteoarthrosis. Curr Opin Rheumatol 10:256–262
8. Radin EL, Paul IL, Rose RM (1977) Current concepts of the etiology of idiopathic osteoarthrosis. Bull Hosp Joint Dis 38:117–120
9. Mankin HJ (1974) The reaction of articular cartilage to injury and osteoarthritis: 1. N Engl J Med 291:1285–1292
10. Mankin HJ (1974) The reaction of articular cartilage to injury and osteoarthritis: 2. N Engl J Med 291:1335–1340
11. Dean DD, Martel-Pelletier J, Pelletier JP, Howell DS, Woessner JF Jr (1989) Evidence for metalloproteinase and metalloproteinase inhibitor imbalance in human osteoarthritic cartilage. J Clin Invest 84:678–685
12. Dean DD (1991) Proteinase-mediated cartilage degradation in osteoarthritis. Semin Arthritis Rheum 20:2–11
13. Pinals RS (1996) Mechanisms of joint destruction, pain and disability in osteoarthritis. Drugs 52:14–20
14. Kraus VB (1997) Pathogenesis and treatment of osteoarthritis. Med Clin North Am 81:85–112
15. Radin EL, Burr DB (1984) Hypothesis: joints can heal. Semin Arthritis Rheum 13:293–302
16. Crane AR, Scarano JJ (1967) Synovial cysts (ganglia) of bone. Report of two cases. J Bone Joint Surg Am 49:355–361
17. Harrison MHM, Schajowicz F, Trueta J (1953) Osteoarthritis of the hip: a study of the nature and evolution of the disease. J Bone Joint Surg Br 35:598
18. Cruickshank B, Macleod JG, Shearer WS (1954) Subarticular pseudocysts in rheumatoid arthritis. J Fac Radiol Lond 5:218
19. Bugnion JP (1951) Lesions du poignet; pseudokystes necrobiotiques, kusts par herniations capsulaires, arthrite chronique degenerative par osteochondrose marginale. Acta Radiol [Suppl] 90:5
20. Resnick D, Niwayama G, Coutts RD (1977) Subchondral cysts (geodes) in arthritic disorders: pathologic and radiographic appearance of the hip joint. AJR 128:799–806
21. Milgram JW (1983) Morphologic alterations of the subchondral bone in advanced degenerative arthritis. Clin Orthop 173:293–312
22. Freund E (1940) The pathological significance of intra-articular pressure. Edinb Med J 47:192–203
23. Landells JW (1953) The bone cysts of osteoarthritis. J Bone Joint Surg Br 35:643–649
24. Rhaney K, Lamb DW (1955). The cysts of osteoarthritis of the hip. A radiological and pathological study. J Bone Joint Surg Br 37:663

25. Ferguson AB (1964) The pathologic changes in degenerative arthritis of the hip and treatment by rotational osteotomy. J Bone Joint Surg Am 46:1337
26. Resnick D, Niwayama G (1995) Degenerative disease of extraspinal locations. In: Resnick D (ed) Diagnosis of bone and joint disorders, 3rd edn. Saunders, Philadelphia, pp 1263–1371
27. Goldenberg DL, Egan MS, Cohen AS (1982) Inflammatory synovitis in degenerative joint disease. J Rheumatol 9:204–209
28. Altman R, Alarcon G, Appelrouth D, Bloch D, Borenstein D, Brandt K et al (1990) The American College of Rheumatology criteria for the classification and reporting of osteoarthritis of the hand. Arthritis Rheum 33:1601–1610
29. Kellgren JH, Lawrence JS (1957) Radiological assessment of osteoarthritis. Ann Rheum Dis 16:494–501
30. Kallman DA, Wigley FM, Scott WW Jr, Hochberg MC, Tobin JD (1990) The longitudinal course of hand osteoarthritis in a male population. Arthritis Rheum 33:1323–1332
31. Lane NE, Nevitt MC, Genant HK, Hochberg MC (1993) Reliability of new indices of radiographic osteoarthritis of the hand and hip and lumbar disc degeneration. J Rheumatol 20:1911–1918
32. Goldberg RP, Zulman JI, Genant HK (1980) Unilateral primary osteoarthritis of the hand in monoplegia. Radiology 135:65–66
33. Goldman JA, Goldman L, Jaffe MS, Richfield DF (1977) Digital mucinous pseudocysts. Arthritis Rheum 20:997–1002
34. Martel W, Snarr JW, Horn JR (1973) The metacarpophalangeal joints in interphalangeal osteoarthritis. Radiology 108:1–7
35. Ehrlich GE (1975) Osteoarthritis beginning with inflammation. Definitions and correlations. JAMA 232:157–159
36. Martel W, Stuck KJ, Dworin AM, Hylland RG (1980) Erosive osteoarthritis and psoriatic arthritis: a radiologic comparison in the hand, wrist, and foot. AJR 134:125–135
37. Watson HK, Ryu J (1984) Degenerative disorders of the carpus. Orthop Clin North Am 15:337–353
38. Aune S (1955) Osteoarthritis of the first carpo-metacarpal joint. Acta Chir Scand 109:449–456
39. North ER, Eaton RG (1983) Degenerative joint disease of the trapezium: a comparative radiographic and anatomic study. J Hand Surg Am 8:160–166
40. Eaton RG, Littler JW (1973) Ligament reconstruction for the painful thumb carpometacarpal joint. J Bone Joint Surg Am 55:1655–1666
41. Lasserre C, Pauzat D, Derennes R (1949) Osteoarthritis of the trapeziometacarpal joint. J Bone Joint Surg Br 31:534–536
42. Gedda K (1954) Studies on Bennett's fracture: anatomy, roentgenology and therapy. Acta Chir Scand [Suppl] 193:39
43. Peter JB, Marmor L (1968) Osteoarthritis of the first carpometacarpal joint. Calif Med 109:116–120
44. North ER, Rutledge WM (1983) The trapezium-thumb metacarpal joint: the relationship of joint shape and degenerative joint disease. Hand 15:201–206
45. Chen C, Chandnani VP, Kang HS, Resnick D, Sartoris DJ, Haller J (1990) Scapholunate advanced collapse: a common wrist abnormality in calcium pyrophosphate dihydrate crystal deposition disease. Radiology 177:459–461
46. Palmer AK, Glisson RR, Werner FW (1984) Relationship between ulnar variance and triangular fibrocartilage complex thickness. J Hand Surg Am 9:681–682
47. Palmer AK, Werner FW (1984) Biomechanics of the distal radioulnar joint. Clin Orthop 187:26–35
48. Ekenstam FWa, Palmer AK, Glisson RR (1984) The load on the radius and ulna in different positions of the wrist and forearm. A cadaver study. Acta Orthop Scand 55:363–365

49. Steyers CM, Blair WF (1989). Measuring ulnar variance: a comparison of techniques. J Hand Surg Am 14:607–612

50. Voorhees DR, Daffner RH, Nunley JA, Gilula LA (1985) Carpal ligamentous disruptions and negative ulnar variance. Skeletal Radiol 13:257–262

51. Gelberman RH, Salamon PB, Jurist JM, Posch JL (1975) Ulnar variance in Kienböck's disease. J Bone Joint Surg Am 57:674–676

52. Palmer AK, Glisson RR, Werner FW (1982) Ulnar variance determination. J Hand Surg [Am] 7:376–379

53. Coleman DA, Blair WF, Shurr D (1987) Resection of the radial head for fracture of the radial head. Long-term follow-up of seventeen cases. J Bone Joint Surg Am 69:385–392

54. Palmer AK (1989) Triangular fibrocartilage complex lesions: a classification. J Hand Surg [Am] 14:594–606

55. Escobedo EM, Bergman AG, Hunter JC (1995) MR imaging of ulnar impaction. Skeletal Radiol 24:85–90

56. Imaeda T, Nakamura R, Shionoya K, Makino N (1996) Ulnar impaction syndrome: MR imaging findings. Radiology 201:495–500

13 Rheumatic Diseases

Herwig Imhof, Franz Kainberger, Irene Sulzbacher,
Thomas Rand

13.1 Pathologic Anatomy and Physiology

Inflammatory arthritis starts in the synovial membrane. The synovial membrane is composed of two layers: an external fibrous and an internal synovial layer. Whereas the first is a complex structure of collagen fibers with hardly any metabolic activity, the synovial layer with its high content of capillaries ensures a fast and extensive reaction to any kind of agent. It is arranged in folds covered by one or two layers of two types of lining cells: the A-cells and the B-cells. The so-called A-cells are derived from bone marrow and are capable of phagocytosis when presented with foreign material. The B-cells are special fibroblasts of mesenchymal origin and synthesize important proteins of the synovial fluid such as glycosaminoglycans. No basal layer separates these lining cells from the underlying synovial stroma that consists of a loose network of collagen fibers with many capillaries and a varying amount of fat cells. The synovium is an immunocompetent tissue and reacts to any agent according to general defense mechanisms (Fig. 13.1) (Leeb et al. 1996).

The articular cartilage consists of five different layers according to the structures of fibers (Fig. 13.2): On the surface is the lamina splendens, which is several micrometers thick and consists of horizontally oriented fine fibers. The second layer is the tangential zone, which consists of tightly packed bundles of individual

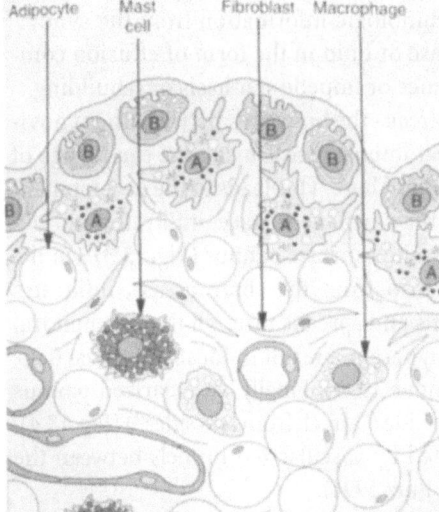

Fig. 13.1. Schematic drawing of synovialis: *A* A-cells, *B* B-cells representing the surface of the synovialis

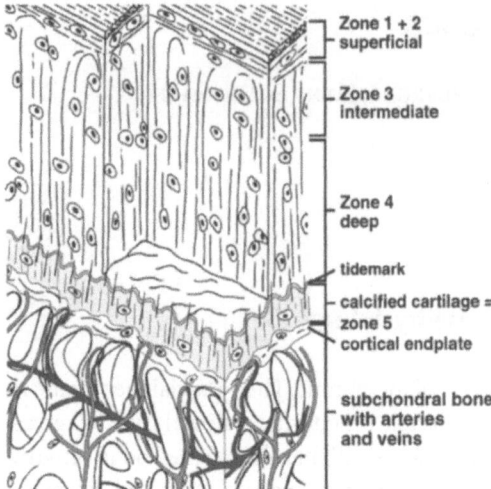

Zone 1 + 2
superficial

Zone 3
intermediate

Zone 4
deep

tidemark

calcified cartilage =
zone 5
cortical endplate

subchondral bone
with arteries
and veins

Fig. 13.2. Schematic drawing of hyaline (articular) cartilage and subchondral region

collagen fibrils. They are arranged parallel to the articular surface and often at right angles to each other. The tangential zone is essential for the integrity of cartilage and is thickest at the periphery and thinnest at the center of the joint. The third zone is the transitional zone. It contains significant amounts of proteoglycans as well as collagen. The collagen fibrils are randomly arranged. The radial zone, the fourth layer, is usually the largest compared with the other layers. The fifth layer is the calcified cartilage. Between the calcified cartilage and radial zone lies the so-called tidemark (Imhof et al. 1997).

Below the fifth layer – the calcified cartilage-layer – the subchondral bone is located. It contains the undulated cortical endplate and the bony trabeculae with bony marrow in between and many of arteries and veins (Bullough 1992; Imhof et al. 1999a;Lane and Weiss 1975).

The synovial fluid is produced by the synovium. It serves as gliding fluid, and transports nourishment, debris and immunologic information from the synovium to the cartilage and vice versa. Increase of fluid in the form of effusion compensates for malalignment and may enhance or impede synthesis or rebuilding.

In pathophysiology the so-called bare areas - the bony area between the synovium and the hyaline cartilage – are of great importance. During the early stage of any form of arthritis, cell proliferation is found here. This leads to the development of granulation tissue, which grows over the cartilage surface, infiltrates and destroys the cartilage and represents the so-called surface pannus (Fig. 13.3). On the other hand, the marrow pannus starts also from the "bare areas", infiltrates through the cortical bone, leads to erosions and spreads through the subchondral bone. Activated osteoclasts and reactive hyperemia result in localized periarticular osteopenia and, later, osteolysis (Hunder 1999). Finally, vascularized pannus tissue infiltrates the cartilage from the bony side ("attack from two sides") (Fig. 13.4). This attack from the bony side is facilitated by vascularized tunnels between the subchondral bone and cartilage (Milz and Putz 1994).

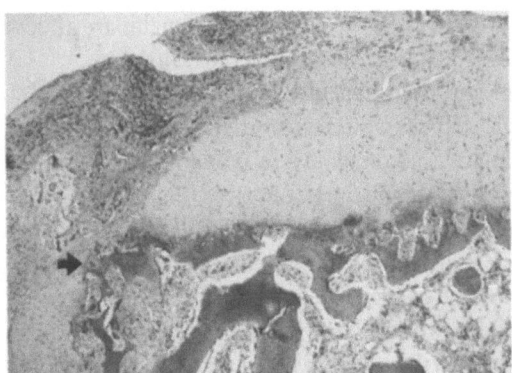

Fig. 13.3. Histologic section of "bare area" (HE staining): infiltration of the subchondral region by inflammatory tissue (*arrow*) through the so-called bare areas. The hyaline cartilage is overgrown and partly destroyed by pannus tissue (= surface-pannus).

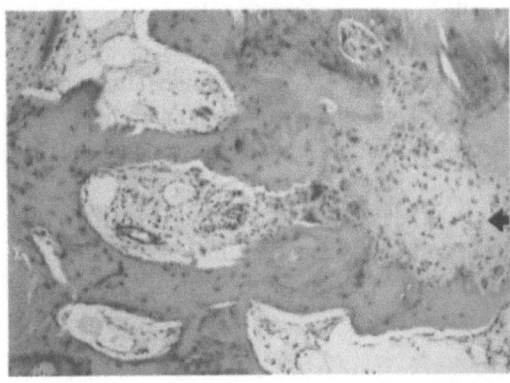

Fig. 13.4. Histologic section of subchondral region (HE staining) infiltration by inflammatory granulation tissue and resorption by osteoclasts (*arrow*)

Rheumatoid arthritis and related diseases are multi-phase processes. Deficient healing will take place resulting in chondroid metaplasia and fibrous-calcified scar tissue. Besides these processes, subchondral osteonecrosis may develop, ending in cystic formations and reactive debris. Finally, degenerative processes may overlay the primary inflammatory base.

13.1.1 Rheumatoid Arthritis and Related Diseases

13.1.1.1 Rheumatoid Arthritis

There is strong evidence that rheumatoid arthritis occurs in genetically predisposed individuals, probably after exposure to as yet unknown antigens. It is believed to be an immune response to such potential antigens as *Candida* or viruses as well as mycobacteria and *Mycoplasma*. These agents may act either directly, through molecular mimicry, or indirectly through other pathways. It is very likely that there are also multiple genes involved. In white populations, this genetic predisposition appears to be associated with major histocompatibility complex antigens of the human lymphocyte antigen (HLA-D) locus. The B-lymphocyte alloantigen HLA-DR4 is present in about 70% of patients with rheumatoid arthritis, compared with 28% of controls. Gender plays a clear role, as females are affected more often than males in a ratio of 3:1 (Stasny 1978; Harris 1990).

Exposure of such a genetically predisposed patient to a putative environmental trigger initiates a cascade of histologic changes which can be described in four stages. At first, proliferation of synovial lining cells accompanied by mononuclear infiltrates resulting in hyperplasia of the synovial membrane can be observed (Fig. 13.5) Secondly, lymphocytes in the stroma organize into germinal-center like aggregates with a predominantly perivascular location. In addition plasma cells surround the aggregates. Neutrophilic granulocytes are located between the synovial lining cells and areas of fibrinoid necrosis can be found in the tips of the synovial fronds. The whole tissue is edematous and swollen. Characteristically the necrotic tissue sloughs into the joint cavity where these fragments are known as rice bodies. In the third stage granulation tissue, rich in macrophages – the so-called pannus – organizes the necrotic and inflammatory parts of the synovium (Fassbaender 1994; Athanasou et al. 1998). Formation of new blood vessels is essential to the process of synovial proliferation (angiogenesis). These new blood vessels support synovial hypertrophy and permit access of inflammatory cells into the joint. Eventual vascular infiltration of the cartilage plays a key role in the erosive disease process of rheumatoid arthritis (Fig. 13.6).

The active synovial inflammatory process and the active pannus itself can directly destroy the cortex in the so-called bare areas at the base of the joints, where synovium and synovial fluid have direct contact with bone. This process leads to the well-known

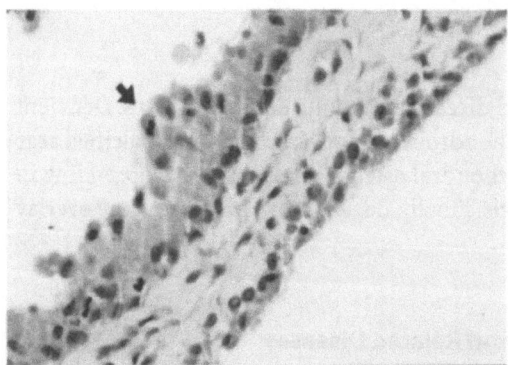

Fig. 13.5. Synovial frond with proliferation of lining cells on one side (*arrow*) (HE staining, histological section)

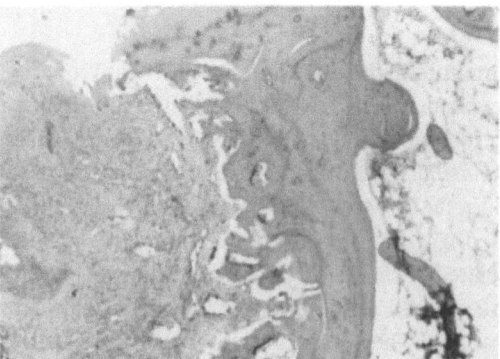

Fig. 13.6. Histological section of aggressive pannus and hyaline (articular) cartilage (HE staining) showing infiltration and destruction of hyaline cartilage by hypervascularized granulation tissue

erosive changes in anatomically typical locations. Synovial cysts may develop as a result of synovial hyperplasia and herniation of inflamed synovial tissue through the overlying fascia. Mature pannus itself is aggressively invasive and contributes, together with intra-articular inflammatory processes, to characteristic joint destruction. Finally the destruction of the underlying cartilage begins by the released proteinases. The inflammatory process continues in the subchondral bone also, where mononuclear cells stimulate changes also seen in osteomyelitis. The cellular infiltration and hyperemia, accompanying edema and immobilization due to pain result in periarticular osteopenia. The end of this relapsing disease is fibrosis of the destructive granulation tissue resulting in joint ankylosis (Netter 1990) (Table 13.1).

The usual pattern of onset is in 80% of cases polyarticular, with the wrist, metacarpophalangeal and proximal interphalangeal joints being affected. Twenty percent of patients have monoarticular disease. The typical peak age of onset is between about 20 and 50 years of age. The articular disease is usually polycyclic and progressive. However, in about 20% of patients it is monocyclic, with remission for at least 1 year after the onset. In a minority it is relentlessly active with an ever-increasing number of joints involved and worsening severity of joint involvement with the passing years. Long-term remission is rare, and probably occurs in less than 5% of patients with disease of 5 or more years duration. Intermittent remission is seen in 10–20% of patients who have periods of clinical quiescent disease that are longer than the periods of active disease. In most patients the extent of disability is determined within the first several years of disease, with slow worsening of functional capacity thereafter. This understanding of the natural history emphasizes the need for early disease recognition and therapeutic intervention (McCarty 1993).

In rheumatoid disease symmetric involvement of wrist, metacarpophalangeal and proximal interphalangeal joints is typical (Fig. 13.7). Quite often not all joints are involved to the same degree. Asymmetric involvement may be due to relative overuse of the more affected joint or because of secondary disease, such as septic arthritis of an already inflamed joint. Due to neuroimmunologic phenomena, patients with rheumatoid disease who suffer from a stroke, polio, etc., have little if any active synovitis.

Table 13.1. Stages of rheumatoid arthritis and associated radiologic findings

Stage	Radiologic findings
Stage I	None (antigen presentation to T-cells)
Stage II	None (lymphoid in synovium cell hyperplasia with angiogenesis)
Stage III	Conventional radiography: soft tissue swelling
	MRI: synovial thickening with edema; contrast medium enhancement due to angiogenesis/fibrovascular tissue
	Doppler US: synovial hyperemia; thickening of synovium
Stage IV	Conventional radiography: juxta-articular osteopenia
	MRI: pannus visualization; joint effusion
Stage V	Conventional radiography: marginal subchondral erosions; joint space narrowing; indistinct carpal margins
	MRI: pannus formation; activity of pannus corresponding to contrast enhancement; cartilage destruction

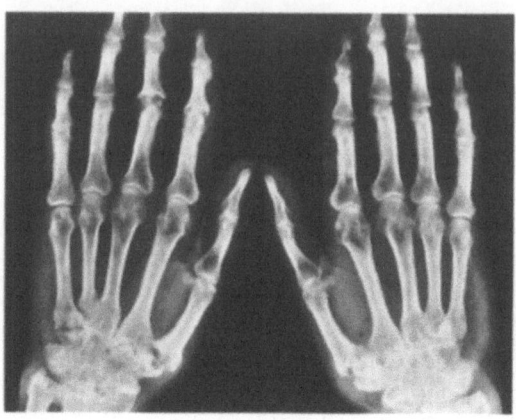

Fig. 13.7. Rheumatoid polyarthritis (dorsovolar radiograph of both hands): there is symmetric inflammatory involvement of metacarpophalangeal, wrist and proximal interphalangeal joints with periarticular osteopenia and diffuse bony and joint destruction in both wrists

Synovitis of the tendon sheath is another important feature of rheumatoid arthritis. It leads to proliferation and hypervascularity with development of rheumatoid nodules – nodules with fibrinoid necrosis, surrounding mononuclear cells and small vessel vasculitis in the acute stage, later with surrounding fibrosing connective tissue. The nodules (Fig. 13.8), which can measure up to 30 mm, may erode into the tendon, leading to their rupture. In some cases the inflamed tenosynovial tissue cannot move through the flexor tendon sheath, resulting in a "trigger finger". Tenosynovitis of the extensor tendons may be accompanied by hyperextension of the metacarpophalangeal joint, flexion of the proximal interphalangeal joint and hyperextension of the distal interphalangeal joint resulting in the so-called buttonhole deformity. On the other hand swan-neck deformity shows flexion in the metacarpophalangeal joint, hyperextension in the proximal interphalangeal joint and flexion in the distal interphalangeal joint (Fig. 13.9).

Due to joint destruction, laxity of ligaments, and shortening (shrinkage) of tendons and joint capsules, severe ulnar deviation of fingers with subluxation in several joints may be found. Synovial proliferation and hypervascularity within the wrist may lead to carpal tunnel syndrome with median nerve compression and thenar atrophy. In the worst cases severe long-standing rheumatoid arthritis can lead to joint erosion and resorption with shrinkage of the complete hand – typical

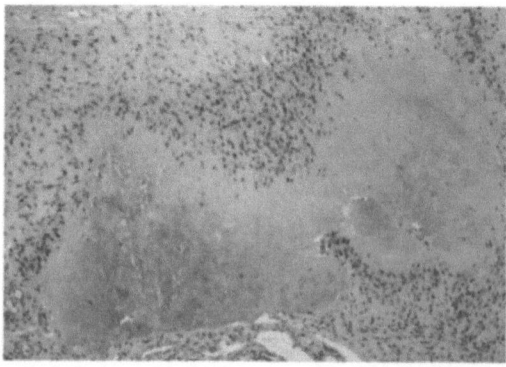

Fig. 13.8. Histological section of a rheumatoid nodule (HE staining) showing central fibrinoid necrosis with surrounding fibrosing connective tissue

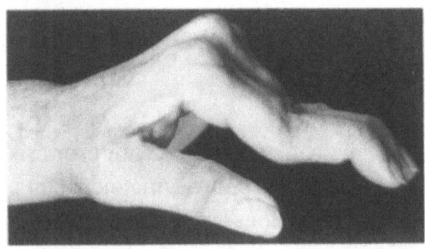

Fig. 13.9. Swan-neck deformity of the finger-joints due to tenosynovitis

signs of arthritis mutilans with complete destruction of distal radius, ulna and carpal bones and ankylosis of the carpal bones as well. Resorption of multiple wrist bones and phalanges may be evident as a profound osteopenia (Fig. 13.7).

13.1.1.2 Juvenile Rheumatoid Arthritis

Also widely known as juvenile chronic arthritis, juvenile rheumatoid arthritis is a term denoting several chronic arthritic conditions of childhood, the cause(s) of which are unknown. Long-standing arthritis is a typical symptom. Similar to rheumatoid arthritis, tenosynovitis, synovitis, pannus development and rheumatoid nodules of the hands and wrists are found in the majority of cases. Typical radiographic findings are symmetric radiodense soft tissue swelling, loss of joint space with bony overgrowth and reactive widening of bone. In the later stages erosions, joint resorption and destruction may be found as in rheumatoid arthritis.

13.1.1.3 Adult-Onset Still's Disease

In contrast to rheumatoid disease the small joints of the fingers are not affected in Still's disease. The wrist and metacarpophalangeal joints show similar radiographic features to rheumatoid disease: destructive polyarthritis with periarticular osteopenia and loss of joint space. The pathophysiologic basis is again synovitis.

13.1.1.4 Jaccoud's Arthritis

Jaccoud's arthritis shows similar deformities to rheumatoid arthritis and systemic lupus erythematosus, but lacks the deforming, erosive joint changes. The acute episode is characterized by a mild synovitis with minimal edema and cellular infiltration of the superficial synovial layers. Within the deeper synovial strata and joint capsule, the collagen fibers undergo a fibrinous change. There is no alteration in joint cartilage or subchondral bone. The synovial and capsular changes may completely regress with no permanent residual sequel.

Chronic recurrent progressive fibrosis of the capsule, periarticular tendons and fascia results in the characteristic digital ulnar deviation and deformities. The joint most frequently involved are the metacarpophalangeal joints. There is normal bone density.

13.1.2 Seronegative Spondyloarthropathies

13.1.2.1 Psoriatic Arthropathy

Psoriatic arthritis is defined as an inflammatory arthritis associated with psoriasis but occurring in the absence of rheumatoid nodules and serum rheumatoid factors. The arthritis may precede the onset or diagnosis of cutaneous lesions of psoriasis in 10–15% of patients. Psoriatic arthritis occurs in 10% of patients with psoriasis. It is found in the age group between 20 and 50 years. There is an equal sex distribution. It is more common in Eurocaucasians and rare in Africans, Chinese and North American Indians. There are various forms of arthritis including distal interphalangeal joint arthritis, symmetric peripheral arthritis and asymmetric oligoarthritis mutilans. Some patients may show peripheral enthesitis without arthritis, a typical feature of all seronegative spondyloarthropathies (ankylosing spondylitis, Reiter's syndrome, enteropathic arthritis, undifferentiated spondyloarthropathy, juvenile spondyloarthropathy, SAPHO disease) (Khan 1992).

The pathologic changes of psoriatic arthritis are essentially similar to those of rheumatoid arthritis but asymmetric. In the synovial joint an initial proliferative synovitis results in pannus formation with prominent fibrosis. Superficial cartilage and small marginal bone erosions occur secondary to the invading pannus (much less than in rheumatoid arthritis). Adjacent to the erosions periostitis results in new bone formation.

At bone-ligament junctions similar erosive and proliferative changes may occur. Prominent fibrous tissue production within the joint cavity may widen the joint, which eventually undergoes metaplasia producing bony ankylosis (Fig. 13.10). In contrast to rheumatoid arthritis psoriatic arthritis shows a distinct lack of intense synovial hyperemia, maintaining normal bone mineralization adjacent to the involved bone.

The most commonly involved joints are the distal interphalangeal and proximal interphalangeal joints. Occasionally, all three articulations of one digit will be involved, producing the "sausage digit" that is virtually a diagnostic sign of psoriatic arthritis. Bony erosions are most common at the joint margins. There is frequently fluffy periosteal new bone formation ("mouse ear" sign) (Fig. 13.11). Progression of the erosions results in a whittling effect of the distal articular end of the phalanx. Rarely the disease ends in severe arthritis mutilans.

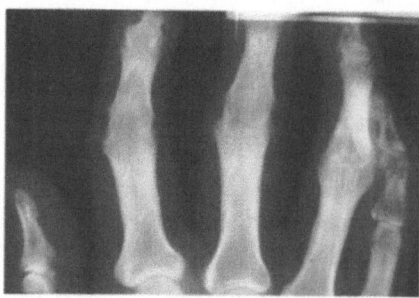

Fig. 13.10. Radiograph (detail) of the fingers of a patient with psoriatic arthropathy, showing complete bony fusion of the proximal interphalangeal joints II, III and IV

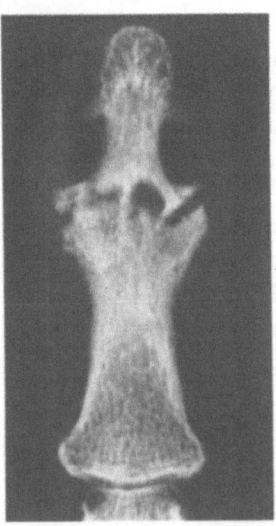

Fig. 13.11. Radiograph of the distal interphalangeal joint in psoriatic arthropathy showing severe erosions with fluffy periosteal new bone formation ("mouse-ear" sign). There is no periarticular osteopenia

13.1.2.2   Reactive Arthritis and Reiter's Syndrome

Reactive arthritis is defined as an aseptic inflammatory arthritis, usually asymmetric and oligoarticular. Reactive arthritis is triggered by microbial infection at a distant site usually in the gastrointestinal or genitourinary tract. The term reactive arthritis is often used when the identity of the triggering organism is known, and it encompasses the more restrictive term Reiter's syndrome, which in its classic form consists of oligoarthritis and conjunctivitis following a nongonoccocal urethritis or cervicitis or an episode of diarrhea. Today incomplete forms of reactive arthritis are more often found than complete ones. The disease is most commonly seen in young sexually active adults, mostly men, when it is triggered by *Chlamydia trachomatis*. However, reactive arthritis is underdiagnosed in women due to the frequently subclinical or asymptomatic chlamydial infection (Toivanen 1993).

The joints involved are usually those of the lower limbs with often asymmetric involvement. The presence of any associated tenosynovitis, enthesitis or "sausage digits" is highly suggestive of the diagnosis. Reactive osteopenia may be seen only in the acute phase. Small marginal erosions on the ulnar side with fluffy, periosteal reactions may be seen.

Rarely mutilation or ankylosis may evolve. There has been an increase in reactive arthritis resulting from immunodeficiencies (e.g., HIV-infection, A-gamma-globulinemia and others).

1.2.3   Ankylosing Spondylitis (Bechterew's Disease)

Ankylosing spondylitis is a chronic inflammatory disorder of undetermined etiology, usually beginning in early adulthood. It primarily affects the axial skeleton, but it can also exhibit some extra-articular features. It is 3 times more common in males.

The inflammation appears to originate in ligamentous and capsular sites of attachment to bones (enthesitis), juxta-articular ligamentous structures, and the synovium, articular cartilage and subchondral bones of involved joints. The site of enthesitis is infiltrated by lymphocytes, plasma cells and polymorphonuclear cells and there is also edema and infiltration of the adjacent marrow space (Van der Linden 1996).

In more than 50% of cases peripheral arthritis may be detected. The joints of the hands are almost never a primary site of inflammation. Erosive changes with proliferative signs in the joints of the wrist, rarely of the metacarpophalangeal, proximal interphalangeal and distal interphalangeal joints, are relatively typical. Accompanying soft tissue swelling with periarticular osteopenia may be seen (Fig. 13.12) (Resnick and Niwayama 1995).

13.1.3   Collagen Disease

13.1.3.1   Systemic Lupus Erythematosus

Systemic lupus erythematosus (SLE) is a genetically determined disease characterized by diverse clinical features. The disease affects women (between the ages of 20 and 50 years) 9 times more frequently than men and is most common in the child-bearing years. Factors that appear to exacerbate the disease are ultraviolet light, certain drugs, post-pregnancy, and marked stress. Articular signs and symptoms occur in up to 90% of patients. The most striking histologic feature are synovitis with so-called fibrinoid necrosis and fibrinoid deposition within the synovium of the joints and tendon sheaths. Due to the also on fibrinoid deposition based vasculitis of small arteries and capillaries Raynaud disease may develop as well . Shrinkage of tendons leads to severe nondestructive deformity in metacarpophalangeal and phalangeal joints and(or) spontaneous rupture of tendons. The disease in usually bilateral, symmetric and most frequently involves the hand (Hughes 1994).

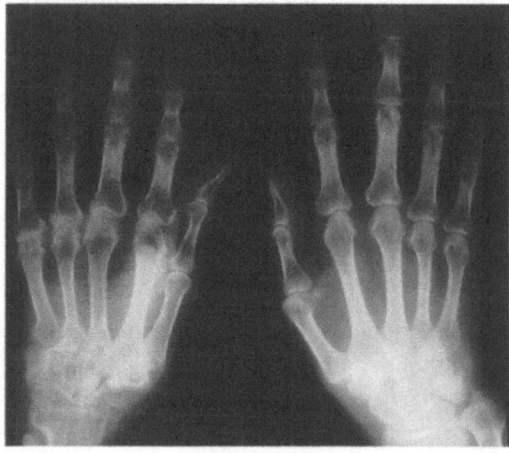

Fig. 13.12. Radiograph of both hands of a patient with ankylosing spondylitis, showing severe right-sided erosive changes in the wrist bones. Additionally there is a moderate periarticular osteopenia

The most prominent clinical and radiologic symptom is the atrophy of the overlying musculature. Occasionally, sheet-like or punctate calcifications can be seen. Changes in the joint space and subchondral bone are rare. Generalized osteoporosis is typical and small degrees of tuftal resorption due to accompanying Raynaud disease is seen. Digital ulnar deviation, buttonhole deformities and swan-neck deformities are characteristic, but usually not permanent in nature.

13.1.3.2   Scleroderma and Mixed Connective Tissue Disease

Sleroderma is a generalized systemic inflammatory connective tissue disease of unknown etiology. The pathologic changes observed are predominantly vascular in nature, consisting of a low-grade inflammatory reaction in the perivascular tissue, with atrophy and fibrosis of adjacent collagen. The result is promotion of fibrous tissue deposition and induration. Synovium reveals inflammatory cellular infiltration with fibrin internally and externally.

The most prominent changes are in the hand. Resorption of soft tissue results in a tapered, conical configuration of the fingertip with retraction of the tip in a proximal manner. In up to 80% of cases resorbing osteolysis of the terminal tufts may be seen (acro-osteolysis). Eventually complete osteolysis of the phalanx may be evident. Soft tissue calcification is seen in up to 20% of patients. The calcification is punctate or sheet-like. The location of these calcifications seems to be related to areas of trauma such as the radial surface of the second digit, and(or) ulnar aspect of forearm, especially in the dominant hand (Le Roy et al. 1988). Generalized osteoporosis is usually due to disuse and immobilization. Rarely, scleroderma-induced vasculitis may result in avascular necrosis.

Articular alterations are variable. Bilateral selective involvement of the first carpometacarpal joint of the wrist with resorption of the first metacarpal base and trapezium is distinctive. Occasionally, intra-articular calcification and manifestations of rheumatoid arthritis, erosive arthritis and psoriasis are seen.

The so-called Thibierge-Weissenbach syndrome is a combination of soft tissue calcification, Raynaud phenomenon and generalized telangiectasia (Fig. 13.13).

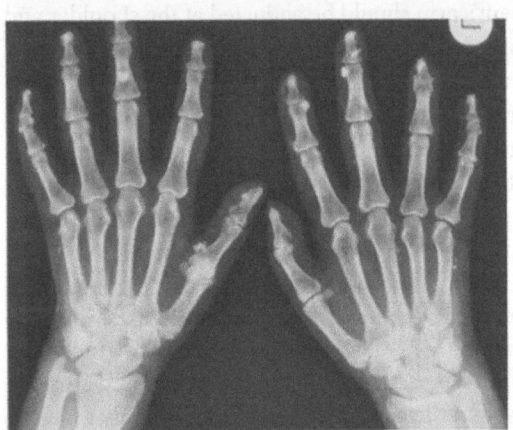

Fig. 13.13. Radiograph of both hands of a patient with scleroderma, showing soft tissue resorption and osteolysis of the fingertips with multiple punctate soft tissue calcifications

CREST syndrome is a term for identifying the major associations in scleroderma: Calcinosis, Raynaud, Esophageal dysmotility, Scleroderma, Telangiectasia. Sharp syndrome (mixed connective tissue disease) is an overlap-syndrome of scleroderma, SLE, dermatomyositis and rheumatoid disease.

13.1.3.3 Dermatomyositis/Polymyositis

A number of classifications of myositis and dermatomyositis have been proposed. The most common forms are dermatomyositis of the adult and the juvenile form, polymyositis and inclusion body myositis. Arthritis of the hand is rarely seen, except as vanishing arthralgia.

13.1.3.4 Rheumatic Fever

A rare disease today, based on an infection with b-hemolytic *Streptococcus*, rheumatic fever leads to systemic inflammatory changes. It is combined frequently with carditis and endocarditis and reactive, relapsing arthritis. In the hand it leads very often to Jaccoud's arthritis (Schmitt and Lanz 1996).

13.2   Investigative Techniques

13.2.1   Conventional and Digital Radiography

Despite continuous advances in cross-sectional imaging techniques during the last decade, conventional radiography still plays a key role in imaging of rheumatic diseases of the hand and wrist (Resnick and Niwayama 1995). Conventional radiographs provide basic and comprehensive information about arthritic changes in the hands. Films should be exposed in a form that documents both bony and soft tissues. Standardization of the positioning of the upper limb and of the direction of the X-ray beam is mandatory to provide sufficient information for the diagnosis of possible malalignment (Wilson et al. 1990). The patient's arm should be abducted at the shoulder and flexed at the elbow to 90°. Criteria of correct positioning are that the styloid process of the ulna is imaged without rotation and that a single line may be drawn along the distal end of the radius, the third metacarpal bone and the third finger (Wilson et al. 1990).

Digital soft-copy visualization results in new problems: use of specific edge-enhancement programs; gray-level of screens; intermission and minimal detail resolution are necessary. Digital radiography is generally performed by means of phosphor storage devices. In an in-house study of our department, it was shown that the better contrast resolution and the optimization of brightness are important parameters of increased image quality with respect to the diagnosis of rheumatic diseases. Since the advent of magnetic resonance imaging (MRI) and high-resolution sonography the importance of plain film imaging for the detection of early pre-erosions and erosions has been reduced. For the same reasons, arthrography of the wrist plays only a limited role in selected cases of surgical planning. Magnification views, especially taken with dedicated techniques and small spot sizes lower than 0.1 mm, have been proven to show even more details of the formation of pre-erosions and small erosions of the articular bone (Genant et al. 1975). The clinical application of this technique, however, has been reduced in view of modern cross-sectional imaging.

On images exposed in a dorsovolar direction not all erosions may be detected. This is especially true for the triquetral, pisiform and hamate bones. Instead of taking additional films in dedicated oblique directions, tomographic techniques like MRI should be performed. With respect to both the precision of measurements in follow-up studies and the radiation exposure, images in a dorsovolar projection are generally regarded to be sufficient for the diagnosis of arthritis of the wrist. Instead of angulated views, documentation of both hands, both feet and all other symptomatic joints should be performed to assess the extent and severity of disease (Freyschmidt 1985; Kainberger et al. 1996; Watt 1995). Image analysis, whether it is performed by means of conventional film or of digital equipment, should in any case include options for optimizing brightness parameters and for magnifying parts of the images.

13.2.2 Sonography

Sonography of the hand and wrist is a technique with the capability of documenting different forms of disease manifestation of the soft tissues. It is of specific importance in all forms of early arthritis to confirm morphologic abnormalities in patients when clinical and radiographic signs are subtle or absent. The main limitation of sonography is the lack of visualization of deeper tissues, especially those within the center of a joint. As a general rule, ultrasound imaging should be performed together with conventional radiography and the sonograms interpreted in context with the radiographic findings.

There is no general agreement in the literature about the technique of investigation. Transducer frequency should be in the range between 7 and 16 MHz to generate high-resolution images of the tendons, nerves, vessels and of the articular structures. Scanning should include transverse and sagittal sections of the volar and dorsal aspects of the wrist (Table 13.2). Color Doppler ultrasound may be useful to identify blood vessels and to assess the vascularity of inflammatory tissues. Flow dynamics should be documented on video or in the form of digital sequential images. It is necessary to differentiate the normal signal of tendons from abnormalities due to artifacts resulting from acoustic fiber anisotropy. If the angle between the emitted sound waves and the tendon is more than 83°–88° higher or lower than the perpendicular sound beam the majority of the reflected waves will not be received by the transducer and tendons will become hypoechoic (Crass et al. 1988). The effect of such anisotropy effects is most noticeable at the wrist (Van Holsbeeck and Introcaso 1991). Evaluation of the ulnocarpal compartment and its surrounding structures are of particular importance in the case of suspected rheumatic disease. The extensor carpi ulnaris tendon is located in intimate relationship with the posteromedial aspect of the distal ulna, the ulnar styloid process and the triquetrum (Fig. 13.14). The median nerve has a fibrillar texture, but is

Table 13.2. Semi-standardized documentation of ultrasound investigation of the wrist in suspected arthritis

Region	Orientation of scan	Anatomic key structures to be defined
Plantar aspect of wrist	Transverse median nerve	Superficial and deep flexor tendons
Dorsum of wrist	Transverse	Extensor tendons
Distal styloid, posterolateral	Sagittal, transverse	Tendon of extensor carpi ulnaris muscle, distal end of ulna, triquetrum, triangular fibrocartilage

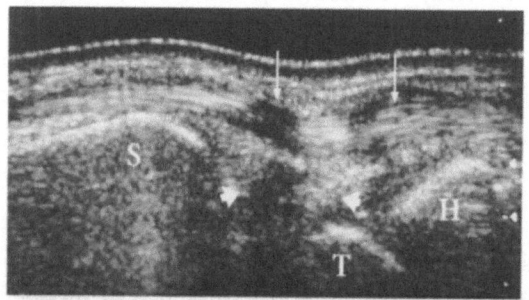

a

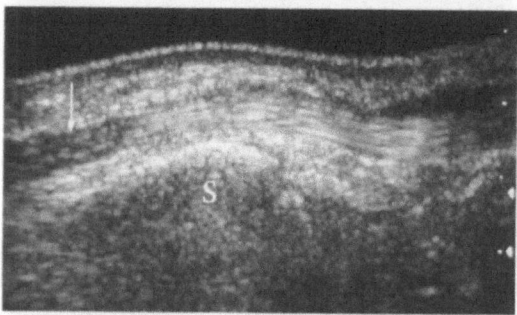

b

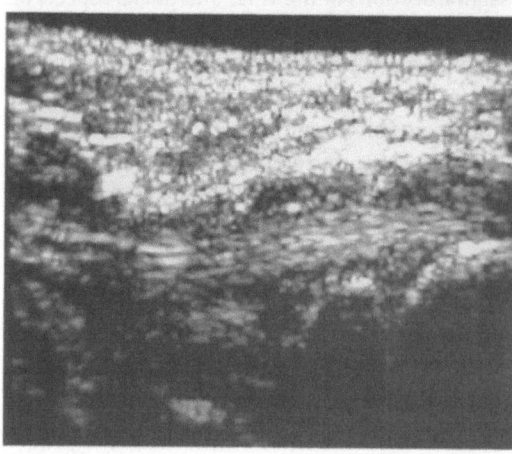

c

Fig. 13.14a–c. Basics in sonographic imaging of the hand. **a** Hyperechoic tendon of extensor carpi ulnaris muscle with hypoechoic foci (*arrows*) due to acoustic anisotropic artifacts. Beneath the tendon, the triangular cartilage complex (*arrowheads*) is visible. *S* ulnar styloid process, *T* os triquetrum, *H* hamate bone. **b** Under angulation of the transducer the anisotropic hypoechoic foci move to a different area of tendon that is now prone to angulated sound waves (*arrow*). **c** In this case of rheumatoid arthritis, beneath tendon structures, hypoechoic transformation of tissue indicating inflammation is found

slightly less echoic than the flexor tendons. It is identified by its anatomic location and its immobility, in contrast to the adjacent flexor tendons that are mobile during flexion movements of the fingers. The triangular fibrocartilage is a hyperechoic structure with ill-defined borders. It is identified beneath the extensor carpi ulnaris tendon on sagittal scans and beneath the flat belly of the pronator teres muscle on transverse scans, respectively (Marcelis et al. 1996; Van Holsbeeck and Introcaso 1991).

13.2.3   MRI

MRI has been proven helpful in the detection of the number and extent of erosions as well as of articular effusion (Sugimoto et al. 1998). To fulfill the requirements of both imaging as many joints as possible and imaging the articular structures with high spatial resolution a standardized protocol has been proven helpful: one or both hands should be imaged with a surface coil from the distal lower arm to the proximal phalanges of the fingers. If possible, dedicated surface coils should be used. The patient should lie in a prone position with the arms elevated. This position, however, cannot be obtained in every patient suffering from advanced arthritis. Coronal images should be obtained with a T1-weighted SE-sequence and a T2*-weighted gradient-echo sequence. Additionally, a T2-weighted axial sequence of the wrist and a T1-weighted coronal sequence after intravenous injection of Gd-DTPA should be obtained to differentiate effusion from various forms of granulation tissue. A T2-weighted fat-suppressed sequence (STIR) may be performed but has the disadvantage of a lower spatial resolution.

13.3   Basic Signs in Imaging

An empirically developed standardized method of film analysis has been proven helpful in the assessment of lesions of the joint and will be followed throughout this chapter (Watt 1995; Freyschmidt 1985; Kainberger et al. 1996). Standardization of the image generation and interpretation process is: logical, and therefore easily understood; systematic, with a resulting reduction of possible errors due to missing unexpected findings; and diagnostic, with respect to describing features in the same way as they pathophysiologically develop (Fig. 13.15). Radiographic signs may be grouped as follows: abnormalities of axis, of the soft tissues, of the joint space, and/or of the bones (Fig. 13.16).

13.3.1   Basic Signs in Conventional Radiology and CT

In rheumatic diseases the number of characteristic radiographic findings is relatively small with not more than 12 features (Table 13.3). Anatomic subtypes of these features and various combinations in their occurrence, however, may lead to

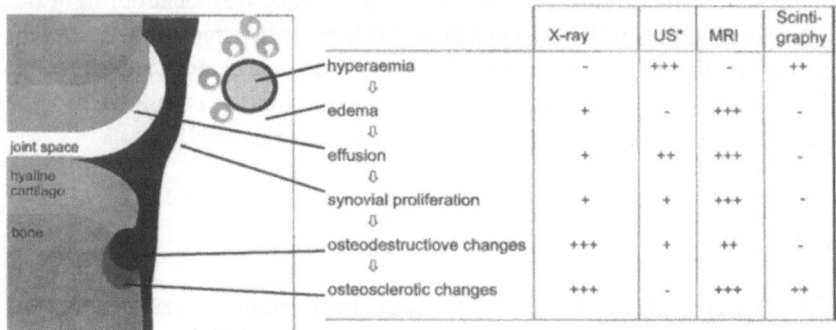

	X-ray	US*	MRI	Scinti-graphy
hyperaemia	-	+++	-	++
edema	+	-	+++	-
effusion	+	++	+++	-
synovial proliferation	+	+	+++	-
osteodestructiove changes	+++	+	++	-
osteosclerotic changes	+++	-	+++	++

*) ultrasound techniques including power Doppler imaging

Fig. 13.15. Comparison of the value of different imaging technologies and pathology. With cross-sectional imaging technologies, earlier stages of rheumatic disease become visible. (Adapted and modified from Kainberger et al. 1996)

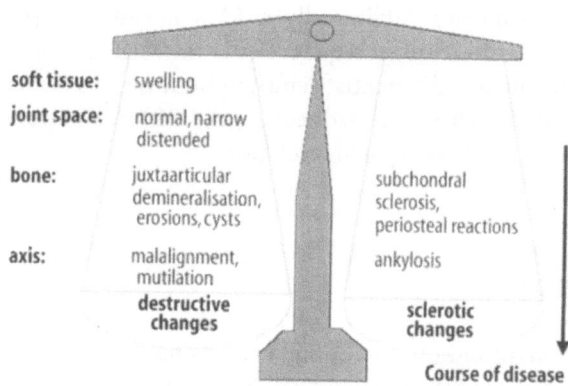

Fig. 13.16. Synopsis of the characteristic radiographic findings in inflammatory arthritis

Table 13.3. Synopsis of radiographic and sonographic signs in rheumatic diseases

Malalignment	Carpoulnar malalignment
	Flexion instability
Soft tissue abnormalities	Swelling
	Calcification or ossification
Joint space abnormalities	Widening
	Narrowing
	Ankylosis
Abnormalities of bone, posterolateral	Juxta-articular demineralization (osteopenia)
	Erosions, pre-erosions, and cysts (marginal, central or juxta-articular)
	Subchondral sclerosis
	Periosteal reaction
	Mutilation

a wide variety of appearances with multiple overlaps with other diseases of the hand and the wrist. Nevertheless, distinct patterns of rheumatic diseases may be observed, their analysis being a valuable aid in radiologic diagnosis. In CT, findings are principally the same as in conventional radiography (Dihlmann 1987).

13.3.1.1 Malalignment

In rheumatic diseases, malalignment results from capsular and ligamentous destruction due to synovial proliferation and is accelerated by imbalance of muscles and tendons. Carpo-ulnar malalignment, generally in the form of ulnar subluxation or scapholunate instability, is the most common type of deviation in patients with rheumatoid arthritis. A typical finding is the dorsal subluxation of the ulna due to destruction of the triangular fibrocartilage complex (TFCC). Biomechanical overload and rupture of the extensor tendons due to rheumatic tenosynovitis may complicate it. Disruption of the normal concavity of the proximal row of carpal bones may occur due to mediopalmar migration of the lunate and the scaphoid along the articular surface of the radius (Fig. 13.17). The scaphoid appears to be shortened and less than 50% of the proximal surface of the lunate covers the distal radius. Of the two types of flexion instability (palmar or volar intercalated segment instability, or VISI, and dorsal intercalated segment instability, or DISI), dorsiflexion instability, with scapholunate dissociation, seems to occur more frequently, especially in cases of longstanding rheumatoid arthritis (Resnick and Niwayama 1995).

13.3.1.2 Soft Tissue Abnormalities

Swelling of the soft tissues of the wrist is a typical and often early sign in various forms of rheumatic diseases (Fig. 13.18). Swelling of the soft tissue covering the

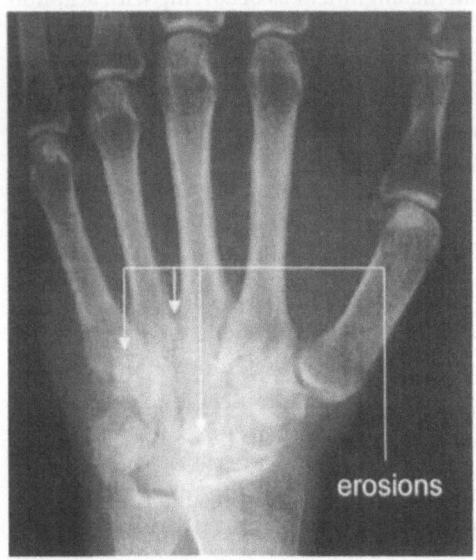

erosions

Fig. 13.17. Erosions and malalignment of the proximal carpal row with typical ulnar transposition of the lunate bone

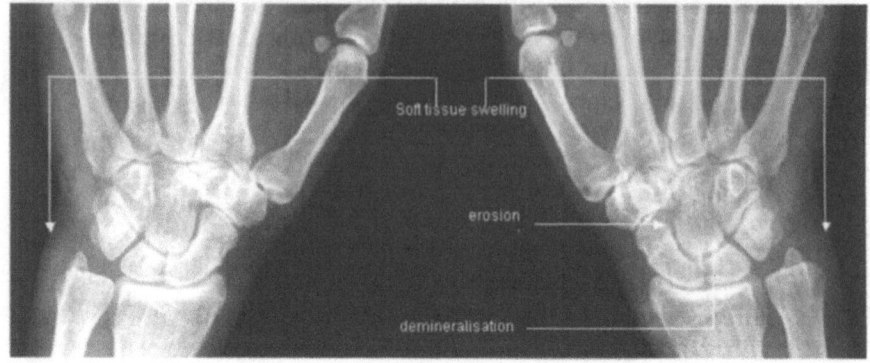

Fig. 13.18. Typical soft tissue swelling, demineralization and erosions in rheumatoid arthritis as visible on conventional radiographs

distal end of the ulna results from inflammation of the extensor carpi ulnaris tendon and sheath. Commonly, this sheath is in direct communication with the radiocarpal compartment of the wrist.

Calcifications or ossifications of soft tissues are rarely observed in systemic rheumatic diseases. They are generally associated with abnormalities in scleroderma, SLE, or severe forms of sarcoidosis.

13.3.1.3 Joint Space Abnormalities

Narrowing of the joint space results from inflammatory chondrolysis mixed with biomechanical overload. In contrast to degenerative or post-traumatic causes, joint space narrowing is visible in symptomatic arthritis in an extensive form with several compartments or the whole wrist involved. Widening of joint spaces is less often observed and mainly results from malalignment as occurring with scapholunate instability.

Fibrous and bony ankylosis indicates the end-stage of severe arthritis with the formation of intra-articular osseous fusions leading to an os carpale by fusion of the midcarpal compartment. Radiocarpal compartmental bony ankylosis is less common, with fibrous ankylosis instead of bony fusion occurring more frequently.

13.3.1.4 Abnormalities of Articular Bones

Arthritic changes of the bones may be observed in the form of a more destructive pattern, a more sclerotic pattern, or a mixed destructive-sclerotic pattern. Signs of destruction, and in many cases progression of disease, include juxta-articular demineralization, pre-erosions or erosions, subchondral cysts, and mutilation. Signs of a sclerotic pattern include sclerosis and ankylosis.

Juxta-articular demineralization (osteopenia): This sign results from hyperemia, the effects of cytokines, reduced mobility of the inflamed painful joint, and metabolic or drug-induced effects (Fig. 13.19). Because of the complex inflammatory, biomechanical, and neurovegetative causative factors the term "osteoporosis" should be avoided (Kainberger et al. 1998). Increased attenuation of the X-ray beam due to soft tissue swelling may enhance the effect of hyperlucency of the bones. Subtle forms of demineralization may be subject to perception errors. They are of particular importance in digital radiography as its signal-to-noise ratio is significantly lower than that of conventional screen-film combinations. Juxta-articular demineralization is generally more pronounced in younger patients and therefore is a common finding in juvenile arthritis.

Pre-erosions, erosions, and subchondral cysts: A pre-erosion is a circumscribed defect of juxta-articular bone prior to the formation of manifest erosions and often precedes the development of manifest erosions. It may occur in the form of subtle defects of the subchondral or cortical bone, slight irregularities of the osseous borders, or as tiny subchondral lucencies of the trabecular bone. As a general rule, all parts of bone are outlined by a more or less thick cortical or subchondral radiodense "white line". If this line is "erased", this, besides an inappropriate exposure technique, indicates damage of any cause, i. e., pre-erosion due to inflammation, degeneration, metabolic joint disease, or trauma. MRI may be helpful to confirm pre-erosions.

Erosions are circumscribed defects of the articular bone. Typically, they are located in the vicinity of capsular insertions and are referred to as "marginal" erosions. In the wrist, another type may be observed: resorptive erosions (Fig. 13.20). These occur beneath inflamed tendon sheaths, commonly at the distal end of the ulna. The cortices appear thin, with resorption of the subperiosteal margin. Associated, sometimes quite subtle, periosteal proliferation may be seen.

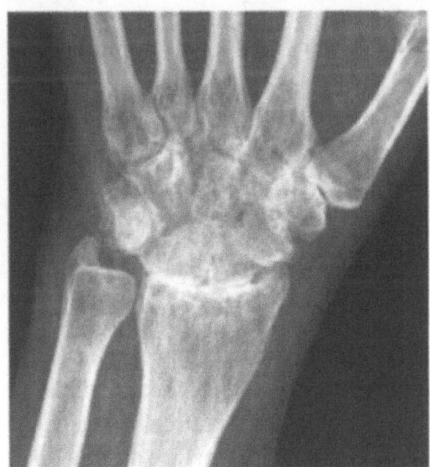

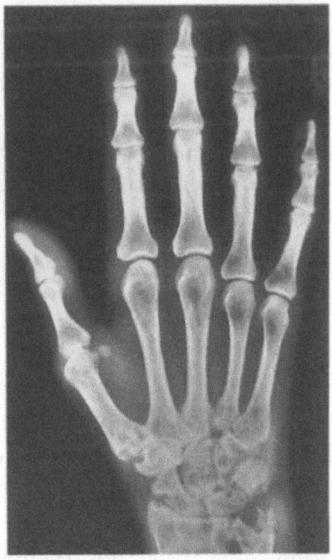

Fig. 13.19. A 20-year-old woman with Still's disease since childhood. There is advanced juxta-articular osteopenia of carpal bones, distal ends of radius and ulna as well as proximal ends of metacarpal bones

Fig. 13.20. Soft tissue swelling and erosions in the wrist due to rheumatoid arthritis

Erosions of the distal end of the ulna result from three forms of synovial proliferation which may occur in isolated form or simultaneously: prominent synovial folds within the prestyloid recess in direct contact with the tip of the ulnar styloid process, synovitis within the inferior radioulnar compartment extending over the distal aspects of the radius and ulna, and tenosynovitis of the extensor carpi ulnaris tendon.

In the inferior radioulnar compartment, findings include shallow surface defects, which progress to become extensive scalloped erosions, and sharply angular surfaces on the distal portions of the radius and ulna. The intimate relationship of the radius and the ulna often leads to secondary compression erosions. Compressive erosions represent a third type of erosive defect and are the result of biomechanical overload. They may be regarded as a sign of severe or end-stage arthritis.

13.3.2 Basic Signs in Sonography

Sonographic key signs of rheumatic disease of the hand and the wrist are tendinitis and tenosynovitis or intra-articular abnormalities in the form of articular effusions, granulation tissue or erosions.

Tenosynovitis is one of the most important features of early rheumatoid disease. Abnormalities of the tendon itself occur in the form of focal areas of thickening or thinning or areas of inhomogeneous texture (De Flaviis and Musso 1995). Tendinitis often occurs together with tenosynovitis. Depending on the amount of effusion or granulation tissue and on the effects of drug therapy the appearance of tenosynovitis varies considerably. Enlarged tendon sheaths are oval or spindle-shaped containing the hyperechoic tendon. Sheaths may contain anechoic or hypoechoic fluid or hypoechoic pannus. Rheumatoid nodules predominantly appear as small, rounded hypoechoic masses.

Tenosynovitis of the flexor tendons may result in carpal tunnel syndrome. Its diagnosis is of therapeutic relevance with regard to successful conservative or surgical treatment. Studying the vascularization of inflamed tissues with a color Doppler application may be useful to support the diagnosis of the inflammatory character of abnormalities. Color Doppler has, however, only in part been proven helpful to quantify disease activity.

13.3.3 Basic Signs in MRI

As with no other imaging modality, the extent and the characteristics of rheumatic diseases can be displayed by MRI. With its high contrast resolution virtually all forms of inflammatory involvement of soft tissues and bones may be differentiated from each other: effusion, synovial thickening, soft tissue edema, contrast enhancement, pannus visualization (surface and so-called marrow pannus), marrow edema, erosion and cartilage destruction.

For differentiating effusion from synovial pannus, the use of fat suppression techniques and of intravenous gadolinium is necessary. Signal enhancement in synovial and subchondral tissue on gadolinium-enhanced T1-weighted images generally implies active inflammation; this technique is beneficial in monitoring therapeutic response (Imhof et al. 1999b). Thus, the evaluation of the synovial layer, cartilage and the subchondral region is possible, and allows early detection of articular disease. Several authors have described the evaluation of inflammatory affections of the hand (Backhaus et al. 1999; Jevtic et al. 1996; Giovagnoni et al. 1998; Jewell and Watt 1996). For the evaluation of disease activity and for measurement of the volume of enhancing pannus, MRI can be useful (Sugimoto et al. 1998; Scutellari and Orzincolo 1998). The finger joints are usually among the first to be affected in rheumatoid arthritis, and they are considered to be the best markers of overall joint damage in the disease (Klarlund et al. 1999). MRI of the finger joints has become possible at clinical MRI units. Quantification of the amount of synovial membrane in the finger joints has been introduced (Klarlund et al. 1999). MRI of small hand joints in patients with early erosive rheumatoid arthritis may have prognostic value for future development of bone-destructive changes (Jevtic et al. 1996).

In particular, with MRI an essential basic understanding of inflammatory processes in rheumatic diseases can be provided. The basic pathologic process in noninfectious inflammatory disease is the proliferation of synovial tissue. Normal synovialis is not visible on standard MRI images. Thickened synovialis and pannus proliferations can be visualized by application of gadolinium-containing contrast agents (Fig. 13.21). Pannus is defined as synovial proliferation that extends over the hyaline cartilage and infiltrates the subchondral region. The MR appearance depends on the disease activity of both structures. Differentiation of synovialis and fluid in the inflammatory joint is based on the enhancement of synovialis and pannus after contrast application. The enhancement depends on the vascularization of the synovialis. After intravenous injection the hypervascular synovialis shows strong contrast enhancement with a maximum after 1.5 min. Later a diffusion process into the synovial fluid and the soft tissue starts. Therefore early investigation after contrast application is necessary for reliable interpretation. However, due to these dynamics only joints of one hand can be investigated when using contrast agent (Sugimoto et al. 1998).

The most important event during the course of rheumatoid arthritis is the transition of synovitis to pannus, which usually represents the beginning of irreparable joint destruction. The evaluation of erosions varies with the course of disease (Jevtic et al. 1996).

MRI for the noninvasive direct demonstration of synovial proliferation and bone erosions is now well established. It has been suggested that an important advantage of MRI over radiography may be the prognostic value due to its ability to show the natural history of active destructive to inactive fibrous pannus (Jevtic et al. 1995a; König et al. 1990).

MRI findings permit the differentiation of subsets of disease (Jevtic et al. 1996) including findings compatible with inflammatory, active, destructive pannus, moderately active pannus (represented by a nodular mass within the erosions and homogenous marked contrast enhancement on the T1-weighted post-contrast images) and inactive fibrous pannus (low signal intensity masses on all sequences).

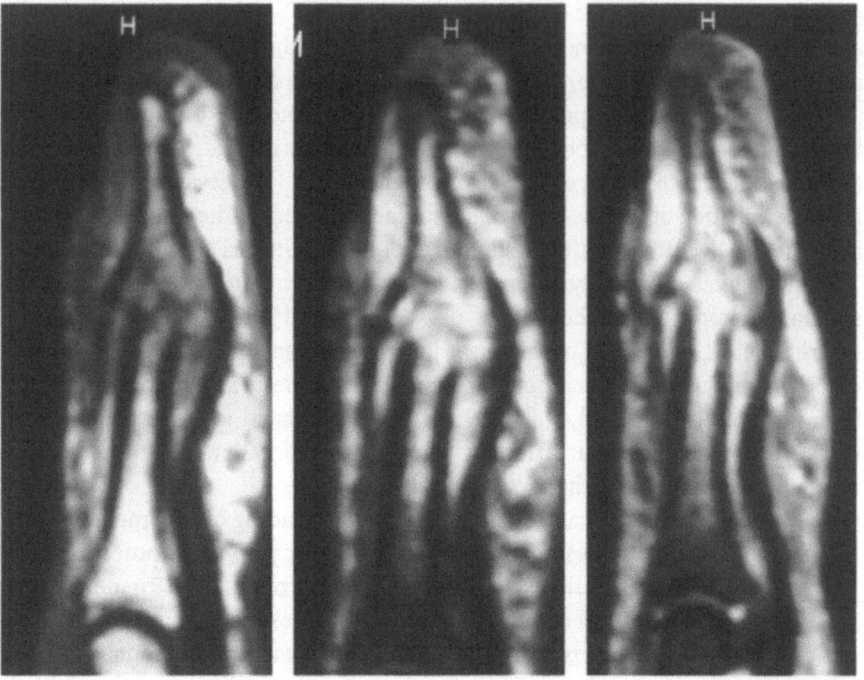

a,b   c

Fig. 13.21a–c. Psoriatic arthritis. **a** T1-weighted image of a digit with hypointense increased soft tissue at the proximal interphalangeal joint. **b** High edematous signal alterations on STIR images. **c** Enhancement of synovial tissue on T1-weighted fat-suppressed images after intravenous contrast application

Quantifying the formation of pannus, the primary target tissue in rheumatoid arthritis treatment, has been considered for assessing disease activity in individual patients. Articular involvement of rheumatoid arthritis can occur in various joints, including the hand. Evaluation of the hands is particularly important because the features they exhibit frequently reflect the patient's overall disease condition. As for the anatomic MRI site for evaluation of rheumatoid arthritis activity, the hands are considered the most appropriate joints. The volume of enhancing pannus (VEP) can be used as an indicator to assess disease activity in individual patients (Sugimoto et al. 1998). Fibrotic pannus is enhanced as well as active pannus when MR images are obtained relatively late after injection. Enhancement of fibrotic pannus is negligible when MRI images are obtained within a few minutes after gadolinium injection, due to the difference in enhancement rate between these types of pannus (König et al. 1990; Yamato et al. 1993). Therefore the synovial enhancement rate can be used to distinguish between active and inactive arthritis (Ostergaard et al. 1994, 1997; König et al. 1990). Volumetric quantification was shown to have a 10% error rate.

Another limitation for the investigation of the hand in noninfectious inflammatory disease is its low specificity. Gadopentatetic acid (Gd-DTPA) accumulates in inflammatory joints. This phenomenon is nonspecific, reflecting varying degrees of hypervascularity, and abnormal vascular permeability has been described in several infectious and rheumatologic inflammatory processes. Thus differentiation between the various rheumatic diseases does not seem possible on the basis of contrast medium enhancement alone. The final MRI diagnosis depends on the morphologic characteristics of the joint disease (Fig. 13.21) (Jevtic et al. 1995b).

Synovial membrane volumes as determined by MRI in finger joints are related to clinical signs of synovitis, but the volumes may vary more than can be accounted for by clinical appearance. Histopathologic evidence of synovitis has been seen in patients in whom the disease is assumed inactive, according to clinical and laboratory evaluation. There may be discrepancies between clinical, laboratory and radiographic assessment of disease activity and severity.

MRI of the finger joints has become possible at clinical MRI units. Synovial membrane volumes are considerably larger in clinically active than in clinically inactive RA joints (Klarlund et al. 1999).

The spin echo T1-weighted precontrast, T2-weighted and especially T1-weighted post-contrast images demonstrate distinct differences in the distribution of inflammatory changes within and adjacent to involved small hand joints (Fig. 13.22). Most applications of MRI have been described for rheumatoid arthritis. Two major subtypes of inflammatory arthritis provide a specific differential diagnosis between rheumatoid and seronegative spondylarthritis (SNSA). Patients with Reiter's syn-

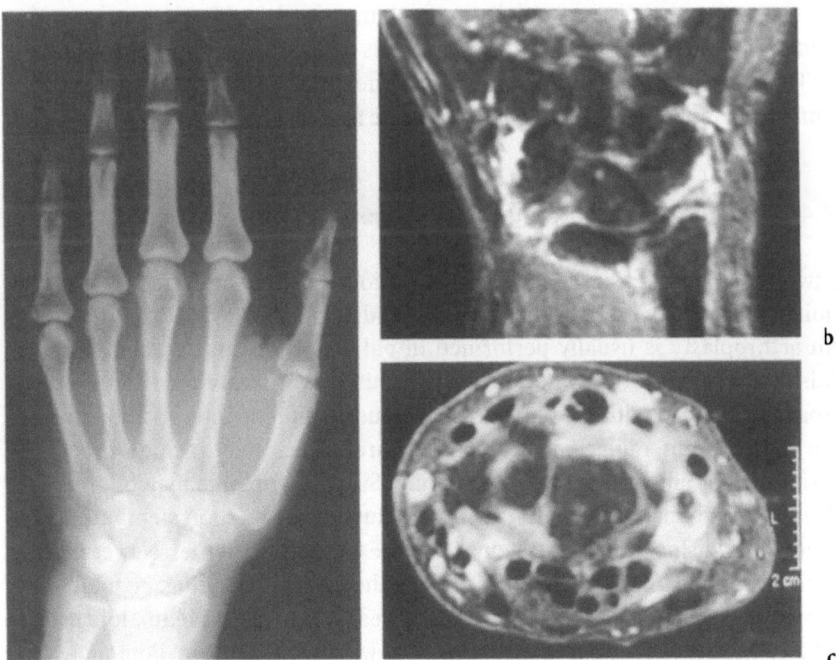

Fig. 13.22a–c. Early manifestation of rheumatoid arthritis. a Plain film radiographs without evidence of inflammation. b Coronal STIR image of the wrist with increased (edematous) signal intensities of periarticular soft tissue c Axial T1-weighted image after intravenous contrast application demonstrating an increased and enhancing layer of synovial tissue

drome and psoriatic arthritis have a distinctive pattern of extra-articular disease involvement. It was also noted that juxta-articular osteopenia on plain film did not correlate with bone marrow edema on MRI. Early diagnosis of and thus differentiation between RA and SNSA is important for management of patients with initial presentation of inflammatory disease in the small hand joints (Jevtic et al. 1995a). For the detection of early erosions T2-weighted sequences with fat-suppression techniques (STIR sequences) have shown promising results. Early erosions appear as hyperintense signal alterations affecting the subchondral area.

Bone lesions are detected earlier by MRI than by conventional radiography. Dynamic contrast-enhanced MRI allows better differentiation between edema of soft tissue as well as of bone marrow and pannus than does a T2-weighted sequence. Compared with T2-weighted imaging a dynamic study yields additional information regarding the differentiation of edema from pannus tissue. The early demonstration of erosions seems to be an important prognostic parameter (Backhaus et al. 1999).

For the evaluation of cartilage three-dimensional gradient echo (3D GE) images have been found to show superior details. However, these studies have been performed for larger joints with thicker cartilage than is found at the wrist and finger joints (Peterfy et al. 1994). Also due to the small size of finger joints evaluation of the subchondral area with standard MR units is limited, and the investigation of cartilage does not appear appropriate.

The assessment of disease activity and volume of enhancing pannus in noninfectious inflammatory disease of the hand has been shown to be possible with MRI. This technique may be the only tool differentiating synovial fluid and inflammatory pannus and is particularly valuable for the detection of early arthritis.

13.3.4   Radiographic Findings after Surgery

The two most popular surgical treatment options for joints affected by arthritis are joint arthroplasty or arthrodesis (Smith and Cristensen 1996).

An arthroplasty is usually performed in patients with limited functional demands that require motion. The affected joint surfaces are resected with the resulting space to be filled with the patient's soft tissues, synthetic interposition materials, or a total joint replacement. Carpal arthroplasties may include prosthetic material such as silicone, rubber or titanium. Silicone implants may migrate and settle into the soft arthritic bone, causing fracture of the fixation stems at the site of bending, or dislocation of the stems from the medullary cavities. Newer models have incorporated metal flanges to protect the sites of bending. A total wrist arthroplasty is performed in patients over 50 years of age with rheumatoid arthritis who require more motion than is available with a wrist fusion. Potential complications include loosening or migration of the fixation stems, dislocation of the proximal and distal components or fracture of the implant.

Arthrodesis is performed after failed arthoplasty or in patients with the need for stability. Arthrodesis techniques vary. Generally a corticocancellous bone graft from the ilium is sculpted to fit the dorsum of the wrist and fixed with screws. If the bone graft reabsorbs around the screws, they may project into the dorsal soft tissues without surrounding bone graft. Frequently a so-called Steinmann pin or Kirschner wire is inserted in a retrograde technique into the distal radius to maintain support until the fusion heals. Postoperative radiographs must be examined for signs of loosening or migration (Figs. 13.23, 13.24).

13.4 Specific Imaging Patterns in Rheumatic Diseases

Despite considerable variations in the anatomic distribution, severity and the cause of disease, rheumatic diseases generally present with certain patterns on plain films, ultrasound images or MRI scans. Successful interpretation of these

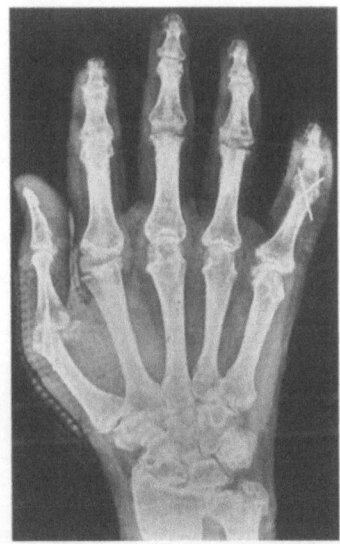

Fig. 13.23. Arthrodesis with K wires (Kirschner wire) in metacarpophalangeal (MCP) I joint and proximal interphalangeal V joint; Swanson spacer in MCP II joint

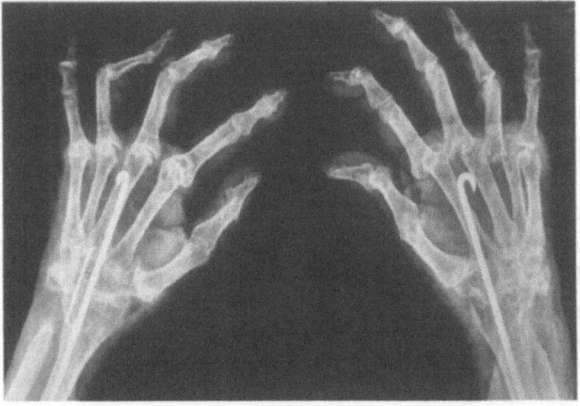

Fig. 13.24. Arthrodesis (Mannerfelt technique) in the advanced stage of rheumatoid arthritis with rush pin and staple

patterns requires the analysis of a number of basic criteria along with information from clinical and laboratory investigations.

For the radiologic evaluation plain film radiographs are definitely necessary and demonstrate characteristic features of joint affections. Sonography has been shown to be helpful in the evaluation of soft tissue affections. With the use of color Doppler techniques, quantification of blood flow might also be used for the evaluation of arthritides. MRI has become a powerful method for imaging of synovitis and soft tissue involvement, and in particular plays an important role in the evaluation of early diagnosis in arthritic disease. Computed tomography (CT) is useful for the evaluation of subtle osseous lesion calcifications; however, it has limited value for the diagnosis of soft tissue pathology.

13.4.1 Rheumatoid Arthritis and Related Diseases

13.4.1.1 Rheumatoid Arthritis

Rheumatoid arthritis (RA) is the most common inflammatory affection of the hand. Its etiology is unknown, but an immunopathologic genesis based on viral infection and comprising chronic and acute stages is under discussion. The IGM-anti IgG autoantibodies that are found in 75% of patients are a nonspecific finding. Rheumatoid factor (RF) is not specific and may be negative in the early course of disease but eventually becomes positive in 90–95% of cases. Females are more commonly affected than males (2:1 or 3:1 ratio).

Clinical diagnosis is established on the ARA criteria (Arnett et al. 1988). Within these, radiographic findings are definitely included, mainly in the form of osteopenia and erosions. Consideration of the results from other imaging techniques, especially MRI, is the subject of continuing discussion. Clinical symptoms and signs include morning stiffness, pain due to capsular distension, periarticular muscle wasting, and tendon constrictions with or without ruptures. Extra-articular manifestations present as subcutaneous or tendon sheath nodules, tenosynovitis or bursitis, pleural effusion, rheumatoid pulmonary nodules and diffuse interstitial pneumonia.

13.4.1.1.1 Imaging Findings

The anatomic distribution of abnormalities plays a key role in establishing a correct diagnosis. Both hands are affected in a relatively symmetric fashion, and the lesions may appear in most of metacarpophalangeal (MCP) joints and the proximal interphalangeal (PIP) joints. Affections of the distal interphalangeal (DIP) joints are less frequent (Martel 1980; Dihlmann 1987; Resnick and Niwayama 1995) (Fig. 13.25).

Soft tissues: The soft tissue component represents a predominant feature of early changes: Synovial hypertrophy, soft tissue edema, accumulation of intra-articular fluid and osteochondral destruction near inflammatory pannus are most evident at specific target sites. Earliest changes most frequently are apparent in the second and third MCP joints and the third PIP joint. Fusiform soft tissue swelling, intra-articular osteopenia,

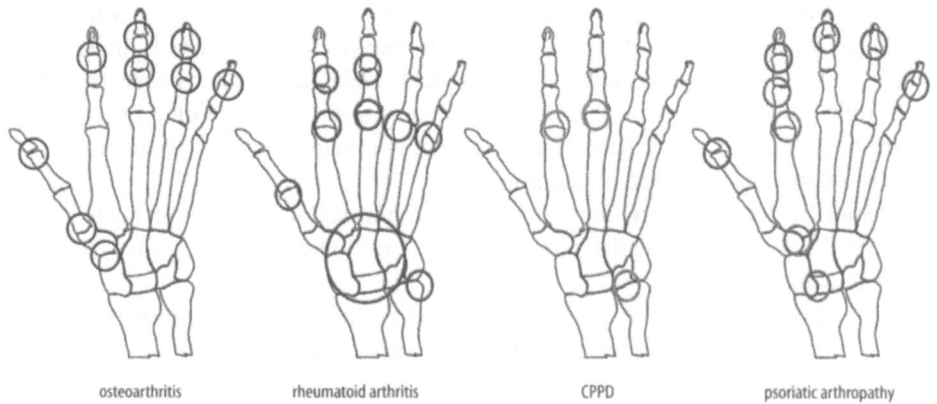

| osteoarthritis | rheumatoid arthritis | CPPD | psoriatic arthropathy |

Fig. 13.25. Schematic drawing showing the anatomic distribution of the four most common rheumatic diseases in the skeleton of the hands

diffuse joint space narrowing and mainly marginal bony erosions represent the typical appearance of RA. Soft tissue swelling may be visible as displaced skin contours and fascial planes or a slight increase in periarticular soft tissue density.

Osteopenia: In the further progression of disease osteopenia is frequently prominent early in the epiphysis and metaphyses. The articular cortex may appear intermittently interrupted due to this acute diminution in bone mass, creating a "dot-dash" appearance. Later, osteopenia will become more generalized (Fig. 13.26). A characteristic feature is indistinctness of the osseous outline corresponding to the insertion of the capsule on the dorsoradial aspect of the proximal portion of the four medial digits. For the metacarpal bones the reduction in subchondral bone is an early sign. A tender periosteal lamellar reaction is commonly found in the adult form of RA (Dihlmann 1987).

Erosions: Erosions are observed at specific sites of predilection, mainly at the "bare areas". These represent those intra-articular areas of the joint which are

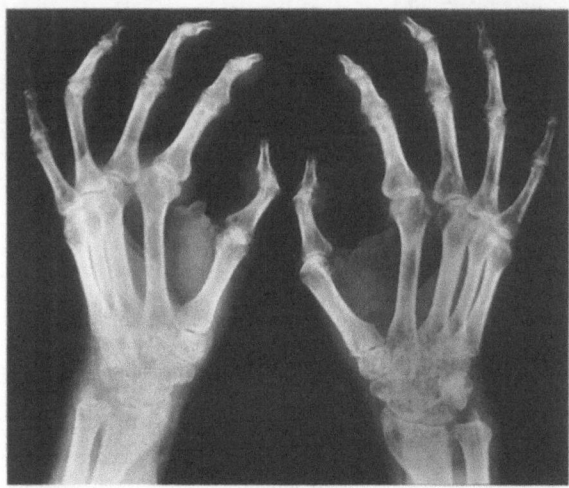

Fig. 13.26. Diffuse demineralization of the carpal bones and the proximal radius without evidence of erosions in early rheumatoid arthritis

not covered with cartilage, and where synovial proliferations (pannus) may therefore may cause the earliest effects on the bone (Monsees et al. 1985; Murphy 1973) (Fig. 13.27). With further destruction of cartilage and bone the articular space will be obliterated and erosions in a central position appear. These radiolucent defects are cysts or pseudocysts that communicate with the articular cavity, and represent a transchondral extension of pannus.

Specific forms of erosions at typical anatomic locations have been described that account for the generally typical radiographic appearance of RA (Dihlmann 1987):

- The radial aspect of the head of the metacarpals is a common site of first manifestation of disease. Erosions are usually marginal and less frequently central.
- Erosions, in their typical form, show a hazy border with the subjacent cancellous bone that indicates continuing inflammatory activity of the disease. Once the inflammatory process has ceased, a tiny sclerotic rim may develop that may be assessed as a radiographic sign of repair (Dihlmann 1987).
- The "radius crypt" is deep erosion of the radius, located at the scapholunate joint (ligament of Testut), that is a reaction of an inflammatory process at the band insertion.
- A small recess of the radiocarpal joint capsule also has a topographic location close to the styloid process, which may cause erosion of the tip of the process in later stages of the disease.
- Inflammation of the extensor carpi ulnaris tendon and the destruction of the distal radioulnar joint causes the "caput ulnae syndrome", which is associated with a palmar luxation of the carpal bones and a dorsal subluxation of the caput ulnae in lateral radiographs.
- On the thumb, characteristic deep erosion occurs at the ulnar site of the distal phalanx and ulnar sites of the first metacarpophalangeal articulation.

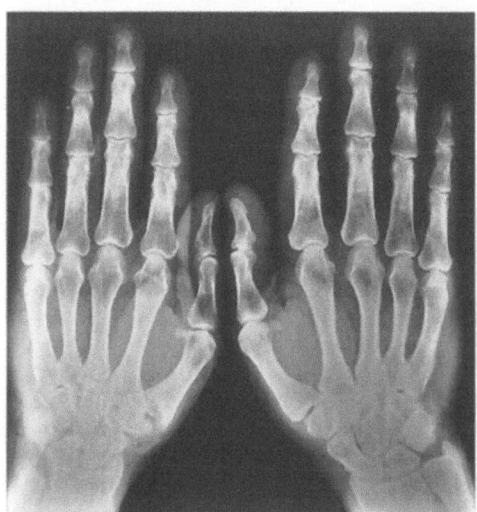

Fig. 13.27. Erosions at the first carpometacarpal joint and the styloid process of the left hand in a patient with an advanced stage of rheumatoid arthritis. Soft tissue swelling at the ulnar side becomes obvious when compared with the right hand

- The radial styloid process and scaphoid exhibit a bare area on the surface of the bone adjacent to the radial collateral ligament. Alterations to the lateral midportion of the scaphoid are characteristic (36%). Erosions and surface irregularities should be distinguished from a normal degree of notching of the scaphoid (Swezey and Alexander 1969).
- At the palmar aspect of the distal radius erosions on the area of fingerlike projections of the palmar and radial recesses may appear as irregular radiolucent shadows overlying the midportion of the distal radius.
- In the triquetral and pisiform bones three locations are common: the proximal medial portion of the triquetrum; the distal medial portion of the triquetrum and the adjacent surfaces of the triquetrum and the pisiform. Note, however, that the pisiform triquetral compartment is seen tangentially in reverse oblique radiographs with the wrist in a semisupinated position.
- Marginal erosion of the trapezium close to the attachment of the radial collateral ligament may occur. Erosion of central portions of the joint can lead to subchondral defects, so-called cysts, or pseudocysts.
- Erosions of the triquetrum and the pisiform bones may be observed at the medial portion of the triquetrum or in the triquetro-pisiform joint. They may be aggravated by biomechanical stress due to direct contact with the distal end of the ulna, which eventually leads to extensive destruction of the involved bones. Sometimes, erosions on the hamate may be observed.

Malalignment: Deformities can be attributed to numerous factors such as inflammatory destruction of intra-articular structures, capsular and ligamentous weakening leading to laxity, tendinitis and tenosynovitis with contracture, rupture and muscular contractions.

The most common luxation types are volar subluxation and ulnar deviation, which give a characteristic appearance to the hand in RA. The boutonniere deformity or swan-neck deformity or changes result in further deformities by subcutaneous rheumatic nodules. Dislocations of the distal radioulnar joint are due to destruction of the capsule and band (Hastings and Evans 1975; Stack and Vaughan-Jackson 1971).

Characteristic deformities of the fingers appear within the course of disease:

- Boutonniere deformity: A collapse deformity of the three joints (MCP, PIP, and DIP) can lead to hyperextension of one joint and reciprocal flexion of the continuous articulation. The PIP joint protrudes upward through the lateral extension of the extensor tendon like a button through a buttonhole.
- Swan-neck deformity: This deformity is due to hyperextension of the PIP joint and flexion of the DIP joint. Synovitis of the flexor tendon sheath, which restricts the interphalangeal joint flexion, is the primary cause of drift.
- A rarer deformity is caused by loosening or disruption of the distal attachment of the extensor tendon to the terminal phalanx, which may result in the development of a typical mallet or drop finger, due to instability of the distal interphalangeal joint.

- The scapholunate ligament is an important stabilizer of the radiocarpal joint. After its destruction the proximal carpal row shifts ulnarly and the distal carpal row together with the metacarpal bones II–V is shifted radially.
- At the thumb, the most frequent deformities are collapse deformities related to disturbance of functions at the first MCP joint, swan-neck deformity related to disturbance of function at the first MCP joint and instability and stiffness or pain.

13.4.1.1.2 Quantification

With respect to modern therapeutic regimens, quantification of RA has to be performed as precisely as possible to determine progression rates. For clinical and scientific purposes a precise grading of joint damage is mandatory to determine progression rates of the disease. Different radiologic scoring systems have been applied to prognosticate and define patient outcomes. A four-step scoring method developed by Steinbrocker in 1949 has been used for many years because of its high feasibility for clinical purposes (Steinbrocker et al. 1949). However, it has been shown to be insufficient with respect to both accuracy and precision and has been replaced by modern and more sophisticated systems. Among them, Larsen's scoring method has been used extensively in European countries whereas in North America a scoring system developed by Sharp and by Genant have been established (Larsen et al.1977; Sharp 1996;).

Despite extensive research activities all scoring modalities show some inherent characteristics that strongly influence their clinical use: First, the technique of taking the X-ray films varies from one institution to another, which, according to Larsen, may be the main cause of imprecision (Larsen 1995). Secondly, familiarity with the disease may differ between radiologists or rheumatologists, with the potential for a high interobserver variability (Sharp 1996). Thirdly, the designs of the various scoring systems do not necessarily fulfill clinical and scientific requirements: e.g., films of patients with early arthritis should be graded in a different fashion from those with advanced abnormalities. Finally, in order to be used in clinical settings the process of scoring should be applied with high feasibility. Many different scoring systems, some of which have been modified by different authors, have been published (Table 13.4) (Rau and Herborn 1995; Van der Heijde 1996; Wassenberg and Rau 1995; Scott et al. 1995). Despite these various attempts consensus has been reached that the quantification of RA principally relies on three approaches: clinical assessment with special focus on feelings of pain and on mobility of affected joints, laboratory investigation with measures indicating inflammatory activity, and radiographic scoring.

13.4.1.2 Juvenile Rheumatoid Arthritis

Juvenile (chronic) rheumatoid arthritis (JRA) resembles a group of related diseases of unknown etiology in childhood in variable symptom complexes, such as

Table 13.4. Different scoring systems for assessment of the severity of rheumatoid arthritis

System Scoring characteristics	
Assign one grade per patient (of historical interest only)	
Steinbrocker et al. (1949)	Scale 0–4
Kellgren (1963)	Scale 0–4
Sievers (1965)	Scale 0–7
Berens and Lin (1969)	Scale 0–5
Assign one grade per joint, sum scores of multiple joints	
Larsen (1975)	Scale 0–5 (modifications 1977, 1978, 1987, 1995)
Gofton et al, (1984)	Scale 0–4
Score two or more features, sum scores of multiple joints	
Bluhm et al. (1983)	Scale 0–5
Genant (1983)	Scale 0–3.5 (by increments of 0.5)
Sharp et al.(1985)	Scale 0–5
Nance et al. (1986)	Scale 0, 2–4 (malalignment included)
Van der Heijde et al.(1989)	Scale 0–5

Still's disease, pauciarticular disease, seronegative polyarticular disease, seropositive polyarticular disease, or juvenile ankylosing spondylitis. Generally predilections are for the large joints.

The radiologic changes may be similar to those of RA or of psoriatic arthropathy, with predominant DIP erosion and fusions. Usually, fewer joints are involved (Ansell and Kent 1977).

For the hand and wrist, MCP and PIP involvement appear similar to adult RA. The radiocarpal joint may be spared with the midcarpal joint involved. A site of specific predilection is the pericapitate region, distinguishing JRA from adult RA. Adult-onset Still's disease is similar in this respect. In JRA, ankylosis is very common in the joints of the hand.

13.4.2 Seronegative Spondylarthropathies

Joint diseases with negative rheumatoid factor, a clinical presence of sacroiliitis and an association with HLA-B27 have been summarized under the term seronegative spondylarthropathies. Similar to RA they involve synovial articulations and tendon insertions. Fundamental differences compared with RA exist, however, not only in the anatomic distribution but also in the arrangement of the radiologic findings that reflect the activity of disease. In contrast to the progressive character of RA, seronegative arthritis is less aggressive with a typical coexistence of osteodestructive and osteoproliferative signs. Soft tissue swelling may be more extensive and involves both articular and periarticular structures; erosions are smaller and often associated with various forms of periostitis or proliferative fibroostitis.

Manifestations at the hand are generally observed in psoriatic arthropathy and may occur less commonly in reactive arthritis or even ankylosing spondylitis.

13.4.2.1   Psoriatic Arthropathy

Psoriatic arthropathy (PA) occurs in 10% of patients with psoriasis. It affects generally young adults, males and females equally. The characteristic distribution is the small joints of the hands and feet. Clinically soft tissue swelling, especially in the small joints of the hand and feet, may involve the entire digit, which gives the appearance of a "sausage digit". Signs of arthropathy are reported to antedate skin findings in 10–15% of cases. A thorough clinical investigation with search for isolated cutaneous manifestation in the anal and the umbilical regions may help to establish the correct diagnosis.

13.4.2.1.1 Imaging Findings

Soft tissue swelling occur at involved joints, either fusiform or involving the entire digit. Abnormal calcifications may develop an ivory phalanx with reactive sclerosis of the tuft. The joints may be widened by fluid but generally are narrowed due to cartilage destruction.

Erosions begin marginally, as in RA, but progress to severe subchondral erosions, occasionally resulting in a pencil in cup deformity, which is characteristic but not pathognomonic for PA.

Phalangeal tuft resorptions and DIP erosive disease are usually seen earlier and involvement may be more severe of PIP or MCP joints (Martell et al. 1980). This pattern helps differentiate PA from RA. Also, any compartment of the wrist may be involved, but generally only after the DIP abnormalities have occurred. Asymmetry is far more common than in RA.

Osteoproliferative changes represent a typical finding in PA and may occur in the form of productive changes, usually in the form of excrescences at and around the joint. Other forms include periosteal reaction at hand phalanges. An enthesiopathy similar to reactive arthritis may also be observed. Ankylosis can commonly appear, especially at the hand.

Ligamentous abnormalities are not a prominent feature; however, phalanges with severe pencil-in-cup deformities may appear.

The differential diagnosis includes reactive arthritis, in which involvement of the hands is generally less prominent than in PA. The periostitis may help to differentiate PA from RA. Lesions may sometimes be indistinguishable from those in RA, but in many cases the more distal distribution in PA may aid in establishing the correct diagnosis. Adult-onset Still's disease with DIP distribution may be indistinguishable from PA. Ankylosing spondylitis predominantly affects large joints with involvement of the sacroiliac joint and the thoracolumbar spine. Erosive osteoarthritis (EOA) affects usually the first carpometacarpal joints or the scaphoid-trapezium-trapezoid joints.

13.4.2.2   Reactive Arthritis and Reiter's Syndrome

Reiter's syndrome consists of the triad of urethritis, conjunctivitis and arthritis. Young adults and males are affected much more commonly than females. The syndrome may be incomplete. The arthropathy only rarely precedes the clinical findings of urethritis or conjunctivitis.

13.4.2.2.1 Imaging Findings

Reiter's syndrome is accompanied by radiographic features, which it shares with other seronegative spondyloarthropathies such as PA and ankylosing spondylitis (Finder et al. 1983; Stadalnik and Dublin 1975).

For the hand and wrist severe and widespread radiographic abnormalities are unusual in Reiter's syndrome. In 10–30% of cases, however, one or more fingers of one or both hands reveal radiographic changes. Fusiform or sausage-like soft tissue swelling, regional or periarticular osteoporosis and joint space narrowing can be evident. The erosive changes are accompanied by fluffy new bone formation. Such proliferation also can involve adjacent sesamoids, producing an enlarged bone contour.

The PIP joints are more frequently involved than the MCP or DIP joints. For the wrist any compartment can be affected, although severe bone destruction is unusual.

13.4.2.3 Ankylosing Spondylitis

Ankylosing spondylitis (AS, Bechterew's disease) is the most common seronegative spondylarthropathy of unknown etiology, involving primarily the axial skeleton and large proximal joints. The hand, however, is less commonly involved and the affections, if evident, are not specific (Resnick 1974).

13.4.3   Collagen Disease

13.4.3.1   Systemic Lupus Erythematosus

In systemic lupus erythematosus (SLE) a deforming, nonerosive arthropathy with a bilateral and symmetric distribution affecting MCP and interphalangeal (IP) joints of all the digits can be observed. The musculoskeletal abnormalities include polyarthritis, deforming nonerosive arthropathy, subchondral cysts, spontaneous tendon weakening and rupture, soft tissue calcification, osteomyelitis, septic arthritis and miscellaneous abnormalities (Weissman et al. 1978; Bywaters 1975). Osteonecrosis at one or more MCP joints can also be observed (Leventhal and Dorfman 1975; Klippel et al. 1979). Further, a RA-like condition may appear and may be coexistent with RA or mixed connective tissue disease. Synovial inflammation may be evident but usually not as severe as in RA. Also joint effusions are not large. Articular findings are usually bilateral and symmetric.

13.4.3.1.1 Imaging Findings

Radiographic findings are soft tissue swelling and periarticular osteoporosis. Cartilaginous and osseous destruction is rare in the absence of osteonecrosis. In the hand, the findings of fusiform soft tissue prominence and "regional osteoporosis" about PIP and MCP joints simulate findings of RA. In addition, well-defined lytic lesions or cysts in periarticular bone may be observed in SLE, but in contrast to RA they are not marginal and the joint space is usually not narrowed. An overlap syndrome may exist, with signs of erosive arthritis in SLE simulating RA.

- Deforming nonerosive arthropathy may appear in patients with SLE (5–40%).
- Hyperextension at the PIP joints and flexion at the DIP joints create a swan-neck deformity. Boutonniere deformities also may appear. Hyperextension at the IP joint of the thumb is characteristic.
- Joint space narrowing and osseous erosion are not prominent and may be used in the differential diagnosis of RA. Rarely, cartilaginous and osseous alterations become evident in SLE.
- Bilateral or unilateral defects on the metacarpal heads occasionally are evident, predominantly on the radial aspect of the bone.
- Osteopenia and cyst formation within the subchondral bone can occur in SLE. Most common sites are the carpus and metacarpal heads.
- Spontaneous rupture of tendons can be observed in patients with SLE; however, in general tendons in weight-bearing positions are affected.
- Osteonecrosis is a well-described feature in SLE and may also appear at the small bones of the hand. The occasional occurrence in unusual sites such as the metacarpal heads should suggest SLE as a potential cause (Fishel et al. 1989).
- Soft tissue calcification is occasionally observed in SLE (Weiberger et al. 1979).
- Alterations of the terminal tufts of the phalanges in SLE include osteosclerosis and resorption and may be significant.

The differential diagnosis includes Jaccoud's arthritis and Ehlers-Danlos syndrome. Thumb deformities in SLE can be extensive. Hyperextension of the IP joint and subluxation at the first carpometacarpal joint are rather characteristic (Hoffman et al. 1991).

13.4.3.2 Scleroderma

Scleroderma affects women more frequently than men and usually appears in the third to fifth decades. The radiographic abnormalities of scleroderma are characteristic (Brun et al. 1983; Yune et al. 1971; Rabinowitz and Twersky 1974; Resnick et al. 1978; Pile et al. 1992; Bunch et al. 1976) (Figs. 13.28, 13.29).

13.4.3.2.1 Imaging Findings

For the hand and wrist lesions are characterized by resorption of the soft tissue, involvement of the fingertips being a common finding (Yune et al. 1971). Further, a bilateral erosive arthritis showing predilection for the DIP joints and to a lesser extent the PIP joints can be observed. Features resemble PA and erosive osteoarthritis. A similar pattern appears also with polymyositis. More characteristic is soft tissue calcification and tuft resorption. Amorphous calcification (together with Raynaud phenomenon and telangiectasia calcification) in patients with scle-

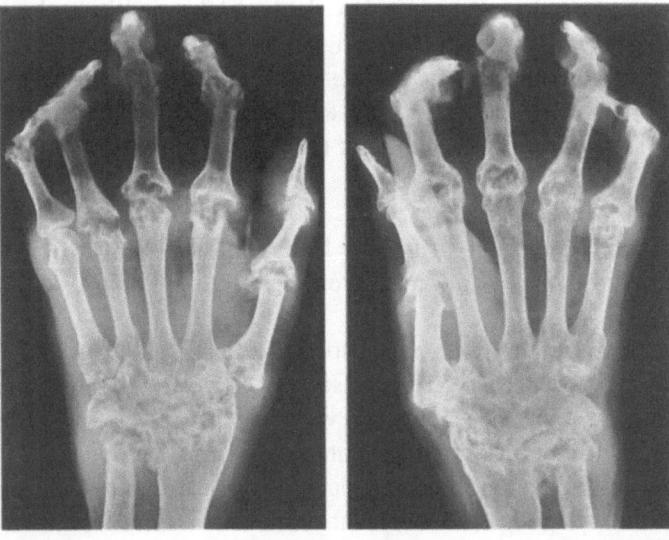

Fig. 13.28.a,b Extensive, large erosions in all joints of the hand, involvement of the carpal bones and the radiocarpal joint with extensive erosions, together with contractions and luxations in all digits, in a patient with scleroderma (**a** left hand; **b** right hand)

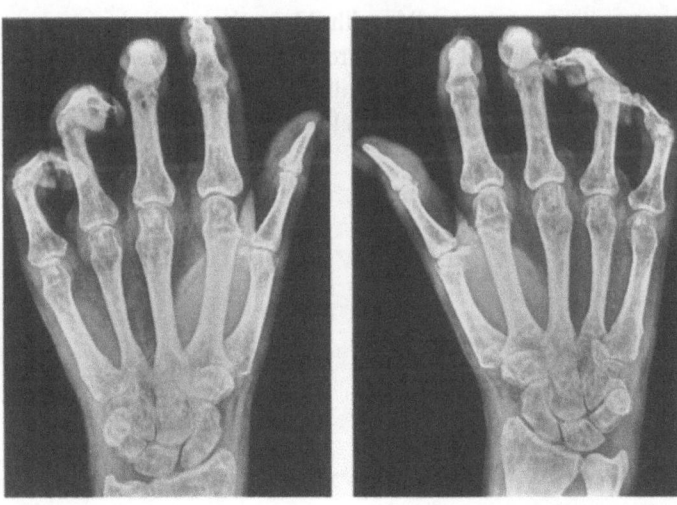

Fig. 13.29a, b. Diffuse demineralization of all bones and contracture of the interphalangeal and distal interphalangeal joints in a patient with scleroderma. No erosions or osseous destruction are evident at this stage. (**a** left hand; **b** right hand)

roderma is most common in the hand and is described as Thibierge-Weissenbach syndrome (Thibierge and Weissenbach 1911). Digital calcification appears in approximately 10–30% of cases and can affect either the subcutaneous or the capsular tissues (Fig. 13.30). Bony erosion occurs in 40–80% of patients. It commences at the tuft and particularly on the palmar aspect of the bone. Continued resorption leads to penciling or sharpening of the phalanx.

Differential diagnosis includes:
- Rheumatoid arthritis: Unlike in RA the MCP joint and wrist articulations are tend to be spared and more prominent findings appear at the DIP joints.
- Psoriatic arthritis: Findings resembling psoriatic arthritis and neuropathic osteoarthritis have also been described. Also intra-articular bony ankylosis has been described at interphalangeal and wrist joints.
- Selective involvement of the first MCP joint can appear in scleroderma.
- Distinctive bilateral resorption of the trapezium and adjacent metacarpal bone is observed with varying degrees of radial subluxation of the metacarpal base.
- Synostosis of carpal bones may appear. Synovial cysts are additional articular manifestations.

13.4.3.3 Mixed Connective Tissue Disease (MCTD, Sharp Syndrome)

MCTD combines overlapping clinical features of scleroderma, SLE, dermatomyositis and RA. The radiographic characteristics of MCTD also underscore the mixed character of the disease. Changes compatible with RA (such as articular erosions, joint space narrowing and periarticular osteoporosis), with scleroderma (such as tuft resorption and soft tissue calcification) and with SLE (such as deforming nonerosive arthropathies) can be observed (Udoff et al. 1977; Szanto 1980).

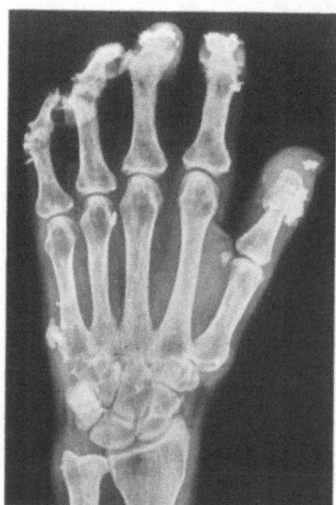

Fig. 13.30. Thibierge-Weissenbach syndrome with soft tissue calcifications along the tendons together with diffuse demineralization and the beginning contracture of the digits. Note also the tuftal resorption at the distal phalanx of the thumb

13.4.3.3.1 Imaging Findings

On radiographs osseous, articular and soft tissue abnormalities can be found in a wide spectrum from nonerosive and nondeforming to osseous erosions and joint deformity. In the hand, most frequent disease manifestations are in the PIP and MCP joints and at the midcarpal and radiocarpal compartments. Manifestations include:
- Osteopenia, joint space narrowing, erosions and changes at the fingertips.
- Soft tissue atrophy, soft tissue calcification, and resorption of the terminal tufts of the phalanges that may simulate the findings of scleroderma.
- Osseous resorption leading to typical "penciling" of the phalanges. The osseous erosions are similar to those in RA; however, manifestation at the DIP joints can be observed. Changes at the fingertips simulate those of scleroderma. The subluxations are typical to those of RA or scleroderma.

13.4.3.4 Rheumatic Fever

Rheumatic fever is a disorder characterized by fever, carditis and polyarthritis. Post-rheumatic fever arthropathy as described by Jaccoud was characterized by muscle atrophy, ulnar deviation with flexion and subluxation at multiple MTC joints, and hyperextension of distal IP joints (Murphy and Staple 1973; Twigg and Smith 1963).

Joint involvement is the most common clinical manifestation of rheumatic fever. The deforming arthropathy that may appear after repeated attacks has been described as Jaccoud's syndrome, or arthritis.

On radiographs the hand abnormalities resemble changes in SLE and other collagen vascular diseases, such as periarticular osteoporosis, but have some characteristics:
- Flexion and ulnar deviation of the MCP joints, particularly the fourth and fifth. The changes may be combined with hyperextension at interphalangeal joints. The reversible nature of the articular deformity is striking. During radiography, pressing the hand against the cassette may result in a normal radiograph. The deformities may become fixed.
- Symptomless and reversible joint deformities, particularly in the hands. Typically ulnar deviation and flexion deformities are evident at the MCP joints.
- Joint space narrowing is rare.
- Hook erosions on the radial and palmar aspect of the metacarpal heads.

Differential diagnosis includes:
- SLE and other collagen vascular diseases and vasculitides, which have similar findings. Deforming nonerosive arthropathies may also be encountered in A-gammaglobulinemia, Ehlers-Danlos syndrome, sarcoidosis and, rarely, RA.
- RA: the appearance of joint space narrowing and osseous erosions complicates the differentiation between these two disorders. The distribution and extent of articular space loss, however, are less widespread and severe in rheumatic fever than in RA. The hook erosions also differ from RA.

References

Ansell BM, Kent PA (1977) Radiological changes in juvenile chronic polyarthritis. Skeletal Radiol 1:129–134

Arnett FC, Edworthy SM, Bloch DA, McShane DJ, Fries JF, Cooper NS, Healey LA, Kaplan SR, Liang MH, Luthra HS (1988) The American Rheumatism Association revised criteria for the classification of rheumatoid arthritis. Arthritis Rheum 31:315–320

Athanasou NA, Quinn J, Woods CG (1998) Immunohistology of rheumatoid nodules and rheumatic synovitis. Ann Rheum Dis 47:398–403

Backhaus M, Kamradt T, Sandrock D, Loreck D, Fritz J, Wolf KJ, Raber H, Hamm B, Burmester GR, Bollow M (1999) Arthritis of the finger joints. Arthritis Rheum 42:1232–1237

Berens DL, Lin RK (1969) Roentgen diagnosis of rheumatoid arthritis. CC Thomas, Springfield, Ill, pp 1–89

Bluhm GN, Smith DW, Mikulaschek WM (1983) A radiologic method of assessment of bone and joint destruction in rheumatoid arthritis. Henry Ford Hosp Med J 31:152–161

Brun B, Serup J, Hagdrup H (1983) Radiological changes of the hands in systemic sclerosis. Acta Derm Venereol 63:349–358

Bullough PG (1992) Atlas of orthopaedic pathology. Gower, London

Bunch TW, O'Duffy JD, McLeod RA (1976) Deforming arthritis of the hands in polymyositis. Arthritis Rheum 19:243

Bywaters EGL (1975) Jaccoud's syndrome. A sequel to the joint involvement in systemic lupus erythematosus. Clin Rheum Dis 1:125

Cassidy JT, Petty RE (1995) Textbook of pediatric rheumatology, 3rd edn. Saunders, Philadelphia

Crass JR, van de Vegte GL, Harkavy (1988) Tendon echogenicity: ex vivo study. Radiology 167:499–501

De Flaviis L, Musso MG (1995) Hand and wrist. In: Fornage B (ed) Musculoskeletal ultrasound. Churchill Livingstone, New York, p 151

Dihlmann W (1987) Arthritis. Gelenke-Wirbelverbindungen. Thieme, Stuttgart, pp 4–94

Fassbender HG (1994) Inflammatory reactions in arthritis. In: Davis ME, Dingle JT (eds) Immunopharmacology of joints and connective tissue. Harcourt/Brace, London

Finder JG, Ellman MH, Jablon M (1983) Massive synovial hypertrophy in Reiter's disease. J Bone Joint Surg Am 65:555

Fishel B, Caspi D, Eventov I, Avrahami E, Yaron M (1989) Multiple osteonecrotic lesions in systemic lupus erythematosus: a reevaluation. J Rheumatol 16:604–610

Freyschmidt J (1985) Gelenkerkrankungen. Springer, Berlin Heidelberg New York, pp 1–24

Genant HK (1983) Methods of assessing radiographic change in rheumatoid arthritis. Am J Med 75 (6A):35–47

Genant HK, Doi K, Mall JC (1975) Optical versus radiographic magnification for fine-detail skeletal radiography. Invest Radiol 10:160–172

Giovagnoni A, Valeri G, Burroni E, Amici F (1998) Rheumatoid arthritis: follow-up and response to treatment. Eur J Radiol 27:25–34

Gofton JP, O'Brien WM, Hurley JN (1984) Radiographic evaluation of erosion in rheumatoid arhtirtis: double blind study of auranofin vs placebo. J Rheumatol 11:768–771

Harris ED Jr (1990) Rheumatoid arthritis: pathophysiology and implications for therapy. N Engl J Med 322:1277–1289

Hastings DE, Evans JA (1975) Rheumatoid wrist deformities and their relation to ulnar drift. J Bone Joint Surg 57:930–936

Hoffman GS, Filie JD, Schumacher HR Jr, Ortiz Bravo E, Tsokos MG, Marini JC, Kerr GS, Ling QH, Trentham DE (1991) Intractable vasculitis, resorptive osteolysis, and immunity to type I collagen in type VII Ehlers-Danlos syndrome. Arthritis Rheum 34:1466–1473

Hughes GRV (1994) Systemic lupus erythematosus. In: Hughes GRV (ed) Connective tissue diseases. Blackwell Scientific, Oxford

Hunder GG (1999) Atlas of rheumatology. Current Medicine, Philadelphia

Imhof H, Breitenseher M, Kainberger F, Trattnig S (1997) Degenerative joint disease: cartilage or vascular disease. Skeletal Radiol 26:398–403

Imhof H, Breitenseher M, Kainberger F, Rand T, Trattnig S (1999a) Importance of subchondral bone to articular cartilage in health and disease. Magn Reson Imaging 10:180–192

Imhof H, Kainberger F, Breitenseher M, Grampp S, Rand T, Trattnig S (1999b) Joints. In: Reimer P, Parizel PM, Stichnoth FA (eds) Clinical MR imaging. A practical approach. Springer, Berlin Heidelberg New York, p 187

Jevtic V, Watt I, Rozman B, Kos-Golja M, Demsar F, Jarh O (1995a) Distinctive radiological features of small hand joints in rheumatoid arthritis and seronegative spondylarthritis demonstrated by contrast-enhanced (Gd-DTPA) magnetic resonance imaging. Skeletal Radiol 24:351

Jevtic V, Rozman B, Watt I, Presetnik M (1995b) Grand round– the use of contrast enhanced MR in the assessment of the therapeutic response to a disease modifying antirheumatic drug. Br J Rheumatol 34:956

Jevtic V, Watt I, Rozman B, Presetnik M, Logar D, Praprotnik S, Tomsic M, Sipek A, Kos-Golja M, Sepe A, Jarh O, Demsar F, Musikic P, Campion G (1996) Prognostic value of contrast enhanced Gd-DTPA MRI for development of bone erosive changes in rheumatoid arthritis. Br J Rheumatol 35 [Suppl 3]:26–37

Jewell F, Watt I (1996) Arthritis – imaging and therapy. Past, present and future. Radiologe 36:646–656

Kainberger F, Czerny C, Trattnig S, Lack W, Machold K, Graninger W (1996) MRI and sonography in rheumatology. Radiologe 36:609–616

Kainberger F, Fischer W, Bohndorf K (1998) Prinzipien der Differentialdiagnose von Gelenkerkrankungen. In: Bohndorf K, Imhof H (eds) Radiologische Diagnostik der Knochen und Gelenke. Thieme, Stuttgart, pp 293–304

Kainberger F, Boegl K, Peloschek P, Graninger W, Adlassnig KP, Imhof H (1999) A computerised scoring system for rheumatoid arthritis. In: Lemke HU, Vannier MW, Inamua K, Farman AG (eds) CARS 99, Springer, Berlin Heidelberg New York, pp 393–397

Kellgren E (1963) Atlas of standard radiographs of arthritis. FA Davis, Philadelphia, pp 1–212

Khan MA (1992) Spondyloarthropathies. Rheum Dis Clin North Am 18:1–276

Klarlund M, Ostergaard M, Lorenzen I (1999) Finger joint synovitis in rheumatoid arthritis: quantitative assessment by magnetic resonance imaging. Rheumatology 38:66–71

Klippel JH, Gerber LH, Pollak L, Decker JL (1979) Avascular necroses in systemic lupus erythematosus. Silent symmetric osteonecrosis. Am J Med 67:83–89

König H, Sieper J, Wolf KJ (1990) Rheumatoid arthritis: evaluation of hypervacsular and fibrous pannus with dynamic MR imaging enhanced with Gd-DTPA. Radiology 176:473–481

Lane, JM, Weiss C (1975) Review of articular cartilage collagen research. Arthritis Rheum 18:553–562

Larsen A (1995) How to apply Larsen score in evaluating radiographs of RA in long-term studies. J Rheumatol 22:1974–1976

Larsen A, Dale K, Eek M (1977) Radiographic evaluation of RA and related conditions by standard reference films. Acta Radiol 18:481–489

Leeb BF, Machold KP, Smolen JS (1996) Diagnose und Therapie der chronischen Polyarthritis. Radiologe 36:657–662

Le Roy EC, Black C, Fleischmajer R (1988) Scleroderma (systemic sclerosis): classification, subsets and pathogenesis. J Rheumatol 15:202–205

Leventhal GH, Dorfman HD (1974) Aseptic necrosis of bone in systemic lupus erythematosus. Semin Arthritis Rheum 4:73–93

Marcelis S, Daenen B, Ferrara MA (1996) Wrist. In: Dondelinger RF (ed) Peripheral musculoskeletal ultrasound atlas. Thieme, Stuttgart, p 92

Martel W, Stuck KJ, Dworin AM, Hylland RG (1980) Erosive osteoarthritis and psoriatic arthritis: a radiologic comparison in the hand, wrist, and foot. AJR 134:125

McCarty DJ (1993) Clinical picture of rheumatoid arthritis. In: McCarty DJ, Koopmann WJ (eds) Arthritis and allied conditions, 12th edn. Lea and Febiger, Philadelphia

McQueen FM, Stewart N, Crabbe J, Robinson E, Yeoman S, Tan PL, McLean L (1998) Magnetic resonance imaging of the wrist in early rheumatoid arthritis reveals a high prevalence of erosions at four months after symptom onset. Ann Rheum Dis 57:350–356

Milz S, Putz R (1994) Lückenbildung der subchondralen Mineralisierungszone des Tibiaplateaus. Osteologie 3:110–118

Monsees B, Murphy WA (1985) Pressure erosions: a pattern of bone resorption in rheumatoid arthritis. Rheumatism 28:820–827

Monsees B, Destouet JM, Murphy WA, Resnick D (1985) Pressure erosions of bone in rheumatoid arthritis: a subject review. Radiology 155:53

Murphy WA, Staple TW (1973) Jaccoud's arthropathy reviewed. AJR 118:300

Nance EP, Kaye JJ, Callahan LF (1986) Observer variation in quantitative assessment of rheumatoid arthritis. I. Scoring erosions and joint space narrowing. Invest Radiol 21:922-927

Netter FH (1990) Rheumatic diseases. In: The CIBA collections of medical illustrations, vol 8, part II. CIBA Geigy, Summit, NJ, p. 176

Ostergaard M, Lorenzen I, Henriksen O (1994) Dynamic gadolinium-enhanced MR imaging in active and inactive immunoinflammatory gonarthritis. Acta Radiol 35:275

Ostergaard M, Stoltenberg M, Lovgreen-Nielsen P, Volck B, Jensen CH, Lorenzen I (1997) Magnetic resonance imaging-determined synovial membrane and joint effusion volumes in rheumatoid arthritis and osteoarthritis: comparison with the macroscopic and microscopic appearance of the synovium. Arthritis Rheum 40:1856–1867

Peterfy CG, van Dijke CF, Janzen DL, Gluer CC, Namba R, Majumdar S, Lang P, Genant HK (1994) Quantification of the articular cartilage in the knee with pulsed saturation transfer subtraction and fat-suppressed MR imaging. Optimization and validation. Radiology 192:485–493

Pile KD, Gendi NST, Mowat AG (1992) Scleroderma with bilateral synovial fistulae. J Rheumatol 19:1150–1158

Rabinowitz JG, Twersky J (1974) Guttadauria M: similar bone manifestations of scleroderma and rheumatoid arthritis. AJR 121:35–42

Rau R, Herborn G (1995) A modified version of Larsen's scoring method to assess radiologic changes in rheumatoid arthritis. J Rheumatol 22:1976

Resnick D (1974) Patterns of peripheral joint disease in ankylosing spondylitis. Radiology 110:523–530

Resnick D, Niwayama G (1995) Rheumatoid arthritis. In: Resnick D, Niwayama G (eds) Diagnosis of bone and joint disorders. Saunders, Philadelphia

Resnick D, Greenway G, Vint VC, Robinson CA, Piper S (1978) Selective involvement of the first carpometacarpal joint in scleroderma. AJR 131:283

Schmitt R, Lanz U (1996) Bildgebende Diagnostik der Hand. Hippokrates, Stuttgart

Scott DL, Houssien DA, Laasonen L (1995) Proposed modification to Larsen's scoring methods for hand and wrist radiographs. Br J Rheumatol 34:56

Scutellari PN, Orzincolo C (1998) Rheumatoid arthritis: sequences. Eur J Radiol 27:31

Sharp JT (1996) Scoring radiographic abnormalities in rheumatoid arthritis. Radiol Clin North Am 34:233–240

Sharp JT, Young DY, Bluhm GB (1985) How many joints in the hand and wrist need to be included in a score of radiologic abnormalities? Arthritis Rheum 28:1326–1335

Sievers K (1965) The rheumatoid factor in definite rheumatoid arthritis: an analysis of 1279 adult patients, with a follow-up study. Acta Rheum Scand Suppl 9:1–121

Simmen BR, Huber H (1994) The wrist joint in chronic polyarthritis: a new classification based on the type of destruction in relation to the natural course and the consequences for surgical therapy. Handchir Mikrochir Plast Chir 26:182–189

Smith DK, Christensen A (1996) Miscellaneous surgical entities of the hand and wrist. In: Gilula L (ed) Imaging of the wrist and hand, 1st edn. Saunders, Pennsylvania

Stack HG, Vaughan-Jackson OJ (1971) The zig-zag deformity in the rheumatoid hand. Hand 3:62–70

Stadalnik RC, Dublin AB (1975) Sesamoid periostitis in the thumb in Reiter's syndrome. J Bone Joint Surg Am 57:279–285

Stasny P (1978) Association of the B-cell alloantigen Drw4 with rheumatoid arthritis. N Engl J Med 298:869–871

Steinbrocker O, Traeger CH, Batterman RC (1949) Therapeutic criteria in rheumatoid arthritis. JAMA 140:659–665

Sugimoto H, Takeda A, Kano S (1998) Assessment of disease activity in rheumatoid arthritis using magnetic resonance imaging: quantification of pannus volume in the hands. Br J Radiol 37:854–860

Swanson AB, Swanson GG (1972) Pathogenesis and pathomechanics of rheumatoid metacarpophalangeal joint. J Bone Joint Surg 54:687

Swezey RL, Alexander SJ (1969) Notching of the carpal navicular. Ann Rheum Dis 28:45–52

Szanto D (1980) MCTD-syndrome (mixed connective tissue disease). ROFO 133:445–454

Thibierge G, Weissenbach RJ (1911) Concretions calcaire et sclerodermie. Ann Dermatol Syphiligr 2:129–138

Toivanen A (1993) z. In: Klippe J, Dieppe PA (eds) Reactive arthritis in rheumatology. Mosby, St Louis, pp z–z

Udoff EJ, Genant HK, Kozin F, Ginsberg M (1977) Mixed connective tissue disease: the spectrum of radiographic manifestations. Radiology 124:613

Van der Heijde DM (1996) Plain X-rays in rheumatoid arthritis: overview of scoring methods, their reliability and applicability. Baillieres Clin Rheumatol 10:435–440

Van der Heijde DMFM, van Reil PL, Nuvar-Zwart IH (1989) Effects of hydroxychloroquine and sulphalazine on progression of joint damage in rheumatoid arthritis. Lancet I:1036–1038

Van der Linden S (1996) Ankylosing spondylitis. In: Kelly WN, Harris ED, Ruddy S, Sledge CB (eds) Textbook of rheumatology, 5th edn. Saunders, Philadelphia

Van Holsbeeck M, Introcaso JH (1991) Musculoskeletal ultrasound. Mosby Year Book, St Louis, pp 289–297

Wassenberg S, Rau R (1995) Problems in evaluating radiographic findings in rheumatoid arthritis using different methods of radiographic scoring: examples of difficult cases and a study design to develop an improved scoring method. J Rheumatol 22:1990–1998

Watt I (1995) Arthritis: basic differential diagnosis. In: Bloem JL (ed) Musculoskeletal imaging. Springer, Berlin Heidelberg New York, pp 57–64

Weinberger A, Kaplan JG, Myers AR (1979) Extensive soft tissue calcification (calcinosis universalis) in systemic lupus erythematosus. Ann Rheum Dis 38:384–390

Weissman BN, Rappoport AS, Sosman JL, Schur PH (1978) Radiographic findings in the hands in patients with systemic lupus erythematosus. Radiology 126:313–320

Wilson AJ, Mann FA, Gilula LA (1990) Imaging the hand and wrist. J Hand Surg [Br] 5:153–167

Yamato M, Tamai K, Yamaguchi T, Ohno W (1993) MRI of the knee in rheumatoid arthritis: Gd-DTPA perfusion dynamics. J Comput Assist Tomogr 17:781

Yochum TR, Rowe LJ (1996) Essentials of skeletal radiology. Williams and Wilkins, Baltimore

Yune HY, Vix VA, Klatte EC (1971) Early fingertip changes in scleroderma. JAMA 215:215–221

14 Bone and Soft Tissue Infections

A.M. Davies

14.1 Introduction

Before the introduction of antibiotics, infections of the hand frequently resulted in severe morbidity, and even on occasion in septicaemia and death [1]. Today prompt detection and diagnosis of infection with appropriate medical and or surgical management will usually ensure a satisfactory clinical outcome. Infections of the hand and wrist may be classified by temporal occurrence (acute or chronic), site (bone, joint, soft tissue or combined) and by causative organism (bacterial, viral, fungal and parasitic). Attention to the clinical history may reveal predisposing factors for infection including prior trauma, remote infection, systemic disease (diabetes and immunosuppression) and occupational exposure [2]. This chapter will cover the common manifestations of the various infections indicating the appropriate use of imaging.

14.2 Pyogenic Infections

14.2.1 Soft Tissue Infection

The most frequently encountered infections of the hand and wrist are confined to the soft tissues, usually as a result of trauma. In the majority of cases imaging may be unnecessary or only be required to exclude involvement of deeper structures (e.g. osteomyelitis). In order to understand the mechanism of spread of infection it is important to have knowledge of the different compartments and their communications.

The nail fold (eponychium) is firmly attached proximally to the base of the terminal phalanx. This is particularly susceptible to infection (paronychia) following minor localized trauma and is the most common infection in the hand. Chronic paronychia is usually seen in diabetic patients, in whom the causative agent is frequently *Candida albicans* [3].

The terminal pulp of the finger may have infection localized to the septated apical spaces immediately beneath the tip of the nail or more generalized within the pulp (felon). The latter, if neglected, will lead to secondary infection of the terminal phalanx with periosteal new bone formation and lysis (Fig. 14.1). A non-pyogenic cause of both paronychia and a felon is herpetic whitlow caused by the herpes simplex virus.

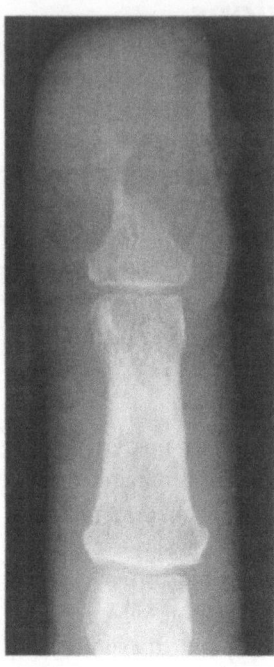

Fig. 14.1. Lysis of the terminal phalanx due to osteomyelitis secondary to neglected soft tissue infection of the pulp

There is a limited thickness of soft tissue coverage for the tendons rendering them susceptible to puncture wounds, particularly in the digital creases. Because there is communication between the flexor sheaths, infection may rapidly spread to the wrist and lower forearm or extend across the hand to involve the tendon sheaths of both the thumb and little fingers ("horseshoe" abscess). Both ultrasound and MR imaging may be used to identify the fluid collection within the tendon sheaths. MR imaging will show the fluid to be hypointense on T1-weighted and hyperintense on T2-weighted and STIR sequences surrounding the low signal intensity tendons. There may be some diffuse synovial thickening that can be distinguished from the fluid using contrast-enhanced T1-weighted images. It is not possible, however, to distinguish between infected and non-infected collections [4]. Despite this limitation, MR imaging is valuable in confirming or excluding other sites of infection, including osteomyelitis, as well as potentially identifying the optimum site for percutaneous aspiration [4]. While imaging is potentially helpful it is important that treatment is not delayed as pyogenic infection of the tendon sheath rapidly leads to adhesions and necrosis. Urgent surgical drainage will be required unless the infection is caught within the first 2 days of onset.

There are four deep spaces in the palm of the hand that may become infected. These are the web space, the palmar spaces (thenar and mid-palmar) and rarely the hypothenar space. The typical web space infection is the collar-stud abscess, so called because two loci of pus communicate via a narrow channel through the deep fascia. The mid-palmar space is deep to the flexor tendons and can become infected by penetrating wounds, extension from the flexor tendons of the middle to little fingers or from distal palmar abscesses extending proximally. Thenar space infections occur by similar mechanisms including penetrating injury, subcutaneous and flexor tendon sheath infections of the thumb and index finger as well as extension of infection from the radial bursa or mid-palmar space. The typical MR appearances of a soft tissue abscess are a well-demarcated fluid collection surrounded by a pseudocapsule. The fluid collection is hypointense on T1-weighted and hyperintense on T2-weighted sequences. The pseudocapsule is hypointense on all sequences. On signal characteristics alone it may be difficult to distinguish an abscess from the commonest of all soft tissue masses seen in the hand and wrist, a ganglion cyst. Infections, however, are usually associated with some inflammatory change in the surrounding soft tissues seen as more diffuse hyperintensity on T2-weighted images.

The dorsum of the hand has no significant anatomical compartments. A localized infection or carbuncle on the dorsum of a finger is known as a whitlow. Because of the limited soft tissue coverage traumatic dorsal infections are often associated with infection of the underlying joint (see below).

14.2.2   Septic Arthritis

The commonest cause of a pyogenic joint infection, septic arthritis, is a human bite. This is something of a misnomer when the metacarpophalangeal joint is involved as the mechanism of injury is usually a clenched fist blow to the biter's mouth. Because the posture of the finger in the extended position differs from that at the point of impact, the puncture wound will appear proximal to the joint [5]. For this reason any wound over the knuckle should be considered as a potential cause of a septic arthritis. The commonest pathogen in septic arthritis is *Staphylococcus aureus* [6]. Another common organism found in human bites is *Eikenella corrodens* and in animal bites, *Pasteurella multocida* [7]. Fortunately, both are sensitive to penicillin.

The radiographic appearances of septic arthritis are initially soft tissue swelling and juxta-articular osteoporosis (Fig. 14.2). This will be followed within days or a couple of weeks with joint space narrowing due to articular cartilage damage. As the underlying bone is laid bare by the destructive process, there will be loss of definition of the articular cortex with ill-defined erosion (Fig. 14.2). The inflammatory process may well extend to produce some periosteal new bone formation along the adjacent tubular bones. In time, if the infective process is not halted, the joint will be destroyed with sclerosis, progressive deformity and secondary degenerative change.

The clinical course of a septic arthritis is usually so rapid that by the time MR imaging is organized it is unlikely to show changes in the absence of any radiographic abnormalities. However, it will reveal the full extent of the inflammatory change and early cartilage destruction. As with synovitis of the tendons, MR imaging cannot definitively distinguish between infective and non-infective causes [8, 9]. To suspect septic arthritis, other features of infection should be present, includ-

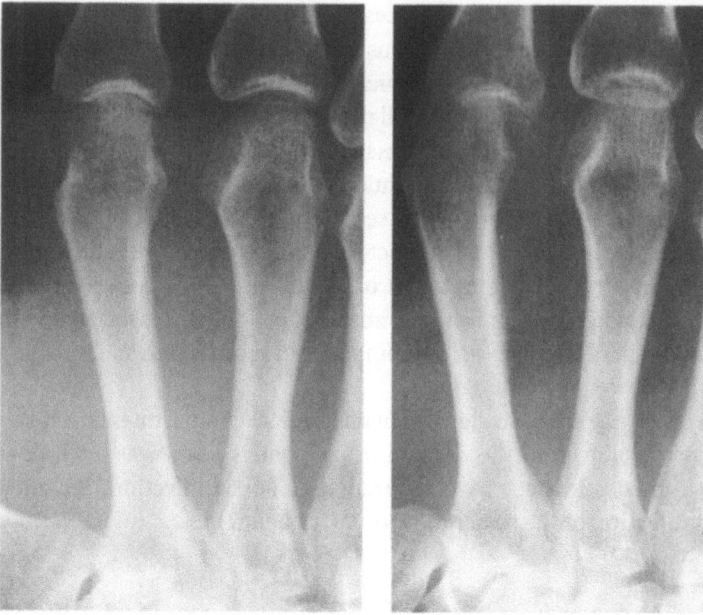

a   b

Fig. 14.2. a Early septic arthritis of the second metacarpal joint indicated by juxta-articular osteopenia and joint space narrowing. **b** The follow-up radiograph obtained 2 weeks later shows rapid progression with articular erosions

ing extensive inflammatory reaction in the surrounding tissues or coexisting osteomyelitis [10, 11].

In the absence of prior trauma, other causes of an inflammatory arthropathy should be considered including tuberculosis, gonorrhoea, brucellosis [12], gout, Reiter's syndrome and rheumatoid arthritis [13]. Where clinical doubt remains aspiration and culture is mandatory.

Septic arthritis of the proximal interphalangeal joint may result in a boutonniere deformity as pus destroys the dorsal capsule and central slip of the extensor mechanism [14].

14.2.3 Osteomyelitis

Osteomyelitis is defined as infection of bone, irrespective of the causative organism. Involvement of the bones of the hand occurs in approximately 10% of all cases of osteomyelitis, and osteomyelitis represents less than 6% of all hand infections [15]. Osteomyelitis in the hand commonly results from trauma including penetrating wounds such as bites, crush or mutilating open injuries, by contiguous spread from an adjacent infection of joint or soft tissue, following surgery, by haematogenous spread and in patients with peripheral vascular disease or systemic illness. The commonest infecting organism is *Staphylococcus aureus*. Many other organisms may be found. Clearly, the clinical presentation is important in determining the infective agent – for example, the well-recognized association between *Salmonella* osteomyelitis and sickle cell anaemia [16].

The initial site of infection will depend on whether the origin is traumatic or atraumatic. In the former, the bones of the fingers and the distal metacarpals are the most commonly affected, whereas, in the absence of trauma or predisposing condition, the distal forearm bones are frequently involved, particularly in the younger age group. Osteomyelitis of the carpal bones usually occurs secondary to septic arthritis of the wrist.

Initial radiographs may be normal or show subtle soft tissue swelling with early demineralization [17]. Within 2–3 weeks bony destruction will develop with periosteal new bone formation (Fig. 14.3). The pattern of bone destruction may be permeative, mimicking tumour, or more well defined indicating the formation of a discrete bone abscess (Figs. 14.3, 14.4). The presence of sequestrum and/or involucrum indicates chronic osteomyelitis [18].

Scintigraphy may be used to detect acute osteomyelitis before changes are visible on radiographs. Technetium and gallium scans alone are nonspecific for infection [19]. Indium-labelled leucocyte scanning is more accurate, with increased specificity and sensitivity if combined with technetium scanning [20]. Bone scintigraphy can also be of value in revealing other sites of infection, as can be found in recurrent multifocal osteomyelitis. This is particularly important in the paediatric age group where multifocal infection is seen in 7% of cases [21].

MR imaging is currently the most sensitive imaging technique available to demonstrate marrow abnormality. The sensitivity of MR imaging for the diagno-

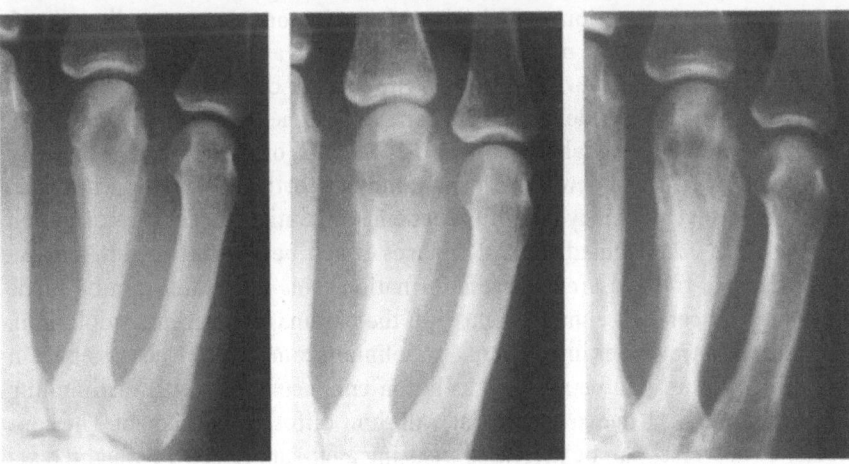

a,b   c

Fig. 14.3a–c. Progression of osteomyelitis of the fourth metacarpal following a human bite injury: at presentation (a) and 1 week (b) and 3 weeks (c) after presentation. Initially the lesion looks more aggressive but by the 3 week film, with the patient on antibiotic treatment, some consolidation is developing

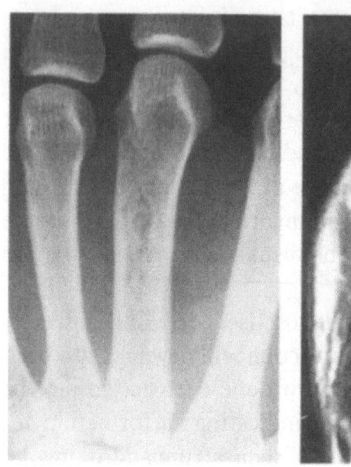
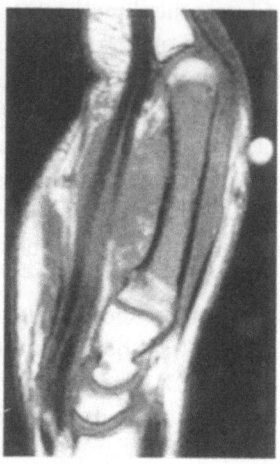

a

b

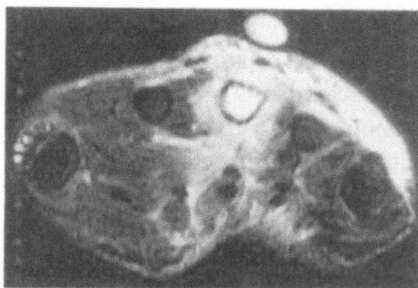

c

Fig. 14.4. Early osteomyelitis of the third metacarpal indicated by minor permeative lysis on the radiograph (a). MR imaging shows florid marrow oedema involving much of the shaft of the metacarpal on the sagittal T1-weighted image (b) and early erosion of the cortex with surrounding soft tissue oedema on the axial T2-weighted fat-suppressed image (c)

sis of osteomyelitis is reported to be 88–100%, with a specificity of 75–100% [22, 23]. MR imaging is superior to CT in that it also demonstrates any adjacent soft tissue involvement and the multiplanar capability will aid surgical planning [22]. The MR imaging findings will depend on the stage of development of the infection. Early on, marrow oedema will appear as ill-defined low signal intensity on T1-weighted and high signal intensity on T2-weighted or STIR images (Fig. 14.4). Subsequently, periosteal new bone formation with cortical breaching will occur. Soft tissue involvement may be diffuse oedema or contiguous abscess formation (Fig. 14.4). On T2-weighted or STIR images it can be difficult to differentiate diffuse oedema from discrete abscess formation. This distinction can be made with the use of contrast enhancement with the paramagnetic agent, gadolinium. Following the intravenous injection of a gadolinium compound an abscess, be it in bone or soft tissue, will be revealed as a non-enhancing area with surrounding enhancement [24]. Oedema, in contrast, will show diffuse enhancement. The conspicuity of abscesses can be increased by using a fat-suppressed T1-weighted sequence following contrast enhancement, which has been found to be more sensitive than three-phase bone scanning and more specific than unenhanced MR imaging in the diagnosis of osteomyelitis [25]. The routine use of gadolinium in MR imaging of all cases of osteomyelitis remains debatable [26].

The rate of progress of osteomyelitis is due primarily to the "virulence" of the organism. The presence of a chronic, indolent infection should suggest a non-pyogenic cause. However, the progress is also mediated in part by the host response. It is for this reason that the same organism may produce varying appearances in different patients. Figures 14.5 and 14.6 illustrate this point by showing two different patients with staphylococcal osteomyelitis of the distal radius. In one the infection is unchecked with rapid progress over a period of 2 weeks (Fig. 14.5). In the other there is the gradual development over several years of a Brodie's abscess due to the host's attempt to contain the infection (Fig. 14.6).

a b

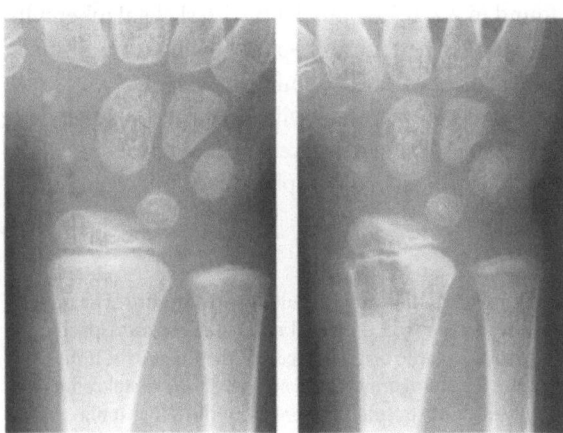

Fig. 14.5a, b. Rapid progression of acute osteomyelitis in the distal radius in a 5-year-old boy. Normal radiograph at presentation (**a**). Eleven days later there is a 1 cm in diameter lytic lesion in the distal radial metaphysis with a faint periosteal reaction (**b**)

a

b

c

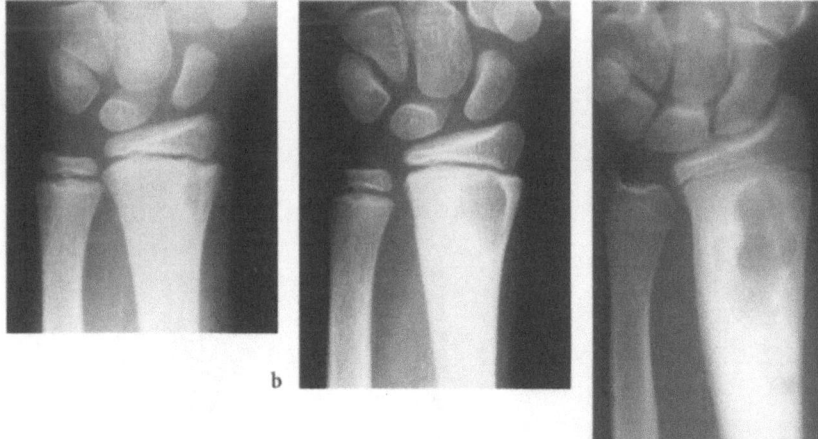

Fig. 14.6a–c. Development of untreated Brodie's abscess in the distal radial metaphysis in a 9-year-old boy: at presentation (**a**), 8 months (**b**) and 5 years later (**c**). The last radiograph shows a typical well-defined medullary abscess cavity with a sinus tract extending through the cortex

14.3 Mycobacterial Infections

14.3.1 Tuberculosis

The causative agents of tuberculosis are bacteria belonging to the so-called *Mycobacterium tuberculosis* complex. These include *Mycobacterium tuberculosis*, *M. bovis*, *M. bovis BCG* and *M. africanum*. *Mycobacterium tuberculosis* is the commonest cause of skeletal tuberculosis. The incidence of skeletal tuberculosis differs between the western world and developing countries. The decline in this disease has been reversed in the past 20 years due to a number of factors. These include antibiotic resistance and increasing infections in immunocompromised individuals. Involvement of the hand and wrist is found in 2.2–6.9% of patients with skeletal tuberculosis. Overall, multifocal bone lesions may be found in approximately 11% of cases. Bone scintigraphy is useful in revealing occult sites of infection (Fig. 14.7).

Tuberculosis of the hand and wrist may present with osteomyelitis/dactylitis, septic arthritis and extensor or flexor tenosynovitis. Because of the chronicity of the disease and variability of appearance it can radiographically mimic many other

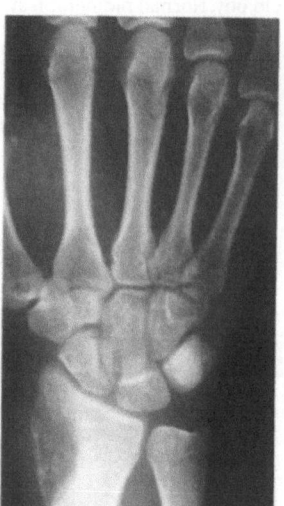

Fig. 14.7a, b. Multifocal tuberculous osteomyelitis. The appearances of the focus in the distal radius (**a**) are non-specific but the patient's ethnic origin suggested the diagnosis. Bone scintigraphy (**b**) showed increased activity in the distal radius and also revealed the occult involvement of the left scapula

a

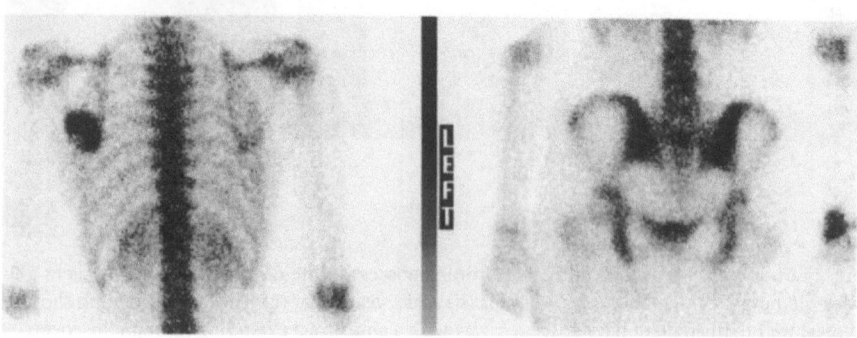

b

conditions including tumours and non-infective arthropathies (Fig. 14.7). It should always be considered in the differential diagnosis of a destructive lesion in the hand, particularly if the patient is from a high-risk group, e.g. from the Asian subcontinent.

The radiographic features of tuberculous osteomyelitis include soft tissue swelling, diffuse demineralization, bony lysis with cavities or honeycombing, marginal osteosclerosis and periosteal new bone formation (Fig. 14.8). Sequestra are said to be an uncommon feature. When the lesion is confined to one or more of the small tubular bones of the hand with florid soft tissue swelling it is known as tuberculous dactylitis. This form is commoner in children and, if associated with marked bony expansion, is known as "spina ventosa" (Fig. 14.8a, b). It is important to recognize that other conditions may present with a dactylitis [27] (Table 14.1). For example, in a patient of Afro-Caribbean origin, sickle cell dactylitis may have a similar presentation.

Tuberculous dactylitis is commoner in children than adults. Conversely, tuberculous arthritis, usually of the wrist joint, is commoner in adults. Contiguous

Table 14.1. Causes of dactylitis (modified from [27])

Pyogenic osteomyelitis (especially *Salmonella*)
Sickle cell anaemia
Tuberculosis (spina ventosa)
Fungal infections (e.g. mycetoma, sporotrichosis)
Leprosy
Tumour (osteoid osteoma, metastasis, Ewing's sarcoma)
Syphilis, yaws
Sarcoidosis

a 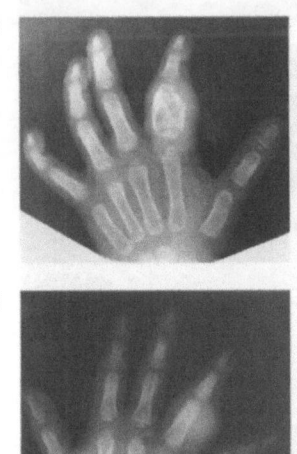 b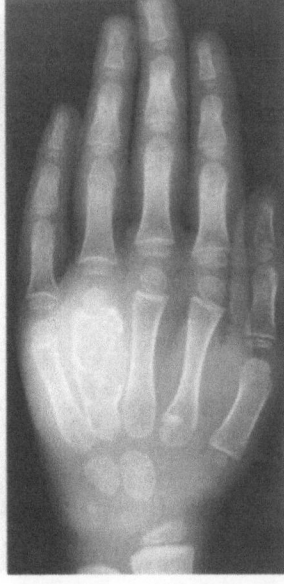

c

Fig. 14.8a–c. Three examples of tuberculous osteomyelitis in children. Classic spina ventosa of the second proximal phalanx (**a**) and fourth metacarpal (**b**). Dactylitis of the fifth metacarpal and fourth digit (**c**)

spread from involved tenosynovium is the most likely route of infection. The earliest radiographic signs are soft tissue swelling and severe articular and juxta-articular osteopenia. As the synovitis progresses there is joint space narrowing with loss of definition of the articular cortex due to fine erosions. This has been described as "like nibbling of cheese" (Fig. 14.9) [28]. If the introduction of antituberculous therapy is delayed until the destructive changes are pronounced, healing may be accompanied by bony ankylosis. Healing may also be associated with calcification, particularly if there is abscess formation (Fig. 14.10). In the early stages tuberculous arthritis may easily be confused with a non-infective arthropathy such as rheumatoid arthritis. It is unlikely to be mistaken for a pyogenic arthritis due to its relatively indolent progress.

Tuberculous tenosynovitis is the most frequent tuberculous infection of the hand. It clinically simulates rheumatoid tenosynovitis. The flexor tendons of the

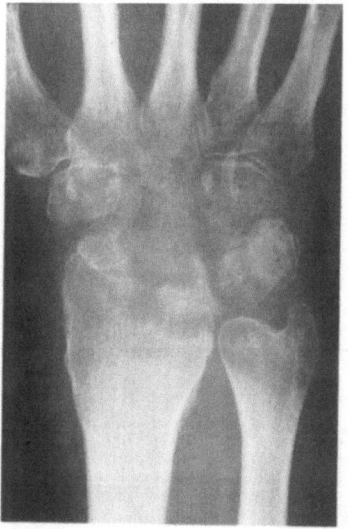

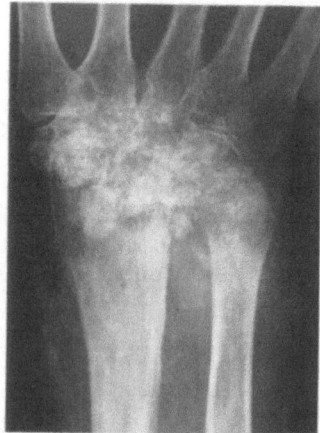

a

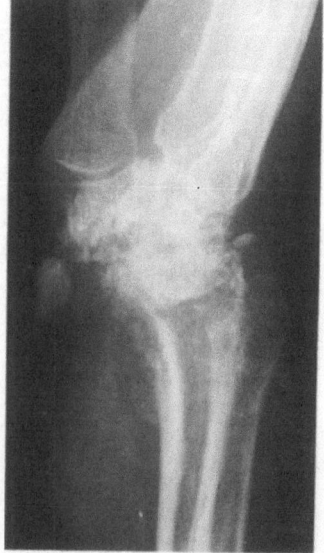

b

Fig. 14.9. Tuberculous arthritis. There is severe articular and juxta-articular demineralization with diffuse erosions of all the carpal bones

Fig. 14.10a, b. Chronic tuberculous arthritis of the wrist joint. Anteroposterior (**a**) and lateral (**b**) radiographs. The appearances are those of a severe chronic inflammatory arthropathy. The correct diagnosis is indicated by the dystrophic calcification within the soft tissue abscess

hand, wrist and forearm are more commonly affected than the extensor tendons (Fig. 14.11). Over 50% of cases are due to *Mycobacterium marinum*. Less common infecting organisms are *Mycobacterium kansasii* and *M. avium-intracellulare*. Discomfort is mild, localized signs of inflammation minimal, and constitutional upset absent. Coexisting pulmonary tuberculosis is rare such that the chest radiograph is almost always normal. Radiographs of the hand are usually normal until late in the disease, when there may be spread to cause a tuberculous arthritis or osteomyelitis. The extent of the disease process can be well demonstrated using either ultrasound or MR imaging (Fig. 14.11) [29, 30].

14.3.2 Leprosy

Hansen's disease is a chronic infection caused by *Mycobacterium leprae*, mainly affecting the peripheral nerves and skin in the cooler parts of the body. In the early 1990s there were about 2.5 million cases of leprosy worldwide, mostly in Asia, Africa and South America. Most cases seen in the developed world are to be found in immigrants. The radiographic changes may be classified into two types. First, there are specific changes resulting from the infection, seen in less than 10% of affected cases. Second, and more common, are changes resulting from trauma and infection in a denervated hand [31, 32].

The specific changes include soft tissue swelling, demineralization, well-defined cyst-like lesions in the epiphyses and metaphyses of the phalanges, prominent phalangeal nutrient foramina, osseous destruction and deformity (Fig. 14.12a). Non-specific bone lesions include acro-osteolysis, osteomyelitis, fractures and bony resorption resulting in the classic "licked lollipop/candystick" appearance (Fig. 14.12b). Similar appearances may be found in other neuropathic conditions such as syringomyelia and congenital insensitivity to pain. Nerve calcifica-

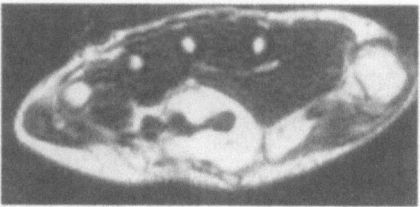

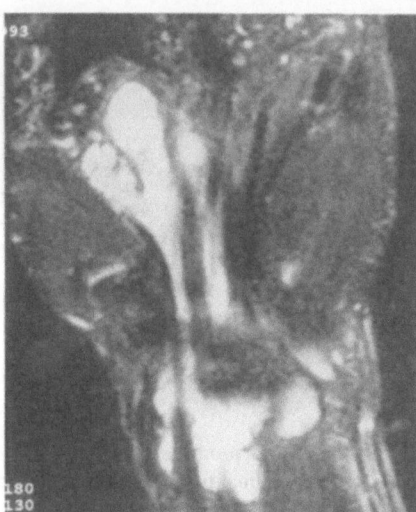

b

a

Fig. 14.11a, b. Tuberculous tenosynovitis of the wrist flexors. The distended synovial sheaths appear hyperintense on both the coronal STIR (a) and axial T2-weighted (b) MR images. On these images alone the condition cannot be distinguished from a chronic tenosynovitis due to other causes

tion in leprosy is mentioned in many textbooks but all would appear to cite the same single case report to substantiate this association [33].

The abnormalities listed above all occur in well-established disease. Early abnormalities of the peripheral nerves can be revealed with ultrasound and MR imaging [34]. These include diffuse nerve enlargement and compression [34]. Most patients with leprosy, however, live in parts of the world where access to sophisticated imaging remains limited.

14.4 Treponemal Infections

14.4.1 Syphilis

In congenital syphilis the spirochete, *Treponema pallidum*, crosses the placenta to infect the fetus. In those that survive, the osseous lesions are typically seen in the long bones, with metaphyseal defects and periosteal new bone formation. Dactylitis may occur (Fig. 14.13) [35]. Acquired syphilis rarely involves the bones of the hand.

14.4.2 Yaws

Yaws is a tropical infection caused by the spirochete *Treponema pertenue*, with bone involvement in the secondary and tertiary forms. The appearances are similar to syphilis with only the tubular bones affected. The radiographic changes include a dactylitis with bone destruction and periosteal new bone formation (Fig. 14.14) [36]. The degree of destruction may result in shortening of the fingers to give a "doigt en lorgnette" appearance [37].

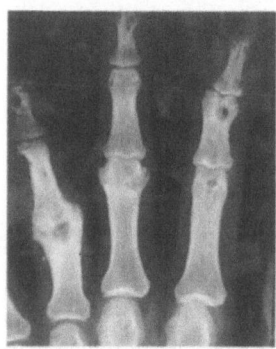 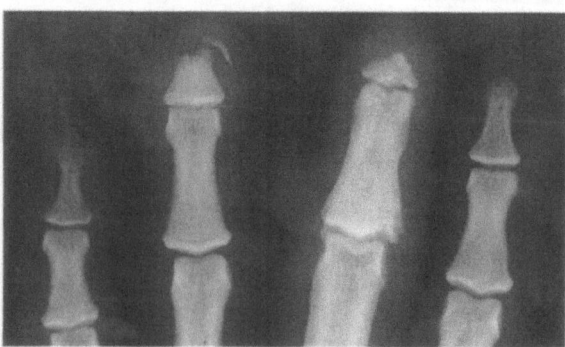

a   b

Fig. 14.12a, b. Leprosy. Specific changes (a) showing cyst-like lesions, prominent nutrient foramina and destruction with deformity of the distal ends of the proximal phalanges. Non-specific acro-osteolysis (b) which may be seen in any neuropathic condition

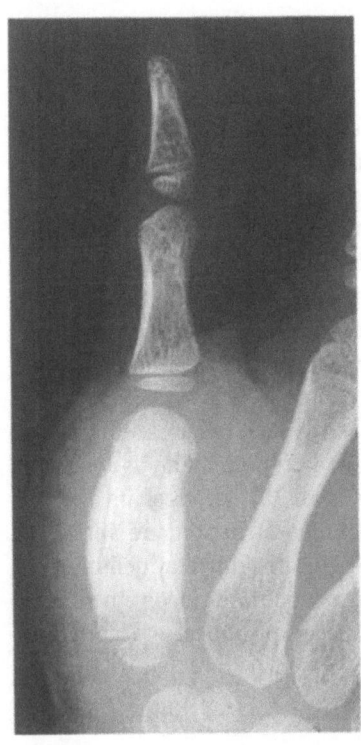

Fig. 14.13. Congenital syphilis affecting the first metacarpal. There is soft tissue swelling and periosteal new bone formation. Similar appearances may be seen with other infections and tumours such as osteoid osteoma

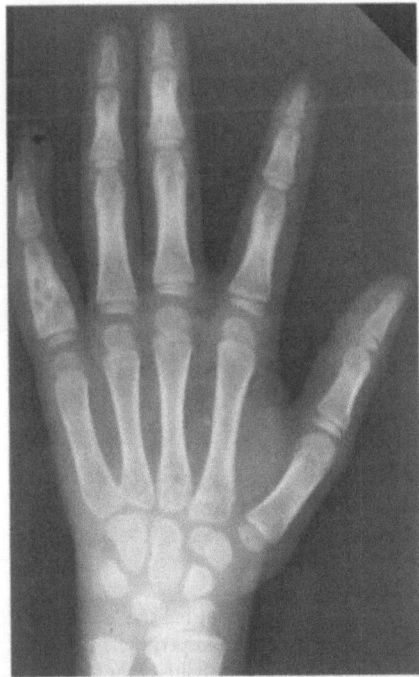

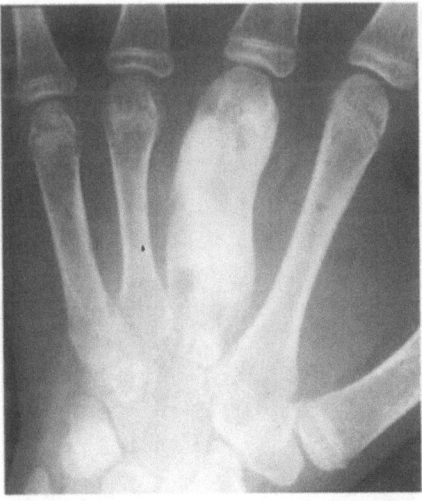

b

Fig. 14.14a, b. Yaws. Secondary yaws showing a dactylitis of the little finger with lysis and expansion of the proximal phalanx (**a**). Tertiary yaws showing expansion and sclerosis of the third metacarpal with several destructive foci (**b**)

a

14.5   Fungal Infections

Fungal infections of the hand may be classified as cutaneous, subcutaneous and deep. Cutaneous fungal infections are relatively common and treated by dermatologists with no requirement for imaging. Subcutaneous or deep fungal infections are rare but should be considered in patients with immunodeficiency, malignancies, chronic renal failure and organ transplantation recipients. Fungal infections that may involve the hand and wrist include blastomycosis [38], actinomycosis [39], coccidiomycosis [40], histoplasmosis [36] and sporotrichosis [41]. The radiographic changes in these infections are frequently non-specific with varying degrees of bone destruction and periosteal new bone formation. A localized fungal osteomyelitis may be mistaken for a sarcoma [42].

Mycetoma is a disease complex that can be caused by both bacteria and fungi. It is a chronic inflammatory cutaneous and subcutaneous granulomatous condition with multiple abscess, fistulae and sinuses. Less than 10% of cases involve the hand. Gross soft tissue swelling is typical, with bone destruction and periosteal new bone formation a late feature (Fig. 14.15) [36]. MR imaging may demonstrate the bone lesions of fungal infections and the extent of soft tissue involvement [43]. The findings are non-specific and the diagnosis is based on clinical and laboratory findings.

14.6   Parasitic Infections

Parasitic infections of the hand and wrist are rare. Occasionally the calcified remnants of dead worms may be identified on radiographs of the hand and upper extremity. These include; cysticercosis, guinea worm and *Loa loa* [12].

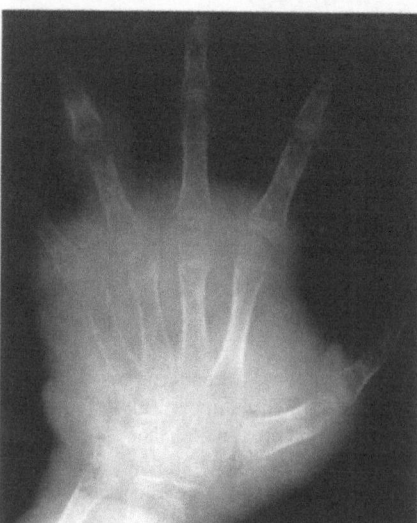

Fig. 14.15. Mycetoma causing soft tissue swelling, demineralization and periosteal new bone formation. There is a dactylitis of the ring finger

14.7 Sarcoidosis

Although the aetiology of sarcoidosis remains unknown many consider that an infective cause is the most likely. Many agents have been considered but none has been substantiated. Virtually all organs and tissues of the body can be involved with non-caseating epitheloid granulomas. Skeletal involvement is encountered in approximately 5% of all cases, with the tubular bones of the hand the commonest site. The middle and distal phalanges are typically involved, with intramedullary lysis variously described as honeycomb or latticework in appearance, and acro-osteolysis (Fig. 14.16). Two less common patterns are localized cyst-like vacuoles and extensive mutilation and destruction of the bone ends. An extremely rare sclerotic form of sarcoid affecting the distal phalanges has also been described [44]. Eccentric soft tissue swelling and soft tissue calcification are also recognized manifestations of sarcoidosis. In any case with suspected bony sarcoid it is advisable to obtain a chest radiograph, although radiographic evidence of pulmonary disease will be absent in 10–20% of cases.

14.8 Paget's Disease

The cause of Paget's disease is unknown although there is circumstantial evidence suggesting a viral aetiology. Hand involvement is uncommon but there is usually little difficulty in correctly identifying the condition as the appearances are identical to that regularly seen in the long bones. Most cases are identified in the sclerotic form. The disease process tends to start proximally within one of the tubular bones and extend distally (Fig. 14.17). Sarcomatous change in Paget's disease of the hand has been described [45].

a

b

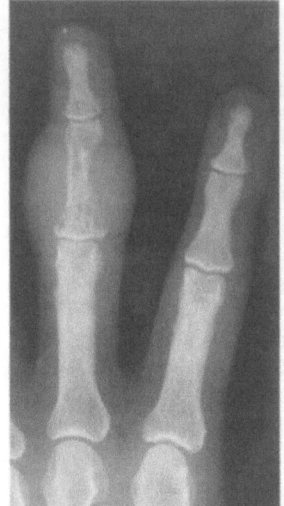 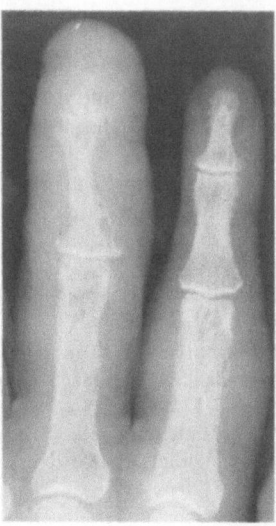

Fig. 14.16a, b. Sarcoidosis. At presentation (a) showing eccentric soft tissue swelling with a honeycomb appearance of the underlying middle phalanx of the middle finger. Fourteen years later (b) showing soft tissue swelling of the index and middle fingers and progression of the disease with terminal phalangeal resorption and further destruction of the middle phalanx of the middle finger. There is now a honeycomb appearance to the proximal phalanges of both digits

a
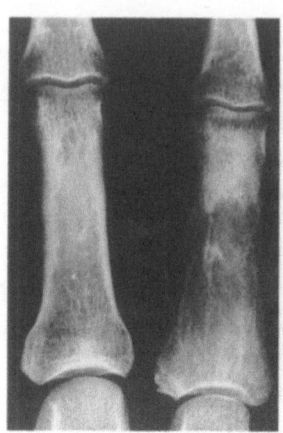
b
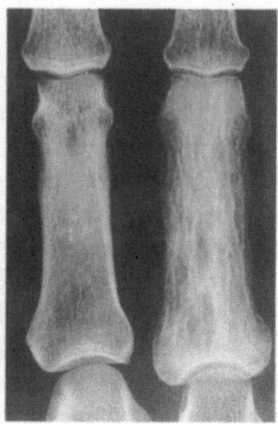

Fig. 14.17a, b. Paget's disease of the proximal phalanx of the ring finger showing the lytic phase (**a**) and sclerotic phase 13 years later (**b**)

14.9   Conclusion

The treatment of infections of the hand evolves as management becomes more sophisticated. The pattern of infection is changing with the increase in worldwide travel and the prolonged survival of immunocompromised patients. Provided the diagnosis is made promptly, imaging is unnecessary in the majority of cases. An early authority on hand infections, the Chicago surgeon Allen Kanavel, summed up the function of clinical management stating; "In almost all cases of serious infection the difficulty is to make a correct diagnosis both as to the nature of the infection and the position of the pus" [46]. The role of imaging is as an adjunct to clinical examination by aiding the process of diagnosis and assessment of the extent of the infection.

References

1. Kono M, Stern PJ (1998) The history of hand infections. Hand Clin 14:511–518
2. Lister G (1993) Inflammation. In: The hand: diagnosis and indications, 3rd edn. Churchill Livingstone, Edinburgh, pp 323–351
3. Jebson PJL (1998) Infections of the fingertip. Hand Clin 14:547–555
4. Beltran J (1995) MR imaging of soft tissue infection. MRI Clin North Am 3:743–751
5. Faciszewski T, Coleman DA (1998) Human bite infections of the hand. Hand Clin 14:683–690
6. Newman JH (1976) Review of septic arthritis throughout the antibiotic era. Ann Rheum Dis 35:198–201
7. Snyder CC (1998) Animal bite infections of the hand. Hand Clin 14:691–711
8. Tehranzadeh J, Wang F, Mesgarzadeh M (1992) Magnetic resonance imaging of osteomyelitis. Crit Rev Diagn Imaging 33:495–534
9. Graif M, Schweitzer ME, Deely D, Matteucci T (1999) The septic versus nonseptic inflamed joint: MRI characteristics. Skeletal Radiol 28:616–620

10. Beltran J, Noto AM, McGhee RB, et al (1987) Infections of the musculoskeletal system: high-field strength MR imaging. Radiology 164:449–454
11. Tang JHS, Gold RH, Bassett LW, Seeger LL (1988) Musculoskeletal infection of the extremities: evaluation with MR imaging. Radiology 166:205–209
12. Poznanski AK (1984) The hand in radiologic diagnosis, 2nd edn. Saunders, Philadelphia, pp 607–636
13. Louis DS, Jebson PJL (1998) Mimickers of hand infections. Hand Clin 14:519–529
14. Murray PM (1998) Septic arthritis of the hand and wrist. Hand Clin 14:579–587
15. Barbieri RA, Freeland AE (1998) Osteomyelitis of the hand. Hand Clin 14:589–603
16. Bennett OM (1992) *Salmonella* osteomyelitis and the hand-foot syndrome in sickle cell disease. J Pediatr Orthop 12:534–539
17. Gold RH, Hawkins RA, Katz RD (1991) Bacterial osteomyelitis: findings on plain radiographs, CT, MR and scintigraphy. AJR 157:365–368
18. Reilly KE, Linz JC, Stern PJ, et al (1997) Osteomyelitis of the tubular bones of the hand. J Hand Surg [Am] 22:644–649
19. Beltran J, McGhee RB, Shaffer PB, et al (1988) Experimental infection of the musculoskeletal system: evaluation with MR imaging and ^{99}Tc-MDP and ^{67}Ga-scintigraphy. Radiology 167:167–172
20. Merkel KD, Brown ML, Dewanjee MK, et al (1985) Comparison of indium-labeled leukocyte imaging with sequential technetium-gallium scanning in the diagnosis of low grade musculoskeletal sepsis. J Bone Joint Surg Am 67:465–476
21. Jaramillo D, Treves ST, Kasser JR (1995) Osteomyelitis and septic arthritis in children: appropriate use of imaging to guide treatment. AJR 165:399–403
22. Gylys-Morin VM (1998) MR imaging of pediatric musculoskeletal inflammatory and infectious disorders. MRI Clin North Am 6:537–559
23. Sammak B, Abd El Bagi M, Al Shahed M, Hamilton D, Al Nabulsi J, Youseff B, Al Thagafi M (1999) Osteomyelitis: a review of currently used imaging techniques. Eur Radiol 9:894–900
24. Dangman BC, Hoffer FA, Rand FF (1992) Osteomyelitis in children: gadolinium-enhanced MR imaging. Radiology 182:743–747
25. Morrison WB, Scweitzer ME, Bock GW, et al (1993) Diagnosis of osteomyelitis: utility of fat-suppressed contrast enhanced MR imaging. Radiology 189:251–257
26. Haddad MC, Sharif HS, Aabed MY, et al (1993) Gadolinium DTPA: value in MR imaging of extraspinal musculoskeletal infections. Eur Radiol 3:527–535
27. Reeder MM (1993) Reeder & Felson's gamuts in radiology, 3rd edn. Springer, Berlin Heidelberg New York, p 245
28. Hodgson AR, Smith TK (1972) Tuberculosis of the wrist. With a note on "chemotherapy". Clin Orthop 83:73–83
29. Riehl J, Schmitt H, Bergmann D, Sieberth HG (1997) Tuberculous tenosynovitis of the hand: evaluation with B-mode ultrasonography. J Ultrasound Med 16:369–372
30. Jaovisidha S, Chen C, Ryu KN, Siriwongpairat P, Pekanan P, Sartoris DJ, Resnick D (1996) Tuberculous tenosynovitis and bursitis: imaging findings in 21 cases. Radiology 201:507–513
31. Faget GH, Mayoral A (1944) Bone changes in leprosy: a clinical and roentgenological study of 505 cases. Radiology 42:1–13
32. Enna CD, Jacobson RB, Rausch RO (1971) Bone changes in leprosy: a correlation of clinical and radiographic features. Radiology 100:295–299
33. Trapnell DH (1965) Calcification of nerves in leprosy. Br J Radiol 38:796–797
34. Gandolfo N, Martinoli C, Bianchi S, Nunzi E, Martolotto M, Giacchino M (1999) Sonographic and MR evaluation of peripheral nerves in leprosy (abstract). Eur Radiol 9(6):C22
35. Cremin BJ, Fisher RM (1970) The lesions of congenital syphilis. Br J Radiol 43:333–341
36. Cockshott WP (1963) Dactylitis and growth disorders. Br J Radiol 36:19–26
37. Jones WP (1972) Doigt en lorgnette and concentric bone atrophy associated with healed yaws osteitis. J Bone Joint Surg Br 54:341–345

38. Gehweiler JA, Capp MP, Chick EW (1970) Observations on the roentgen patterns in blasto-
    mycosis of bone. A review of cases from the Blastomycosis Cooperative Study of the Veter-
    ans Administration and Duke University Medical Center. AJR 108:497–510
39. Mendelsohn BG (1965) Actinomycosis of a metacarpal bone. Report of a case. J Bone Joint
    Surg Br 47:739–742
40. Dalinka MK, Dinnenberg S, Greendyke WH, Hopkins R (1971) Roentgenographic features
    of osseous coccidiomycosis and differential diagnosis. J Bone Joint Surg Am 53:1157–1164
41. Comstock C, Wolson AM (1975) Roentgenology of sporotrichosis. AJR 125:651–655
42. Monsanto EH, Johnston AD, Dick HM (1986) Isolated blastomycotic osteomyelitis: a case
    simulating a malignant tumor of the distal radius. J Bone Joint Surg Am 11:896–898
43. Sharif H, Clark DC, Aabed M, et al (1991) Mycetoma: comparison of MR imaging with CT.
    Radiology 178:865–870
44. Bonakdarpour A, Levy W, Aegerter EE (1971) Osteosclerotic changes in sarcoidosis. AJR
    113:646–649
45. Friedman AC, Orcutt J, Madewell JE (1982) Paget's disease of the hand: radiographic spec-
    trum. AJR 138:691–693
46. Kanavel A (1939) Infections of the hand. Lea and Febiger, Philadelphia, pp 17–410

15 Imaging of Soft Tissue Tumors of the Hand and Wrist

Luc H. L. De Beuckeleer, Arthur M. De Schepper,
Damienne de la Kethulle de Ryhove, Hiroshi Nishimura

15.1 Introduction

Although numerous different soft tissue masses may affect the hand or wrist, their overall prevalence is rather low. A few, however, have a propensity to affect that region more frequently. Most common benign tumors of the hand and wrist are giant cell tumors of the tendon sheath, fibrolipohamartoma, angioma and glomus tumor [12]. Pseudotumoral lesions which are more frequently found at the hand or wrist are ganglion, Dupuytren's contracture, epidermoid cyst and de Quervain tenosynovitis. No malignant lesion has a particularly high prevalence at the hand or wrist [23, 48, 51]. The epidemiologic and imaging characteristics of these tumors and pseudotumors will be discussed extensively.

The most common soft tissue mass of the hand and wrist is the ganglion cyst. Since the findings on ultrasonography are mostly pathognomonic, MR imaging is seldom performed in this particular case. Benign tumors and pseudotumoral lesions outnumber malignant ones. In our series of 1,350 soft tissue tumors examined by MR imaging, 9.9% of the lesions of the hand and wrist were malignant and 61.9% benign [21]. In another series, consisting of pathology files of 28,833 soft tissue tumors, 12.3% of tumors of the hand and wrist were malignant and 76.5% benign [48]. Pseudotumoral lesions in the two series constituted 28.2% and 11.2% respectively.

Any soft tissue mass must be evaluated firstly with radiography. Most often, a nonspecific density is seen. Intralesional calcifications, scalloping or even destruction of adjacent bones may be detected (Fig. 15.1). Sometimes, an underlying bony abnormality such as an osteochondroma or hypertrophic callus, responsible for a palpable mass, may be seen [23, 48, 51].

The role of ultrasonography is limited, since most lesions are hypoechoic and do not have characteristic features. However, in the case of a ganglion, ultrasound is mostly effective in detection and characterization. In the postoperative follow-up, ultrasonography may enable recurrent masses to be detected accurately [7].

MR imaging has generally been acknowledged as the method of choice for local staging of soft tissue masses. Many soft tissue masses have a set of characteristic features on T1- or T2-weighted images (Table 15.1), a characteristic shape or enhancement pattern and are often found in a typical location or age group [22, 23]. Therefore, some lesions such as lipoma, giant cell tumor of the tendon sheath, ganglion and Dupuytren's contracture may be identified correctly [12]. However, the ability of MR imaging in grading soft tissue masses remains controversial [6, 16, 22, 56, 81]. Some authors have proposed that MR imaging

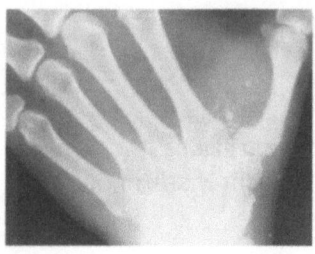

a

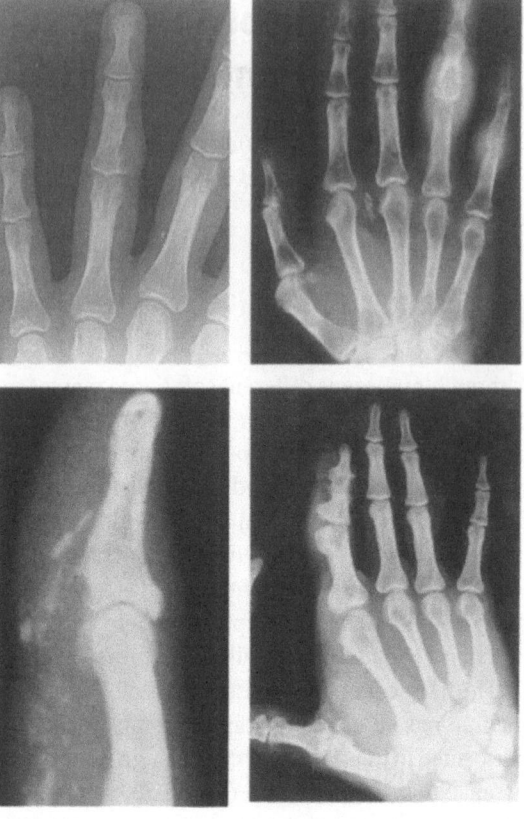

b,c

d,e

Fig. 15.1. a Soft tissue hemangioma at the thenar of the left hand. A mass with increased density is seen at the thenar. Well-circumscribed, rounded calcifications of varying size correspond to intralesional phleboliths. A pressure erosion is seen at the ulnar-sided cortex of the first metacarpal bone. **b** Soft tissue chondroma in the left hand of a 16-year-old girl. Radiography of the left hand shows a pressure erosion at the radial aspect of the middle phalanx of the fourth digit. Note also a soft tissue mass with intermediate density, causing a bulging of the cutaneous structures. **c** Gout in a 65-year-old man. There is a low-density soft tissue mass at the proximal interphalangeal joint of the fourth finger. Note the presence of a well-circumscribed osteolytic lesion in the base of the middle phalanx of the fourth digit, corresponding to an intraosseous tophus. The proximal interphalangeal (PIP) joint is not narrowed and mineralization is maintained. Erosive and osteophytic changes at the PIP joint of the fifth digit, also accompanied by a low-density soft tissue mass, correspond to a tophus. **d** Dystrophic calcifications in the left hand of a 65-year-old woman. Irregular, linear and amorphous calcifications are seen at the flexor compartment of the third finger in a patient with panniculitis calcificans (by permission of Prof. Dr. K. Verstraete, University of Ghent, Belgium). **e** Macrodystrophia lipomatosa in a 25-year-old man. Anteroposterior view of the right hand shows marked overgrowth of the distal end of the second metacarpal bone and of the phalangeal bones, and symphalangism of the middle and distal phalangeal bone of the index finger. There is a global increase in the soft tissues of the second finger (by permission of Dr. F. Vanhoenacker, University Hospital Antwerp, Belgium)

can reliably differentiate between benign and malignant tumors in the majority of soft tissue tumors located in the hand or wrist [8, 68]. This may be due to the high prevalence of benign lesions in this region, which furthermore often have distinctive MR features. In contradistinction with benign lesions, malignant masses generally more often affect older patients, are larger and more heterogeneous, are often situated deeper, have irregular boundaries, enhance heterogeneously and show intratumoral necrosis. Sometimes, extension to adjacent bones or a neurovascular bundle may be present (Fig. 15.2). Therefore, any mass

Table 15.1. Signal intensities on T1- and T2- weighted MR images

---

High signal intensity on T1-weighted image + intermediate signal intensity on T2-weighted image
Lipoma
Liposarcoma
Lipoblastoma
Hibernoma
Elastofibroma
Fibrolipohamartoma
Metastasis of melanoma (melanin)
Clear cell sarcoma (melanin)

High signal intensity on T1-weighted image + high signal intensity on T2-weighted image
Hemangioma
Lymphangioma
Subacute hematoma
Small arteriovenous malformation

Low signal intensity on T1-weighted image + high signal intensity on T2- weighted image
Cyst
Myxoma
Myxoid liposarcoma
Sarcoma

Low to intermediate signal intensity on T1-weighted image + low signal intensity on T2-weighted image
Desmoid and other fibromatoses
Pigmented villonodular synovitis
Morton's neuroma
Fibrolipohamartoma
Giant cell tumor of tendon sheath
Acute hematoma (few days)
Old hematoma
Xanthoma
High-flow arteriovenous malformation
Mineralized mass
Scar tissue
Amyloidosis
Granuloma annulare
High-grade malignancies

Intermediate signal intensity on T1-weighted image + high signal intensity on T2-weighted image
Neurogenic tumor
Desmoid

---

fitting the above-mentioned criteria should be viewed with major concern. However, since the compartments of the hand, fingers and wrist are small, many of the lesions will be of limited size at the time of detection by the patient or by the referring physician. For this reason, a small high-grade malignancy may present with regular borders, may enhance homogeneously lacking intratumoral necrosis, and may be limited to one compartment, thereby demonstrating a "benign-looking" appearance on MR images (Fig. 15.3). Thus, any lesion that cannot reliably be characterized should be evaluated by further diagnostic investigation.

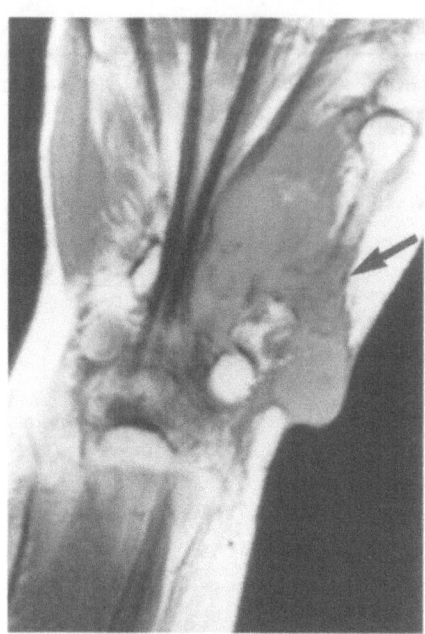

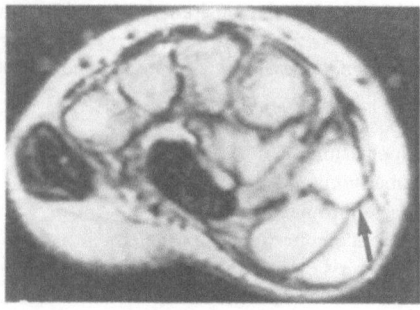

a

b

Fig. 15.2a, b. Synovial sarcoma in a 47-year-old woman. Coronal T1-weighted image (a) shows a huge inhomogeneous mass, slightly hyperintense to muscle. A well-circumscribed area of intermediate signal intensity at the base of the fifth metacarpal bone corresponds to involvement of the adjacent bone (*arrow*). On the axial T2-weighted image (b), the lesion is more inhomogeneous. Intralesional areas with high signal intensity correspond to cystic components (*arrow*)

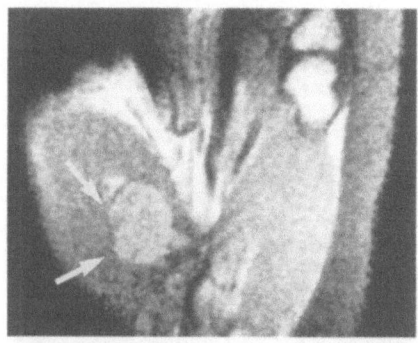

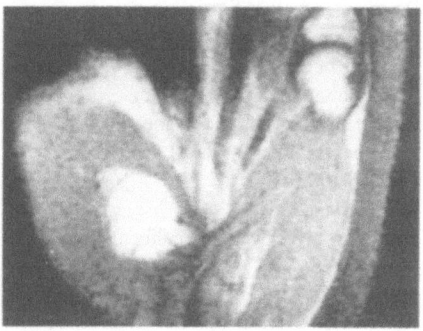

a

c

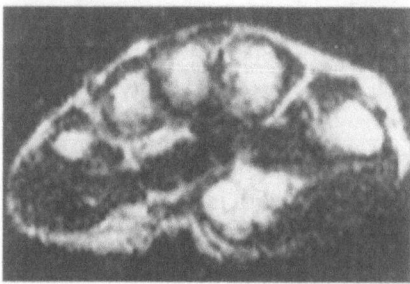

b

Fig. 15.3a–c. Clear cell sarcoma in the hand of a 25-year-old woman. Coronal T1-weighted image of a nodular mass at the thenar (*arrows*) (a). The lesion is hyperintense compared with the adjacent muscles. On the axial T2-weighted image, a hyperintense mass with intralesional septa is seen (b). On the coronal gadolinium-enhanced T1-weighted image, the lesion shows homogeneous, strong enhancement (c)

Since, as mentioned already, many masses are of limited size, it is possible to use a small field of view and a large matrix, resulting in a high spatial resolution [90]. Furthermore, the development of dedicated small loop coils with an inner diameter of less than 4 cm ensures a considerable increase in image quality and allows the detection of even detailed anatomic structures, thereby enabling better delineation of the lesion from adjacent tissues (Fig. 15.4).

15.2 Benign Tumoral Lesions

15.2.1 Giant Cell Tumor of the Tendon Sheath

Giant cell tumor of the tendon sheath (GCTTS), also called localized nodular tenosynovitis, is the second most common mass of the hand after the ganglion [7, 30, 42, 53, 55]. It shares histopathologic features with pigmented villonodular syn-

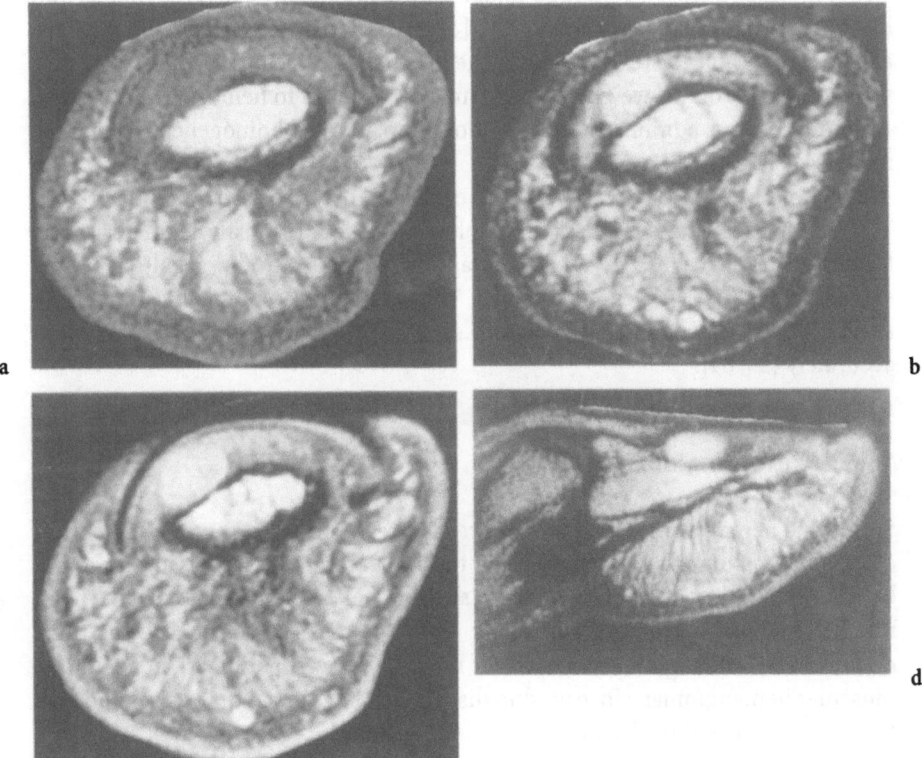

a
b
c
d

Fig. 15.4a–d. Glomus tumor of the left thumb in a 52-year-old patient, suffering from pain elicited by pressure or changes of temperature. Axial T1-weighted image of the distal part of the thumb demonstrates a subungual tumor with intermediate signal intensity and unsharp delineation from adjacent structures (a). T2-weighted image at the same level shows a well-delineated homogeneous mass with high signal intensity (b). After intravenous administration of gadolinium contrast, strong, homogeneous enhancement is seen (c, d). The subungual location is well demonstrated on both axial (c) and sagittal slices (d). (By permission of Dr. P. Flandroy and Dr. M. Baghaie, Centre Hospitalier Universitaire de Liège, Belgium)

ovitis [39]. It is found mostly in adults, with a peak incidence between 30 and 50 years of age[19, 42]. The lesion is more commonly situated at the palmar than at the dorsal side of the first three fingers [42].

Clinically, most patients present with an asymptomatic slowly enlarging mass that is attached to deeper structures, i.e., the tendon sheath or the joint capsule [19, 42]. The lesion may become painful when adjacent soft tissue structures are compressed or on movement [30, 39, 68]. Therapy consists of resection. Local recurrences are seen in 7–27% of cases [7, 39].

On radiography, a pressure erosion or periosteal reaction may be present, thereby resembling a periosteal chondroma [40]. Rarely, intraosseous extension may be detected [82].

On MR imaging, a well-delineated mass is seen. Often, the mass envelops – at least partially – the tendon sheath of the flexor digitorum tendon. On T1-weighted images the lesion is homogeneous and has intermediate signal intensity (Fig. 15.5a). On T2-weighted images the lesion is more heterogeneous and has predominantly low signal intensity [19, 39, 53, 68, 84] (Fig. 15.5b). Intralesional hemorrhage may be responsible for the internal derangements. The areas of low signal intensity on T2-weighted image may correspond to hemosiderin deposits. After intravenous administration of gadolinium, marked homogeneous enhancement is seen [19, 53] (Fig. 15.5c).

Desmoid tumors may present with the same signal intensities on both T1- and T2-weighted sequences [19, 22, 53]. Histologically, they are mostly characterized as lesions with low cellularity and abundant collagenous stroma, resulting in low signal intensity on T2-weighted images. The extent and anatomic location of the two lesions differs significantly, thereby enabling them to be differentiated more accurately [53, 84].

15.2.2 Hemangioma

Soft tissue hemangiomas have a high prevalence, representing approximately 7% of all benign tumors. Hemangioma is the most common soft tissue tumor in babies and children [2, 3, 29]. There is a slight female predominance. Unlike juvenile hemangiomas, most intramuscular hemangiomas are detected in the third decade. Most hemangiomas referred for radiologic investigation are in fact intramuscular hemangiomas, since no skin discoloration occurs in these cases and, due to the mass effect of the lesion, clinical findings may be confusing [54].

Hemangiomas contain a variable amount of nonvascular elements, such as lipomatous tissue, connective tissue, thrombus, hemosiderin and fibrous tissue [60, 68]. Hemangiomas are classified, depending on the predominant vessel type, as capillary, cavernous, arteriovenous or venous.

MR imaging is the modality of choice for evaluating these lesions. On T1-weighted images, a poorly delineated mass with intermediate signal intensity is seen. Intralesional linear or curvilinear areas of high signal intensity correspond to intralesional fat [54, 60, 68, 70] (Figs. 15.6a, 15.7a). On T2-weighted images, a

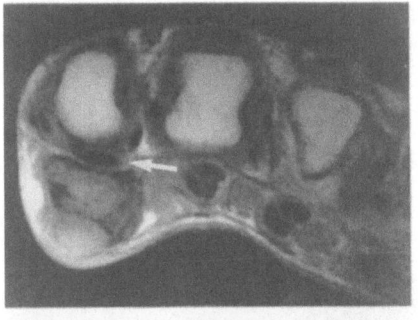

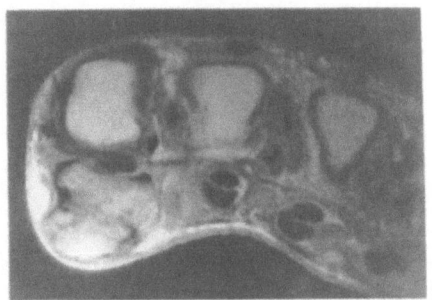

a

c

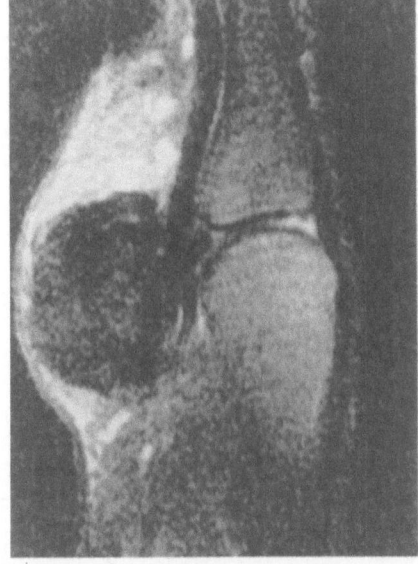

b

Fig. 15.5a–c. Giant cell tumor of the tendon sheath in the left hand of a 63-year-old woman. Axial T1-weighted image of a mass at the superficial flexor tendon of the fifth finger demonstrates a homogeneous lesion with intermediate signal intensity (**a**). Note that the deep flexor tendon is not involved (*arrow*). On the sagittal fat-saturated T2-weighted image, the mass is hypointense (**b**). On the axial gadolinium-enhanced T1-weighted image (**c**), the lesion shows strong enhancement

hemangioma presents as a well-delineated, lobulated mass with areas of high signal intensity corresponding to slowly flowing intralesional blood and areas of intermediate signal intensity which represent muscular or fatty components [60, 68, 70] (Figs. 15.6b, 15.7b).

Differentiation from a lipoma may be difficult in some cavernous hemangiomas in which the lipomatous component predominates, showing high signal intensity on T1-weighted images and intermediate signal intensity on T2-weighted images [54].

Except for small lesions (<2 cm), all hemangiomas are more or less heterogeneous on T1- and T2-weighted images. MR imaging may demonstrate intralesional fluid-fluid levels, corresponding to intratumoral hemorrhage [70] (Figs. 15.7b, 15.8). Phleboliths may present as small dots of signal void on MR images. T1-weighted images after intravenous administration of gadolinium show moderate to strong enhancement of the lesion (Fig. 15.6c). The type of enhancement depends on the intratumoral blood flow [22, 54].

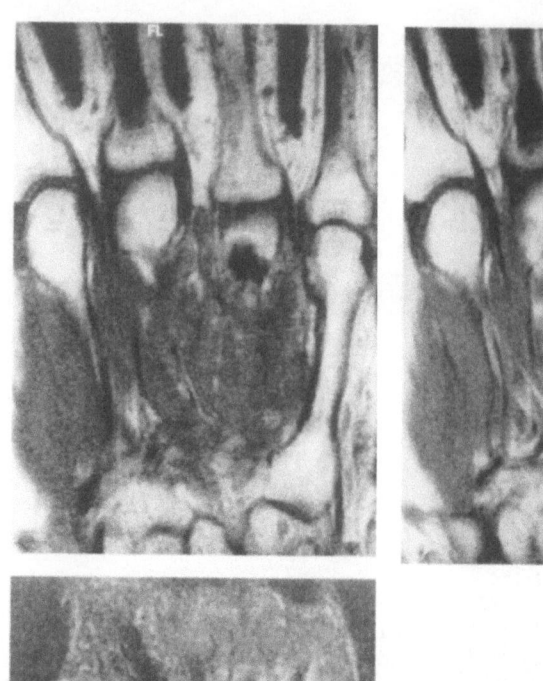

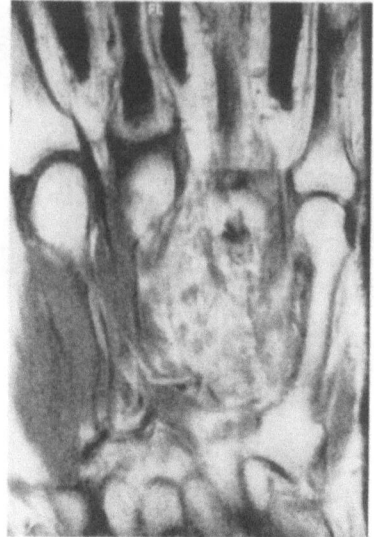

a

c

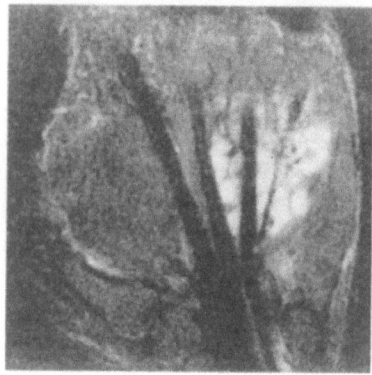

b

Fig. 15.6a–c. Hemangioma in a 46-year-old woman. Coronal T1-weighted image of a capillary hemangioma at the level of the metacarpal bones, predominantly having the same signal intensity as muscle (**a**). On the STIR image, small fatty components of the lesion are demonstrated as low-intensity areas (**b**). After intravenous administration of gadolinium contrast, strong enhancement is seen (**c**)

15.2.3 Lipoma

A lipoma is a benign soft tissue mass composed of mature adipocytes, almost indistinguishable from subcutaneous fat. It is a soft tissue tumor with a high prevalence. However, only 5% of all lipomas of the upper extremity are located within the hand [4]. The preferential location is the thenar or hypothenar eminence or the median part of the palmar aspect of the hand [68] (Fig. 15.9). Most frequently, lipoma affects patients in the fifth to sixth decade.

Lipomas present with a slowly growing, asymptomatic mass. Pain and paresthesias may occur if the mass is situated in the deep palmar space, thereby eliciting a carpal tunnel syndrome [4].

On radiography, a mass with low to intermediate density may be seen. CT reveals a homogeneous, well-delineated mass with low density (from −60 to −130 HU). After injection of iodinated contrast, no enhancement is seen. Sometimes, thin fibromuscular septa traversing the mass may be detected [58].

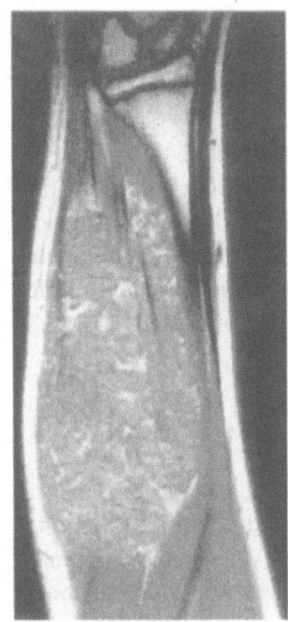

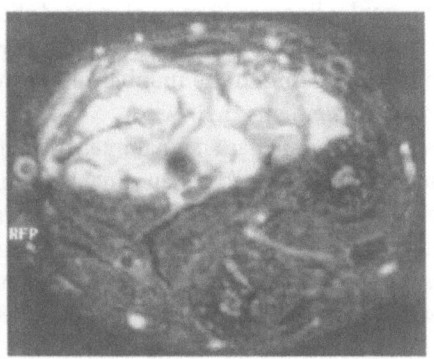

Fig. 15.7a, b. Cavernous hemangioma at the right wrist/forearm of a 16-year-old boy. On coronal T1-weighted image, a voluminous mass with intermediate to high signal intensity is seen; vascular components have equal signal intensity to skeletal muscle whereas adipose constituents have high signal intensity (**a**). On the axial fat-saturated T2-weighted image, the lesion has predominantly high signal intensity. Note the presence of multiple fluid-fluid levels, corresponding to hemorrhagic intralesional areas (**b**)

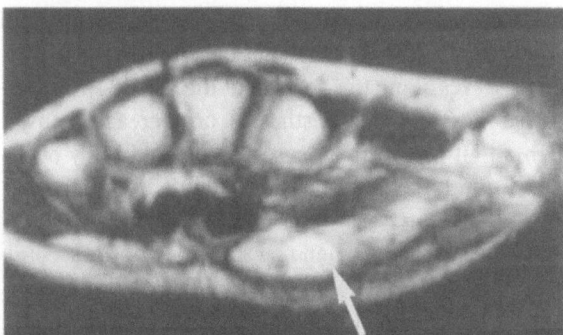

Fig. 15.8. Cavernous hemangioma in a 27-year-old woman. Axial T2-weighted image shows an inhomogeneous mass with multiple fluid-fluid levels (*arrow*), corresponding to hemorrhagic areas. The supernatant corresponds to serous fluid, whereas the dependent low signal intensity component is composed of sedimented blood degradation products

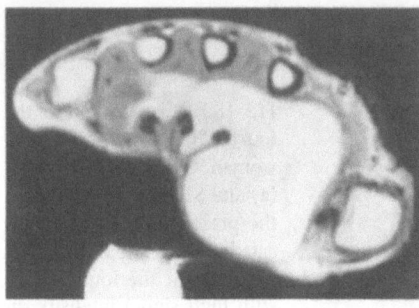

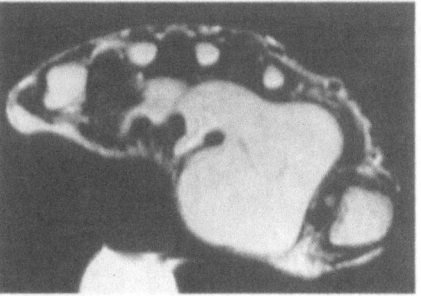

Fig. 15.9a, b. Lipoma. Axial T1-weighted image of the wrist (**a**). A huge lesion at the palmar aspect of the wrist extends between the flexor tendons of the fingers. The lesion has high signal intensity, similar to that of subcutaneous fat. On a T2-weighed image at the same level, a homogeneous mass with the same signal intensity as subcutaneous tissue is seen (**b**)

On ultrasonography, lipomas have an elongated shape and are mostly oriented parallel to the skin. The ultrasonography findings are widely variable (from hypo- to hyperreflective) according to the number of internal interfaces between fatty and connective tissue elements [34].

On MR imaging, a lipoma has a signal intensity comparable to that of normal fat on all sequences and shows no enhancement after intravenous administration of gadolinium contrast [60, 68] (Figs. 15.9, 15.10). Fat-saturated or STIR sequences may contribute to the diagnosis of these lesions (Fig. 15.10b). On gadolinium-enhanced fat-saturated T1-weighted images, thin enhancing intralesional strands corresponding to fibro-connective septa are sometimes demonstrated.

15.2.4   Fibrolipohamartoma

Fibrolipohamartoma has been designated also as lipomatous hamartoma, neural fibrolipoma, intraneural lipoma, fibrofatty overgrowth and fatty infiltration of a nerve. It is an extremely rare tumor, affecting children and young adults. The mass is composed of different elements such as fatty and fibrous tissue which surround the nerve and infiltrate the epineurium and perineurium [49, 58, 60].

Mostly, patients present with a slowly growing soft tissue mass at the palmar aspect of the hand, wrist or forearm. Usually, the lesion is located along the median nerve, although occasional involvement of other nerves has been reported such as the radial and ulnar nerves or the nerves along the dorsum of the foot [24]. Neural fibrolipohamartoma usually gives rise to pain, paresthesias, or decreased sensation or muscle strength [49]. In about one third of cases, associated bony overgrowth and macrodactyly, a condition known as macrodystrophia lipomatosa, is seen [28, 75].

On radiography, the tumor may be suspected when macrodactyly of the second or third digit is seen in a symptomatic patient [49, 58]. CT and MR imaging enable identification of the neural origin of the lesion, by demonstrating multiple tortu-

a   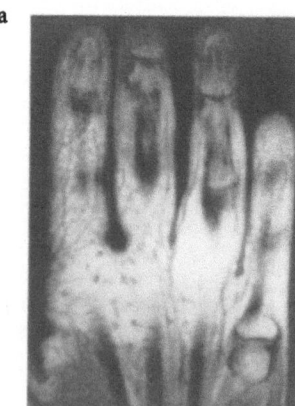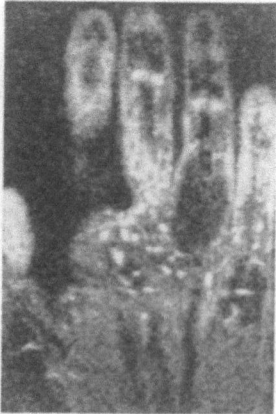   b

Fig. 15.10a, b. Lipoma of the fourth digit in a 64-year-old woman. Coronal T1-weighted (a) and STIR (b) images show the presence of a well-delineated mass at the flexor compartment of the fourth digit, with high signal intensity on T1-weighted and low signal intensity on STIR images, proving the lipomatous nature of the lesion

ous tubular structures representing thickened nerve bundles and fibrous strands within a predominantly lipomatous mass [58, 60]. These structures show low signal intensity on both T1- and T2-weighted images according to their fibrous content [13, 24, 57, 88] (Fig. 15.11).

15.2.5   Glomus Tumor

A glomus tumor is a hamartoma arising from the neuromyoarterial apparatus. This lesion accounts for 1.2% of the tumors of the hand. Theoretically, these tumors may be found in any location of the body, but up to 75% are found in the hand and up to 65% of these in the subungual region. Multiple lesions are seen in approximately 2.3% of cases [17]. Other regions that may be involved are the wrist, the forearm and the foot [54]. Glomus tumor affects patients between 20 and 40 years of age and there is a female predominance [54].

Clinical signs are the presence of a reddish-blue nodule which is electively painful, exacerbating on pressure or with changes of temperature [17, 54, 59, 70].

On radiography, a small mass may be seen at the dorsal aspect of the finger, associated with a small erosion of the adjacent bone in 14–60% of cases [17]. On ultrasonography, a solid homogeneous, hyporeflective mass is noted at the subungual region [7, 17]. Experienced operators are able to detect lesions as small as 3 mm in diameter. Doppler ultrasonography may be able to demonstrate high-flow intratumoral shunts [7]. In the past, arteriographic study of the painful digit was

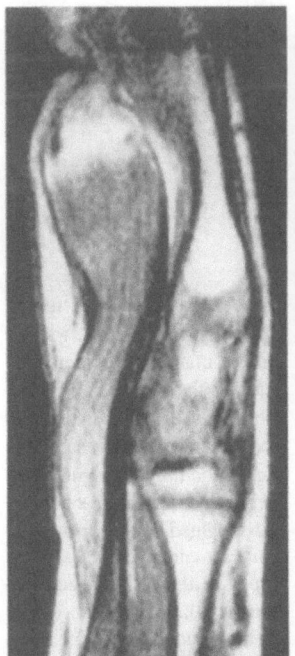
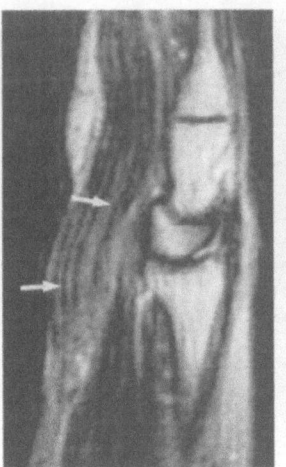
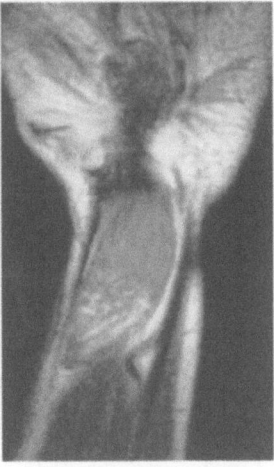

b,c

Fig. 15.11a–c. Fibrolipohamartoma at the median nerve in a 6-year-old boy. Sagittal T1-weighted image (a). T2-weighted image at the same level (b). Coronal T1-weighted image (c). A mass with predominantly fatty content is present. Intervening nerve fibers (*arrows*) are seen as tortuous tubular structures with intermediate signal intensity on different sequences

a

the first choice examination, showing an entangled arteriovenous anastomosis in large tumors. Smaller tumors were sometimes missed [17]. Nowadays, this technique may be substituted by MR angiography (Fig. 15.12).

In the past, there have been many attempts to demonstrate these small fingertip lesions. Most MR studies published in the early 1990s were able to demonstrate a high signal intensity lesion on T2-weighted images [15, 27, 59]. However, spatial resolution was low. Nowadays, high-resolution MR imaging allows the detection of lesions 2 mm diameter. On T1-weighted images, the normal glomus body has low signal intensity. On T2-weighted images, very high signal intensity is seen. After intravenous injection of gadolinium contrast, strong enhancement is seen. Glomus tumors present with intermediate signal intensity on T1- and very high signal intensity on T2-weighted images (Fig. 15.4a, b). After intravenous administration of gadolinium, moderate to strong enhancement is seen, depending on the subtype of the tumor (solid and myxoid versus vascular respectively) [27] (Fig. 15.4c, d). Often, the lesion is delineated by a small hypointense capsule on both T1- and T2-weighted images. On gadolinium-enhanced T1-weighted images, rupture of the capsule may be detected.

The differential diagnosis includes ganglion and hemangioma. A ganglion can be differentiated from a glomus tumor on gadolinium-enhanced T1-weighted im-

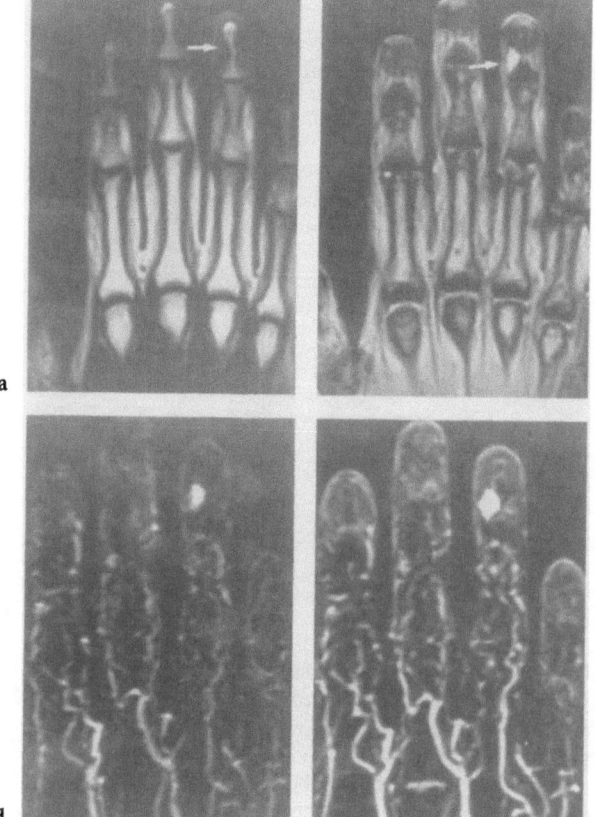

a

b

c,d

Fig. 15.12a–d. Glomus tumor. T1-weighted (a) and T2-weighted (b) images of a glomus tumor of the soft tissues neighboring the distal phalanx of the fourth finger, with low signal intensity on the T1-weighted and very high signal intensity on T2-weighted image (*arrow*). On contrast-enhanced MR angiography in the early (c) and late phases (d), strong enhancement of the tumoral mass, consisting of telangiectatic "lakes", is seen

ages, since only its periphery enhances. Hemangiomas share the signal intensity characteristics of a glomus tumor, but are most often flatter, more superficially located, and are not painful.

15.2.6 Neurogenic Tumors

Most frequent subtypes of neurogenic tumors encountered in the hand or wrist are neurinomas (schwannomas) and neurofibromas. Neurinomas predominantly affect patients between 20 and 50 years of age. Neurofibromas constitute about 5% of all soft tissue tumors [43]. Most are solitary and affect patients in their third decade. The majority of lesions (60–90%) are not associated with neurofibromatosis type I [67].

On clinical examination, a subcutaneous painless mass is detected. Upon pressure, pain may be elicited. Mostly, a neurogenic tumor is a firm but compressible mass that can be moved freely underneath the skin.

On MR imaging, these tumors have intermediate signal intensity on T1-weighted images and are often almost indistinguishable from adjacent muscle [60, 67]. On proton-density weighted images, the mass is hyperintense compared with muscle. On T2-weighted sequences, the lesion has very high signal intensity (Fig. 15.13a, b). The detection of a capsule, visualized as a low-intensity rim, has been proposed as a useful parameter in differentiating neurinomas from neurofibromas, the former having a capsule, the latter lacking one [52, 67]. It has also been suggested that the relationship between the nerve and the tumor is a useful differ-

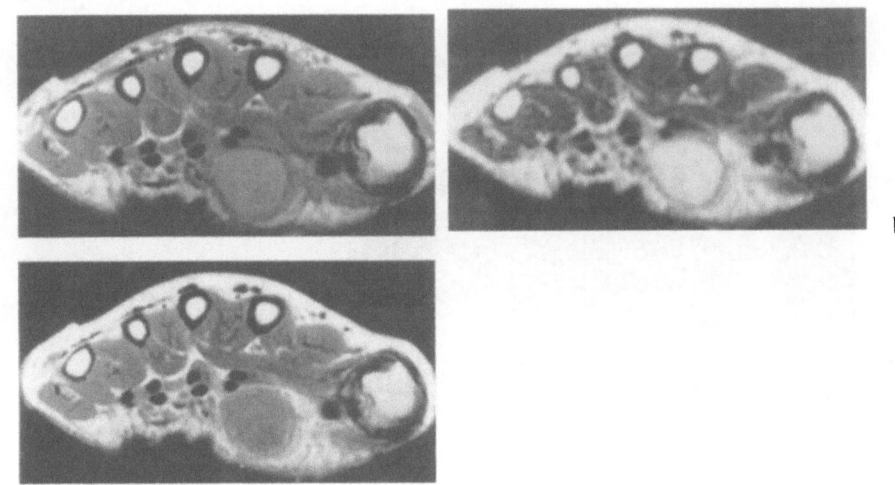

a

b

c

Fig. 15.13a–c. Benign neurogenic tumor at the median nerve in a 73-year-old man. Axial T1-weighted (**a**) and T2-weighted (**b**) images and T1-weighted image after gadolinium contrast injection (**c**), demonstrate a mass with slightly increased signal intensity on T1- (**a**) and high signal intensity on T2-weighted (**b**) images. A hypointense rim is seen at the periphery of the lesion on T2-weighted images. After intravenous gadolinium administration, moderate peripheral enhancement is seen

ential diagnostic tool. A majority of schwannomas were considered to be located along a side of the nerve, whereas the parent nerve was either trapped within the tumor or was obliterated and no longer discernible in the case of a neurofibroma (Fig. 15.14). In our opinion, these parameters have no additional value in differentiating these two masses, since detection of these features, even on images in a longitudinal plane, remains difficult.

Approximately two third of the lesion enhance heterogeneously on gadolinium-enhanced T1-weighted images, whereas the other third shows homogeneous enhancement [67] (Fig. 15.13c).

A so-called target sign has been reported to be characteristic of neurofibroma. On T2-weighted images, the target appearance is reflected by a peripheral area of high signal intensity and a central area of low signal intensity. Histopathologically, the peripheral zone is constituted by a hypocellular area with hydrated, loose connective tissue, whereas the central part consists of dense, collagenous and fibrotic tissue [52, 67]. In our experience, sensitivity of this parameter for differentiating neurofibroma from neurinoma is low but specificity indeed high.

15.2.7 Soft Tissue Chondroma

Soft tissue chondroma, also called extraskeletal chondroma or chondroma of soft parts, is a well-defined nodule of cartilage, originating in the soft tissues. It is a rare soft tissue tumor, accounting for only 6% of all tumors of the hand and wrist [51]. However, the hand and wrist is the most frequent localization since approximately

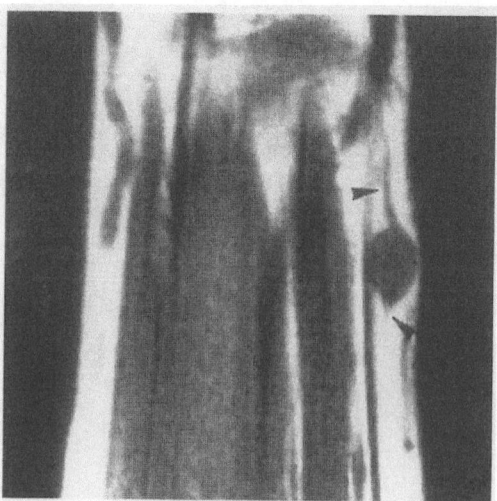

Fig. 15.14. Schwannoma of the radial aspect of the wrist. On the coronal T1-weighted image, a round soft tissue mass with low to intermediate signal intensity is seen within the subcutaneous fat. Note the continuity of the mass with a linear structure (*arrowheads*) that was interpreted as the radial nerve. (Reprinted with permission of Dr. A. Capelastegui, Osatek, Hospital de Galdacano, Basque Country, Spain [12])

55% of all soft tissue chondromas are located there [25, 46, 47]. It affects patients from 1 to 85 years of age, presenting with a slowly growing soft tissue mass. Most lesions are attached to a tendon, tendon sheath, joint capsule or periosteum.

On radiography, a well-defined soft tissue mass may be detected. Intralesional calcifications are present in 33–70% of the lesions. Extrinsic pressure erosions on adjacent bone may be seen (Fig. 15.1b). On MR imaging, soft tissue chondroma has intermediate signal intensity on T1- and high signal intensity on T2-weighted images (Fig. 15.15). Intratumoral areas of low signal intensity correspond to intralesional calcifications [51].

15.2.8 Pigmented Villonodular Synovitis

Pigmented villonodular synovitis is a benign proliferation of synovial origin. Mostly, it is located in large joints or bursae. Involvement of the wrist occurs in

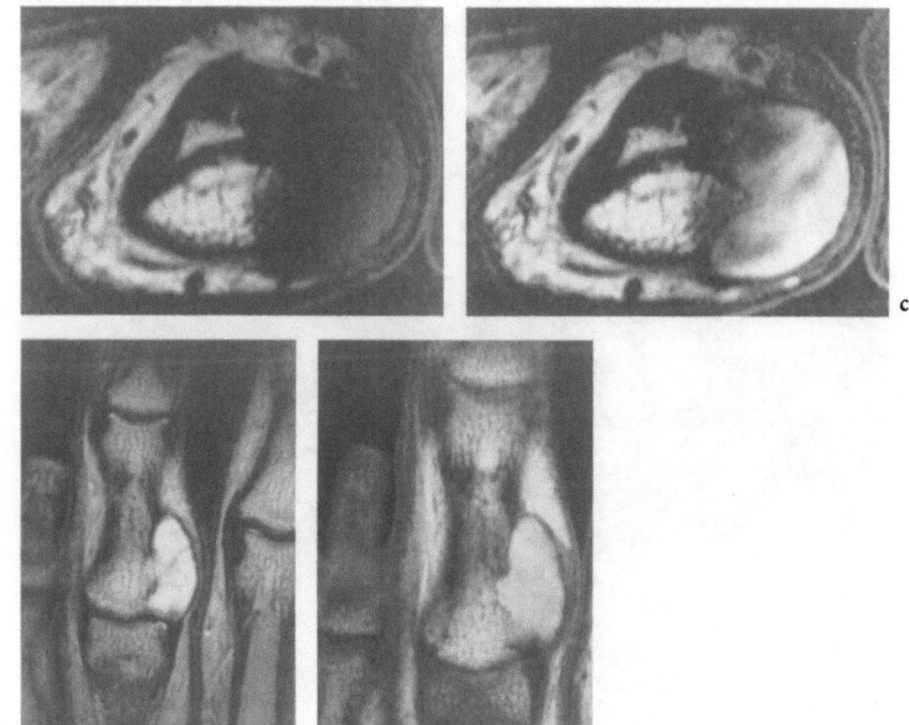

Fig. 15.15a–d. Soft tissue chondroma in the left hand of a 16-year-old girl (same patient as Fig. 15.1b). On the axial fat-saturated T1-weighted image, a homogeneous mass with intermediate signal intensity is seen (a). On the coronal fat-saturated T2-weighted image, a well-delineated mass with high signal intensity is seen. Note the presence of some intralesional low signal intensity septa and a pressure erosion at the radial aspect of the base of the middle phalanx of the fourth digit (b). On the axial fat-saturated (c) and coronal non-fat-saturated (d) T1-weighted images after intravenous administration of gadolinium contrast, strong enhancement is seen

only 2% of lesions [83]. Histopathologically, the lesion consists of dense connective and fibrous tissue, giant cells, lipid-laden foam cells, and hemosiderin secondary to repeated intralesional bleeding. Most frequently, it affects adults between 30 and 40 years of age. Men are affected slightly more often than women. The clinical picture consists of an insidious onset of monoarticular swelling, accompanied by pain [84].

On radiography or CT, pressure erosion on adjacent bones, narrowing of the joint space and subchondral cyst formation may be present [40] (Fig. 15.16). Ultrasonography may reveal a nonspecific, heterogeneous, articular mass. On MR imaging, the lesion has characteristic features. It presents as a hypertrophic, heterogeneous synovial process with areas of low signal intensity on all sequences, most obvious on T2-weighted images (Figs. 15.16, 15.17). These areas correspond to intratumoral deposits of hemosiderin, secondary to repeated hemorrhage [3, 45, 53, 60, 84]. Hemosiderin deposits cause local changes in susceptibility and are therefore best appreciated on gradient echo images. On gadolinium-enhanced T1-weighted images, strong enhancement is noted [53] (Fig. 15.17c).

Differential diagnosis on MR imaging includes other causes of hemorrhagic synovitis such as chronic trauma, hemophilia and rheumatoid arthritis. However, these entities may be easily distinguished, since clinical history and laboratory findings are substantially different.

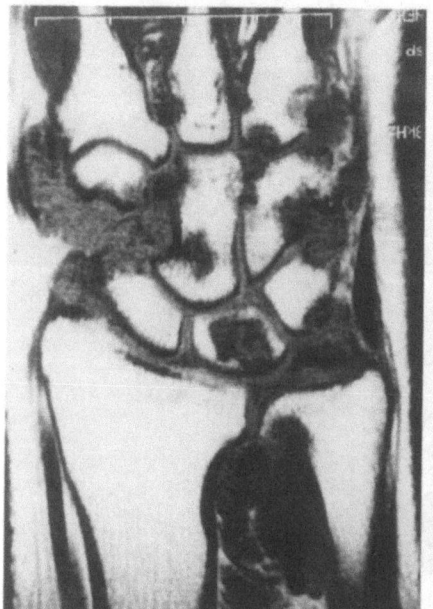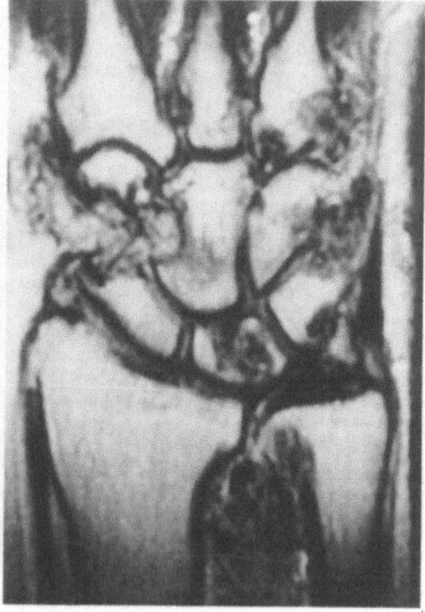

a   b

Fig. 15.16a, b. Pigmented villonodular synovitis. Coronal T1-weighted (a) and T2-weighted images (b) of many lesions distributed at some intermetacarpal, carpometacarpal, the radiocarpal, the ulnocarpal and some intracarpal joints of the wrist. The lesions are hypointense on both sequences. Note the erosion of adjacent bones. (By permission of Dr. F. Deckers, Medisch Instituut Sint Augustinus, Wilrijk, Belgium)

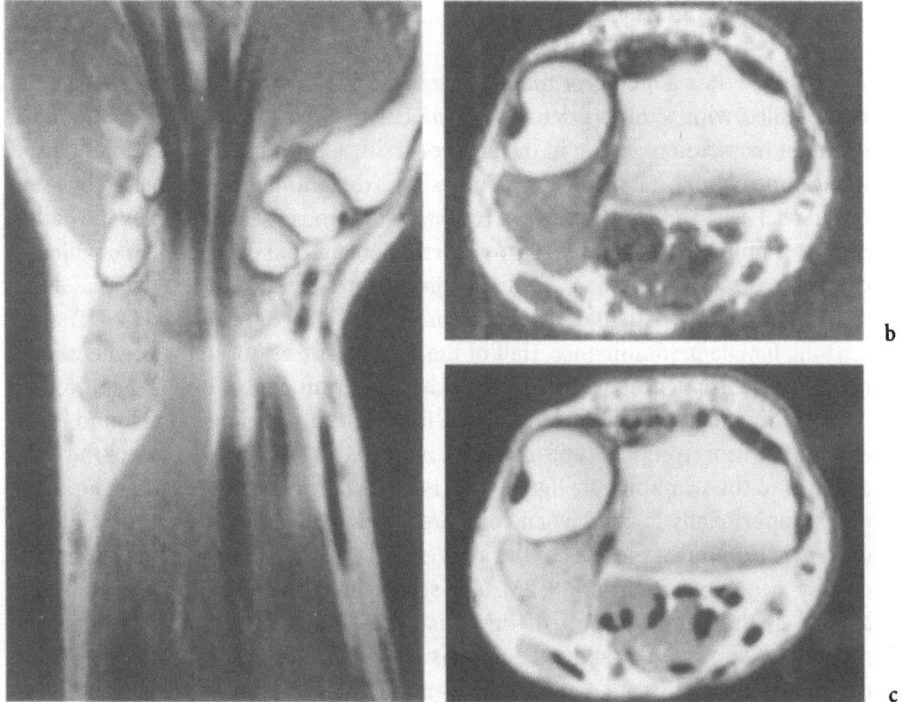

a

b

c

Fig. 15.17a–c. Pigmented villonodular synovitis in a 56-year-old man. Coronal T1-weighted (**a**) and axial T2-weighted images (**b**). An inhomogeneous mass with small intralesional hypointense areas corresponding to hemosiderin deposits is seen. Note the predominantly low signal intensity on the T2-weighted image (**b**). The connection with the joint space and the extent of the lesion are well visualized. On the axial T1-weighted image after intravenous administration of gadolinium contrast, strong homogeneous enhancement is seen (**b**)

15.3   Pseudotumoral Lesions

Tumorlike lesions are a common problem in daily clinical practice. Affected patients present with mass lesions which turn out, after radiologic or histopathologic investigation, to be pseudotumoral lesions. Most common pseudotumoral lesions in the hand and wrist are ganglia, accessory muscles, de Quervain 's tenosynovitis, epidermoid inclusion cyst, Dupuytren's disease and gout. We will not discuss other disorders presenting with articular or peri-articular inflammation at length, since they are discussed elsewhere in this book. Furthermore, some nontumoral conditions associated with calcification or ossification of the soft tissues, such as scleroderma or collagen vascular disease, are not described since they mostly do not present as mass lesions, thereby excluding confusion with neoplasms.

15.3.1   Ganglion Cyst

A ganglion cyst is a mono- or multiloculated cystic lesion in the juxta-articular soft tissues filled with a thick, gelatinous or mucinous fluid [32, 53, 66]. It is the most common mass lesion arising in the hand or wrist, accounting for 50–70% of all soft tissue tumors of the hand and wrist. The lesion is discontinuously delineated by pseudosynovial cells and supported by a compressed fibrous pseudocapsule. The pathogenesis is unknown and trauma, chronic irritation, mucoid degeneration of adjacent connective tissue and synovial herniation have been suggested as etiologic factors.

Most frequently, patients between 20 and 40 years of age are affected [36]. There is a strong female predominance. Half of the patients are asymptomatic, whereas the others suffer from chronic wrist pain, tenderness or functional impairment [65].

According to their location and origin, four subtypes of ganglia are found [7, 36, 66, 73]. The most frequent type (60–70%) is located at the dorsal aspect of the wrist adjacent to the scapholunate ligament. It is formed by two components. The larger one is superficially located when compared with the extensor tendons, while the deep part is found at the level of the joint capsule. The two components communicate by a tortuous pedicle [68, 85]. The second most common type (15–20%) is located at the palmar aspect of the wrist, most often between the flexor carpi radialis tendon and the abductor pollicis longus tendon. It probably arises from the radioscaphoid, scapho-trapezial, scapholunate or metacarpotrapezial joint. Ten percent of ganglia are small lesions (<10 mm) arising from the tendon sheath of the flexor digitorum tendons (palmar retinaculum) or within the tendons. Rarely, ganglia arise from the dorsal aspect of the interphalangeal joints, often secondary to a Heberden arthritis, and are referred to as mucous cysts. The latter mostly affect older patients between the fifth and seventh decades [74].

Mostly, no abnormality is seen on radiography. Rarely, ossification of a ganglion cyst may occur [78]. Ultrasonography may be effective in the detection and characterization of ganglia [37]. Usually, a ganglion presents as a well-defined hyporeflective mass with posterior acoustic enhancement. However, the technique is operator-dependent and requires high-resolution probes.

On MR imaging, a ganglion presents as a well-delineated homogeneous mass. The high protein concentration results in T1 shortening, rendering this cystic lesion isointense to muscle on T1-weighted images. Therefore, it may be detected on T1-weighted images only when visible mass effect on neighboring structures is present. On T2-weighted images, homogeneous high signal intensity is seen [3, 8, 53, 60, 68, 84] (Fig. 15.18). On gadolinium-enhanced T1-weighted images, a thin enhancing rim is seen at the periphery of the lesion. Rarely, hemorrhage, trauma, or infection may occur, mystifying the characteristic MR appearance of this lesion.

15.3.2   Gout

Gout is a common metabolic disorder in which the body overproduces uric acid. Monosodium urate crystals are deposited in peri-articular, subcutaneous, syn-

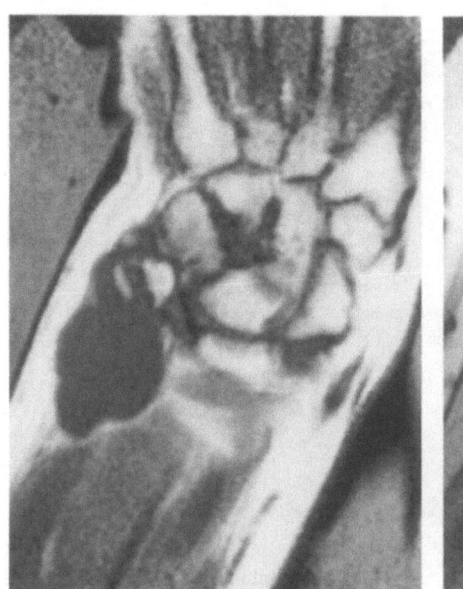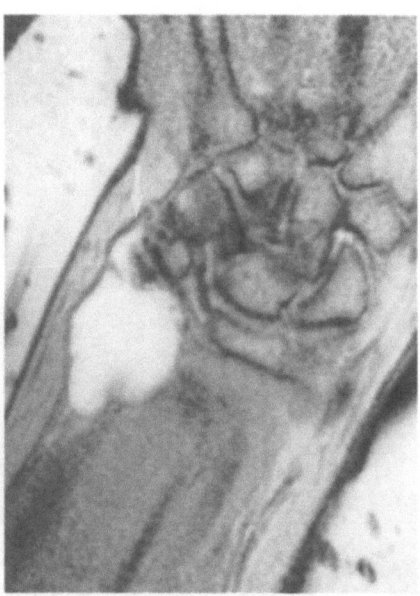

a   b

Fig. 15.18a, b. Ganglion in a 56-year-old man. Coronal T1-weighted image shows a hypointense lesion at the ulnar side of the wrist, with a stalk to the joint (a). On the coronal T2-weighted image, the extent of the hyperintense lesion is better seen (*arrow*) (b). (By permission of Dr. H. Dijkstra, Dr. P. Van Wiechen, and Prof. Dr. P.M. Parizel, Ignatius Ziekenhuis Breda, The Netherlands)

ovial, tendinous and articular sites. Patients are mostly middle-aged men presenting with a mono-articular arthritis. Most frequently, the first metatarsophalangeal joint is involved. Occasionally, the small joints of the hand are involved, mostly in patients who developed gout at a younger age. After multiple episodes of gouty arthritis, palpable multinodular swellings (tophi) may become apparent. A tophus is a mass consisting of urate crystals or amorphous urate and inflammatory reaction. Exceptionally, tophi may be the first manifestation of gout [92].

On radiography, eccentric, asymmetric soft tissue calcifications are seen. Well-defined marginal erosions of the subchondral bone with "overhanging edges" may be demonstrated. Tophi are seen as soft tissue densities. Since gout presents with characteristic clinical signs and biochemical data, MR imaging is seldom performed. However, when tophi are inflamed, or when articular disease has subsided, a clinical misinterpretation of infection or neoplasm may occur. MR images may then be obtained. On MR imaging, tophi have an intermediate signal intensity on T1-weighted images, and a variable signal intensity on T2-weighted images [72]. On gadolinium-enhanced T1-weighted images, strong homogeneous enhancement is seen [92] (Fig. 15.19). MR imaging is able to detect subclinical tophaceous deposits, not readily apparent on physical examination or radiography [69]. Differential diagnosis should include rheumatoid arthritis and other crystal deposition arthropathies.

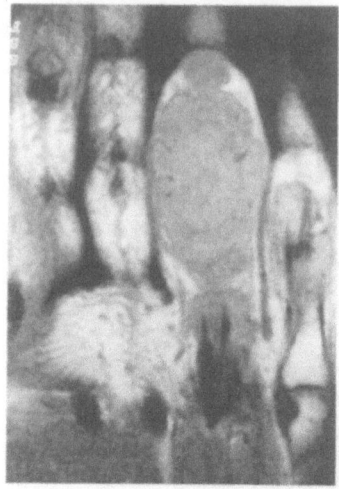 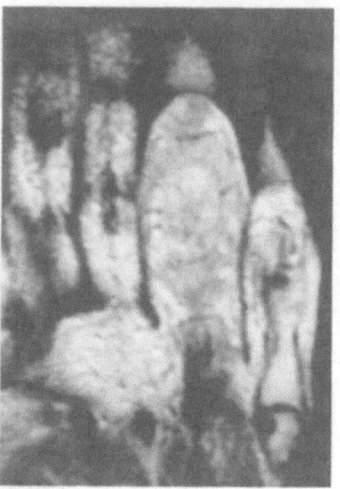

a   b

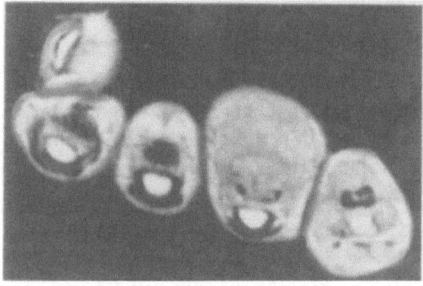

Fig. 15.19a–c. Gout in a 65-year-old man (same patient as Fig. 15.1c). On the coronal T1-weighted image, huge tophi are seen at the proximal interphalangeal joint of the fourth finger. The lesions have intermediate signal intensity (**a**). Coronal T2-weighted image shows an inhomogeneous mass with hyper- and hypointense areas (**b**). On the axial gadolinium-enhanced T1-weighted image, the lesion shows strong, homogeneous enhancement (**c**)

c

15.3.3 Tuberculosis

Tuberculous tenosynovitis is a rare manifestation of musculoskeletal involvement of systemic tuberculosis, affecting 1% of patients with osteoarticular tuberculosis. It most often involves the flexor tendon compartment of the wrist and the radioulnar bursa [38, 76]. On clinical examination, local pain, swelling and limitation of motion of the fingers and wrists is noted.

About 50% of patients with musculoskeletal tuberculosis have no concomitant pulmonary tuberculosis. Furthermore, since most patients have no fever and laboratory data are normal, tuberculous tenosynovitis may be clinically difficult to differentiate from soft tissue tumors. On radiography, a soft tissue swelling with or without intralesional calcifications may be seen. Osteopenia is frequently present. In late-stage disease, associated changes such as bone involvement or destruction of adjacent cartilage may occur.

On MR imaging, various patterns of disease may be seen: synovial fluid distending the tendon sheath with a normal-looking tendon inside, thickened synovial tissue with deformed tendons, or peritendinous soft tissue masses. Synovial fluid has low to intermediate signal intensity on T1- and high signal intensity on T2-weighted images. Low signal intensity areas on T2-weighted images may correspond to tissue debris, caseous material, fibrosis or calcification. When the tendon itself is involved, it may be thickened – secondary to infiltration by caseous tissue – or thinned because of partial rupture.

The differential diagnosis of tuberculous tenosynovitis includes pyogenic infection, which is usually more destructive to bones and adjacent joint spaces, fungal tenosynovitis, and rheumatoid or gouty arthritis. Rheumatoid arthritis, however, is accompanied by bony erosions whereas gout is characterized by the presence of tophaceous deposits [38].

15.3.4   Sarcoidosis

Sarcoidosis is a chronic systemic disease, characterized by the development of granulomas. Bony alterations in the hand consist of cortical atrophy and granulomatous replacement of the medullary bone of the proximal and middle phalanges or phalangeal acrosclerosis. The soft tissues of the hand and wrist are rarely involved. Sarcoid arthropathy primarily affects small joints, presenting as a symmetric polyarthritis. Sarcoid tenosynovitis is extremely rare and affects chiefly the flexor digitorum tendons. Cutaneous and subcutaneous granulomas as the first manifestation of sarcoidosis are also a rare occurrence [71].

15.3.5   Tenosynovial Osteochondromatosis

Synovial chondromatosis is characterized by cartilaginous metaplasia of the synovium. Late-phase osteochondromatosis is characterized by the release of these cartilaginous areas which are then recognized as mineralized loose bodies within a joint or a tendon sheath [60]. Most patients are middle-aged men who present with swelling, stiffness or pain of the affected joint or tendon sheath.

On radiography, faint calcified intra-articular nodules are frequently seen. On MR imaging, a lobulated mass with intermediate signal intensity on T1- and very high signal intensity on T2-weighted images is seen. Intralesional signal voids correspond to calcified loose bodies. MR imaging may help in determining the extent of the process (Fig. 15.20).

15.3.6   Accessory Muscles

Accessory muscles are congenital anatomic variants that may clinically simulate a more ominous mass lesion. Most common accessory muscles of the hand and wrist are the accessory palmaris longus muscle, the accessory abductor pollicis minimi muscle, the extensor digitorum brevis muscle, and the anomalies of the flexor digitorum muscles [77, 80]. Clinically, a mass with anomalous localization is noted. Sometimes, pain or paresthesias may occur secondary to compression of adjacent nerves; e.g., variants of the palmaris longus muscle or accessory flexor

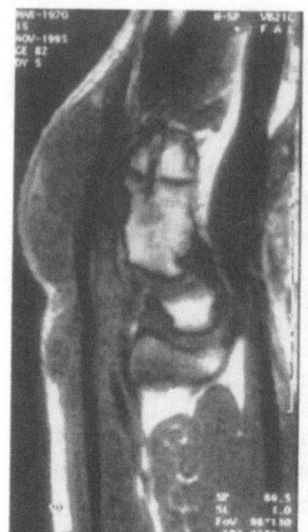
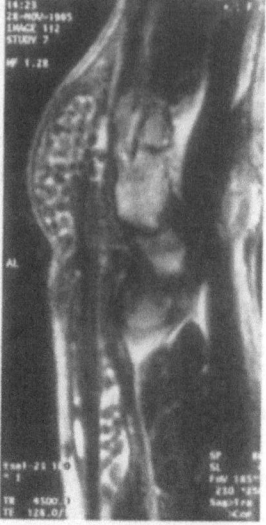
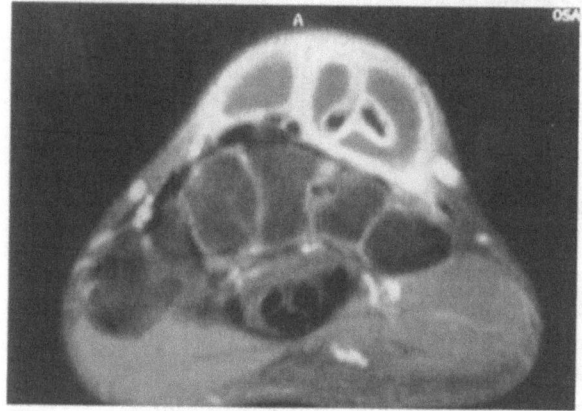

Fig. 15.20a–c. Tenosynovial osteochondromatosis. On the sagittal T1-weighted image, a mass lesion with intermediate signal intensity is seen at the extensor compartment of the wrist (**a**). On the sagittal T2-weighted image, the lesion has high signal intensity, corresponding to fluid. Numerous intralesional dots of low signal intensity correspond to cartilaginous bodies (**b**). After intravenous administration of gadolinium contrast, strong enhancement of the synovial membrane of the tendon sheaths of the third and fourth extensor tendon compartment is seen (**c**). (Reprinted with permission of Dr. A. Capelastegui, Osatek, Hospital de Galdacano, Basque Country, Spain [12])

digitorum superficialis muscle may be associated with symptoms of median or ulnar nerve entrapment (Fig. 15.21).

Accessory muscles have a non-aggressive behavior on MR imaging and are isointense to muscles on all imaging sequences [60]. Recognition of these MR characteristics obviates the need for biopsy [3].

15.3.7   Foreign Body Reaction

After a penetrating trauma, foreign bodies may be removed by the patient or by a physician. If the foreign body is not recognized or not retrieved, it will be retained and will generate a foreign body granuloma. Most patients complain of pain, discomfort or a palpable mass.

On radiography, a radio-opaque retained foreign body may sometimes be seen easily. For non-radio-opaque objects, ultrasonography may be helpful [9].

On MR imaging, small foreign bodies may be demonstrated as low signal intensity structures within the subcutaneous space (Fig. 15.22). A long-standing foreign body will present as a well-encapsulated multiloculated cystic mass with heterogeneous signal intensities. Usually, a definitive diagnosis will be made only peroperatively [61].

15.3.8 Epidermal Inclusion Cyst

Epidermal inclusion cysts are the third most common mass at the hand. They are cystic lesions lined with epithelial cells and filled with keratin [63]. Their etiopathology remains in doubt, but since they occur frequently in manual laborers, a traumatic etiology with introduction of epidermis into the subcutaneous tissue seem plausible. According to another theory, embryonic epithelial cell rests are thought to become stimulated by trauma.

Patients present with painless, fluctuating masses in the palm or at the distal fingers. In a subungual location, epidermal inclusion cysts are frequently accompanied by a secondary bone erosion.

On CT or MR imaging, a well-delineated soft tissue mass is seen. Signal intensities vary as a function of its content [50].

15.3.9 De Quervain's Disease

De Quervain's disease, also called de Quervain's tenosynovitis, presents histopathologically as a myxoid degeneration of the intercellular matrix of the tendon sheath of the abductor pollicis longus tendon and the extensor pollicis brevis tendon. Inflammatory signs are often absent. Therefore, the terms "tenosynovitis" or "stenosing tenovaginitis" are misnomers [14]. Affected patients present with tenderness or swelling at the radial styloid.

On MR imaging, abnormal accumulation of fluid is seen within the tendon sheath on T2-weighted images [3]. The involved tendons may be thickened and their signal intensity increased at the level of the radial styloid.

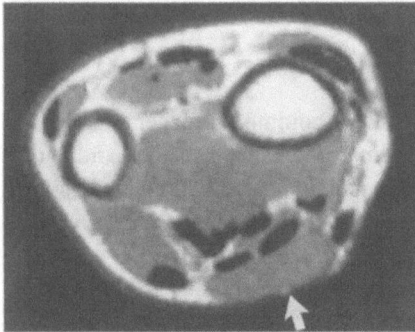

Fig. 15.21. Accessory muscle in a 13-year-old boy. On the axial gadolinium-enhanced T1-weighted image, an anomalous structure is seen within the subcutaneous tissues (*arrow*), with the same signal intensity as the other muscles. It is an anatomic variant of the palmaris longus muscle (nontendinous variant)

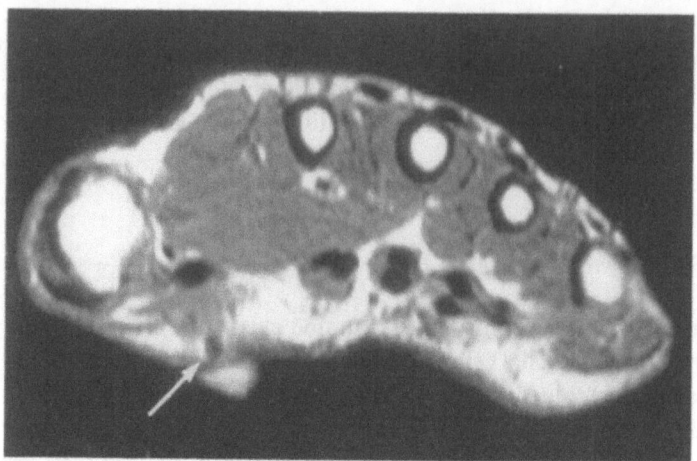

Fig. 15.22. Foreign body granulomatous reaction of the palmar aspect of the hand. On the axial proton density image, an abnormality of the subcutaneous fat is seen at the palmar aspect of the hand, under the external marker placed to identify the location of the palpable mass. Note the presence of a small focus of hypointensity (*arrow*), corresponding to a foreign body. The patient did not recall a traumatic event. (Reprinted with permission of Dr. A. Capelastegui, Osatek, Hospital de Galdacano, Basque Country, Spain [12])

15.3.10 Macrodystrophia Lipomatosa

Macrodystrophia lipomatosa is one of the commonest causes of limb overgrowth, varying in degree from macrodactyly to hemihypertrophy. It represents a congenital non-hereditary overgrowth of all mesenchymal elements, particularly of fibroadipose tissue. Localized overgrowth is usually unilateral and affects one or more adjacent digits, chiefly the third and second [18, 35, 89] (Fig. 15.1e). The bone marrow, periosteum, muscles, nerve sheaths and subcutaneous fat may be involved.

On radiography, affected bones are broad and elongated. MR imaging shows extreme amount of lipomatous tissue in the affected areas. Bony hypertrophy and cortical thickening may also be seen [89].

15.3.11 Dupuytren's Contracture

Dupuytren's contracture or palmar fibromatosis is a common disorder affecting 1–2 % of the general population, involving the palmar aponeurosis of the hand and its extensions. Initially, the disease manifests as a small nodular subcutaneous lesion in the palm of the hand at the level of the distal palmar crease. Later, it progresses to formation of a collagenous cord, oriented parallel and superficial to the flexor tendons. The overlying skin thickens and retracts. Finally, disabling flexion contractures are seen on physical examination. The fourth ray is most commonly involved.

On MR imaging, cordlike structures arising from the aponeurosis are seen as hypointense bands on T1- and T2-weighted images. These lesions terminate as fine strands in the subcutaneous tissue or with the formation of a small nodule. These associated nodules, seen in two thirds of patients, mostly have intermediate signal intensity on T1- and T2-weighted images (Fig. 15.23). Some intralesional dots of low or high signal intensity may be shown. Yacoe et al. [91] evaluated 13 nodular lesions of patients with Dupuytren's contracture and concluded that the signal intensities correlated with the cellularity of the lesions. Nodules with low signal intensity on T2-weighted images correspond to lesions with a lower cellularity which are believed to recur less frequently (18%) than more cellular ones (70%) [91].

15.4   Malignant Tumoral Lesions

Since most of soft tissue sarcomas of the hand and wrist are rather slow growing, small masses at the time of presentation, surgical treatment without amputation

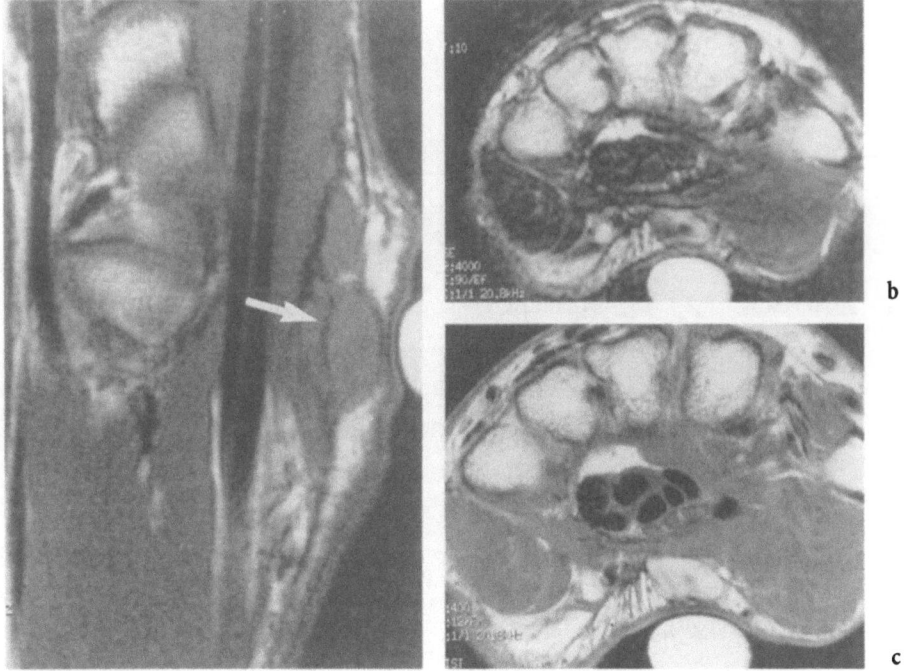

Fig. 15.23a–c. Dupuytren's contracture in the right hand of a 28-year-old man. On the sagittal T1-weighted image, a well-circumscribed ovoid mass with intermediate signal intensity is seen at the palmar aspect of the hand/wrist (*arrow*) (a). The mass is located at the palmar aponeurosis. On the axial T2-weighted image, the lesion has predominantly low to intermediate signal intensity (b). After intravenous administration of gadolinium, strong enhancement is seen (c). (By permission of Dr. W. Van Rompaey, Medisch Instituut Sint Augustinus, Wilrijk, Belgium)

may be effective to achieve local control. However, patients are still too frequently operated on for "shelling out of a lump" that afterwards, on histopathologic examination, turns out to be a sarcoma. These apparently unexpected encounters are mostly treated with an incomplete excision. Therefore, one or more recurrences will occur, making repeat operations or even amputation mandatory.

Since most patients with a soft tissue sarcoma of the hand are young adults, and since they have no major complaints except for a small painless mass without functional deficit, soft tissue sarcomas present clinically as "a wolf in sheep's clothing". Therefore, the rule of thumb that any deep-seated tumor that is firm and 5 cm or larger should be considered to be possibly malignant until proven otherwise is a good approach for these lesions. However, any lesion that is smaller and more superficially located should not be assumed to be benign (Figs. 15.3, 15.24). In contrast to Kransdorf and Murphey, who advocate a less aggressive policy, we believe that any mass that cannot be characterized reliably should be biopsied, keeping definitive surgical treatment options in mind [33,51]. We subscribe to this point of view the more so because soft tissue tumors of the hand and wrist are

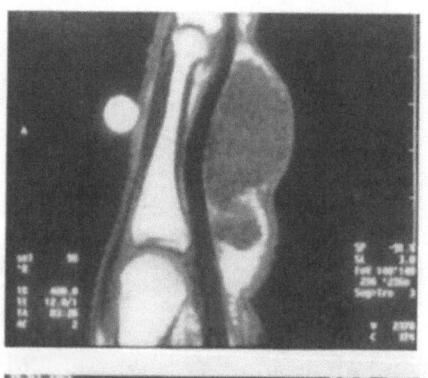
a

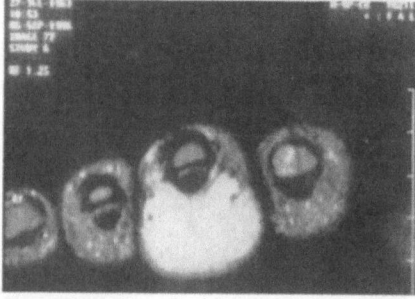
b

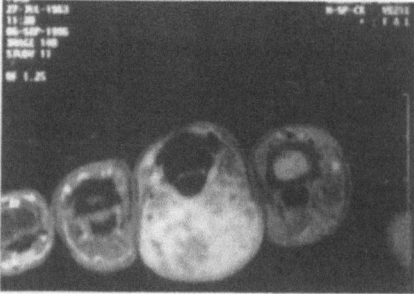
c

Fig. 15.24a–c. Myxoid liposarcoma of the third finger. On the sagittal T1-weighted image, a well-defined, superficially located mass is seen at the extensor compartment of the third digit. The extensor tendon and the proximal phalanx are not involved. The mass has intermediate signal intensity (a). On the axial T2-weighted image, the lesion has predominantly high signal intensity (b). No perilesional edema is seen. After intravenous administration of gadolinium contrast, diffuse, heterogeneous enhancement is noted (c). (Reprinted with permission of Dr. A. Capelastegui, Osatek, Hospital de Galdacano, Basque Country, Spain [12])

generally small at presentation, since they are located in small anatomic compartments that are rapidly functionally impeded by any mass lesion and thus subject to early detection by the patient. Furthermore, it is generally accepted that small soft tissue tumors in extremities, outside the hand, are approached by wide excisional biopsy. The difficulty with this procedure in tumors of unknown origin of the hand or wrist is that significant tumor spread in adjacent important structures may occur. Therefore, any lesion exceeding 3 cm in diameter should be evaluated by incisional biopsy without jeopardizing definitive treatment options [79].

15.4.1 Synovial Sarcoma

Synovial sarcoma is the fourth most common sarcoma of the soft tissues, accounting for approximately 6–10% of all soft tissue sarcomas [64, 84]. It arises in para-articular regions, mostly in close association with tendon sheaths, bursae or joint capsules. Most frequently, it affects young adults between 15 and 35 years of age [53, 84]. Rarely, synovial sarcoma is located at the hand and wrist (8.5% of all cases), thereby more frequently encountered at the carpus than at the fingers [64]. Patients present with a slow-growing, often painful soft tissue mass. Paresthesias or numbness may occur if neural structures are involved [53, 84].

On radiography or CT, small densities caused by calcification or ossification may be present at the periphery of the lesion in 20–30% of cases [11]. Bone remodeling, erosion, periosteal reaction, or even bone invasion, may be present [11].

MR imaging shows a heterogeneous mass with intermediate signal intensity on T1-weighted images and high signal intensity on T2-weighted images (Fig. 15.2). Small areas of increased signal intensity on T1- and T2-weighted images, seen in approximately 45% of cases, correspond to intratumoral hemorrhage. Intralesional fluid-fluid levels, although nonspecific and infrequently seen (15–25%), can be a striking feature. Internal septations may also be present. Especially in small lesions, the mass may have well-defined margins and may be homogeneous on all sequences, resulting in its misdiagnosis as a benign lesion [6, 8, 41, 62, 64].

In the differential diagnosis on MR imaging of a mass with heterogeneous aspect and infiltrative margins, in close proximity to a joint, tendon or bursa, malignancy is the most likely consideration. Small, multilocular lesions may be confused with hemangiomas or ganglion cysts, but unlike these are mostly more sharply delineated and less heterogeneous.

15.4.2 Clear Cell Sarcoma

Clear cell sarcoma or malignant melanoma of the soft parts is a rare tumor of the soft tissues, accounting for 1% of all soft tissue sarcomas [52]. This tumor is mostly associated with a tendon or aponeurosis [26]. It affects young adults between 20 and 40 years of age. There is a female predominance [26, 52]. The lesion is mostly located at the lower limbs, especially foot and ankle, but may also arise from the hand or forearm. Unlike other sarcomas, it metastasizes to the lymph nodes and has an extremely bad prognosis [26, 52].

On MR imaging, a well-circumscribed mass is seen. On T1-weighted images, the lesion has intermediate signal intensity equal to that of adjacent muscle or slightly higher than muscle. The melanocytic differentiation of the cells may contribute to the relatively high signal intensity of this tumor on T1-weighted images (Fig. 15.3a). On T2-weighted images, a more heterogeneous mass is seen [26] (Fig. 15.3b). Intratumoral necrosis is only seldom present. After intravenous administration of gadolinium, strong homogeneous enhancement is noted [5, 20, 26] (Fig. 15.3c).

15.4.3   Neurofibrosarcoma and Malignant Schwannoma

Both neurofibrosarcoma and malignant schwannoma are "malignant peripheral nerve sheath tumors", accounting for 5–10% of all soft tissue sarcomas. In 25–70% of all cases, there is association with neurofibromatosis type I [31, 44]. In these cases, a strong male preponderance is seen [52, 67]. Approximately 3% of the lesions arises in the wrist or hand [44].

Patients with a malignant peripheral nerve sheath tumor present with pain or symptoms of a sensory or motor nerve deficit such as paresthesias and weakness. However, most patients have nonspecific complaints. Sudden enlargement of a known soft tissue mass (neurofibroma) in a patient with neurofibromatosis type I should prompt immediate diagnostic investigation [52, 67].

MR imaging findings are nonspecific. On T1-weighted images, the mass has equal to slightly increased signal intensity compared with muscle (Fig. 15.25a). On T2-weighted images, the mass has very high signal intensity [10] (Fig. 15.25b). The internal architecture of the mass may be anarchic due to intratumoral hemorrhage or necrosis [10, 67]. On gadolinium-enhanced T1-weighted images, heterogeneous enhancement is seen.

15.5   Post-therapeutic Surveillance

Local recurrences of malignant or aggressive soft tissue tumors are frequent (up to 50% of cases) [86]. High frequency of recurrences is related to the presence of satellite lesions in the pseudocapsule and of skip metastases beyond the reactive zone within the compartment of origin.

Although ultrasonography provides a safe, rapid and accurate method for localizing recurrent, superficial soft tissue masses and then guiding needle biopsies to acquire cytologic material for a definite diagnosis, ultrasonographic examination is limited because of the small field of view and the difficulty in penetrating thickened postoperative or irradiated skin [1].

Therefore we still use the "easy-to-follow" and reliable algorithm for post-therapeutic follow-up proposed by Vanel et al. [86, 87] and recently confirmed in a

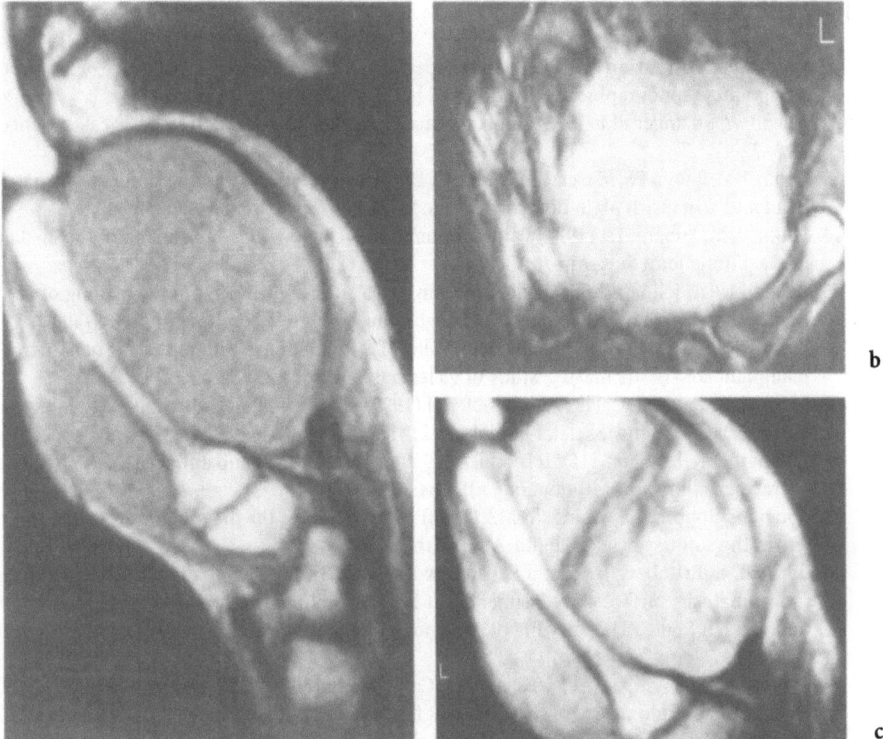

a

b

c

Fig. 15.25a–c. Neurofibrosarcoma in a 17-year-old boy. Sagittal T1-weighted image of a voluminous mass with intermediate signal intensity at the palmar aspect of the hand (**a**). The mass is
hyperintense on the coronal gradient echo T2*-weighted image (**b**). After intravenous administration of gadolinium contrast, strong enhancement is seen (**c**)

study reporting on the application of a dynamic contrast-enhanced MR technique
with subtraction for detecting recurrent soft tissue tumors. The procedure starts
with a fat-saturated T2-weighted sequence or fat-suppressed sequence with inversion recovery technique (STIR). If there is a mass lesion with low signal intensity
or a high signal intensity lesion without a mass, a recurrence is not probable
because low signal intensity mostly refers to fibrotic (scar) tissue while high signal
intensity lesions without a mass can be a consequence of (radiation-induced)
inflammatory changes. When a high signal intensity mass is found, T1-weighted
images before and after gadolinium injection are performed. If the mass enhances,
a recurrence is highly probable; if not one is dealing with a hematoma or a hygro-
ma. However standard contrast-enhanced MR imaging cannot differentiate a recurrent tumor from a rare inflammatory pseudotumor. Dynamic contrast-enhanced MR imaging with subtraction is able to make this differentiation because
signal intensity of active tumor increases rapidly whereas inflammatory changes
enhance only after 3–9 min.

References

1. Alexander A, Nazarian L, Feld R (1997) Superficial soft tissue masses suggestive of recurrent malignancy: sonographic localization and biopsy. AJR 169:1449-1451
2. Allen PW, Enzinger FM (1972) Hemangioma of skeletal muscle: analysis of 89 cases. Cancer 29:8-22
3. Azouz EM, Babyn PS, Mascia AT, Tuuha SE, Decarie JC (1998) MRI of the abnormal pediatric hand and wrist with plain film correlation. J Comput Assist Tomogr 22:252-261
4. Babins DM, Lubahn JD (1994) Palmar lipomas associated with compression of the median nerve. J Bone Joint Surg Am 76:1360-1362
5. Benedikt RA, Jelinek JS, Kransdorf MJ, Moser RP, Berrey BH (1994) MR imaging of soft-tissue masses: role of gadopentetate dimeglumine. J Magn Reson Imaging 4:485-490
6. Berquist TH, Ehman RL, King BF (1990) Value of MR imaging in differentiating benign from malignant soft-tissue masses: study of 95 lesions. AJR 155:1251-1255
7. Bianchi S, Martinoli C, Fikry Abdelwahab I (1999) High-frequency ultrasound examination of the wrist and hand. Skeletal Radiol 28:121-129
8. Binkovitz LA, Berquist TH, McLeod RA (1990) Masses of the hand and wrist: detection and characterization with MR imaging. AJR 154:323-326
9. Bonatz E, Robbin ML, Weingold MA (1998) Ultrasound for the diagnosis of retained splinters in the soft tissue of the hand. Am J Orthop 27:455-459
10. Burk DL Jr, Brunberg JA, Kanal E, Latchaw RE, Wolf GL (1987) Spinal and paraspinal neurofibromatosis: surface coil MR imaging at 1.5 T. Radiology 162:797-801
11. Cadman NL, Soule EH, Kelley PJ (1965) Synovial sarcoma: an analysis of 134 tumors. Cancer 18:613-627
12. Capelastegui A, Astigarraga E, Fernandez-Canton G, Saralegui I, Larena JA, Merino A (1999) Masses and pseudomasses of the wrist: MR findings in 134 cases. Skeletal Radiol 28:498-507
13. Cavallaro MC, Taylor JAM, Gorman JD, Haghighi P, Resnick D (1993) Imaging findings in a patient with fibrolipomatous hamartoma of the median nerve. AJR 161:837-838
14. Clarke MT, Lyall HA, Grant JW, Matthewson MH (1998) The histopathology of de Quervain's disease. J Hand Surg [Br] 23:732-734
15. Constantinesco A, Arbogast S, Foucher G, Vinée P, Choquet P, Brunot B (1994) Detection of glomus tumor of the finger by dedicated MRI at 0.1 T. Magn Reson Imaging 12:1131-1134
16. Crim J, Seeger L, Yao L, Chandnani V, Eckhardt J (1992) Diagnosis of soft tissue masses with MR imaging: can benign masses be differentiated from malignant ones? Radiology 185:581-586
17. Dalrymple NC, Hayes J, Bessinger VJ, Wolfe SW, Katz LD (1997) MRI of multiple glomus tumors of the finger. Skeletal Radiol 26:664-666
18. D'Costa H, Hunter JD, O'Sullivan G, O'Keefe D, Jenkins JPR, Hughes PM (1996) Magnetic resonance imaging in macromelia and macrodactyly. Br J Radiol 69:502-507
19. De Beuckeleer L, De Schepper A, De Belder F, et al (1997) Magnetic resonance imaging of localized giant cell tumour of the tendon sheath (MRI of localized GCTTS). Eur Radiol 7:198-201
20. De Beuckeleer LH, De Schepper A, Vandevenne JE, et al (2000) MR imaging of clear cell sarcoma (malignant melanoma of the soft parts): a multicenter correlative MR-pathology study of 21 cases and literature review. Skeletal Radiol (in press)
21. de la Kethulle de Ryhove D, De Beuckeleer LH, De Schepper AM (1999) L'imagerie par résonance magnétique des tumeurs des tissus mous de la main et du poignet. J Radiol z
22. De Schepper AM, De Beuckeleer LH (1999) Imagerie des tumeurs des parties molles. In: Encyclopédie médico chirurgicale, radiodiagnostic – neuroradiologie – appareil locomoteur. Elsevier, Paris, p 31-750-A-10
23. De Schepper AM, Parizel PM, Ramon F, De Beuckeleer L, Vandevenne JE (1997) Imaging of soft tissue tumors. Springer, Berlin Heidelberg New York
24. Declercq H, De Man R, Van Herck G, Tanghe W, Lateur L (1993) Case report 814. Fibrolipoma of the median nerve. Skeletal Radiol 22:610-613

25. Degryse HR, Aparisi F (1997) Extraskeletal cartilaginous and osseous tumors. In: De Schepper AM, Parizel PM, Ramon F, De Beuckeleer L, Vandevenne JE (eds) Imaging of soft tissue tumors. Springer, Berlin Heidelberg New York, pp 299–316

26. Degryse HR (1997) Lesions of uncertain origin. In: De Schepper AM, Parizel PM, Ramon F, De Beuckeleer L, Vandevenne JE (eds) Imaging of soft tissue tumors. Springer, Berlin Heidelberg New York, pp 325–344

27. Drapé JL, Idy-Peretti I, Goettmann S et al (1995) Subungual glomus tumors: evaluation with MR imaging. Radiology 195:507–515

28. Enzinger FM, Weiss SW (1995) Benign lipomatous tumors. In: Soft tissue tumors. Mosby, St Louis, pp 384–390

29. Enzinger FM, Weiss SW (1995) Benign tumors and tumorlike lesions of blood vessels. In: Soft tissue tumors. Mosby, St Louis, pp 579–626

30. Enzinger FM, Weiss SW (1995) Benign tumors and tumorlike lesions of synovial tissue. In: Soft tissue tumors. Mosby, St Louis, pp 735–756

31. Enzinger FM, Weiss SW (1995) Malignant tumors of the peripheral nerves. In: Soft tissue tumors. Mosby, St Louis, pp 889–928

32. Ferrara MA, Marcelis S (1997) Ultrasound examination of the wrist. J Belge Radiol 80:78–80

33. Fleegler EJ (1994) An approach to soft tissue sarcomas of the hand and upper limb. J Hand Surg [Br] 4:411–419

34. Fornage BD, Tassin GB (1991) Sonographic appearances of superficial soft tissue lipomas. J Clin Ultrasound 19:215–220

35. Hildebrandt JW, Olson P, Paratainen H, Griffiths HJ (1993) Macrodystrophia lipomatosa. Orthopedics 9:1075–1077

36. Hoglund M, Tordai P, Muren C (1994) Diagnosis of ganglions in the hand and wrist by sonography. Acta Radiol 35:35–39

37. Jacobson JA (1999) Musculoskeletal sonography and MR imaging. A role for both imaging methods. Radiol Clin North Am 37:713–735

38. Jaovisidha S, Chen C, Nam Ryu K, et al (1996) Tuberculous tenosynovitis and bursitis: imaging findings in 21 cases. Radiology 201:507–513

39. Jelinek JS, Kransdorf MJ, Shmookler BM, Aboulafia AA, Malawer MM (1994) Giant cell tumor of the tendon sheath: MR findings in nine cases. AJR 162:919–922

40. Jelinek JS, Kransdorf MJ, Utz JA et al (1989) Imaging of pigmented villonodular synovitis with emphasis on MR imaging. AJR 152:337–342

41. Jones BC, Sundaram M, Kransdorf MJ (1993) Synovial sarcoma: MR imaging findings in 34 patients. AJR 161:827–830

42. Karasick D, Karasick S (1992) Giant cell tumor of tendon sheath: spectrum of radiologic findings. Skeletal Radiol 21:219–224

43. Kransdorf MJ (1995) Benign soft-tissue masses in a large referral population: distribution of specific diagnoses by age, sex, and location. AJR 164:395–402

44. Kransdorf MJ (1995) Malignant soft-tissue masses in a large referral population: distribution of specific diagnoses by age, sex, and location. AJR 164:129–134

45. Kransdorf MJ, Jelinek JS, Moser RP, et al (1989) Soft-tissue masses: diagnosis using MR imaging. AJR 153:541–547

46. Kransdorf MJ, Meis JM (1993) From the archives of the AFIP. Extraskeletal osseous and cartilaginous tumors of the extremities. Radiographics 13:853–884

47. Kransdorf MJ, Murphey MD (1997) Extraskeletal osseous and cartilaginous tumors. In: Kransdorf MJ, Murphey MD (eds) Imaging of soft tissue tumors. Saunders, Philadelphia, pp 317–350

48. Kransdorf MJ, Murphey MD (1997) Imaging of soft tissue tumors. Saunders, Philadelphia

49. Kransdorf MJ, Murphey MD (1997) Lipomatous tumors. In: Kransdorf MJ, Murphey MD (eds) Imaging of soft tissue tumors. Saunders, Philadelphia, pp 57–63

50. Kransdorf MJ, Murphey MD (1997) Masses that may mimic soft tissue tumors. In: Kransdorf MJ, Murphey MD (eds) Imaging of soft tissue tumors. Saunders, Philadelphia, pp 373–420

51. Kransdorf MJ, Murphey MD (1995) MR imaging of musculoskeletal tumors of the hand and wrist. MRI Clin North Am 3:327–344

52. Kransdorf MJ, Murphey MD (1997) Neurogenic tumors. In: Kransdorf MJ, Murphey MD (eds) Imaging of soft tissue tumors. Saunders, Philadelphia, pp 235–274

53. Kransdorf MJ, Murphey MD (1997) Synovial tumors. In: Kransdorf MJ, Murphey MD (eds) Imaging of soft tissue tumors. Saunders, Philadelphia, pp 275–316

54. Kransdorf MJ, Murphey MD (1997) Vascular and lymphatic tumors. In: Kransdorf MJ, Murphey MD (eds) Imaging of soft tissue tumors. Saunders, Philadelphia, pp 126–31

55. Llauger J, Palmer J, Roson N, Cremades R, Bagué S (1999) Pigmented villonodular synovitis and giant cell tumors of the tendon sheath: radiologic and pathologic features. AJR 172:1087–1091

56. Ma L, Frassica F, Scott E, Fishman E, Zerhouni E (1995) Differentiation of benign and malignant musculoskeletal tumors: potential pitfalls with MR imaging. Radiographics 15:349–366

57. Marom EM, Helms CA (1999) Fibrolipomatous hamartoma: pathognomonic on MR imaging. Skeletal Radiol 28:260–264

58. Marques MC, Garcia H (1997) Lipomatous tumors. In: De Schepper AM, Parizel PM, Ramon F, De Beuckeleer L, Vandevenne JE (eds) Imaging of soft tissue tumors. Springer, Berlin Heidelberg New York, pp 191–199

59. Matloub HS, Muoneke VN, Prevel CD, Sanger JR, Yousif NJ (1992) Glomus tumor imaging: use of MRI for localization of occult lesions. J Hand Surg [Am] 17:472–475

60. Miller T, Potter HG, McCormack RR Jr (1994) Benign soft tissue masses of the wrist and hand: MRI appearances. Skeletal Radiol 23:327–332

61. Monu JUV, McManus CM, Ward WG, Haygood TM, Pope TL Jr, Bohrer SP (1995) Soft tissue masses caused by long-standing foreign bodies in the extremities. AJR 165:395–397

62. Morton MJ, Berquist TH, McLeod RA, Unni KK, Sim FH (1991) MR imaging of synovial sarcoma. AJR 156:337–340

63. Murphy GF, Elder DE (1991) Non-melanocytic tumors of the skin. Atlas of tumor pathology. Armed Forces Institute of Pathology, Washington, DC

64. Nakajima H, Matsushita K, Shimizu H, et al (1997) Synovial sarcoma of the hand. Skeletal Radiol 26:674–676

65. Nakamichi K, Tachibana S (1993) Ultrasonography in the diagnosis of carpal tunnel syndrome caused by an occult ganglion. J Hand Surg [Br] 18:174–175

66. Päivänsalo M, Jalovaara P (1991) Ultrasound findings of ganglions of the wrist. Eur J Radiol 13:178–180

67. Parizel PM, Simoens WA, Matos C, Verstraete KL (1997) Tumors of peripheral nerves. In: De Schepper AM, Parizel PM, Ramon F, De Beuckeleer L, Vandevenne JE (eds) Imaging of soft tissue tumors. Springer, Berlin Heidelberg New York, pp 271–298

68. Peh WC, Truong NP, Totty WG, Gilula LA (1995) Pictorial review: magnetic resonance imaging of benign soft tissue masses of the hand and wrist. Clin Radiol 50:519–525

69. Popp JD, Bidgood WD, Edwards NL (1996) Magnetic resonance imaging of tophaceous gout in the hands and wrists. Semin Arthritis Rheum 25:282–289

70. Ramon F (1997) Tumors and tumorlike lesions of blood vessels. In: De Schepper AM, Parizel PM, Ramon F, De Beuckeleer L, Vandevenne JE (eds) Imaging of soft tissue tumors. Springer, Berlin Heidelberg New York, pp 211–227

71. Rivera-Sanfeliz G, Resnick D, Haghighi P (1996) Sarcoidosis of hands. Skeletal Radiol 25:786–788

72. Ruiz ME, Erickson SJ, Carrera GF, Hanel DP, Smith MD (1993) Monoarticular gout following trauma. J Comput Assist Tomogr 17:151–153

73. Seidman GD, Margles SW (1993) Intratendinous ganglia of the hand. J Hand Surg [Am] 18:707–710

74. Shapiro PS, Seitz WH Jr (1995) Non-neoplastic tumors of the hand and upper extremity. Hand Clin 11:133–160

75. Silverman TA, Enzinger FM (1985) Fibrolipomatous hamartoma of nerve: a clinicopathologic analysis of 26 cases. Am J Surg Pathol 9:7–14

76. Sueyoshi E, Eutani M, Hayashi K, Kohzaki S (1996) Tuberculous tenosynovitis of the wrist: MRI findings in three patients. Skeletal Radiol 25:569–572

77. Sundaram M, Sharafuddin MJA (1995) MR imaging of benign soft-tissue masses. MRI Clin North Am 3:609–628
78. Tehranzadeh J, Anavim A, Lin F (1998) Radiographically ossified ganglion cyst of a finger in a swimmer. Skeletal Radiol 27:705–707
79. Terek RM, Brien EW (1995) Soft tissue sarcomas of the hand and wrist. Hand Clin 11:287–305
80. Timins ME (1999) Muscular anatomic variants of the wrist and hand: findings on MR imaging. AJR 172:1397–1401
81. Totty WG, Murphy WA, Lee JKT (1986) Soft-tissue tumors: MR imaging. Radiology 160:135–141
82. Uriburu IJF, Levy VD (1998) Intraosseous growth of giant cell tumors of the tendon sheath (localized nodular tenosynovitis) of the digits: report of 15 cases. J Hand Surg [Am] 23:732–736
83. Valer G, Ramirez G, Massons J, Lopez C (1997) Synovite villonodulaire hémopigmentée du poignet. Rev Chir Orthop 83:164–167
84. Van Goethem JWM, Shahabpour M. Synovial tumors. In: De Schepper AM, Parizel PM, Ramon F, De Beuckeleer L, Vandevenne JE (eds) Imaging of soft tissue tumors. Springer, Berlin Heidelberg New York, pp 255–270
85. Vandevenne JE, Vanhoenacker F, Hauben E, De Schepper AM (1997) Nosologie des kystes para-articulaires. In: Le genou traumatique et dégénératif. Sauramps Médical, Paris, pp 293–303
86. Vanel D, Shapeero L, Guinebretière J, Lecesne A, Genin J (1997) Posttreatment assessment of soft tissue tumors. In: De Schepper AM, Parizel PM, Ramon F, De Beuckeleer L, Vandevenne JE (eds) Imaging of soft tissue tumors. Springer, Berlin Heidelberg New York, pp 375–381
87. Vanel D, Shapeero LG, Tardivon A, Western A, Guinebretiere GM (1998) Dynamic contrast-enhanced MRI with subtraction of aggressive soft tissue tumors after resection. Skeletal Radiol 27:505–510
88. Walker CW, Adams BD, Barnes CL, Roloson GJ, Fitz-Randolph RL (1991) Case report 667. Skeletal Radiol 20:237–239
89. Wang YC, Jeng CM, Marcantonio DR, Resnick D (1997) Macrodystrophia lipomatosa: MR imaging in three patients. Clin Imaging 21:323–327
90. Weiss KL, Beltran J, Shamam OM, Stilla RF, Levey M (1986) High-field MR surface-coil imaging of the hand and wrist. I. Normal anatomy. Radiology 160:143–146
91. Yacoe M, Bergman G, Ladd A, Hellman B (1993) Dupuytren's contracture: MR imaging findings and correlation between MR signal intensity and cellularity of the lesions. AJR 8:813–817
92. Yu JS, Chung C, Recht M, Dailiana T, Jurdi R (1997) MR imaging of tophaceous gout. AJR 168:523–527

16   Primary Osseous Tumors of the Hand

Henk-Jan van der Woude, Johan L. Bloem

16.1   Introduction

Primary tumors of bone are among the most uncommon of all types of neoplasms. Because of the diversity of these tumors, ranging from benign to high-grade malignant, with associated different types of treatment, it is important to aim at an accurate diagnosis. Radiology plays an important role in this respect, while good interactive communication with orthopedic surgeons and pathologists is required.

In general, local symptoms and results of physical examination are of minor importance in achieving the correct diagnosis. Osteoid osteoma may be one of the exceptions, with its typical pain manifestation during the night, responding well to salicylate medication. Moreover, laboratory studies do not contribute greatly to the diagnosis of bone tumors in general.

Conventional radiographs, despite the development of modern imaging modalities such as magnetic resonance (MR) imaging, are still of pivotal importance in the diagnostic approach to tumors of bone. The definitive diagnosis of bone lesions, which is usually based on histopathologic analysis of tissue acquired by biopsy or resection, is frequently not possible in the absence of adequate radiographs and data on patient-specific features, such as the patient's history and age. For instance, the differentiation between benign and malignant tumors of cartilaginous origin demands a strong integration of radiologic and pathologic information. Together with the radiographic features of a bone lesion, it is important to consider the location of the lesion in the body and the location of the lesion in a particular bone to restrict the differential diagnosis.

After a differential diagnosis has been made, proper locoregional staging may be necessary, including the assessment of the exact position and size of the tumor within a bone, and its relation to a joint and/or neurovascular structures. It is well known that in this respect MR imaging is far superior to other imaging modalities including computed tomography (CT), bone scintigraphy and angiography [4]. In particular the combination of longitudinal T1-weighted spin-echo images (determination of intraosseous tumor extent and joint involvement) and axial T2-weighted (turbo) spin-echo images (extraosseous tumor extent, invasion or encasement of neurovascular bundles) is highly accurate. Staging procedures should always be performed before biopsy, to avoid the confusing influences of biopsy-related edema and hemorrhage. In selected cases, MR imaging features, such as morphologic appearance, presence of fluid-fluid levels, certain signal intensities (fat, blood) and enhancement characteristics after administration of intravenous Gd-DTPA, may contribute to a specific diagnosis.

16.2   Bone Tumors of the Hand

16.2.1   Incidence

Tumors of the carpals and hand are rare, as illustrated by the figures of large bone tumor registries. For instance, in series from the Mayo Clinic, primary bone tumors, either benign or malignant, located in the carpals or hand were encountered in 203 of 7,975 cases (2.5%) [15]. In the series of the Netherlands Committee on Bone Tumors (NCBT), malignant tumors, benign tumors and tumor-like lesions were located in carpals, metacarpals or phalanges in 385 of 6,873 cases (5.6%) [10]. Benign lesions constituted the great majority in both series: 174 of 203 (86%) and 340 of 385 (88%) in the Mayo Clinic and the Netherlands, respectively [10, 15]. Moreover, the vast majority of primary bone tumors of the hand, both benign and malignant, consist of lesions of cartilaginous origin. Malignant bone tumors are equally distributed in metacarpals and phalanges (21 and 24 patients respectively, NCBT); none were found in the carpals. Benign bone tumors were, by far, most frequently encountered in the phalanges (180 patients, NCBT) relative to the metacarpals and carpals (60 and 14 patients respectively, NCBT) [9]. Manifestations of the most common malignant and benign tumors of the hand are discussed below.

16.2.2   Malignant Primary Bone Tumors of the Hand

As shown above, bone tumors of the hand are malignant in less than one sixth of all cases. These malignant tumors are almost always *chondrosarcomas.*

16.2.2.1   Chondrosarcoma

Chondrosarcomas are malignant mesenchymal tumors that are characterized by the formation of cartilage by the tumor cells. Usually, chondrosarcomas develop without the presence of a precursory lesion. On the other hand, chondrosarcomas can develop secondarily from a benign, pre-existing enchondroma or osteochondroma. A substantially higher risk (up to 35%) of developing secondary chondrosarcoma exists in patients with multiple enchondromas (M. Ollier). Chondrosarcomas are further subdivided based on the histologic grade of malignancy (grades I–III).

In the series of the NCBT, the number of central chondrosarcomas in the hand was equally distributed in the metacarpals and phalanges. The tumors mainly arose in elderly patients, predominantly women (Fig. 16.1). Most of the chondrosarcomas were grade I. These tumors were never encountered in the carpal area.

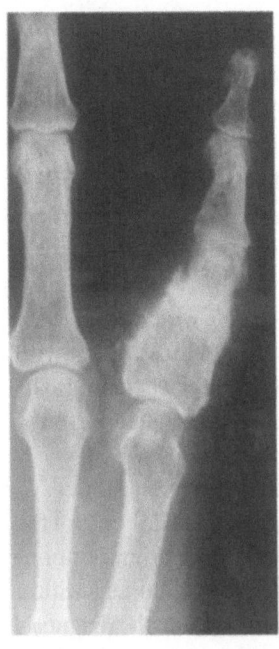

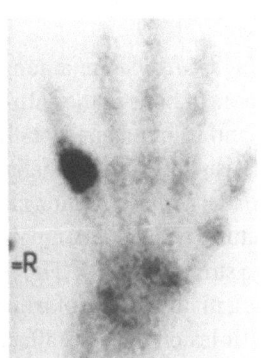

b

Fig. 16.1a, b. A 70-year-old woman with progressive swelling of the fifth digit of the right hand. Plain radiograph (a) displays a lucent lesion within the proximal phalanx with calcifications. There is some expansion. The pattern of bone destruction is partially geographic and otherwise moth-eaten with partial irregular destruction of cortical bone. 99mTc bone scintigraphy (b) shows very high uptake of the tracer at the proximal phalanx of the fifth digit. Biopsy followed by amputation of the fifth digit revealed *chondrosarcoma*

a

Peripheral chondrosarcoma, secondary to an osteochondroma in the hand, was found incidentally only [10].

Conventional radiographs are usually sufficient for the diagnosis of a cartilaginous tumor. Chondrosarcomas are typically osteolytic lesions with varying amounts of calcification, usually showing a geographic pattern of destruction with some expansion. The radiographic pattern is, however, influenced by the histologic degree of malignancy. The slowly progressive grade I chondrosarcoma can usually not be distinguished from its benign counterpart, enchondroma. Presence or absence of cortical destruction and the size of the lesions may be important features for radiographic differentiation. A considerable soft tissue swelling may be present [13].

The common manifestation of a chondrosarcoma on MR images is a lobulated lesion with intermediate signal intensity on T1-weighted images and high to very high signal intensity on T2-weighted images. A septal-nodular enhancement pattern can be found both in enchondroma and in low-grade chondrosarcoma on T1-weighted Gd-DTPA-enhanced images. Recently, dynamic contrast-enhanced gradient echo images were found to be helpful in the differentiation between benign and malignant cartilaginous tumors. Absence of enhancement during the dynamic sequence with a high temporal resolution favors the diagnosis of enchondroma, whereas early and progressive enhancement relative to arterial enhancement favors low-grade malignancy [5].

Histologically proven chondrosarcomas are usually resected, while curettage is used in patients with enchondroma. In selected cases, so-called borderline chondrosarcomas may also be treated by careful curettage, in combination with cryosurgery or application of phenol and bone grafting.

16.2.2.2   Other Malignant Bone Tumors of the Hand

Osteogenic sarcoma and *Ewing's sarcoma* are among the most frequently encountered primary malignant tumors of bone in the entire skeleton; however, manifestation of these tumors in the hand is found anecdotally only [6, 8]. The radiographic appearance of these tumors is usually evidently malignant, with ill-defined margins, a moth-eaten or permeative pattern of destruction and frequently an associated soft tissue mass. Radiographic features should be compared with clinical information, as *osteomyelitis* may present in a similar manner (Fig. 16.2).

Hemangioendothelioma is a malignant vasoformative tumor, which occurs very rarely. It is usually a purely lytic lesion that may affect any part of the skeleton, with a tendency toward the axial skeleton. The small bones of hand and feet may also be affected. Multifocal lesions, especially in contiguous bones, may be demonstrated in about one third of cases (Fig. 16.3).

Although *myeloma* and *metastasis* are the most common primary and secondarily malignant bone tumor respectively, particularly in older patients, the bones of the hand are almost never affected. However, in the case of a known primary tumor (especially kidney, lung, breast or colon) and a bone lesion in the hand with a malignant radiographic appearance, it is always necessary to exclude the diagnosis of metastasis [7]. Metastases to the bone can be misdiagnosed as osteomyelitis [17].

16.2.3   Benign Primary Bone Tumors of the Hand

Benign bone tumors of the hand are far more common than malignant tumors, as shown previously. The vast majority of such lesions are again formed by tumors of cartilaginous origin, particularly *enchondroma, juxtacortical chondroma* and *osteochondroma*.

Tumors or tumor-like lesions such as *osteoid osteoma, giant cell tumor* or *aneurysmal bone cyst* are much less prevalent but can be encountered in the metacarpal bones and phalanges. Moreover, there are various benign tumors that are found incidentally in the bones of the hand. There are also lesions that are found almost exclusively in the phalanges of the hand, including *glomus tumor* and *epidermoid*.

16.2.3.1   Enchondroma

Enchondromas are benign neoplasms, characterized by the formation of mature cartilage arising in the bone metaphysis as a solitary or multiple primary lesions (Fig. 16.4). The absolute incidence is not well known, as enchondromas are usually coincidental findings and do not cause symptoms. Enchondromas are seen at almost all ages; the median age is approximately 35 years. The phalanges in the hand are the main site for enchondromas. Multiple enchondromas present in a single patient in a predominantly unilateral distribution is known as Ollier's disease [9], whereas multiple enchondromas combined with multiple hemangiomas of the skin is known as Maffucci's syndrome (Fig. 16.5). Because of the reported malignant transformation

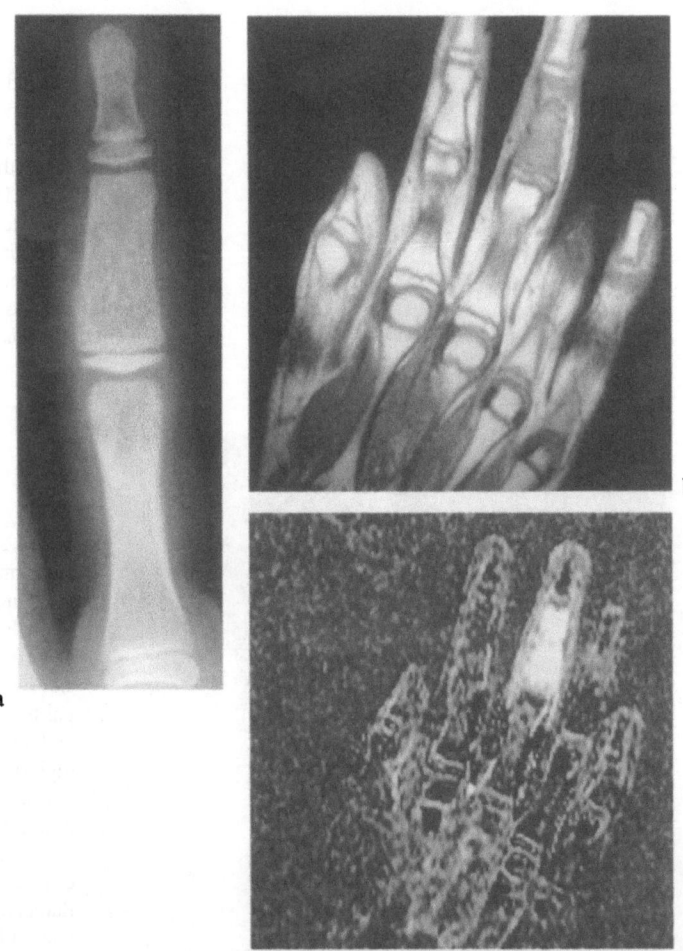

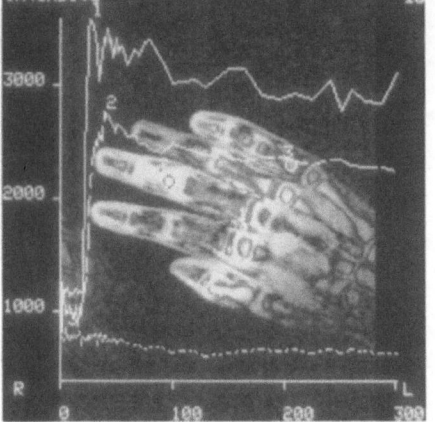

Fig. 16.2a–d. A 12-year-old boy with a painful and swollen digit. Plain radiograph (**a**) displays a permeative bone structure of the mid-phalanx. MR images show a lesion with intermediate signal intensity on coronal T1-weighted image (**b**), intense enhancement on coronal dynamic contrast-enhanced sequence with subtraction (**c**). The pattern of enhancement (**d**) is rapidly progressive with early wash-out according to time-signal intensity curve 2 (curve 1 represents arterial signal, curve 3 represents reference tissue). Because of the clinical presentation and the site of the lesion, radiologic diagnosis was osteomyelitis. Biopsy revealed *small cell osteogenic sarcoma*

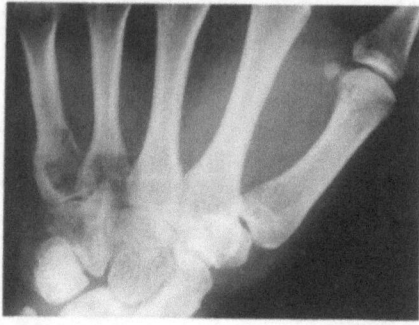

Fig. 16.3. A 28-year-old man with progressive complaints of pain and swelling of the left hand. Plain radiographs demonstrate lucent lesions at the base of both metacarpal bones IV and V of the left hand. There is interruption of the cortical bone; the lesions are partially not well defined. Differential diagnosis: lesions of vascular origin, enchondromas or giant cell tumors. Open biopsy was performed, which revealed *hemangioendothelioma*

a

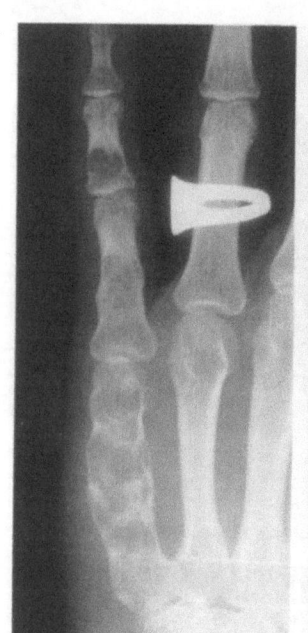

b

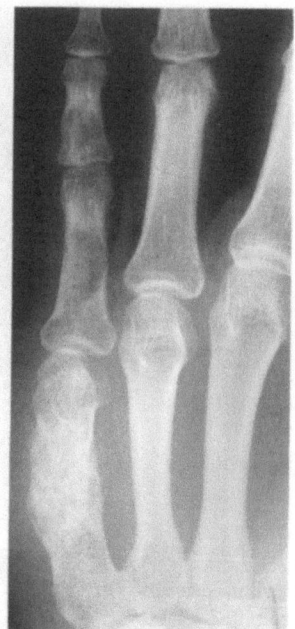

Fig. 16.4a, b. A 21-year-old man with multiple lesions of the fifth finger, without any symptoms. Plain radiographs show more or less uniform lucent lesions within the fifth metacarpal bone and in the proximal and mid-phalanx of the fifth digit (**a**). The lesions cause expansion and endosteal thinning of the cortical bone. There is some lobulation and discrete calcifications are appreciated. Radiologic diagnosis is consistent with *multiple enchondromas*. This was confirmed after surgery and curettage of the fifth metacarpal bone was performed (**b**)

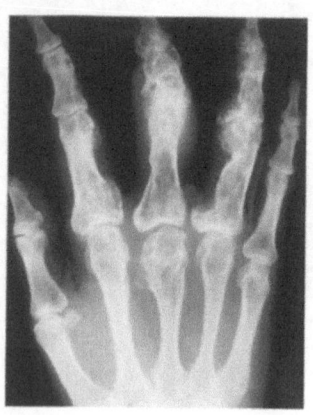

Fig. 16.5. A 47-year-old woman with multiple lesions in both hands. There are multiple lucent lesions within the distal metacarpal bones and in various phalanges of both hands, consistent with enchondromas as part of *Maffucci's syndrome*. Several surgical interventions occurred which revealed chondrosarcoma grade II of the right third digit, and chondrosarcoma grade I in the proximal and mid-phalanx of the left fourth digit

into chondrosarcoma or osteogenic sarcoma, active or painful cartilaginous lesions after termination of growth should be examined thoroughly.

Conventional radiography is usually well suited to render the diagnosis, combined with data on the patient's age, presence or absence of symptoms and lesional size. The lesions are usually lucent and sharply demarcated and some expansion is almost always found with thinning of the cortical bone. In contrast to locations elsewhere in the body, calcifications are frequently lacking in enchondromas of the small bones. The lobulated morphology and septal-nodular static enhancement features on MR imaging studies of enchondromas show overlap with low-grade chondrosarcomas; however, as stated previously, fast dynamic contrast-enhanced gradient-echo sequences may assist in the differentiation between enchondroma and low-grade chondrosarcoma.

16.2.3.2   Juxtacortical Chondroma

Juxtacortical chondroma is also frequently encountered in the small bones of the hand. It is a benign cartilage tumor located adjacent to and frequently partly embedded in the shaft of a tubular bone. As in the group of enchondromas, the age range is wide. Most often the chondroma of the phalanges is appreciated in the proximal third of the shaft. Radiographically, there is a soft tissue mass adjacent to the diaphysis of the metacarpal bone or phalanx, causing a variable indentation. Sometimes there is a thin bony shell covering the lesion on the outside.

16.2.3.3   Osteochondroma

Osteochondroma is a bony protrusion covered by a cartilaginous cap of variable thickness. Growth of osteochondromas can take place during enchondral growth and is normal. Growth of osteochondromas among adults should raise suspicion of malignant transformation to chondrosarcoma. Most patients presenting to an orthopedic surgeon with osteochondroma are in the second or third decade of life. Conventional radiographs are usually adequate for localization and diagnosis of osteochondromas. Typically, the cortical bone of the stalk of the osteochondroma is continuous with the cortex of the underlying bone. T2-weighted turbo spin echo MR images are optimal for assessment of the thickness of the cartilage cap. It is not possible to differentiate radiologically between benign osteochondroma and well-differentiated peripheral chondrosarcoma. Again, dynamic contrast-enhanced images may help, provided that the enchondral growth is finished. Osteochondromas are encountered in the hand; however they are much less prevalent than enchondromas. When an osteochondroma-like lesion is involved in small bones, such as the phalanges, it is likely to be a reactive process [10].

16.2.3.4   Osteoid Osteoma

Osteoid osteoma is a small benign tumor that consists of a central nidus of highly vascularized osteoblastic tissue, surrounded by a reactive (sclerotic) zone. It is a tumor of the first three decades that constitutes approximately 4% of all bone tumors. The bones of the hand are a relatively prominent location. Although asymptomatic osteoid osteomas are known to exist [2], usually there is rather severe pain, associated with the nidus, which is worst at night. Typically, salicylate medication gives definite relief of pain. In most cases, plain radiographs are sufficient for making the diagnosis. The typical case consists of a lucent lesion, 1–1.5 cm in size, with calcifications based on the nidus noted centrally. Usually there is a zone of dense, reactive sclerosis surrounding the lucent lesion. Frequently, a solid periosteal reaction is appreciated. Non-visualization of the nidus does occur. In these cases, CT is very helpful for demonstrating the nidus (Fig. 16.6). CT is also superior for guiding treatment, which aims at removal of the complete nidus. Currently, CT-guided thermocoagulation is a very efficient and cost-effective technique to treat osteoid osteomas at almost all sites within the skeleton, including the (small) bones of the hand. MR imaging allows visualization of the nidus, particularly on T2-weighted images with fat suppression. Moreover, frequently fairly high amounts of intraosseous and soft tissue edema and inflammatory reaction are seen.

16.2.3.5 Giant Cell Tumor

Giant cell tumors are relatively rare benign but aggressive bone tumors, demonstrating a high recurrence rate after removal of the lesion. Most tumors occur within the age range 15 to 45 years. The tumor is by far most commonly appreciated around the knee. The bones of the hand are only rarely involved; among these, the lesion occurs most frequently in the metacarpal bones [11, 13]. Almost all giant cell tumors local-

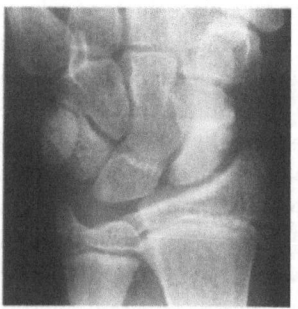
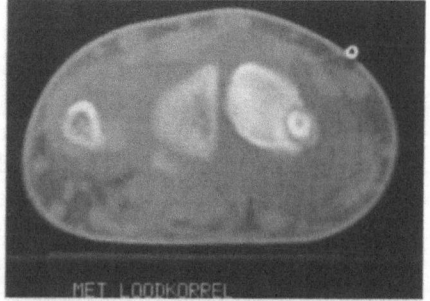
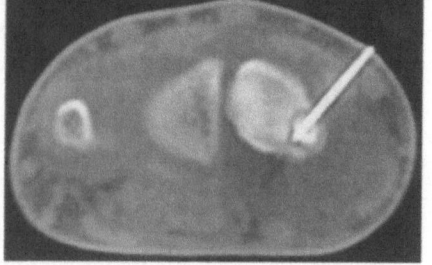

Fig. 16.6a–c. Well-defined lesion in the navicular bone of the left hand with sclerotic margin, peripheral lucent zone and lucent center. Furthermore, there is increased reactive sclerosis surrounding the lesion (a). A similar structure is seen on the axial CT image (b). The image was typical of *osteoid osteoma*, which was treated with percutaneously performed, CT-guided thermocoagulation (c)

ized in tubular bones are found in the epi-metaphyseal or epi-meta-diaphyseal area. The common radiographic manifestation consists of a predominantly osteolytic lesion, showing a geographic pattern of bone destruction (Figs. 16.7, 16.8). Usually internal ridges are seen and the margins are smooth. In the majority of cases there is regular destruction of the cortical bone. MR imaging is most helpful for demonstration of potential extension into the soft tissues. Due to the presence of highly vascularized tissue, giant cell tumors show a rather uniform rapidly progressive pattern of enhancement during a dynamic contrast-enhanced sequence, followed by wash-out (Fig. 16.7). This is also a helpful feature in the detection of recurrences, as opposed to postoperative reactive changes that may occur [16]. Giant cell tumors of bones in the hand are more likely to recur than those that arise elsewhere, so adequate surgical therapy is indicated with thorough follow-up [12, 14].

16.2.3.6 Aneurysmal Bone Cyst

Aneurysmal bone cysts may have the same radiographic features as giant cell tumors but usually there is more expansion and demarcation by a thin bony shell. Moreover, aneurysmal bone cysts are commonly prevalent in a younger population (median age, 14 years). Aneurysmal bone cysts are tumor-like lesions including multiple cavities filled with blood. These cavities with blood-blood levels are very well appreciated on native T1-weighted or T2-weighted MR images, on both sequences expressed by a high signal intensity. Within the hand, the metacarpal bone is the most frequent localization, usually in the metadiaphyseal region [1]. Aneurysmal bone cyst may also be present as a secondary in conjunction with another primary bone tumor, for instance giant cell tumor, chondroblastoma or fibrous dysplasia (Fig. 16.7).

16.2.4 Tumors or Tumor-Like Lesions Related to the Phalanges of the Hand

16.2.4.1 Giant Cell Reaction of Bone

Giant cell reaction of bone is a rare reactive process, occurring predominantly in the phalanges of hand, which can mimic a bone tumor radiographically. Most frequently it is seen in the terminal phalanx of a finger, presenting as an osteolytic lesion with sharp and sclerotic borders (Fig. 16.9). Usually there is some expansion and partial disappearance of the cortical bone. Soft tissue swelling may coexist. At this particular localization, a *glomus tumor* or an *epidermoid cyst* may have a similar radiographic appearance.

16.2.4.2 Epidermoid Cyst

Epidermoid cysts are non-neoplastic bone lesions, consisting of a single cavity lined by epithelium. Cysts of the terminal phalanx, which is one of the preferential sites, are thought to have a traumatic origin. Sometimes there is an associated

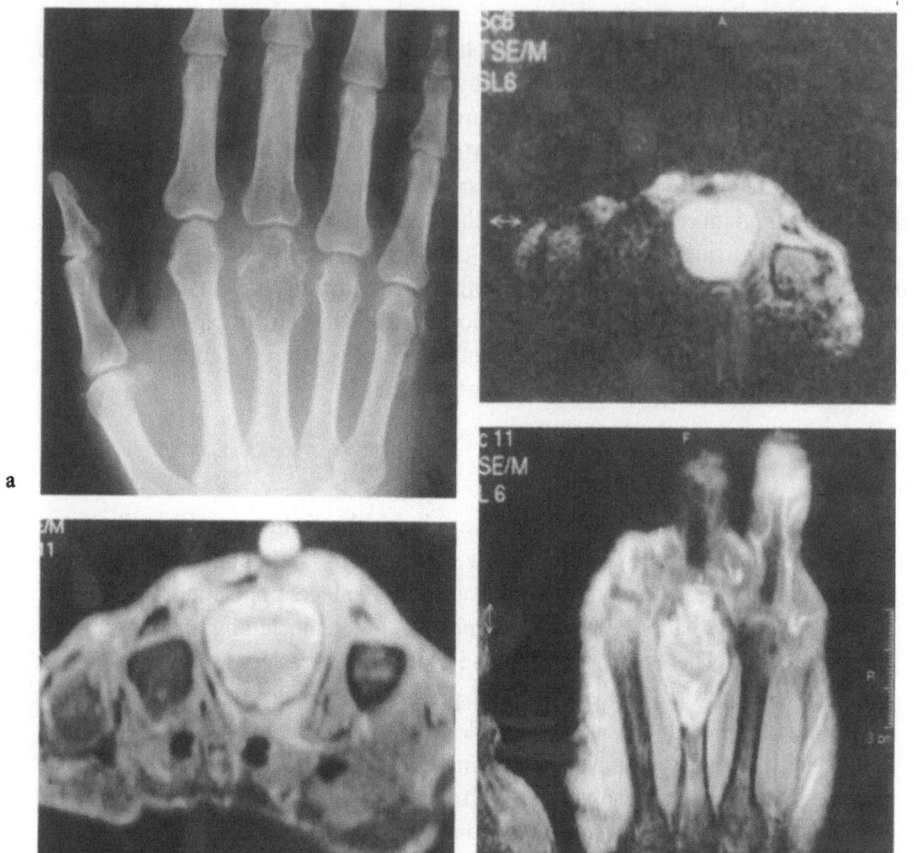

Fig. 16.7a-d (16.7e, f and legend on next page)

swelling. Radiographically, the lesion causes a sharply demarcated osteolytic defect with expansion and sometimes interruption of the cortex (Fig.16.10). As shown above, the differential diagnosis includes a giant cell reaction of bone and enchondroma.

16.2.4.3 Glomus Tumor

A glomus tumor is a benign tumor which originates from a neuromyoarterial plexus in the subcutaneous tissue. These so-called glomus bodies are, among others, particularly found in the soft tissues of the tip of fingers and occasionally in the bone marrow compartment of the terminal phalanx. Therefore, a primary intraosseous glomus tumor manifestation is very rare; more frequently erosion of bone secondary to a soft tissue glomus tumor is depicted. In the case of an intraosseous glomus tumor, a sharply demarcated punched-out osteolytic lesion is appreciated.

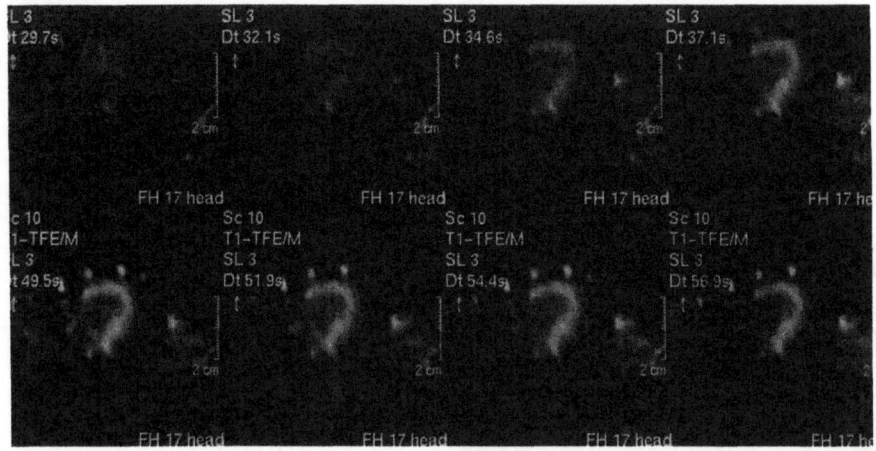

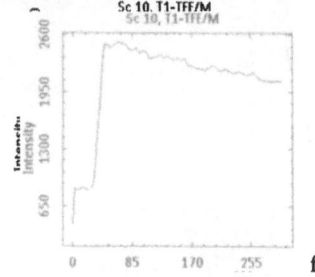

Fig. 16.7a–f. A 59-year-old man with increasing swelling of the right hand. Plain radiograph (**a**) shows an expansive lucent and multilocular lesion within the third metacarpal bone of the right hand. The margins are sharp and there is thinning of the cortical bone. MR images (**b–f**) reveal an expansive lesion with very high signal intensity on T2-weighted image with fat-selective presaturation (**b**), at least partially consistent with the presence of blood. Fluid levels are appreciated (**c**) and static enhancement on coronal image is according to a multilocular pattern (**d**). Dynamic contrast-enhanced sequence with subtraction demonstrates early (**e**) and rapidly progressive enhancement of the lesion (time-signal intensity curve) with early wash-out (**f**). The combination of the radiographic and MR characteristics indicates a diagnosis *of giant cell tumor* with secondary *aneurysmal bone cyst*, which was confirmed histologically on material obtained by biopsy

16.2.5 Other (Incidental) Benign Bone Tumors or Tumor-Like Lesions of the Hand

Osteoblastoma is also called giant osteoid osteoma and is mainly seen in young patients between 10 and 20 years of age. The pattern of complaints with pain throughout the day differs from osteoid osteoma. Incidentally, this tumor is encountered in a metacarpal bone or phalanx [11]. Radiographically, the tumor has an osteolytic appearance, with varying amounts of ossification and a geographic pattern of bone destruction. Especially in the carpus and tubular bones of the hand, marked expansion can be seen. Presence of internal septa and ridges depicted in osteoblastoma of the hand may mimic giant cell tumor or aneurysmal bone cyst.

Chondroblastoma of the bones of the hand is extremely rare [3]. This primary bone tumor is of cartilaginous origin and mainly occurs in the second and third decades of life. Radiographically, there is usually an osteolytic appearance, with

a

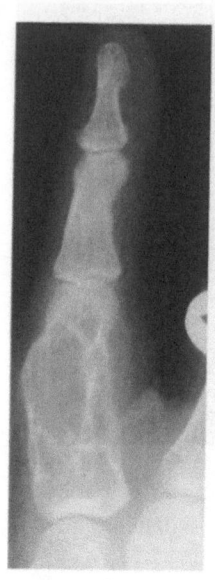
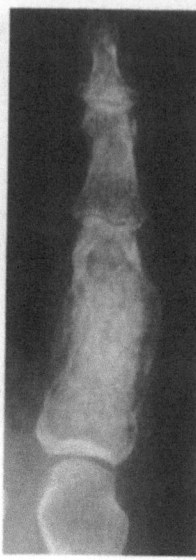

b

Fig. 16.8a, b. A 39-year-old man with swelling of the proximal phalanx of the left fifth digit. Plain radiograph exhibits an expansive lucent lesion with internal sclerotic ridges (a). There is regular cortical destruction with some soft tissue swelling. Differential diagnosis: giant cell tumor or enchondroma. Curettage with bone plasty was performed (b); histologic diagnosis was *giant cell tumor*

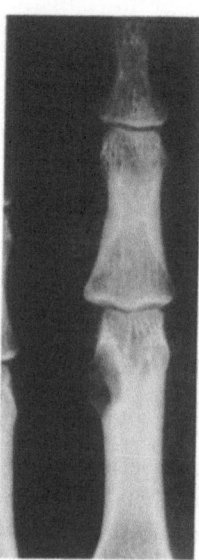
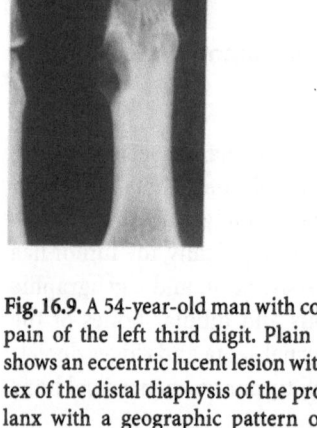

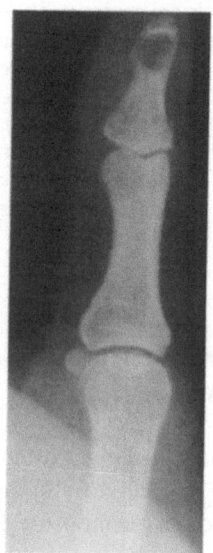

Fig. 16.9. A 54-year-old man with complaints of pain of the left third digit. Plain radiograph shows an eccentric lucent lesion within the cortex of the distal diaphysis of the proximal phalanx with a geographic pattern of bone destruction. The lesion is well demarcated. Differential diagnosis: eccentric chondroma or giant cell granuloma. Histologic diagnosis after curettage revealed *giant cell granuloma*

Fig. 16.10. A 43-year-old woman with progressive swelling of the distal phalanx of the left thumb. Plain radiograph depicts a well-defined lucent lesion, showing regular destruction of the cortical bone. Differential diagnosis: epidermoid cysts, glomus tumor or enchondroma. Histologic diagnosis: *epidermoid cyst*

more or less lobulated contours. The tumor is invariably related to a growth plate. Usually there is regular cortical destruction and a regular periosteal reaction. Commonly, there is rather extensive edema and inflammation related to the tumor, which can be demonstrated with MR imaging (high signal intensity on T2-weighted images).

Brown tumors can occur in any bone, including metacarpal bones, due to pronounced focal bone resorption as part of a metabolic disorder (hyperparathyroidism) which causes levels of calcium in the serum and urine to be increased and phosphate in the serum to be decreased. These tumors present as osteolytic lesions with sharp, though non-sclerotic, margins. Expansion, especially in small tubular bones may occur. The lesion may be confused with a giant cell tumor in an epi-metaphyseal area. Biochemical tests will confirm the former diagnosis.

Fibrous dysplasia is a benign tumor-like lesion, which is most frequently encountered in the first three decades, either as a solitary focus or in a polyostotic form. Fibrous lesions rarely occur in the hand. Most lesions display an osteolytic radiographic appearance in a metadiaphyseal or diaphyseal area. Ground-glass appearance may be present but this is not a sensitive sign. The destruction pattern of bone is always geographic. Depending on the presence or absence of calcification or ossification and on the rate of expansion, fibrous dysplasia may resemble giant cell tumor, aneurysmal bone cyst or enchondroma.

Hemangioma is a rare benign disorder that may occur in soft tissues or bone. Most of these lesions do not cause any symptoms. Radiographic features include the extent of trabecular and cortical bone. Most hemangiomas are found in the ribs, spine or skull. Occasionally, a phalanx of the hand is involved (Fig. 16.11).

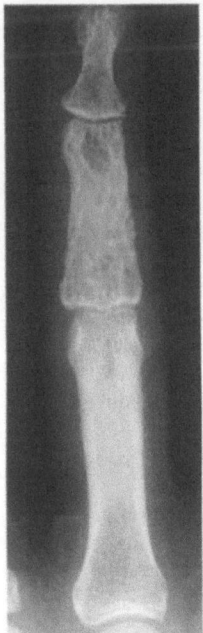

Fig. 16.11. A 61-year-old woman with mild complaints of the mid-phalanx of the third right digit. Plain radiograph depicts a lucent lesion with vertically oriented internal ridges. The radiologic diagnosis of *hemangioma* was confirmed histologically after biopsy

16.3   Concluding Remarks

Intraosseous bone lesions in the hand are almost always enchondromas, which may occur at any age, usually without any symptoms. In older patients, enchondroma-like lesions causing symptoms or demonstrating alterations over time should be considered with suspicion, and low-grade chondrosarcoma should be excluded. MR imaging, especially dynamic contrast-enhanced sequences, may be helpful to this end. The prevalence of malignant bone tumors of the hand other than chondrosarcoma is very low.

Osteoid osteoma and giant cell tumor are among the less rare benign bone lesions of the hand. Osteoid osteoma has typical clinical features and is best depicted for diagnosis and guiding of treatment with spiral CT. Giant cell tumors of the hand are almost exclusively found in the metacarpal bones. The radiographic pattern is nonspecific; however, rapidly progressive enhancement with early plateau phase or wash-out using a dynamic contrast-enhanced MR sequence may be of help, and also for the (early) detection of recurrent tumor. Sometimes fluid-fluid levels may be appreciated, indicating presence of an aneurysmal bone cyst, which can be primary or secondary.

References

1. Apaydin A, Ozkaywak C, Yilmaz S, et al (1996) Aneurysmal bone cyst of metacarpal. Skeletal Radiol 25:76–78
2. Basu S, Basu P, Donell JK, (1999) Painless osteoid osteoma in a metacarpal. J Hand Surg [Br] 24:133–134
3. Bliss DG, Mann RJ (1985) Chondroblastoma of a metacarpal. Report of a case and review of the literature. Clin Orthop 194:211–213
4. Bloem JL, Taminiau AHM, Eulderink F, Hermans J, Pauwels EJK (1988) Radiologic staging of primary bone sarcoma: MR imaging, scintigraphy, angiography and CT correlated with pathologic examinations. Radiology 169:805–810
5. Geirnaerdt MJA, Hogendoorn PCW, Bloem JL, Taminiau AHM, van der Woude HJ (2000) Fast contrast-enhanced MR imaging of cartilaginous tumors. Radiology 214:539–546
6. Kedar A, Bialik V, Fishman J (1984) Ewing sarcoma of the hand: literature review and a case report of nonsurgical management. J Surg Oncol 25:25–27
7. Kobus RJ, Leinberry C, Kirkpatrick WH (1992) Metastatic renal carcinoma in the hand: treatment with preoperative irradiation and ray resection. Orthop Rev 21:983–984, 990–995
8. Liu Y, Chen WY (1998) Ewing's sarcoma of the metacarpal bone of the hand: a case report. J Hand Surg [Am] 23:748–752
9. Miyawaki T, Kinoshita Y, Iizuka T (1997) A case of Ollier's disease of the hand. Ann Plast Surg 38:77–80
10. Mulder JD, Schutte HE, Kroon HM, Taconis WK (1993) Radiologic atlas of bone tumors. Elsevier, Amsterdam
11. Olbourne NA, Saad MN, Clement R (1974) Benign osteoblastoma of the metacarpal bone. Hand 6:198–203
12. Pardo-Montaner J, Pina-Medina A, Barcelo-ALcaniz M (1998) Recurrent metacarpal giant cell tumour treated by en bloc resection and metatarsal transfer. J Hand Surg [Br] 23:275–278

13. Roberts PH, Price CH (1977). Chondrosarcoma of the bones of the hand. J Bone Joint Surg Br 59:213–221
14. Singhai RM, Mukhopadhyay S, Tanwar RK, Pant GS, Julka PK (1994) Case report: giant cell tumour of metacarpals: report of three cases. Br J Radiol 67:408–410
15. Unni KK (1996) Dahlin's bone tumours: general aspects and data on 11087 cases, 5th edn. Lippincott-Raven, Springfield, Ill
16. van der Woude HJ, Verstraete KL, Hogendoorn PCW, Taminiau AHM, Bloem JL (1998) Fast dynamic contrast-enhanced subtraction MR imaging in patients with musculoskeletal tumors. Radiology 208:821–828
17. Wu KK, Guise ER (1978) Metastatic tumors of the hand: a report of six cases. J Hand Surg [Am] 3:271–276

17   Instability of the Wrist

M. Maas, M. P. J. F. Ritt

17.1   Introduction

Movement of the hand relative to the forearm shows a unique combination of motions – flexion-extension, radial-ulnar deviation and even some rotation – while adequate stability is still maintained. Therefore, the human wrist is unlike any other joint in the body. It is not a simple hinge joint or ball-socket joint and does not have an ideal mechanical equivalent. It consists of eight carpal bones, each with their own unique center or axis of rotation, forming a multiple intercalated kinematic chain capable of providing a large range of motion while resisting external forces and torques. However, like any kinematic system, this design also has its potential flaws. Normal wrist function requires precise interaction of bony architecture and soft tissue constraints. Disruption of this delicate functional interdependency between the geometry of bones and soft tissues, by either fracture or ligament injury, may create varying degrees of carpal instability precluding adequate long-term function of the wrist.

Instability of the wrist following injury to its ligaments was first suggested in 1943 by Lambrinudi and coworkers [1, 2]. They popularized the concept of the wrist as a "link" mechanism in which the radius, the proximal carpal row and the distal carpal row constitute the individual links. The link mechanism is stable in tension but collapses with axial compression. In 1961, Landsmeer [3] further developed this concept, emphasizing the role of the proximal carpal bones as intercalated segments, but the concept of post-traumatic carpal instability was not clearly formulated for purposes of diagnosis and treatment until the Hunterian lecture "Carpal instability and the fractured scaphoid" by Sir Geoffrey Fisk [4, 5] in 1968. The true impact of carpal instability on post-traumatic wrist pain was most lucidly explained in 1972 when coworkers Linscheid and Dobyns [6] published their classic work on "Traumatic instability of the wrist". In this study both fracture and ligament damage were implicated as potential causes of carpal instability and the "slider-crank" analogy to explain the scaphoid's role in preventing intercarpal collapse was introduced. The basic and now fundamental concepts of dorsiflexion (DISI) and volar (=palmar) flexion (VISI) intercalated segmental instability were proposed in this work and have served wrist surgeons as basic principles for patient assessment over the past 25 years.

17.2   Definition and Classification

According to the International Wrist Investigators' Workshop, carpal instability is defined as a condition represented by the inability to maintain, or an actual loss of, normal alignment of carpal bones under physiologic loads. Its corollary is that instability alters normal carpal kinematics. Alternatively, for clinical use, it can be defined as a condition in which normal anatomic relationships are present but through some provocative maneuver, such as external stress, muscle contracture, or positioning, an abnormal relationship can be demonstrated. Once this stress positioning or contracture stops, the parts (usually bones) can be returned to their normal anatomic positions. Such abnormal positions are called subluxation if they are not extreme enough to fit the definition for a "dislocation" or a "fracture-dislocation". Radiologically, the abnormal carpal position or arc of motion can be documented using non-stress and stress (provocative) maneuvers with various imaging techniques to confirm the diagnosis.

Classifications of carpal instabilities using different concepts of wrist kinematics have been described by Taleisnik [7] (a modification of Navarro's [8] traditional columnar wrist concept), Weber [9] (radial and ulnar column), Lichtman [10] (oval ring concept), McMurtry et al. [11] (intrinsic and extrinsic disruption) and the Mayo Clinic group [12] amongst others. Each classification emphasizes a certain aspect of wrist function important in understanding the complex function of the wrist. In an attempt to be able to give a complete analysis of carpal instability, Larsen et al. [13] and Hodge et al. [14] proposed a standardized analysis to assist in the diagnosis, give guidelines for treatment and ensure unity when comparing treatment results. Using this analysis, instability should be presented with information in six categories describing its chronicity, constancy, etiology, location, direction and pattern. Consensus about a classification of carpal instability patterns is needed but has not yet been reached.

For clinical use, wrist instabilities can be classified into three groups depending on their anatomic location:

1. Carpal instability:
   The abnormal alignment is located between adjacent carpal bones or between carpal bones and the radius. This is by far the most common type of instability in the wrist
2. Carpometacarpal instability:
   The abnormal alignment is located between the carpus and the metacarpus,
3. Radioulnar instability:
   The abnormal alignment is located between the distal radius and ulna (DRUJ).

In daily practice, parameters used for further definition are:
- *localization* of the pathology,
- *pattern* of instability,
- *degree* of instability.

17.3   Imaging

Several radiologic modalities are used in the evaluation of wrist instability, including plain radiography, cinematography (video fluoroscopy), CT and MRI [15]. Where appropriate, all these modalities will be discussed when dealing with the separate pathologic entities in the following paragraphs.

Arthrography is considered less helpful: it is semi-invasive, it does not provide information about the exact location and size of the ligament defect and there are one-way leaks possible leading to false negative results. The actual techniques of the various modalities are discussed elsewhere in this book and are therefore considered beyond the scope of this chapter. However, a few words concerning cinematography are necessary.

The normal movements of each carpal bone separately as well as their intercarpal relationships are complex. When performing fluoroscopy of the wrist, the movements of the scaphoid, the lunate and the capitate are the main issues of interest. In order to analyze the pathologic movements, it is mandatory to be familiar with the normal movements [16, 17]. When performing this investigation both wrists should be evaluated for comparison. First the hand is placed in a posteroanterior (PA) position in which both radial and ulnar deviation is performed. In the lateral projection some tilting of the wrist is obligatory in order to see the radiocarpal joint optimally. In this projection both radial and ulnar deviation as well as dorsal and palmar flexion are performed. Finally, some axial stress as well as dorsopalmar translation of the wrist is applied, in order to exclude any dynamic pathology. When taping this dynamic fluoroscopy on video it is possible to discuss the findings in a multidisciplinary setting, which is recommended.

17.4   Carpal Instability

17.4.1   Location of Instability

According to the *localization* of the pathology the following categories can be made (Fig. 17.1):

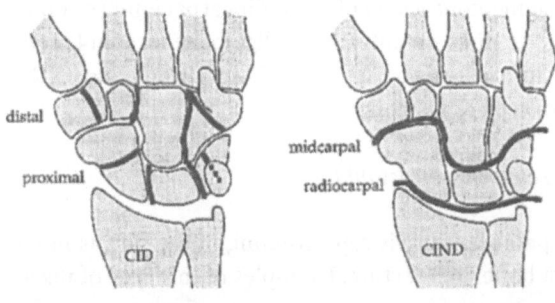

Fig. 17.1. Localization of the pathology in dissociative and nondissociative instability

17.4.1.1   Carpal Instability Dissociative (CID)

In carpal instability dissociative (CID) there is instability between carpals of the same row. Depending on which row is affected, the CID type can be subdivided into a proximal row CID and a distal row CID.

In proximal row CID, there are two possible locations of dissociation. There can be dissociation between the scaphoid and lunate (SL dissociation) or between the lunate and the triquetrum (LT dissociation). SL dissociation is more frequent but may be difficult to diagnose in the acute stage. Both entities are discussed below.

In the distal row CID can occur in combination with a fracture-dislocation and instability of the ossa metacarpalia. The pattern of collapse runs longitudinally and can be subdivided into: axial-radial (AR), axial-ulnar (AU) or a combination of both. However, these types of instability are very rare and always caused by high-energy trauma with extensive soft tissue damage.

17.4.1.2   Carpal Instability Nondissociative (CIND)

In carpal instability nondissociative (CIND) the relationship between carpals within a row is undisturbed but the instability is between two rows, either at the radiocarpal or the midcarpal joint level.

Depending on which level of articulation is affected, the CIND type can be subdivided into radiocarpal, midcarpal or combined. In the radiocarpal type, the carpus can be tilted dorsally relative to the radius (DISI), dorsally translated (DT) or proximally migrated (PM), after a distal radius fracture. Ulnar translation (UT) of the carpus is rarely caused by trauma, but frequent in rheumatoid arthritis.

A midcarpal type can be caused by a ligamentous lesion between, for example, the triquetrum (proximal row) and the hamate and capitate (distal row). Typically, and much more frequently, however, midcarpal instability is caused by a severe ligamentous laxity without any preceding trauma, e.g., in young females.

The so-called CLIP syndrome (capitate-lunate instability pattern) as described by Louis et al. [18] is an example of a combination of a radiocarpal and a midcarpal CIND type of instability.

17.4.1.3   CIC: Combined or Complex CID/CIND Instability

Combinations of these types of carpal instability are not uncommon. For example a perilunar luxation causes a ligamentous lesion of the radiocarpal joint (radiolunate, radiocapitate ligaments), as does an intercarpal ligament (scapholunate, lunotriquetrum). This results in a combined CID (SL dissociation) and CIND (ulnar translation of the lunate) type of instability.

17.4.1.4   Adaptive Carpus or Pseudocarpal Instability

Adaptive carpus or pseudocarpal instability is repositioning of the carpus in response to some change in wrist bone architecture. Examples of this type of instability are DISI or DT in response to dorsiflexion malunion of the distal radius, DISI in response to a healed malunion of the scaphoid or VISI in response to lack of healing of the lunate in Kienböck's disease. The immediacy and degree of response to these bony deformities also depend on the degree of ligamentous laxity, which is also an important ingredient in many of the true instabilities.

17.4.1.5 Rotational Instability

Recently, it has been suggested from cadaver studies that specific ligamentous injuries may lead to a rotational type of instability, which has received little attention in the literature [19]. Future studies will address this possible type of instability.

17.4.2 Pattern of Instability

The division in patterns of instability is not a diagnostic one but purely a description of certain positional abnormalities as seen on radiographs. The most common patterns are:

17.4.2.1 Dorsal Intercalated Segment Instability (DISI)

In dorsal intercalated segment instability there exists a dorsiflexed lunate. In SL dissociation this is combined with a palmar flexion of the scaphoid. By definition the angle between the axis of the scaphoid and the lunate, measured on a standard lateral radiograph, should be between 30° and 60° with an average of 47° (Fig. 17.2A). In a DISI pattern, the SL angle exceeds 70° (Fig. 17.2B). The cause lies within the proximal row, so it is a CID type of instability.

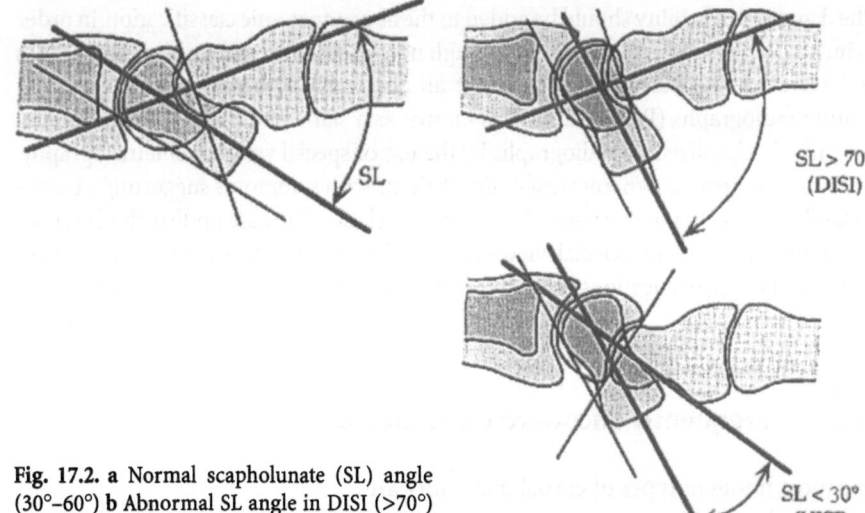

Fig. 17.2. a Normal scapholunate (SL) angle (30°–60°) b Abnormal SL angle in DISI (>70°) and VISI (<30°)

17.4.2.2 Volar (=Palmar) Intercalated Segment Instability (VISI)

In volar (=palmar) intercalated segment instability the lunate is palmar flexed. When the lunate is palmar flexed together with the rest of the proximal row, e.g., in a dislocated distal radius fracture, it is a CIND type of instability. Alternatively, when the lunate is flexed together with the scaphoid only and the triquetrum is tilted dorsally, e.g., in LT dissociation, it is a CID type of instability. However, this stance can also be found in midcarpal instability and this is again a CIND type of instability. This perhaps demonstrates best the limitations of this descriptive type of classification.

Less common patterns are:

17.4.2.3 Ulnar Translation (UT)

In ulnar translation the carpus is ulnarly translated. This occurs, for example, in rheumatoid arthritis.

17.4.2.4 Dorsal Translation (DT)

In dorsal translation the whole carpus is dorsally displaced relative to the radius. This occurs, for example, in dorsal fractures of the distal radius.

17.4.2.5 Proximal Migration (PM)

Proximal migration occurs in, for example, Madelung's deformity.

17.4.3 Degree of Instability

The degree of instability should be added to the above anatomic classification, in order to include anything from potential, although not yet obvious, malpositioning, to gross and severe damage and displacement. If an abnormal positioning can be seen on routine radiographs (PA/lateral) this is known as a static instability. If the instability can only be visualized on radiographs by the use of special views or cinematography, then this is known as dynamic instability. Patients with symptoms suggesting a carpal instability in which intercarpal and radiocarpal relationships are undisturbed on routine radiographs or on special views (e.g., in hyperlaxity) are categorized as predynamic. Finally, dislocations or fracture-dislocations form a separate category.

17.5 Frequently Encountered Pathology

The most frequent types of carpal instability are:
  · SL dissociation

- LT dissociation
- Midcarpal instability.

17.5.1   Scapholunate (SL) Dissociation

17.5.1.1   Clinical Presentation

Most typically this type of lesion is acquired with a fall backward on the hyperextended hand, twisting the wrist. Depending on several factors a wide variety of fractures or dislocations can occur, such as a distal radius fracture, scaphoid fracture, or a perilunate type of fracture-dislocation. When there is only a lesion of the ligaments attached to the scaphoid, the correct diagnosis is often easily overlooked, especially in the early stage. An SL dissociation can lead to carpal instability and eventually to post-traumatic arthritis.

17.5.1.2   Physical Examination

The physical examination reveals localized pain dorsally over the SL joint and a positive stress test according to Watson.

17.5.1.3   Radiologic Findings

Three types of radiologic findings can be distinguished:

Type I: SL dissociation with dynamic carpal instability. Standard PA and lateral radiographs are normal, and no increased SL joint interval, no abnormal axis of scaphoid or lunate are found. Video fluorography, however, can show a diastases of the SL joint in the motion tract between radial and ulnar deviation, where there is a normal position at the maximal deviation. MRI may find ligamentous tears; however, the use of a special device to stress the intercarpal SL ligament may be needed [15,20].

Type II: SL dissociation with static carpal instability (DISI). Standard PA radiographs reveal a widening of the SL joint interval (>3 mm) when compared with other joint spaces on the wrist and the opposite SL joint (Fig. 17.3). On the lateral radiograph a dorsal tilting of the lunate is shown (DISI stance) with a palmar flexion of the scaphoid (Fig. 17.4). The latter may also be visible on the PA view as the typical ring sign of the scaphoid (Figs. 17.5, 17.6). The angle between the axis of scaphoid and lunate is increased. MRI shows ligamentous discontinuity of the SL ligament, with signs of synovitis.

Type III: SL dissociation with carpal instability and secondary arthritis (SLAC wrist; scapholunate advanced collapse). Standard radiographs show osteo-arthritic changes at the radiocarpal joint. These changes may be located only at the styloid process of the radius or the entire radioscaphoid joint. Also in the later stages there may be osteoarthritic changes, or additional changes at the lunate as well as progressive proximal migration of the capitate with widening of the SL joint interval (Figs. 17.7, 17.8).

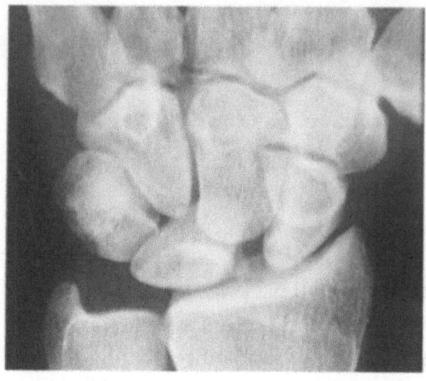

Fig. 17.3. Posteroanterior radiograph shows widening of the SL joint interval

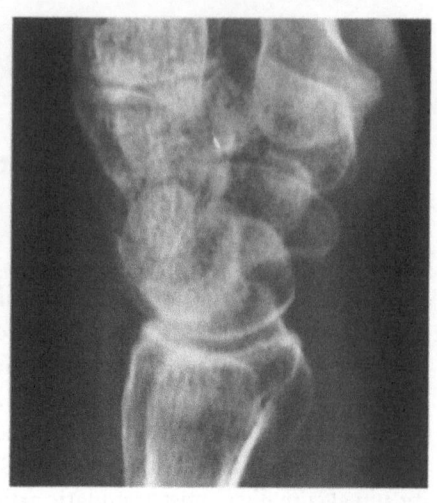

Fig. 17.4. Lateral radiograph showing DISI stance

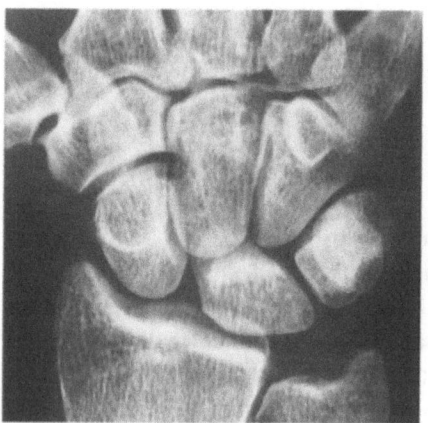

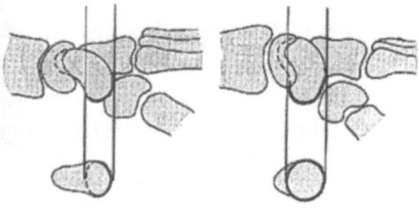

Fig. 17.5. Palmar flexion of the scaphoid may also be visible on the posteroanterior view as the typical ring sign of the scaphoid

Fig. 17.6. Ring sign

17.5.1.4   Surgery

The surgical therapy depends on the type of SL dissociation and the time interval between injury and diagnosis. In type I and II an attempt should be made to repair the SL ligament. The quality of the remaining tissue and therewith the feasibility of a repair can be easily assessed using arthroscopy. In type II, a correct repair can only be done if the tilting of the lunate and scaphoid can be redressed. Capsulodesis using dorsal capsular tissue or a ligament reconstruction using one of the various techniques can be performed in type I and II, should the ligament remnants render a repair impossible. The main goal of these repairs is to avoid the palmar flexion of the

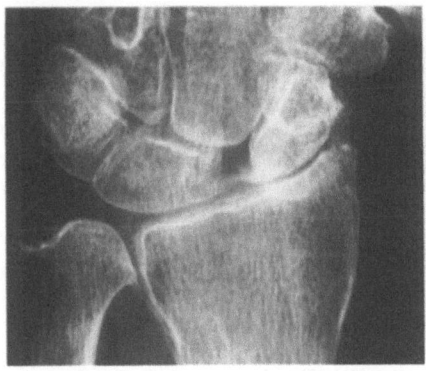 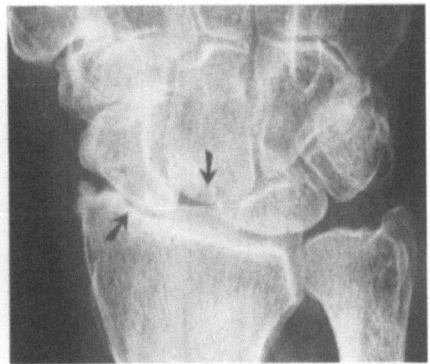

Fig. 17.7. Posteroanterior radiograph shows widening of the SL joint and radiocarpal osteoarthritis

Fig. 17.8. Posteroanterior radiograph showing an advanced stage of scapholunate advanced collapse (SLAC) wrist. There is proximal migration of the capitate and secondary arthritis

scaphoid. In type II several types of intercarpal arthrodesis have been described, e.g., scaphoid-capitate and scaphoid-trapezium-trapezoid arthrodesis. A fusion between scaphoid and lunate appears in more than one aspect ideal, but is very rarely performed due to extremely high non-union rates. In type III several salvage procedures are available such as lunate-capitate-triquetrum-hamate (LCTH) fusion taking out the scaphoid, proximal row carpectomy, and radiocarpometacarpal arthrodesis.

17.5.2   Scaphoid Non-union

A similar type of instability can occur after a scaphoid non-union has developed. Again a classification into three types can be made, in type III leading to a so-called SNAC wrist (scaphoid non-union advanced collapse) (Fig. 17.9). The treatment is, accordingly, to try to establish union in type I and the same salvage procedures as described above for type III.

17.5.3   Lunotriquetral (LT) dissociation

17.5.3.1   Clinical Presentation

An LT dissociation may be caused in several ways: a fall with the wrist in hyperextension, ulnar deviation and intercarpal supination can cause a classic perilunar dislocation emanating from the radial side in which LT dissociation occurs in type III; a perilunar dislocation emanating from the ulnar side when the wrist is forced into hyperextension, radial deviation and intercarpal pronation (type I to III according to Viegas et al. [21]); a degenerative type of LT lesion in the ulnocarpal abutment syndrome.

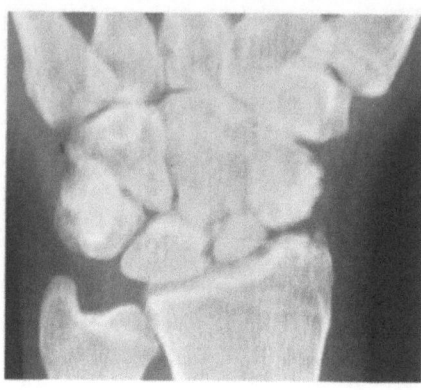

Fig. 17.9. Scaphoid non-union advanced collapse (SNAC) wrist

17.5.3.2 Radiologic Findings

A classification of LT lesions could be presented as follows:

Type I: Partial or total LT lesion without carpal instability. Standard PA radiographs reveal no abnormality. Supplementary investigations are necessary, such as stress function films, arthrography or cinematography. However, arthroscopy, with midcarpal inspection, most likely is the modality of choice.

Type II: LT dissociation with dynamic VISI deformity (with or without ulna plus). Standard PA radiographs are normal. Radiographs in maximal deviation or cinematography show a dynamic VISI instability pattern.

Type III: LT dissociation with static VISI deformity. Standard PA radiographs show palmar flexion of the scaphoid and lunate while the triquetrum is dorsiflexed. The angle between lunate and triquetrum on the lateral view is less than 0°. There is a reduction in the distance between triquetrum and caput ulnae (Meyerbach's sign). Finally, there is a "step-off" of the proximal and distal carpal arch of the proximal carpal row at the LT junction.

17.5.3.3 Surgery

Preferably a LT ligament repair should be performed on the condition that enough tissue is available for repair and the VISI stance can be corrected. However, a longstanding VISI deformity and patients who perform heavy manual labor are contraindications for ligament repair. In case there is an ulna plus variance, an ulnar shortening should be performed in addition to the ligament repair.

17.5.4 Midcarpal Instability

There are two types of midcarpal instability: intrinsic and extrinsic [22].

The *intrinsic* type is caused by hyperlaxity without any trauma. The ligaments fail in constraining the normal interaction between distal and proximal carpal row.

17.5.4.1   Clinical

A typical finding is the so-called supination deformity, in which the hand is dropped palmarly at the radiocarpal joint level, with slight supination stance relative to the forearm. In passive or active ulnar deviation the whole proximal carpal row suddenly flips up and the deformity is corrected with a loud audible clunk, the so-called catch-up clunk according to Lichtman et al. [23].

17.5.4.2   Radiology

Conventional radiographs are normal. Cinematography of the wrist is the modality of choice in demonstrating this midcarpal instability [18, 19].

17.5.4.3   Surgery

The therapy is mostly conservative.

Extrinsic midcarpal instability is caused by a distal radius fracture with a dorsally tilted radiocarpal joint surface. Due to gradual attenuation of ligaments a DISI stance develops together with palmar tilting of the capitate. This deformation aligns the axes of the forearm and hand in a pathologic way. Therapy consists of correction osteotomy of the radius.

17.5.5   Carpometacarpal Instability

Carpometacarpal instability is an abnormal condition occurring between the metacarpal(s) and the distal row which results in the inability to maintain normal anatomic relationship(s) under physiologic loads. All carpometacarpal (CMC) joints may be involved, either isolated or together, or some may be involved with fractures, subluxations or dislocations of the adjacent carpal bones. The dislocations are more often dorsal but can be palmar, radial or ulnar. The direction of the dislocation is defined by the direction of displacement of the distal segment. Isolated CMC I instability with dorsoradial subluxation is quite common in postmenopausal women, and is degenerative in origin. It often progresses to osteoarthritis with gross joint changes. At the CMC II and III joint it is usually related to carpometacarpal bossing. When present at the CMC IV and/or V joints it is most commonly a frank fracture-dislocation after a high-energy injury. When combined with adjacent carpal instabilities, these conditions will fall into the longitudinal (axial) instability group (see above).

Recurrent symptoms of painful grip with variable clinical findings are the subtle signs of a simple sprain or CMC instability type I. Carpometacarpal stress tests may be positive.

Conventional radiography may very well be normal, though osteoarthritic changes may be found. However, CT, MRI or scintigraphy are of more value in detecting early osteoarthritis. When a subluxation or dislocation is present CT is the modality of choice. Multiplanar reconstruction will aid in delineating the extent of the pathology.

17.5.6   Radioulnar Instability

During rotation of the forearm, the radius rotates around the ulna and simultaneously translates in axial and transverse direction relative to the ulna. The joint surfaces of the distal radioulnar joint (DRUJ) are incongruent and, because of this, the contact area is very small, especially in full pronation or full supination. In both positions there is a tendency for luxation of the radius: palmarly in pronation and dorsally in supination. Intrinsic stability is largely provided by the articular disc or triangular fibro-cartilage (TFC), which is part of the triangular fibro-cartilage complex (TFCC) that is also of key importance in providing stability to the carpus [22]. This articular disc has its origin at the medial rim of the distal radius and inserts at the base of the styloid process of the ulna. During rotation of the forearm the radius also translates in axial direction relative to the ulna: distally in pronation and proximally in supination. Normal configuration of the radius and the radiocapitellar contact prohibits abnormal migration of the radius proximally. In addition, the articular disc and interosseous membrane prohibit excessive translation after a comminuted radial head fracture, after radial head excision and in an Essex-Lopresti fracture-dislocation.

Finally, the stability of the DRUJ is also reliant on the anatomy of the radius and ulna and their mutual interdependency. Every change in shape and length has its impact on the DRUJ, causing limited range of motion or even instability or dislocation [22].

Bowers [24] has proposed a classification which combines aspects of clinical presentation, provocative motion (pronation or supination), and anatomic abnormalities. It can be used as a guide for surgical treatment. Four groups of instabilities are distinguished:

I: Insufficiency of soft tissue constraints. This category includes lesions of the ulnar and radial attachments of the TFC (I-A), the ulnocarpal ligaments (I-B), the entire TFCC (I-C) and the dorsal capsular ligaments (I-D).

II: Intra-articular deformity. This category is subdivided into sequelae of fracture-dislocation of the sigmoid notch (II-A) and ulnar head (II-B).

III: Combination of intra-articular deformity and insufficiency of stabilizing ligaments. A typical example is DRUJ instability after Colles' fracture and TFC avulsion with or without ulnar styloid fracture.

IV: Extra-articular deformity. The DRUJ is normal or shows TFC insufficiency. Subdivisions of this category are malunion of the radius or ulna (IV-A), length discrepancy of the radius or ulna (IV-B) and combinations involving both bones (IV-C).

17.5.6.1   Clinical and Radiographic Evaluation

Inspection of the abnormal wrist in various positions of the forearm rotation and during active pronation and supination will reveal abnormalities such as swelling, prominence of the ulnar head, or restricted range of motion. Laxity or destabilization of the DRUJ may be demonstrated by provoking dorsopalmar translation. The "piano-key sign" may be elicited by depressing the ulnar head and watching it spring back.

Standard lateral radiographs are used to detect static dorsal or palmar (sub)luxation of the DRUJ. However, these may not be very sensitive. CT scans are ideal for evaluation of the articular surfaces of the DRUJ and detecting subluxation. Both wrists should be scanned together in both pronation and supination. MRI shows promising results in detecting TFC pathology [25–28]. Arthroscopy appears to be the most reliable tool for detecting and assessing lesions of the TFC. These may either be visualized directly or apparent if palpation of the TFC demonstrates absence of the trampoline effect due to loss of normal TFC tension.

17.5.7 Classification of Wrist Instability

Based on the above, we propose the following classification for wrist instability to be used in clinical practice:

1. Carpal instability dissociative (CID)

   1.1 Proximal carpal row CID

Unstable scaphoid fracture	DISI
Scapholunate dissociation	DISI
Lunotriquetral dissociation	VISI

   1.2 Distal carpal row CID

Axial-radial (AR) dislocation	RT/PM
Axial-ulnar (AU) dislocation	UT/PM

   1.3 Combined proximal/distal CID

2. Carpal instability nondissociative (CIND)

   2.1 Radiocarpal CIND

Palmar ligament rupture	DISI/UT
Dorsal ligament rupture	VISI/DT
In adaptive carpus (see below)	

   2.2 Midcarpal CIND

Ulnar MCI from palmar ligament damage	VISI
Radial MCI from palmar ligament damage	VISI
Combined UMCI/RMCI with palmar ligament damage	VISI
MCI from dorsal ligament damage	DISI

   2.3 Combined radiocarpal/midcarpal CIND

   Capitate-lunate instability pattern (CLIP)

3 Combined or complex CID/CIND instability (CIC)

Perilunate instability with radiocarpal instability	DISI/UT
Perilunate instability with axial instability	AxUI/UT
Radiocarpal with axial instability	AxRI/UT
Scapholunate dissociation with UT	DISI/UT

4 Adaptive carpus

Malposition with distal radius malunion	DISI or DT
Malposition with scaphoid non-union	DISI
Malposition with lunate malunion	DISI or VISI
Malposition with Madelung's deformity	UT/DISI/PT

5 Rotational instability

PM	= proximal migration
UT/RT/DT/PT	= ulnar/radial/dorsal/palmar translation
DISI	= dorsal intercalated segment instability
VISI	= volar (=palmar) intercalated segment instability
AxUI	= axial-ulnar instability
AxRI	= axial-radial instability

References

1. Gilford WW, Bolton RH, Lambrinudi C (1943) The mechanism of the wrist joint with special reference to fractures of the scaphoid. Guy's Hosp Rep 92:52–59
2. Lambrinudi C (1943) Paper read at the British Orthopaedic Association
3. Landsmeer JMF (1961) Studies in the anatomy of articulation. I: The equilibrium of the "intercalated" bone. Acta Morphol Neerl Scand 3:287–303
4. Fisk GR (1968) Hunterian Lecture read at the Royal College of Surgeons of England, 7 May 1968
5. Fisk GR (1970) Carpal instability and the fractured scaphoid. Ann R Coll Surg Eng 46:63–76
6. Linscheid RL, Dobyns JH, Beabout JW, Bryan RS (1972) Traumatic instability of the wrist: diagnosis, classification and pathomechanics. J Bone Joint Surg Am 54:1612–1632
7. Taleisnik J (1985) The wrist. Churchill Livingstone, New York, pp 39–49
8. Navarro A (1985) Luxaciones del carpo. An Fac Med (Montevideo, Uruguay, 1921) 6:113; cited after Taleisnik J (1985) The wrist. Churchill Livingstone, New York pp 229–238
9. Weber ER (1984) Concepts governing the rotational shift of the intercalated segment of the carpus. Orthop Clin North Am 15:193–207
10. Lichtman DM, Martin RA (1988) Introduction to the carpal instabilities. In: Lichtman DM (ed) The wrist and its disorders. Saunders, Philadelphia, pp 244–250
11. McMurtry RY, Paley D, Ebrahim N (1992a) Unified classification of carpal disruptions. Correspondence newsletters of the International Wrist Investigators' Workshop
12. Dobyns JH (1990) Classification of wrist instabilities. AAOS course: The wrist: problems and challenges. AAOS, Newport Beach
13. Larsen CF, Amadio PC, Gilula LA, Hodge JC (1995) Analysis of carpal instability: I. Description of the scheme. J Hand Surg [Am] 20:757–764
14. Hodge JC, Gilula LA, Larsen CF, Amadio PC (1995) Analysis of carpal instability: II. Clinical applications. J Hand Surg [Am] 20:765–776

15. Smith DK (1995) MR imaging of normal and injured wrist ligaments. MRI Clin North Am 3(2):229–248
16. Maas M, Dijkstra PF, Bos KE, Groenevelt F (1991) Cineradiography of normal and painful wrists. Radiology 181:343
17. Maas M, Dijkstra PF, Bos KE, Groenevelt F (1997) Dynamics of the painful wrist; a videofluoroscopic approach. Eur Radiol 7:S 440
18. Louis DS, Hankin FM, Greene TL, Braunstein EM, White SJ. 1984;Central carpal instability-capitate lunate instability pattern. Diagnosis by dynamic displacement. Orthopedics 7:1693–1696
19. Ritt MJPF, Stuart PR, Berglund LJ, Linscheid RL, Cooney WP, An KN (1995) Rotational stability of the carpus relative to the forearm. J Hand Surg [Am] 20:305–311
20. Tjin A Ton ER, Pattynama PMT, Bloem JL, Obermann WR (1995) Interosseous ligaments: device for applying stress in wrist MR imaging. Radiology 196:863–864
21. Viegas SF, Patterson RM, Peterson PD, Pogue DJ, Jenkins DK, Sweo TD, Hokanson JA (1990) Ulnar-sided perilunate instability; an anatomic and biomechanic study. J Hand Surg [Am] 15:268–278
22. Adams BD, Berger RA, Short WH, Viegas SF (1998) Instability of the wrist, including the distal radioulnar joint. Instructional course. AAOS, New Orleans
23. Lichtman DM, Schneider JR, Swafford AR, Mack GR (1981) Ulnar midcarpal instability: clinical and laboratory analysis. J Hand Surg [Am] 6:515–523
24. Bowers WH (1991) Instability of the distal radioulnar joint. Hand Clin 7:311–327
25. Gabl M, Lener M, Pechlaner S, Judmaier W (1996) The role of magnetic resonance imaging in the detection of lesions of the ulnocarpal complex. J Hand Surg [Br] 21:311
26. Sugimoto, et al (1994) Triangular fibrocartilage in asymptomatic subjects: investigation of abnormal MR signal intensity. Radiology 191:193
27. Totterman SM, et al (1996) Lesions of the triangular fibrocartilage complex: MR findings with a three dimensional gradient recalled echo sequence. Radiology 199:227
28. Totterman SMS, Miller RJ (1995) MR Imaging of the triangular fibrocartilage complex. MRI Clin North Am 3(2):213–228

18   Trauma of the Hand and Wrist

CARLO MASCIOCCHI, ALESSIA CATALUCCI, ANTONIO BARILE,
CARLO FALETTI

18.1   Introduction

The hand and wrist are common sites for trauma, resulting in various bony, capsular, ligamentous and tendinous injuries. Traumatic injuries of the wrist are very frequent and occur at every age. Some lesions happen characteristically in a specific decade of life. Bone mineralization, which could be considered age-related, and ligamentous resistance and compliance, together with the mechanism of the trauma determine the resulting lesion [1–5]. Thus, metaphyseal fractures and slipping epiphysis typically occur in children. Both carpal dislocations and fracture-dislocations typically occur in young adults. Fractures, dislocations and fracture-dislocations of the distal extremity of radius and ulna usually occur in the elderly.

The radiological examination is essential for a correct diagnosis, which needs to be prompt in order to avoid complications and disability due to unappreciated lesions. The standard wrist examination should include at least two views, projected perpendicular to each other: a posteroanterior (PA) radiograph and a lateral one. If needed, other specialised radiographic views may be used to obtain more details of a specific region of interest, even if this could be difficult to obtain in case of multiply injured adults or children [6–8]. Magnetic resonance imaging (MRI) or even computed tomography (CT) may be helpful in selected cases [9, 10].

Moreover, trauma imaging requires that the main anatomical variants of the wrist are known and recognised. The scaphoid and the triquetrum, more frequently than the other bones of the wrist, can be bipartite. The main supernumerary bones are the os triangularis, between the ulnar styloid and the triquetrum; the os styloideum, between trapezium, capitate and the base of the second and third metacarpal bones; the "central bone", between trapezium, capitate and scaphoid; and the os hamuli, corresponding to the hook of the hamate [11].

18.2   Wrist

18.2.1   Fractures of the Distal Extremity of Radius and Ulna

Fractures of the distal extremity of radius and ulna account for 12–15% of all fractures. They are observed at every age, even though in the elderly the fractures are attributable to less severe trauma [12]. They are caused by a fall on the hand in dorsal flexion or, less frequently, in ventral flexion. The type of fracture is also conditioned by the radial or ulnar flexion of the hand at the moment of impact [6]. Distal radial fractures are observed most frequently. These are often associated with ulnar fractures. Isolated distal ulnar fractures are rare (Fig. 18.1) [2].

Distal radial fractures are classified as articular or extra-articular, depending on the fracture course. They can be compound or not, with the distal fragment dorsally or, less frequently, ventrally dislocated.

Extra-articular fractures of the distal radius can be diagnosed on standard PA radiographs as a transverse line, 1–3 cm beyond the articulating surface. An abnormal orientation of the radial glenoid can be observed. Frequently, a fracture of the distal ulna can be seen (Fig. 18.2). On the lateral radiograph, the distal fragment could appear dorsally located, with the characteristic deformation similar to a fork (the so-called silver-fork fracture or Colles' fracture) (Fig. 18.3), or ventrally located (Goyrand's fracture). The latter occurs when the hand is flexed at the moment of the impact.

Articular fractures are diagnosed when the articulating surface of the distal radius is interrupted (Fig. 18.4). Often a transverse fracture at the level of the metaphysis is observed from which one or more vertical fracture lines go up to the radial glenoid (the so-called T fracture because the fracture appears as an upside down "T"). Rarely, there is only one isolated oblique or vertical fracture. The vertical fracture lies in either the sagittal or frontal plane; often it lies in both. Frequently, a distal ulnar fracture is an associated feature.

On the basis of both location and morphology, articular fractures are classified into: complex articular fractures (T fractures); marginal fractures, anterior or posterior; and cuneiform fractures, internal or external.

T fractures appear on the AP radiograph as a vertical line of fracture that cuts across a second transverse line, 1–3 cm beyond the articular surface. If the vertical

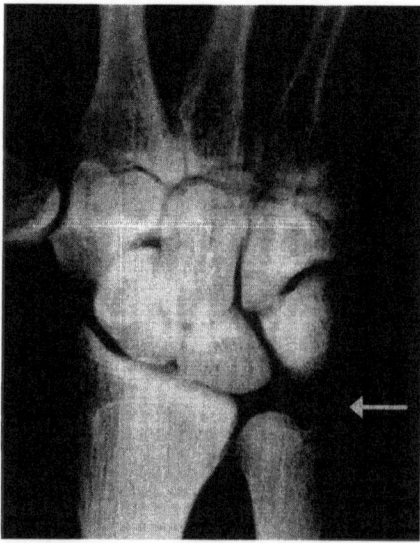

Fig. 18.1. Isolated fracture of the ulnar styloid (*arrow*)

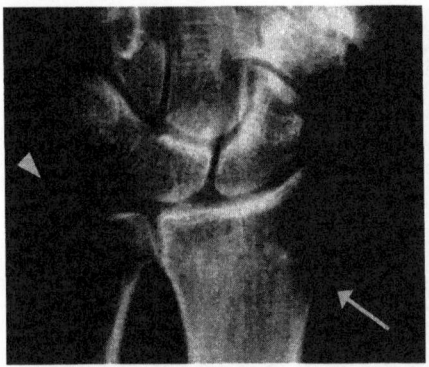

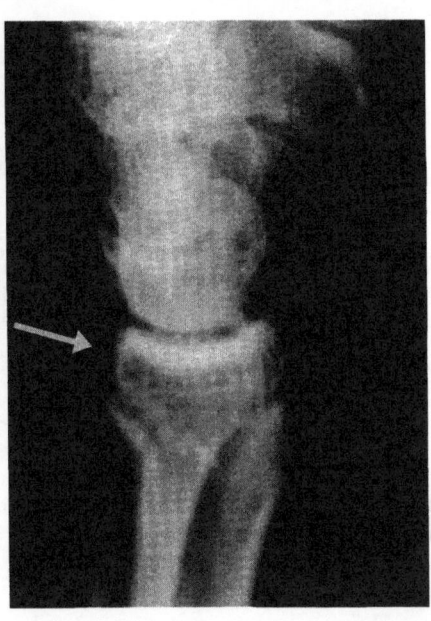

Fig. 18.2a, b. Extra-articular distal radial fracture. The anteroposterior (AP) radiograph (a) shows the transverse radiolucent line (*arrow*) and the associated fracture of the ulnar styloid (*arrowhead*); the lateral radiograph (b) shows the radial distal fragment slightly ventrally dislocated (*arrow*)

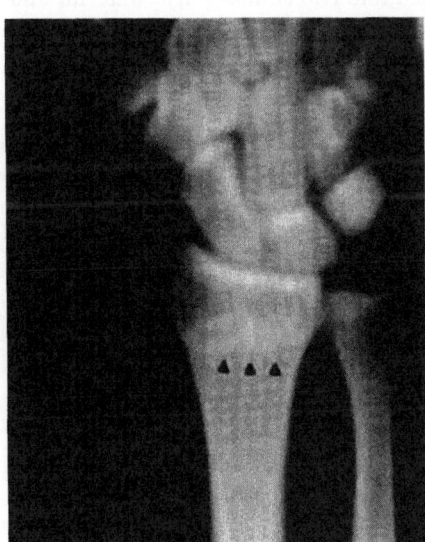

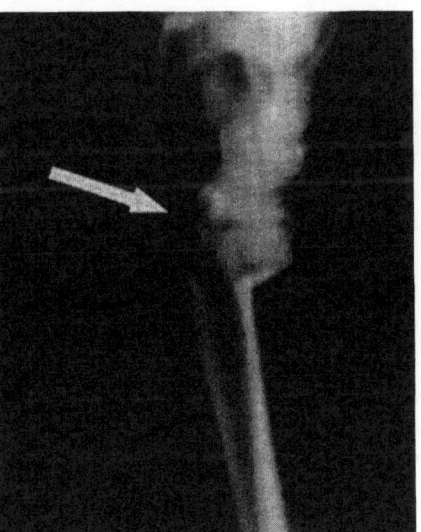

Fig. 18.3. AP (a) and lateral (b) radiographs showing a silver-fork fracture (Colles' fracture, *arrowheads*). The dorsal dislocation of the distal fragment (*arrow*) is well evident

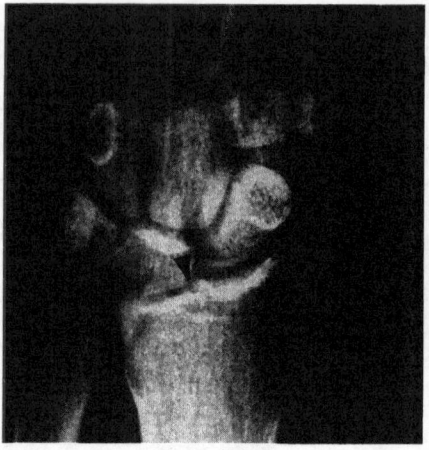

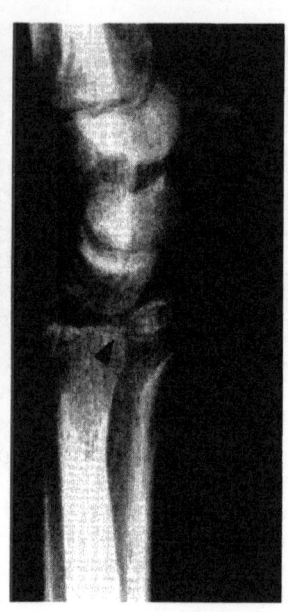

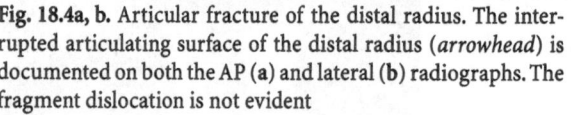

Fig. 18.4a, b. Articular fracture of the distal radius. The interrupted articulating surface of the distal radius (*arrowhead*) is documented on both the AP (a) and lateral (b) radiographs. The fragment dislocation is not evident

line is medial, the distal fragment is divided into two similar parts: anterior and posterior, if the vertical fracture lies in the frontal plane; internal and external if the vertical fracture lies in the sagittal plane. If the fracture line is not medial, the distal fragment is divided into two unequal parts. When the internal fragment is smaller than the external one, it is due to a direct impact on the radial epiphysis by the lunate. Sometimes a third central fragment is present. Particularly severe trauma can result in a comminuted fracture. On the lateral radiograph it is possible to appreciate different degrees of fragment dislocations, usually posteriorly.

Marginal fractures can be anterior or posterior; the latter (Rhea-Barton's fracture) often occur together with dorsal carpal dislocation. In this case, overlapping of both the scaphoid and lunate on the radial epiphysis is evident on the AP radiograph, besides the single vertical fracture extending from the radial metaphysis to the posterior articular surface. An anterior marginal fracture (Letenneur's fracture) is frequently associated with palmar dislocation of the carpal condyle; the fracture appears on the AP radiograph from the radial metaphysis to the anterior articular surface. The anterior fragment can be single or multiple (comminuted anterior marginal fracture).

Cuneiform fractures appear on the AP radiograph as a vertical line interrupting the articular surface; the isolated radial styloid fracture is a type of cuneiform fracture (Fig. 18.5). Involvement of the soft tissue is particularly helpful in diagnosing this type of fracture. In fact, the dislocation or the cancellation of either the fat pad besides the scaphoid bone (AP radiograph) or the fat pad of the pronator muscles (lateral radiograph) should raise the suspicion of an underlying fracture [4]. The fracture line may be unrecognisable on the standard radiological views, particularly when it lies externally.

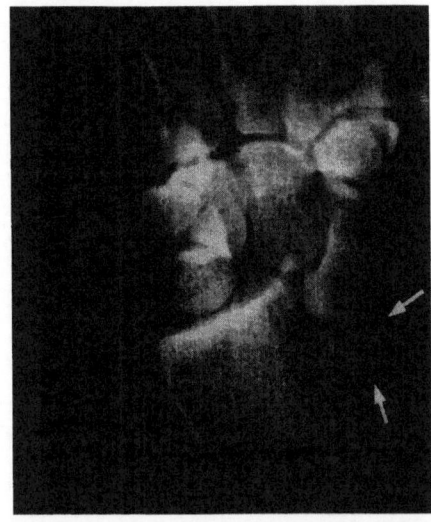

Fig. 18.5. Cuneiform fracture involving the radial styloid process. The AP radiograph shows the lateral dislocation of the main fragment (*arrows*). An associated carpal dislocation is clearly revealed

A very rare fracture is the *depressed fracture*, caused by the impact of the scaphoid against the radial styloid. It is recognisable on the AP radiograph as a double contour of the radial articular surface.

Metaphyseal fractures and *slipping epiphyses* are the most frequent traumatic injuries of the wrist in children [13, 14]. In the case of a metaphyseal fracture, the fracture line lies under the growth plate. It can be either complete or incomplete. The latter is observed more frequently.

An incomplete metaphyseal fracture may appear on plain film as a transverse linear thickening, or, often, as bending or enlargement of the cortical bone, the so-called torus fracture. In the case of a "greenstick fracture", both the break in continuity of the cortical bone on one side and the cortical bending on the opposite side are recognisable on the radiographs (Fig. 18.6).

a

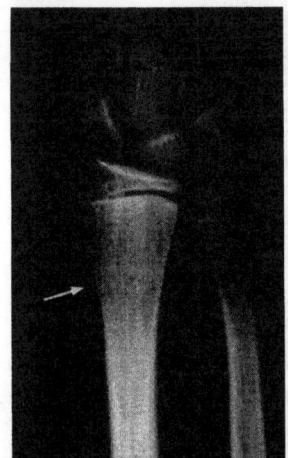 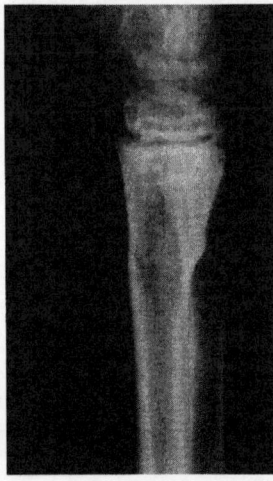

b

Fig. 18.6a, b. Greenstick fracture. The AP radiograph (a) shows cortical bone bending (*white arrow*); on the lateral radiograph (b), the break in continuity of the cortical bone on the ventral side (*arrowhead*) and the cortical bending on the dorsal side (*arrow*) are recognisable

The *slipping epiphysis* occurs at the level of the growth plate. The classification of the slipping epiphysis according to Salter and Harris includes five types of fractures. In type I, the fracture line lies in the growth plate. In type II, the fracture line extends from the growth plate into the metaphysis, so a triangular fragment may be evident. Type III is an articular fracture with a vertical line through the epiphysis. In type IV, the vertical or oblique fracture line extends through both the epiphysis and metaphysis. Type V is similar to a depressed fracture at the level of the growth cartilage. Types I and II occur more frequently in the wrist. It may be very difficult to diagnose these lesions on the radiographs, and it is very important to evaluate the presence of signs of soft tissue involvement (the dislocation/cancellation of either the fat pad besides the scaphoid bone or the pronator muscles).

18.2.2 Dislocations and Fracture-Dislocations of the Distal Extremity of the Radius and Ulna

Very strong traumatic forces cause dislocations and fracture-dislocations of the distal extremity of the radius and ulna [2, 15]. It is possible to distinguish radiocarpal dislocations and distal radioulnar dislocations.

Radiocarpal dislocations are generally associated with marginal fractures of the distal epiphysis of the radius. AP radiographs show the overlapping of the scaphoid and lunate on the radial epiphysis, and the frequently associated fracture, which is confirmed on the lateral view.

Dislocation or subluxation of the distal radioulnar joint (DRUJ) includes the displacement of the radius, and the attached carpus, in relation to the ulna; however, the conventional terminology refers to the position of the ulna in relation to the radius (Fig. 18.7) [16]. Dysfunction of this joint may be associated with various

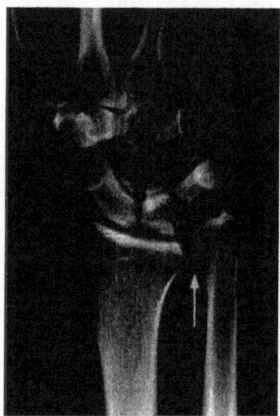
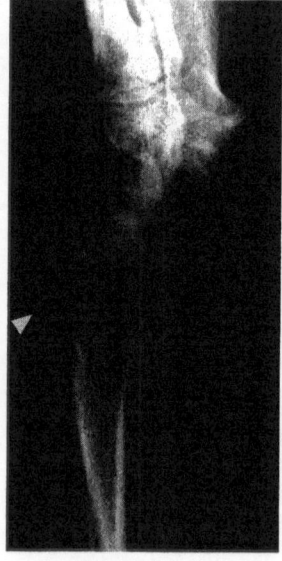

Fig. 18.7a, b. Distal radioulnar joint (DRUJ) dislocation. The AP radiograph (**a**) shows the distal radius and ulna to be not congruent (*arrow*). The dorsal dislocation of the distal ulna (*arrowhead*) is evident on the lateral radiograph (**b**)

bone and soft tissue injuries. DRUJ dislocations are generally associated with a diaphyseal fracture of the radius, frequently between the medial and the distal diaphysis (the so-called Galeazzi's lesion) [17]. In the case of DRUJ dislocation, radiographic examination of the forearm is required; the lateral radiograph usually shows the dorsal ulnar dislocation. The scientific literature reports the usefulness of CT in the diagnosis of DRUJ subluxation [16, 18]. Several methods to measure DRUJ subluxation have been proposed and the "modified radioulnar line" method has been reported to have the highest accuracy rate (about 90%) (Fig. 18.8). These measurements may also be made with MRI, though a false positive diagnosis could be made on MRI with non-standard positioning [19, 20].

18.2.3   Lesions of the Triangular Fibrocartilage Complex

Traumatic lesions of the triangular fibrocartilage complex (TFCC) are relatively common in younger patients. They can be especially disabling in gymnasts, golfers, boxers and ball-handling athletes [21, 22]. The TFCC, which is composed of several distinct anatomical structures, extends from the ulnodistal aspect of the radius to the ulnar styloid process, hamate, triquetrum and the base of the fifth metacarpal bone. The triangular fibrocartilage (TFC), a disk-like structure, is the main component of the TFCC; the dorsal and volar radioulnar ligaments, the meniscus homologue, the ulnar collateral ligament, the extensor carpi ulnaris tendon sheath, and the ulnolunate and ulnotriquetral ligaments comprise the remainder of the TFCC [23]. It acts as a cushion to absorb compressive forces transmitted across the carpal bones to the head of the ulna and stabilises the distal radioulnar joint and the carpal bones.

Traumatic lesions, which are more common in younger patients, may be classified according to their location within the TFC [24]. A class IA lesion is a tear or perforation of the TFC occurring as a 1–2 mm long defect, located 2–3 mm medial to its radial insertion (this portion of the TFC is avascular so this lesion does not heal) (Fig. 18.9). A class IB lesion is an avulsion of the TFC from the distal ulna and may be associated with a fracture of the ulnar styloid, and DRUJ instability (Fig. 18.10): it may heal, as it involves a vascularized segment of the TFC. A class IC lesion is a rare lesion consisting of the distal avulsion of the ulnolunate or the ulnotriquetral

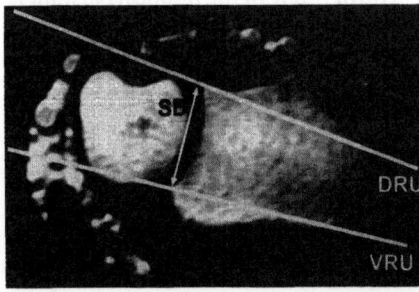

Fig. 18.8. Modified radioulnar line method to diagnose DRUJ subluxation. When the DRUJ is congruent, the ulnar head lies between lines *DRU* (dorsal radioulnar line) and *VRU* (ventral radioulnar line). Subluxation is diagnosed when the maximal width of the dorsally or ventrally subluxed ulna is larger than one-quarter the sigmoid notch diameter (*SD*)

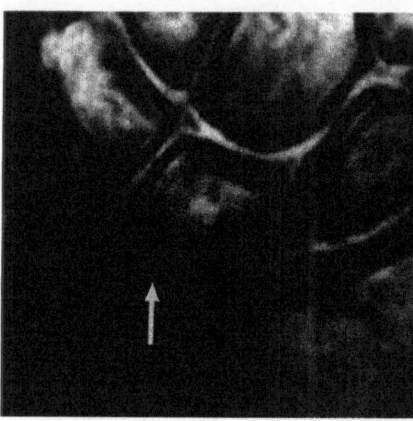

Fig. 18.9. Coronal GE T2-weighted image showing a class IA lesion of the triangular fibrocartilage complex (TFCC). The triangular fibrocartilage (TFC) tear (*arrow*) occurs medial to
its radial insertion

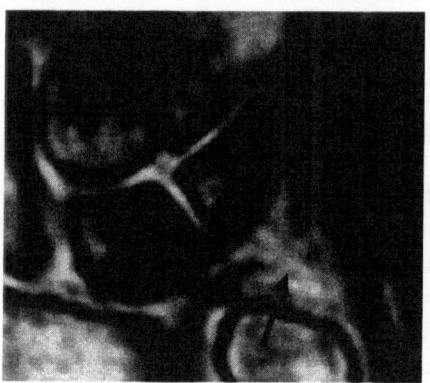
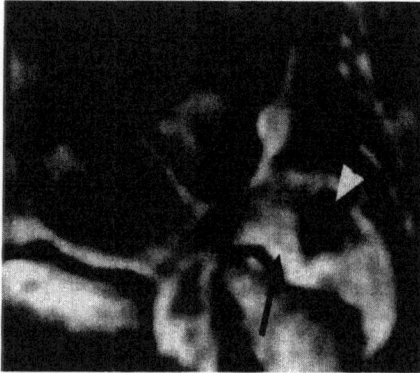

a   b

Fig. 18.10. A class IB lesion: the coronal GE T2-weighted images (**a, b**) reveal the TFC avulsion
from its ulnar insertion (*arrow*). The fractured ulnar styloid is also well evident (*arrowhead*); the
proximal fragment appears hypointense and it is compatible with necrotic phenomena

ligament. A class ID lesion is an avulsion of the TFC from its attachment on the
radius at the sigmoid notch, and may be associated with a distal radius fracture
(Fig. 18.11).

Arthrography of the wrist (all three compartments) has been advocated to detect
tears of the TFC and the lunotriquetral and scapholunate interosseous ligaments
[25–27]. Some authors [28,29] maintain that arthrography of the radiocarpal joint is
sufficient for the evaluation of interosseous ligaments and TFC. A significant limitation of arthrography is the poor correlation between intercompartmental communication and clinical sign and symptoms [30]. It may be of value for demonstrating
lunotriquetral ligament and TFC tears in patients with ulnar-sided wrist pain [30,
31]. However, it is an invasive method as there is the potential for a contrast allergy
reaction and furthermore joint distension may cause discomfort for several hours.
Using a correct technique with a dedicated coil, employing high-resolution three-
dimensional gradient recalled echo sequences, MRI has demonstrated high accura-

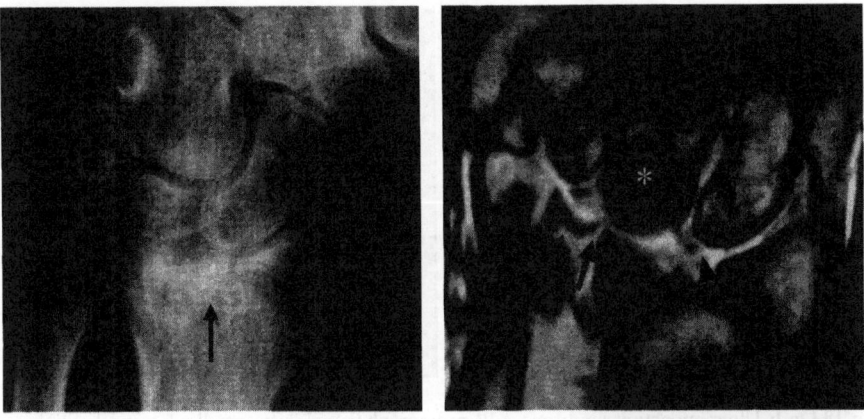

a

b

Fig. 18.11. AP radiograph (a) showing the articular fracture of the distal radius (*arrows*). The MR examination confirms the fracture and reveals the associated lesions. The coronal GE T2-weighted image (b) reveals both the lesion of the TFC and the avulsion from its radial insertion (*arrows*) (class ID lesion). Bone marrow oedema of the lunate (*asterisk*), due to the traumatic involvement, is also evident as well as the lesions of the scapholunate and the lunotriquetral ligaments (*arrowheads*). The sagittal T1-weighted image (c) confirms the volar dislocation of the lunate (trans-radial perilunate dislocation)

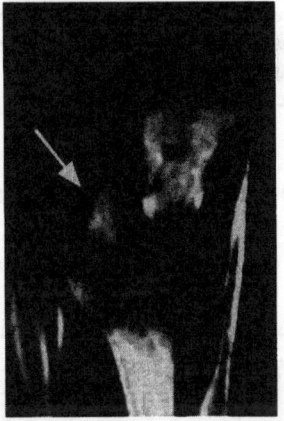

c

cy (80–100%), compared with arthrography and arthroscopy, in the diagnosis of full-thickness tears or perforation of the TFC [32–34]. MRI provides adequate spatial resolution for visualisation of most of the components of the TFCC [35, 36].

18.2.4   Ulnar Impaction Syndrome

Ulnar impaction syndrome is commonly observed in gymnasts due to repetitive axial loading, in the case of positive ulnar variance [37–39]. In fact, a small increase in the ulnar length relative to the distal radius results in an increase in the forces transmitted across the ulna. This predisposes these subjects to degeneration and perforation of the TFCC and to degeneration of the articular cartilage of the distal ulna, proximal lunate and/or proximal surface of the triquetrum and disruption of the lunotriquetral ligament [40]. MRI findings in this condition (signal abnormality within the lunate, ulnar head and tear of the TFCC) may be present prior to the development of radiographic findings (subchondral lucency or sclerosis within the distal ulna, the proximal ulnar aspect of the lunate or the proximal radial aspect of the triquetrum) [41] (Fig. 18.12).

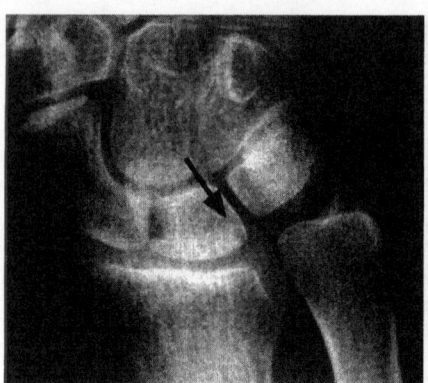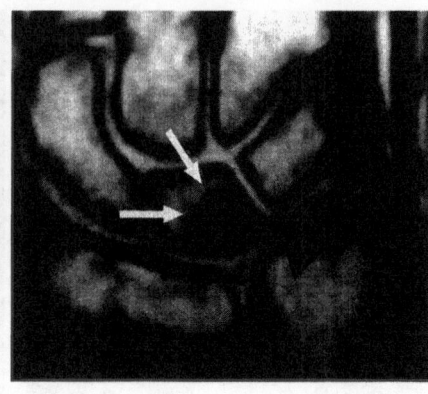

a   b

Fig. 18.12a, b. Ulnar impaction syndrome. A PA radiograph (b) exhibits a small subcortical radiolucency at the proximal ulnar corner of the lunate (*arrow*) and ulnar positive variance. The GE
coronal image (b) reveals the signal abnormality within the proximal and medial portion of the
lunate, with signal characteristics consistent with a subchondral sclerosis or fibrosis due to ischemic damage (*white arrows*); a tear of the radial portion of the TFC (*arrowhead*) is also evident

18.2.5   Carpal Fractures and Fracture-Dislocations

18.2.5.1   *Isolated Carpal Fractures*

Isolated carpal fractures, with the exception of fractures of the scaphoid, are not
frequently seen, and generally occur together with a dislocation [3, 42].

The most frequently fractured carpal bone is the *scaphoid*. Scaphoid fractures
usually occur in young adults and are caused by a fall on the hyperextended,
radially tilted wrist [43]. About 65% of scaphoid fractures occur through the waist
(Fig. 18.13) and 15% through the proximal pole (Fig. 18.14) [42]. About 17% of
scaphoid fractures occur at the level of the tubercle. These are avulsion fractures,
caused by the action of the annular ligament (Fig. 18.15). In children, fractures
(avulsion) of the distal pole account for 75% of scaphoid fractures and are followed in frequency by waist fractures (20%) and proximal pole fractures (5%)
[14]. The distal site of the fracture (about 6%) has a better prognosis because it is
more vascularized (Fig. 18.16). Stress fractures of the scaphoid waist are reported
in sportsmen practising activities involving repetitive loading of the wrist in dorsiflexion (e.g. gymnasts and shot-putters) [44]. Most scaphoid fractures are transverse or slightly oblique to the axial plane and are usually best seen on either a PA
or semipronated oblique radiographs or a PA view with ulnar deviation.

Soft tissue alterations are almost always seen. Therefore, the radiographic evidence of either the dislocation or the cancellation of the fat pad next to the scaphoid
may induce the radiologist to suspect the presence of a fracture of either the radial
styloid, the first metacarpal bone, or the scaphoid bone [4]. Non-displaced scaphoid
fractures, in fact, may frequently escape detection on plain film and require CT or
MRI examination for immediate diagnosis (Fig. 18.17). A prompt diagnosis is essential because missed scaphoid fractures have a significantly high incidence of non-

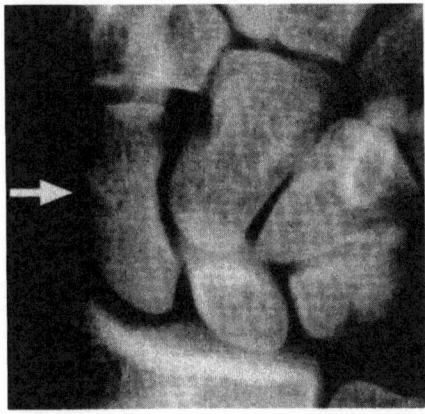

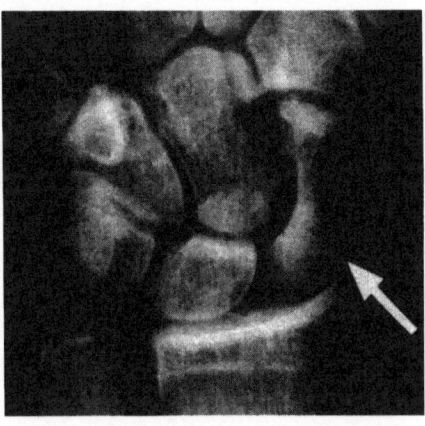

Fig. 18.13. The AP radiograph in ulnar deviation exhibits the horizontal fracture of the scaphoid at the waist (*arrow*)

Fig. 18.14. Fracture of the scaphoid through the proximal pole (*arrow*) revealed by the AP radiograph in ulnar deviation

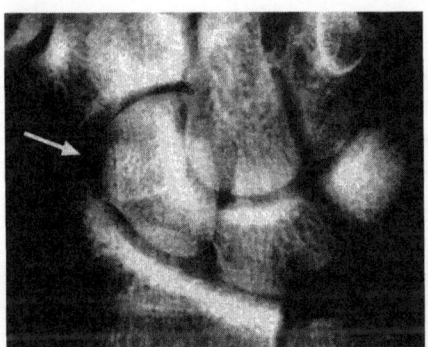

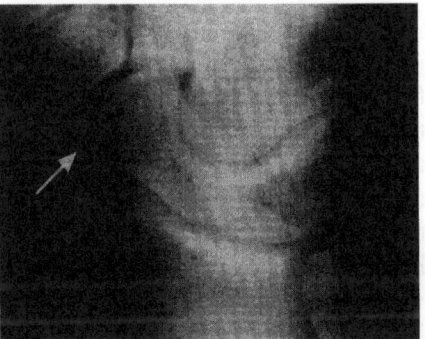

a

b

Fig. 18.15a, b. Avulsion fracture of the tubercle of the scaphoid. The detached fragment (*arrow*) is better revealed on the oblique projection (**b**) than on the AP radiograph (**a**)

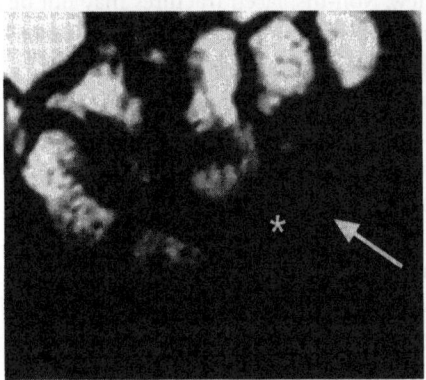

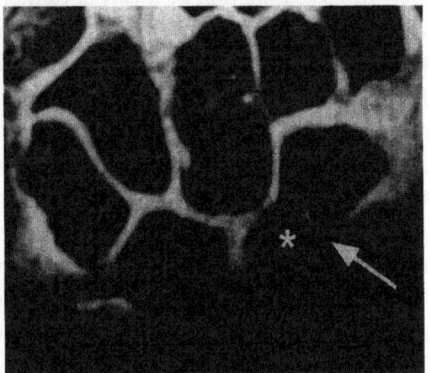

a

b

Fig. 18.16a, b. Fracture of the scaphoid at the waist. The signal intensity of the proximal fragment on both the FSE T1-weighted (**a**) and GRE T2-weighted (**b**) images is consistent with ischemic phenomena (*asterisk*)

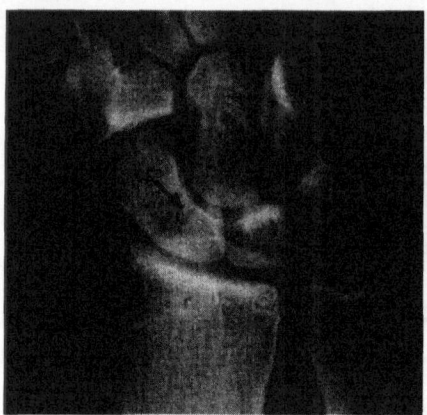
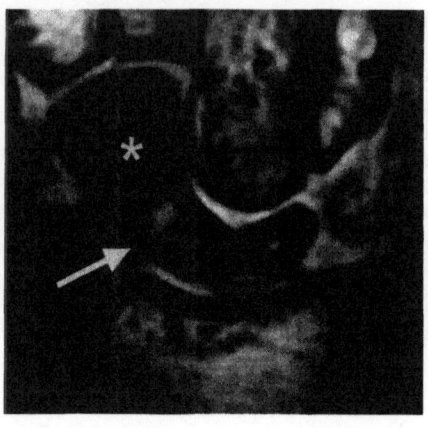

a   b

Fig. 18.17a, b. Non-displaced fracture of the scaphoid. The AP radiograph (a) shows a subtle radiolucent line through the proximal portion of the waist (*arrow*). The oblique coronal GE T2-weighted image (b) exhibits the low signal intensity within the lunate, compatible with bone marrow oedema (*asterisk*), and the hyperintense fracture line through the waist (*arrow*)

union [45] (Fig. 18.18). CT and MRI of the wrist are usually performed to diagnose a fracture, delineate associated bone displacement or angulation and to assess fracture healing including the prediction of the healing potential of the scaphoid fracture [46]. At MRI, a scaphoid fracture is diagnosed by the presence of a low signal intensity fracture line or diffuse bone marrow oedema [47] (Fig. 18.19). If a dislocation of the fractured fragments is present it could be associated with ligamentous lesions. MRI allows the diagnosis of these additional lesions too.

Another difficult diagnosis is that of the fracture of *the hook of the hamate*. This fracture usually occurs at the base of the hook and results from a force directed against the hypothenar eminence. It is typical in golfers or tennis players, caused by repetitive impact of the handle of the racket against the hook of the hamate [48]. The PA view can give evidence of the fracture; however, the diagnosis usually requires an oblique lateral view in 20° supination or a carpal tunnel view. Non-displaced fractures may not be visible on these views and, if the patient cannot fully hyperextend the wrist, the carpal tunnel view may not reveal the fracture at the base of the hook. CT is often necessary for the diagnosis and MRI can also demonstrate the bone marrow oedema in the case of fracture [49, 50]. The os hamuli proprium and congenital absence of the hook of the hamate are normal variants that may cause misdiagnosis of fractures. Long-standing fractures of the hook of the hamate may be associated with non-union, osteonecrosis, decreased grip strength, rupture of the tendons of the fourth and fifth fingers or neuropathy of the deep branch of the ulnar nerve [48, 51].

The *lunate*, which is the fulcrum of the carpal condyle, is contained in a fibrous niche formed by strong ligaments of the wrist. It is frequently exposed to traumatic forces that may be damaging to its vascularization. In fact, the aseptic necrosis of the lunate, or Kienböck syndrome, is a frequently seen lesion in young males even though repetitive microtrauma cannot justify the aseptic necrosis in all cases. Ulnar negative variance may be a predisposing factor [6] (Figs. 18.20, 18.21). Luna-

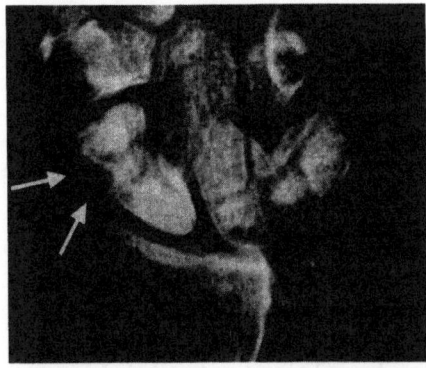

Fig. 18.18. Pseudoarthrosis of the scaphoid. An AP radiograph shows a scaphoid fracture at the waist (*arrows*) with non-union of the fragments and diffuse sclerosis

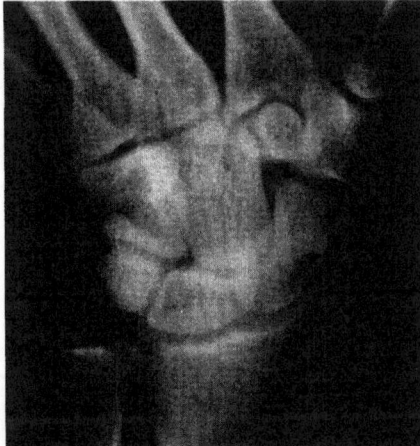

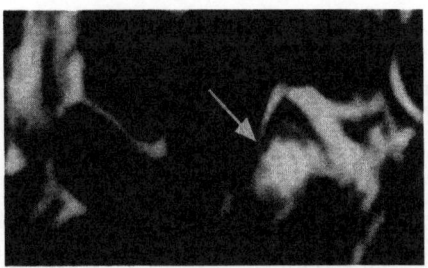

b

a

Fig. 18.19a, b. Occult scaphoid fracture. An AP radiograph in ulnar deviation (**a**) reveals no fracture. A coronal STIR image (**b**) demonstrates a diffuse pattern of increased signal intensity throughout of the scaphoid, consistent with bone marrow oedema (*white arrow*)

te fractures occur less frequently than lunate dislocations. They can occur at the level of the body, caused by the compressive action of both the radius and the capitate, or at one horn, caused by a mechanism of ligamentous avulsion. Fractured horns are better diagnosed on lateral radiographs (Fig. 18.22). Fractures of the *triquetrum* are the next most frequent type of fracture in the wrist after scaphoid fractures. Usually they occur on the dorsal pole at the insertion site of the medial collateral ligament (avulsion fissure) and are usually well evident on the lateral radiograph [6]. Fractures of the triquetrum are frequently associated with carpal dislocation [1].

Fractures of the *pisiform* are caused by both direct trauma and violent tension of the anterior cubital tendon, which inserts on the hook of the hamate. In fact, the pisiform is a sesamoid of this tendon, and fracture of the hook of the hamate is often associated with a fracture of the pisiform. It should be evident on plain radiographs on the 45° oblique semisupination view [1, 5].

Fractures of the *trapezium* are rare; they are often associated with fractures of the first metacarpal bone [52].

Fractures of the *trapezoid* and *capitate* (Fig. 18.23) are also rare [2].

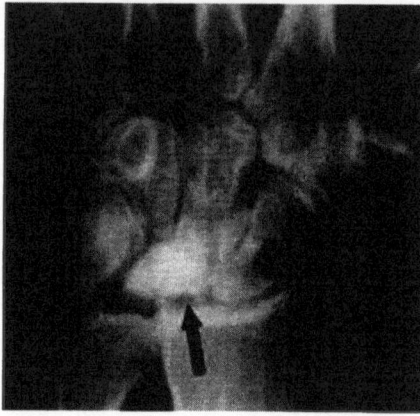

Fig. 18.20. Kienböck syndrome. The AP radiograph reveals the sclerosis of the lunate due to necrosis (*arrow*)

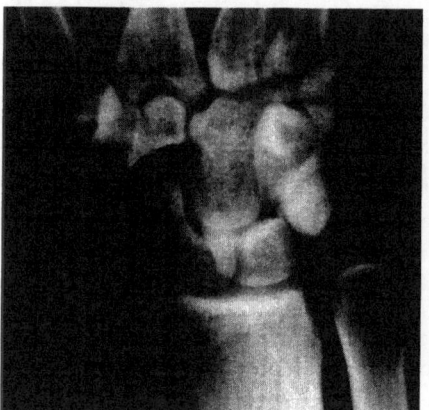

a

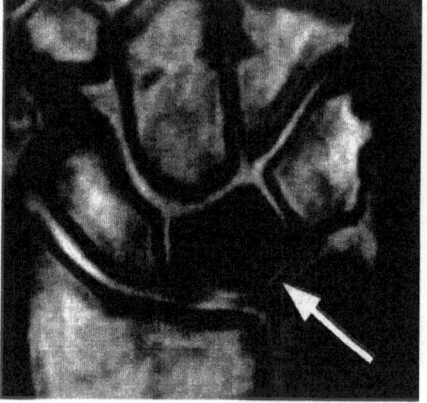

b

Fig. 18.21a, b. Kienböck syndrome. The AP radiograph (a) demonstrates a regular appearance of the lunate. The coronal GE T2-weighted image (b) reveals a diffuse signal abnormality within the lunate (*arrow*), which is compatible with avascular necrosis

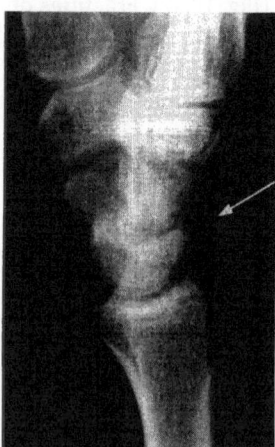

Fig. 18.22. A lateral radiograph reveals the bony detachment from the dorsal horn of the lunate (*arrow*)

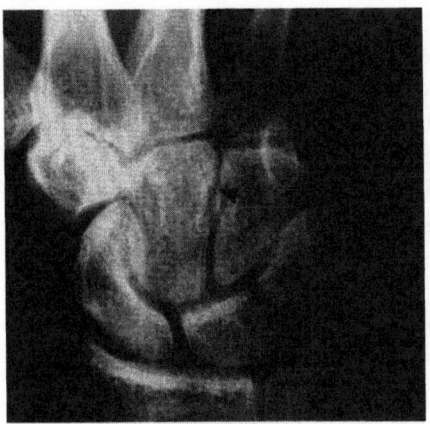
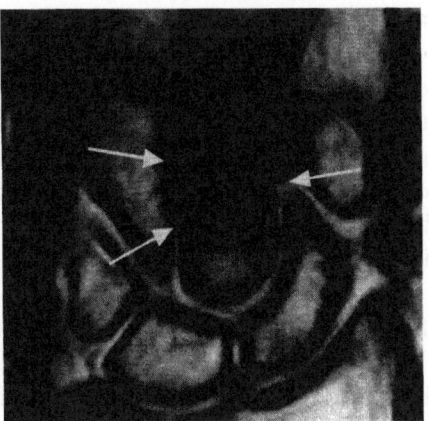

a

b

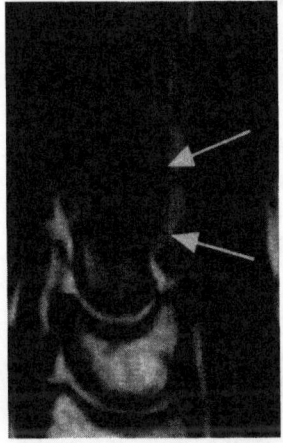

c

Fig. 18.23a, b. Fracture of the capitate. The AP radiograph (a) reveals an irregular profile of the capitate (*arrow*). The MR coronal (b) and sagittal (c) images demonstrate the diffuse signal intensity within the capitate and the complex fracture (*white arrows*)

18.2.5.2   Dislocations and Fracture-Dislocations of the Carpus

18.2.5.2.1 Radiological Approach

Carpal dislocations and fracture-dislocations are rare traumatic lesions of the wrist and occur more frequently in the third decade of life [1, 5]. Gilula proposed a systematic approach to analyse carpal fractures, dislocations and fracture-dislocations on the PA view [7]. In fact, it is possible to recognise on this projection three fairly smooth radiographic arcs to define normal carpal bone relationships. The first arc follows the main convex curvatures of the proximal surfaces of the scaphoid, lunate and triquetrum carpal bones; the second arc follows the distal concave curvatures of these same bones; the third arc outlines the main proximal curvatures of the capitate and the hamate. A broken arc strongly suggests abnormality at that site (disruption of the joint from ligamentous tears or carpal bone fractures). Interruption of the third arc suggests the fracture or dislocation of the capitate, interruption of the first or second arc suggests the fracture or dislocation of the scaphoid, and interruption of all three arcs suggests a more complex lesion. The lateral view, because of the overlap of osseous structures, is not useful for evaluating certain anatomical detail. However, the lateral view allows the evaluation of the intercarpal alignment as well as the alignment of the wrist relative to the distal forearm and hand. The main relationship to be discerned on the lateral view is between the metacarpals, capitate, lunate and radius. The capitate is rigidly fixed to the third metacarpal bone. The convexity of the capitate head should be centred in the distal concavity of the lunate, which should fit into the concavity of the distal radius.

18.2.5.2.2 Terminology of Fracture-Dislocations

Recognition of the position of the lunate with respect to the capitate and the distal radius allows naming of the type of carpal dislocation or fracture-dislocation. Carpal dislocations are generally divided into "lunate" and "perilunate" types [5, 7]. The reference for the normal anatomical position is the distal radial articular surface. If the lunate is centred over the distal radius, unlike the remaining carpal bones (localised by the capitate, which is the rigid midpoint of the distal row), there is a "perilunate" dislocation. The lunate is dislocated if it is displaced from the distal radial articular surface and the other carpal bones are centred over the distal radius; if neither the capitate nor the lunate is centred over the distal radius, there is a "midcarpal" dislocation. The words "dorsal" or "ventral" may indicate the direction of the dislocated bones. When there is a fracture as well as a dislocation, the term "trans" before the fractured bone can be used (e.g. a scaphoid fracture with a perilunate dislocation is called "trans-scaphoid perilunate dislocation"); if there is a fracture of the radial or ulnar styloid or of a metacarpal bone, the term is "transradial", or "transulnar" or "transmetacarpal" [7]. Fracture of the capitate associated with both a fracture of the scaphoid and carpal perilunate dislocation is known as Fenton's syndrome [53].

18.2.5.2.3 Mechanism of Injuries

Carpal bone injuries result most commonly from forceful dorsiflexion of the wrist, caused by falls on the outstretched hand [5–7, 54]; the specific abnormality that occurs is related to the position of the hand at the time of the impact, i.e. whether it is extended or flexed, medially or laterally deviated.

The lunate, on the top of the proximal arc, is suddenly and violently struck. Embedded between the head of the capitate and the radial glenoid, the lunate is forced towards the palmar border and dislocates anteriorly with different degrees of rotation. The lunate dislocation begins at the level of lunotriquetral head. In fact the triquetrum is connected more strongly to the capitate than to the lunate. Therefore, when the latter is pushed anteriorly, the regular connection between lunate and triquetrum is lost [5]. If the ligaments between lunate and scaphoid yield, the lunate remains united to the radius, the carpus dislocates posteriorly to the lunate (volar dislocation is exceptional) and "perilunate dislocation" occurs [5] (Fig. 18.24). The scaphoid can slip against the radial styloid resulting in a scaphoid fracture. In fact, the scaphoid acts as a bridge between the proximal and the distal carpal rows, moving as two separate units. When the wrist is hyperextended, the distal radius articular surface, with its dorsal portion, fixes the lunate and meets the midportion of the scaphoid bone. In radial deviation of the hand the radial styloid impinges on the distal part or distal to the scaphoid bone. With a fall on the hyperextended hand, the body weight passing down the radius may break one of these bony structures (Fig. 18.25). There is some evidence that the more distally on the hand the force is exerted, the greater the chance of carpal fractures or fracture-dislocations rather than just fractures of the distal radius [7]. These two dislocations and scaphoid fracture are frequent traumatic lesions because the distal scaphoid ligaments are more resistant than the proximal ones. If scaphoid fracture occurs with displacement of one of the two fragments and dislocation of the distal carpal row behind the lunate occurs, it is called a transscaphoid-perilunate dislocation [55]. If the ligaments of the scaphoid distal pole are damaged the carpus dislocates behind the lunate and the scaphoid, and the rare periscapholunate dislocation occurs.

With stress enough to separate the carpal bones (usually at the level of the lunate), the scaphoid must tear either its proximal attachment to the lunate or its distal one to the trapezium and trapezoid or fracture at the waist. It has been reported that perilunate dislocation precedes the lunate dislocation [56]. With increasing hyperextension force, the lunate may be pushed ventrally by the capi-

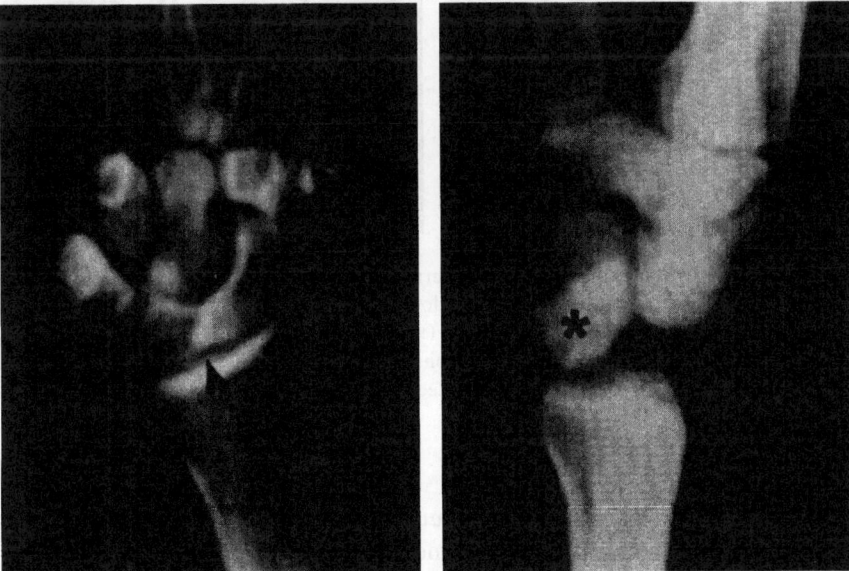

a   b

Fig. 18.24a, b. Perilunate dislocation. The AP radiograph (**a**) reveals the interruption of both the first and the second radiographic arcs (*arrowheads*), suggesting the loss of normal carpal bone relationships. The lateral radiograph (**b**) demonstrates the carpus dislocated posteriorly to the lunate (*asterisk*)

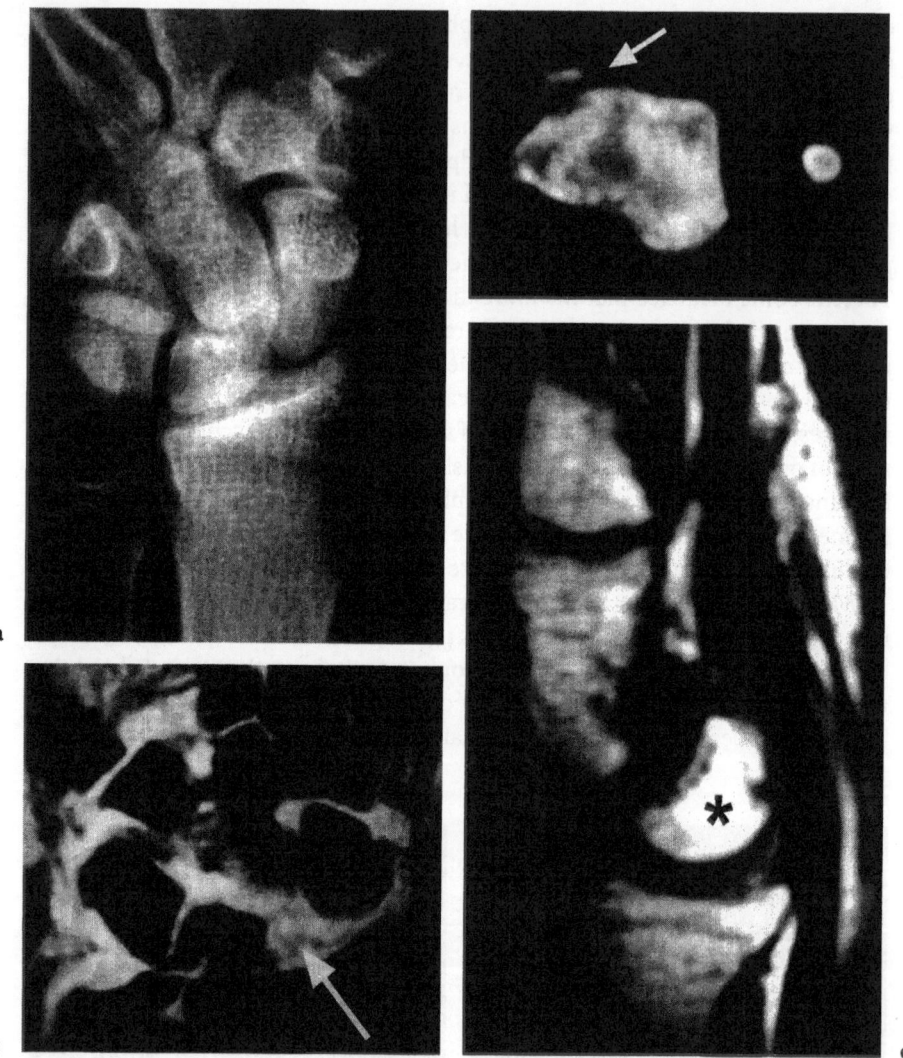

Fig. 18.25. The AP radiograph (**a**) shows the interruption of both the first and the second radiographic arcs; a negative ulnar variance is also documented. The axial CT image (**b**) reveals the cortical detachment of the dorsal radial styloid (*white arrow*). The MR GE T2-weighted coronal image (**c**) demonstrates the rupture of the scapholunate ligament (*arrow*); the sagittal FSE T1-weighted image (**d**) confirms the carpus dislocated posteriorly to the lunate (*asterisk*) (transradial perilunate dislocation)

tate, thus converting a perilunate into a lunate dislocation. If the dislocation exists between the lunate and the perilunate bones but neither the lunate nor the capitate is centred over the radius, the condition may be called "midcarpal" dislocation.

Carpal instability, which is a malalignment of the carpal bones with abnormal intercarpal motion, usually develops secondary to ligament damage or rupture. It is discussed in Chapter 17.

18.3   Hand

Traumatic injuries of the hand have particular importance because they may cause serious functional limitation with reduction of working ability. Men are affected more than women. It is possible to distinguish metacarpal and phalangeal fractures, metacarpophalangeal dislocations, and interphalangeal dislocations.

18.3.1   Fractures of Metacarpal Bones and Phalanx

Metacarpal and phalangeal fractures are usually documented on plain film, using the standard PA and lateral projections; sometimes oblique projections are needed to demonstrate fractures or small bony detachments [2, 4, 6].

Metacarpal fractures may occur at different levels: the proximal or distal epiphysis, diaphysis or metaphysis. Fractures involving the base of the first metacarpal bone, diaphysis of the fourth and fifth metacarpal bones and the distal metaphysis of the fifth metacarpal bone are characteristic.

Fractures of the base of the first metacarpal bone can be intra- or extra-articular. Bennett's fracture (or fracture-dislocation) is an intra-articular fracture. The fracture line is oblique with dorsopalmar and radioulnar direction, with two fragments and dislocation of the distal one, resulting in a shortened metacarpal bone; a comminuted fracture at this level is known as Rolando's fracture. Extra-articular fractures are more frequent. The fracture line never reaches the articulating surface of the metatarsal bone.

Diaphyseal fractures of the metacarpal bones can be transverse or spiral, depending on the type of the trauma. Strong pressure on the metacarpal heads may cause a transverse fracture, usually observed at the second, third and fourth metacarpal bones. A fall on the ulnar side of the hand with twisted fingers may cause a spiral fracture, which is typical in skiers, and usually occurs at the second, third and fifth metacarpal bones (Fig. 18.26).

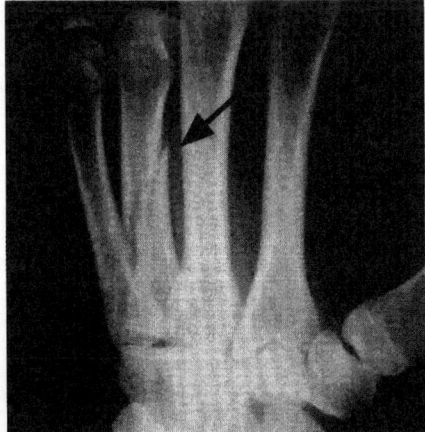

Fig. 18.26. Spiral fracture through the forth metacarpal bone (*arrow*)

Metaphyseal fractures are usually transverse and are caused by either direct or indirect trauma on the epiphysis with flexed fingers; fracture of the fifth distal metacarpal metaphysis is typical of boxers.

Epiphyseal fractures are almost always comminuted secondary to direct trauma.

In case of *phalangeal fractures*, the fracture line is variable and can be transverse, oblique or longitudinal, at the level of diaphysis, epiphysis or both. Phalangeal fractures are about 3 times more frequent than metacarpal fractures, especially considering avulsion fissures of the base. The most frequent phalangeal fractures occur at the ungual phalanges (Fig. 18.27). They are often comminuted and are caused by a direct crushing trauma. Fractures of the middle and proximal phalanges are usually diaphyseal. Avulsion fissures are frequently observed, especially at the level of the distal insertion of the extensor tendons.

18.3.2   Carpometacarpal Dislocation

Carpometacarpal dislocations are caused by violent trauma. A correct radiological examination needs at least the two standard and orthogonal projections. In fact, both the anterior and posterior metacarpal dislocations are confirmed on the lateral view. The AP radiograph only shows a shortened carpal-metacarpal complex, with alteration of the articular space [6].

18.3.3   Metacarpal-Phalangeal Dislocation

Metacarpal-phalangeal dislocation is caused by direct trauma on the palmar aspect of the hyperextended fingers; the articular capsule is always torn (Fig. 18.28). The position of the sesamoid bones, if present, shows the degree of dislocation. If they remain at the level of the metacarpal head, the dislocation is incomplete; if they overturn posteriorly to the metacarpal head, the dislocation is complete.

a 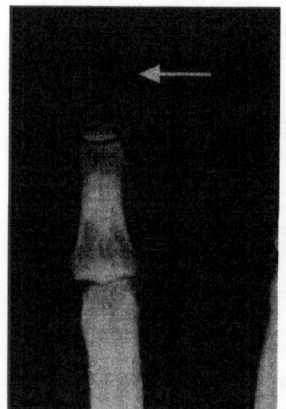 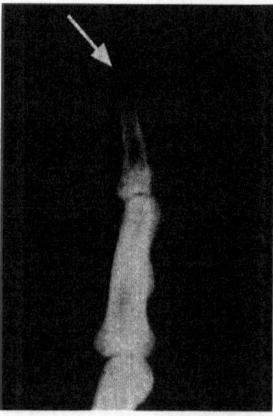 b

Fig. 18.27. AP (a) and lateral (b) radiographs showing a comminuted fracture of the ungual phalanx of the ring finger (*white arrows*)

a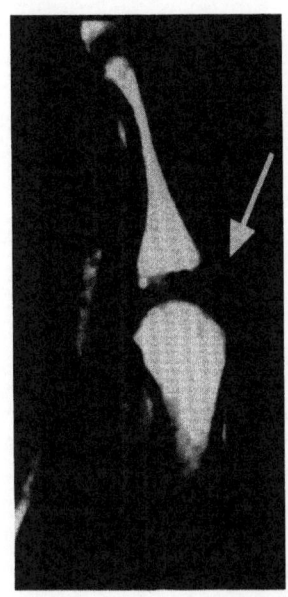

b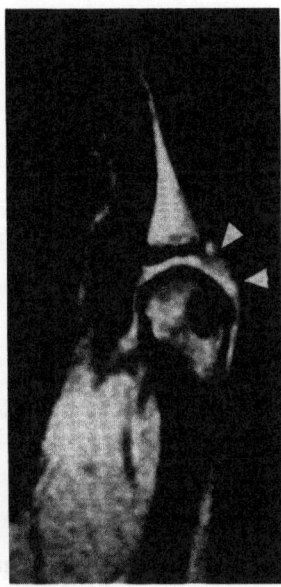

Fig. 18.28. The MR sagittal SE T1-weighted (a) and GE T2-weighted (b) images demonstrate a capsular swelling of the third metacarpophalangeal joint (*white arrow*). The axial TME T2-weighted image (c) better documents the joint effusion (*arrowheads*)

18.3.4 Interphalangeal Dislocation

Interphalangeal dislocation frequently occurs distally, caused by a violent stress in hyperextension. On the posteroanterior view, the articulating rim is not recognisable due to the overlapping of the proximal and distal phalangeal extremities; the lateral projection shows the phalangeal dislocation, which is usually dorsal [6] (Fig. 18.29).

In children, traumatic injuries of metacarpal bones and phalanges are usually caused by crushing trauma. As in the wrist, they are divided into metaphyseal fractures and epiphyseal detachments, which are usually type I and II.

18.3.5 Injury of the Ulnar Collateral Ligament of the Thumb

Rupture of the distal aspect of the ulnar collateral ligament at the first metacarpophalangeal joint is frequently seen in sportsmen following a fall on the outstretched hand and in motor vehicle accidents [57, 58]. The ulnar collateral ligament maintains the lateral stability of the first metacarpophalangeal joint. A violent abduction force may tear it from its insertion site at the medial base of the proximal phalanx [59]. If the distal portion of the torn ligament undergoes proximal retraction such that it lies superficial to the adductor aponeurosis, the latter prevents good healing. This situation is known as the Stener lesion and occurs in about 30–60% of these lesions [60–62]. If untreated, the Stener lesion leads to chronic instability with pain and eventual degenerative arthritis [63]. It can be diagnosed radiographically only if a displaced fracture fragment off the base of the proximal phalanx accompanies the avulsed ligament. MRI of the thumb requires high-resolution images with a small field of view (about 8 cm) [64, 65].

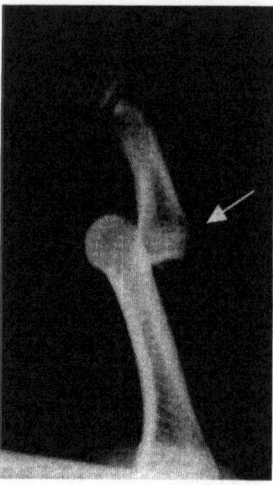

Fig. 18.29. Interphalangeal dislocation. The lateral radiograph demonstrates the posterior dislocation of the second phalanx of the third finger (*arrow*)

18.3.6   Disruption of the Flexor Tendon Mechanism of the Hand

The flexor digitorum superficialis (FDS) tendon lies, within the forearm and the wrist, ventral to the flexor digitorum profundus (FDP) tendon. At the level of the proximal third of the proximal phalanx the FDS tendon splits and passes around the FDP tendon: the two FDS slips reunite deep to the FDP tendon and insert onto the proximal third of the middle phalanx. The FDP tendon inserts onto the base and proximal third of the distal phalanx. The most common tendon injury of the hand is avulsion of the FDP tendon from its insertion at the base of the distal phalanx [66]. The injury involves a hyperextension force applied to an actively flexed finger. This is frequently the ring finger [67]. Unless there has been an associated avulsion fracture, however, the level of retraction of the tendon is difficult to determine clinically and radiographical-ly. MRI may prevent unnecessary surgery by confirming an intact tendon. MRI may also be useful to demonstrate both the level of the retracted tendon, when it has been avulsed, and the level of rupture and location of the tendon ends [68] (Fig. 18.30).

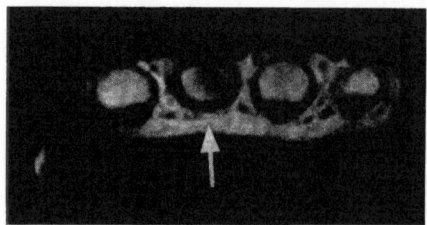
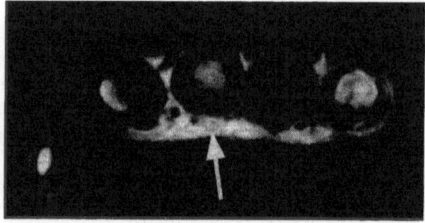

a   b

Fig. 18.30a, b. Rupture of the flexor tendon of the third finger. MR contiguous axial images (**a, b**) at the level of the midportion of the proximal phalanx reveal the absence of the FDP tendon (*white arrows*)

References

1. Martucci E, Rimondi E (1985) Classificazione descrittiva delle lussazioni e fratture-lussazioni del carpo. Chir Org Mov 70:347–354
2. Gui L (1975) Fratture e lussazioni, vol 3. Aulo Gaggi Editore, Bologna, pp 323–458
3. O'Brien ET (1984) Acute fractures and dislocations of the carpus. Orthop Clin North Am 15:237–258
4. Resnick D, Niwayama G (1981) Physical injury. In: Diagnosis of bone and joint disorders, vol 3. Saunders, Philadelphia, pp 2240–2326
5. Rimondi E, Ravazzolo G, Martucci E, Luppi B (1987) Diagnosi radiografica delle lussazioni e delle fratture-lussazioni del carpo. Radiol Med 74:504–511
6. Rimondi E, Albisinni U, Sabalat S, Galli G (1990) Lesioni traumatiche del polso e della mano: studio radiologico convenzionale. In: Albisinni U (ed) Diagnostica per immagini in traumatologia. Aulo Gaggi Editore, Bologna, pp 379–418
7. Gilula LA (1979) Carpal injuries: analytic approach and case exercise. AJR 133:503–517
8. Obermann WR (1996) Wrist injuries: pitfalls in conventional imaging. Eur J Radiol 22:11–21
9. Kerr R, Kingston S (1997) Imaging of sport injuries of the wrist and hand. In: Karasick D, Schweitzer E (eds) Seminars in musculoskeletal radiology, vol 1. Thieme, New York, pp 5–27
10. Totterman SMS, Miller RJ (1996) MRI of the wrist and hand. In: Gilula LA, Yin Y (eds) Imaging of the wrist and hand. Saunders, Philadelphia, pp 471–478
11. Kohler A, Zimmer EA (1986) Limiti del normale ed inizio del patologico nella diagnostica radiologica dello scheletro. Ambrosiana, Milan, pp 144–203
12. Brown DE, Lichtman DM (1984) The evaluation of chronic wrist pain. Orthop Clin North Am 15:183–192
13. Albisinni U, Bungaro P (1990) Introduzione allo studio radiologico convenzionale delle lesioni traumatiche. In: Albisinni U (ed) Diagnostica per immagini in traumatologia. Aulo Gaggi Editore, Bologna, pp 15–48
14. Lovallo JL, Simmons BP (1994) Hand and wrist injuries. In: Stanitski CL, Delee JC, Drez D Jr (eds) Pediatric and adolescent sports medicine. Saunders, Philadelphia, pp 262–278
15. Yeager BA, Dalinka MK (1985) Radiology of trauma to the wrist: dislocations, fracture-dislocations and instability patterns. Skeletal Radiol 13:120–131
16. King GJ, McMurtry RY, Rubinstein JD, Ogston NG (1986) Computerized tomography of the distal radio-ulnar joint: correlation with ligamentous pathology in a cadaveric model. J Hand Surg 11:711–717
17. Reckling FW (1982) Unstable fracture-dislocations of the forearm (Monteggia and Galeazzi lesions). J Bone Joint Surg Am 64:857–862
18. Wechsler RJ, Wehbe MA, Rikfin MD, Edeiken J, Branch HM (1987) Computed tomography diagnosis of distal radioulnar subluxation. Skeletal Radiol 16:1–5
19. Nakamura R, Horii E, Imaeda T, Nakao E (1996) Criteria for diagnosing distal radioulnar joint subluxation by computed tomography. Skeletal Radiol 25:649–653
20. Staron RB, Feldman F, Haramati N, et al (1994) Abnormal geometry of the distal radioulnar joint: MR findings. Skeletal Radiol 23:369–372
21. Linscheid RL, Dobyns JH (1985) Athlete injuries of the wrist. Clin Orthop 198:141–151
22. Taleisnik J (1987) Pain on the ulnar side of the wrist. Hand Clin 3:51–68
23. Mikic ZD (1989) Detailed anatomy of the articular disc of the distal radioulnar joint. Clin Orthop 245:123–132
24. Palmer AK (1989) Triangular fibrocartilage complex lesions: a classification. J Hand Surg 14:594–606
25. Levinsohn EM, Palmer AK, Coren AB, Zinberg E (1987) Wrist arthrography: the value of the three compartment injection technique. Skeletal Radiol 16:539–544
26. Levinsohn EM, Rosen ID, Palmer AK (1991) Wrist arthrography: value of the three-compartment injection method. Radiology 179:231–239
27. Tirman RM, Weber ER, Snider LL, Koonce TW (1985) Midcarpal wrist arthrography for detection of tears of the scapholunate and lunotriquetral ligaments. AJR 144:107–108

28. Manaster BJ (1991) The clinical efficacy of triple-injection wrist arthrography. Radiology 178:267–270
29. Romaniuk GS, Butt WP, Coral A (1995) Bilateral three-compartment wrist arthrography in patients with unilateral wrist pain: findings and implications for management. Skeletal Radiol 24:95–99
30. Metz VM, Mann FA, Gilula LA (1993) Three-compartment wrist arthrography: correlation of pain site with location of uni- and bidirectional communications. AJR 160:819–822
31. Manaster BJ, Mann RJ, Rubenstein S (1989) Wrist pain: correlation of clinical and plain film findings with arthrographic results. J Hand Surg [Am]14:466–473
32. Schweitzer ME, Brahme SK, Hodler J et al (1992) Chronic wrist pain: Spin-echo and short tau inversion recovery MR imaging and conventional and MR arthrography. Radiology 182:205–211
33. Zlatkin MB, Chao PC, Osterman AL et al (1989) Chronic wrist pain: evaluation with high resolution MR imaging. Radiology 173:723–729
34. Golimbu CN, Firooznia H, Melone CP Jr, et al (1989) Tears of the triangular fibrocartilage of the wrist: MR imaging. Radiology 173:731–733
35. Totterman SMS, Miller RJ (1995) Triangular fibrocartilage complex: normal appearance on coronal three-dimensional gradient-recalled-echo MR images. Radiology 195:521–527
36. Totterman SMS, Miller RJ, McCance SE, Meyers SP (1996) Lesions of the triangular fibrocartilage complex: MR findings with a three-dimensional gradient-recalled-echo sequence. Radiology 199:227–232
37. Mandelbaum BR, Bartolozzi AR, Davis CA, Teurlings L, Bragonier B (1989) Wrist pain syndrome in the gymnast. Pathogenetic, diagnostic and therapeutic considerations. Am J Sports Med 17:305–317
38. Albanese SA, Palmer AK, Kerr DR, et al (1989) Wrist pain and distal growth plate closure of the radius in gymnasts. J Pediatr Orthop 9:23–28
39. Tolat AR, Sanderson PL, DE SL, Stanley JK (1992) The gymnast's wrist: acquired positive ulnar variance following chronic epiphyseal injury. J Hand Surg [Br] 17:678–681
40. Palmer AK, Werner FW (1984) Biomechanics of the distal radioulnar joint. Clin Orthop 187:26–35
41. Imaeda T, Nakamura R, Shionoya K, Makino N (1996) Ulnar impaction syndrome: MR imaging findings. Radiology 210:495–500
42. Cooney WP III, Linscheid RL, Dobyns JH (1996) Fractures and dislocations of the wrist. In: Rockwood CA Jr, Green DP, Buchols RW, Heckman JD (eds) Fractures in adults. Lippincott-Raven, Philadelphia, pp 745–867
43. Fisk GR (1970) Carpal instability and the fracture scaphoid. Ann R Coll Surg Engl 46:63–76
44. Hanks GA, Kalenak A, Bowman LS, Sebastianelli WJ (1989) Stress fractures of the carpal scaphoid. J Bone Joint Surg Am 71:938–941
45. Eddeland A, Eiken O, Hellgren E, Ohlsson NM (1975) Fractures of the scaphoid. Scand J Plast Reconstr Surg 9:234–239
46. Sakuma M, Nakamura R, Imaeda T (1995) Analysis of proximal fragment sclerosis and surgical outcome of scaphoid non-union by magnetic resonance imaging. J Hand Surg [Br] 20:201–205
47. Hunter JC, Escobedo EM, Wilson AJ, et al (1997) MR imaging of clinically suspected scaphoid fractures. AJR 168:1287–1293
48. Futami T, Aoki K, Tsukamoto Y (1993) Fractures of the hook of the hamate in athletes. 8 cases followed for 6 years. Acta Orthop Scand 64:469–471
49. Norman A, Nelson J, Green S (1985) Fractures of the hook of hamate. Radiographic signs. Radiology 154:49–53
50. Oneson SR, Scales LM, Erickson SJ, Timins ME (1996) MR imaging of the painful wrist. Radiographics 16:997–1008
51. Hartford JM, Murphy JM (1996) Flexor digitorum profundus rupture of the small finger secondary to nonunion of the hook of hamate: a case report. J Hand Surg [Am] 21:621–623
52. Palmer AK (1981) Trapezial ridge fractures. J Hand Surg 6:561–564

53. Fenton RL (1956) The naviculo-capitate fracture syndrome. J Bone Joint Surg Am 38:681–684
54. Hill NA (1970) Fractures and dislocations of the carpus. Orthop Clin North Am 1:275–284
55. O'Brien ET (1984) Acute fractures and dislocations of the carpus. Orthop Clin North Am 15:237–258
56. MacAusland WR (1944) Perilunar dislocation of the carpal bones and dislocation of the lunate bone. Surg Gynecol Obstet 79:256–266
57. Campbell JI, Feagin JA, King P, Lambert KL, Cunningham R (1922) Ulnar collateral ligament injury of the thumb: treatment with glove spica cast. Am J Sports Med 20:29–30
58. Posner MA, Retailaud J (1992) Metacarpophalangeal joint injuries of the thumb. Hand Clin 8:713–732
59. Noszian IM, Dinnhauser LM, Orthner E, Straub GM, Csanady M (1995) Ulnar collateral ligament: differentiation of displaced and non-displaced tears with US. Radiology 194:61–63
60. Lane LB (1991) Acute grade III ulnar collateral ligament ruptures: a new surgical and rehabilitation protocol. Am J Sports Med 19:234–238
61. Stener B (1962) Displacement of the ruptured ulnar collateral ligament of the metacarpophalangeal joint of the thumb. J Bone Joint Surg 44:869–879
62. Luis DS, Huebner JJ, Hankin FM (1986) Rupture and displacement of the ulnar collateral ligament of the metacarpophalangeal joint of the thumb. J Bone Joint Surg 68:1320–1326
63. Arnold DM, Cooney WP, Wood MB (1992) Surgical management of chronic ulnar collateral ligament insufficiency of the thumb metacarpophalangeal joint. Orthop Rev 21:583–588
64. Hinke DH, Erickson SJ, Chamoy L, Timins ME (1994) Ulnar collateral ligament of the thumb: MR findings in cadavers, volunteers and patients with ligamentous injury (gamekeeper's thumb). AJR 163:1431–1434
65. Hergan K, Mittler C, Oser W (1995) Ulnar collateral ligament: differentiation of displaced and non-displaced tears with US and MR imaging. Radiology 194:65–71
66. McCue FG III, Bruce JF Jr (1994) Hand and wrist. In: De Lee JC, Drez D Jr (eds) Orthopaedic sports medicine. Principles and practice. Saunders, Philadelphia, pp 913–1017
67. Steinberg DR (1992) Acute flexor tendon injuries. Orthop Clin North Am 23:125–137
68. Scott JR, Cobby M, Taggart I (1995) Magnetic Resonance Imaging of acute tendon injury of the finger. J Hand Surg 20:286–288

19   MR Imaging of Carpal Tunnel Syndrome

Elisabeth Dion

Carpal tunnel syndrome is the most frequent entrapment neuropathy. It affects the median nerve where it passes through the fibro-osseous carpal tunnel. The disease occurs predominantly in patients between 35 and 60 years of age. Women are affected 2–5 times more often than men. Up to 50% of cases are bilateral [1].

Clinical presentation includes sensory findings that range from minimal hyperesthesia, discomfort, paresthesias, burning pain and numbness to complete anesthesia, often worse at night. According to the median nerve distribution, the thumb, index, middle fingers, and radial half of the ring finger are affected.

Sensory fibers predominate at the level of the carpal tunnel and will be responsible for the initial findings. Progression of the disease is marked by a progressive weakness of the thenar muscles (abductor pollicis brevis muscle especially) but there is no sensory abnormality of the thenar eminence, which is supplied by the cutaneous branch of the median nerve outside the carpal tunnel [2].

On *physical examination,* different provocative tests have been used; Tinel's sign consists in paresthesias elicited by gentle percussion over the median nerve. Median nerve entrapment can also be depicted by Phalen's test, consisting in initiation of paresthesias in the median distribution provoked by extreme wrist flexion (Phalen's test) or extreme extension (reversed Phalen's test) [3].

Electrodiagnostic tests in carpal tunnel syndrome are reported to have 85–90% accuracy with a false negative rate of 10–15% . The most sensitive electrodiagnostic manifestation is an abnormality in either latency, conduction time or amplitude of the transmitted signal, of sensory conduction across the wrist. Signs of poor prognosis include considerably prolonged conduction (2–3 times normal) and absence of sensory or motor conduction [4–6].

Morphologic evaluation of the carpal tunnel is seldom carried out, probably because, in the vast majority of cases, it will not influence the therapeutic decision. Ultrasonography and magnetic resonance (MR) imaging share the advantage of the soft tissue depiction; MR imaging adds its ability in the analysis of the bone and joint elements and its documented reproducibility [7]. Diagnostic assessment of nerve compressive syndromes is based on clinical features and electrophysiologic testing, and the role of imaging is limited to assessing difficult or atypical cases, or when a mass is suspected on clinical grounds [8].

19.1   MRI Carpal Tunnel Anatomy (Figs. 19.1, 19.2)

19.1.1   Carpal Tunnel

The bony carpus forms the floor and wall of the tunnel and the flexor retinaculum the rigid roof. The flexor retinaculum or transverse carpal ligament appear as a low signal intensity structure and attaches to the tubercle of the scaphoid, the ridge of the trapezium and the ulnar aspect of the hook of the hamate and pisiform (Fig. 19.1d). The proximal fibers of the volar carpal ligament contribute to the roof of the carpal tunnel, although this contribution is not as significant as that of the thicker flexor retinaculum [1].

The flexor pollicis longus tendon invested in its own sheath is located on the radial aspect of the flexor tendons within the carpal tunnel. The eight flexor tendons, four superficialis and four profundus of the second, third, fourth and fifth fingers are located in the same synovial sheath. The tendons appear as low signal

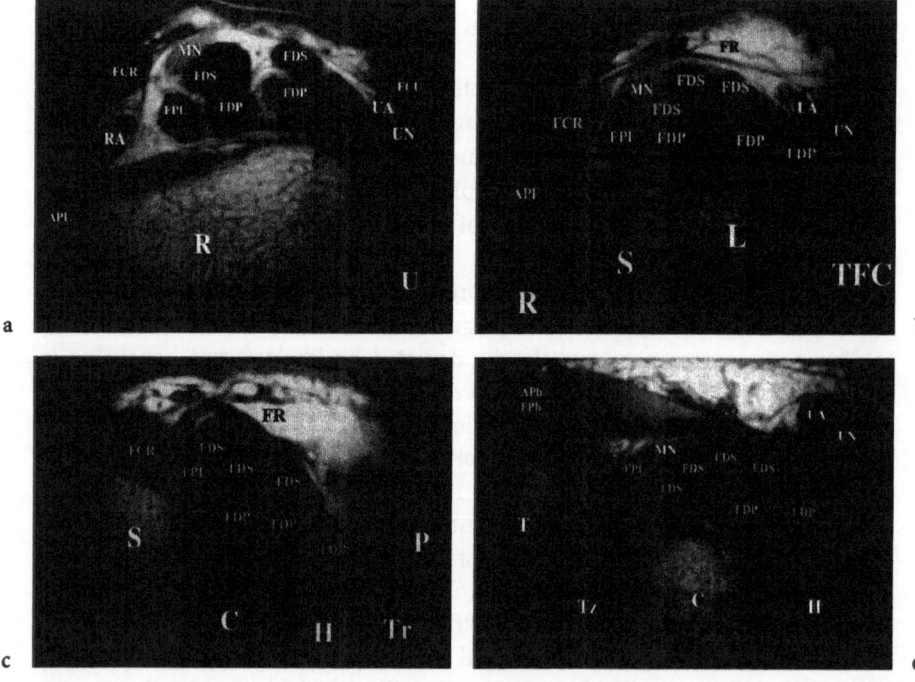

Fig. 19.1a–d. Spin-echo T1-weighted axial images of the carpal tunnel. **a** Proximal section through the distal radius. **b** Section through the radial styloid and lunate. **c** Section through the pisiform. **d** Distal section through the hook of the hamate and the beak of the trapezium. *U* ulna, *R* radius, *C* capitate, *H* hamate, *L* lunate, *P* pisiform, *S* scaphoid, *T* trapezium, *Tr* triquetrum, *Tz* trapezoid, *ER* extensor retinaculum, *FR* flexor retinaculum, *TFC* triangular fibrocartilage, *PA* palmar aponeurosis, *APb* abductor pollicis brevis, *FPb* flexor pollicis longus tendon, *API* and *APL* abductor pollicis longus, *FCU* flexor carpi ulnaris tendon, *FCR* flexor carpi radialis tendon, *FDP* flexor digitorum profundus tendon, *FDS* flexor digitorum superficialis tendon, *FPI* and *FPL* flexor pollicis longus, *RA* radial artery, *UA* ulnar artery, *UN ulnar nerve*, *MN* median nerve

intensity structures in all sequences. Tendon sheaths are of intermediate signal intensity and are only a few millimeters thick [9, 10].

Morphologic changes in the carpal tunnel during motion in healthy subjects have been shown by Skie and Yoshioka [3, 11]. At the proximal level (level of the pisiform), during 45° extension of the wrist, the anteroposterior diameter decreases significantly while the transverse diameter increases slightly, but overall the cross-sectional area decreases in extension. At the distal level (hamate level), in extension, the cross-sectional area of the tunnel increases [3].

19.1.2   Median Nerve

The median nerve in a neutral position of the wrist is anterior to the flexor digitorum superficialis tendons, on the deeper aspect of the flexor retinaculum between the flexor tendon of the middle finger and the flexor carpi radialis [12] (Fig. 19.3).

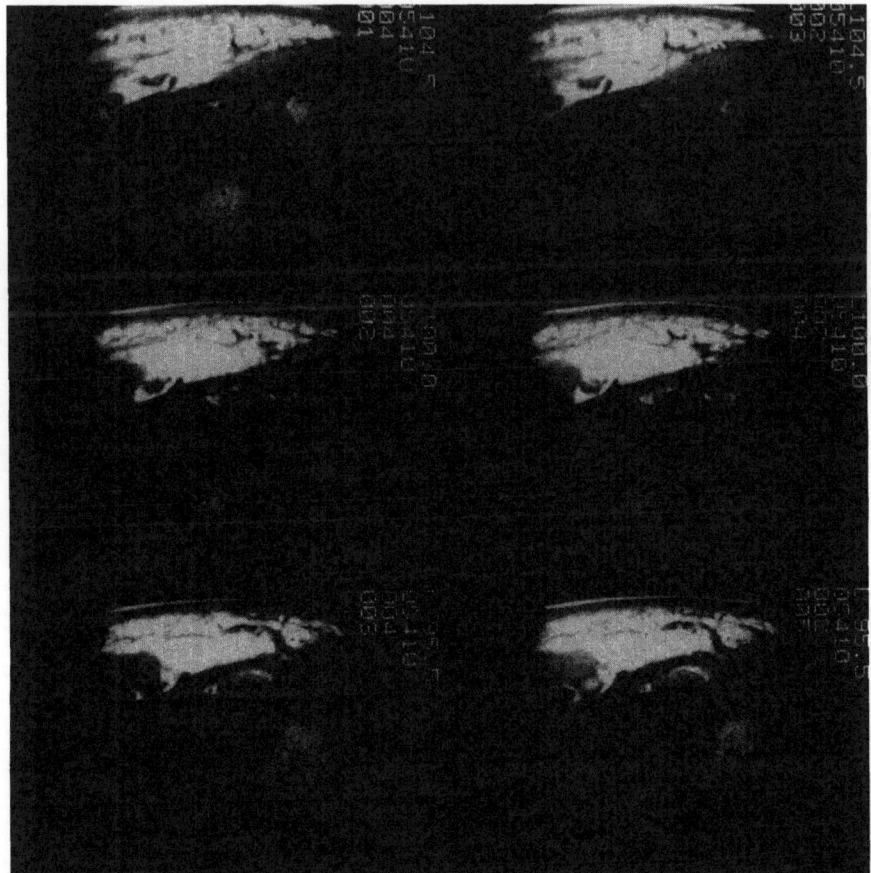

Fig. 19.2. Contiguous axial T1-weighted sections through the carpal tunnel: distal (*top left*) to proximal (*bottom right*)

The median nerve is round or oval at the level of the distal radius; its shape is elliptical at the level of the pisiform and hamate. The median nerve is of low signal intensity on T1- and intermediate on T2-weighted images [13, 14] (Fig. 19.1). Variations shape of the nerve are frequent, as are those of the level of division of the palmocutaneous branch. Evaluation of its size (Table 19.2) is used to diagnose compression. Those measurements (Figs. 19.4, 19.5) should take into consideration normal variants and positional variations.

19.2　Median Nerve

In wrist flexion, the median nerve can be between the flexor digitorum superficialis tendons of either the index finger and thumb or the middle and ring finger [1, 3].

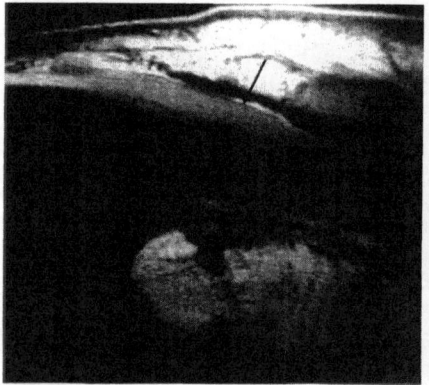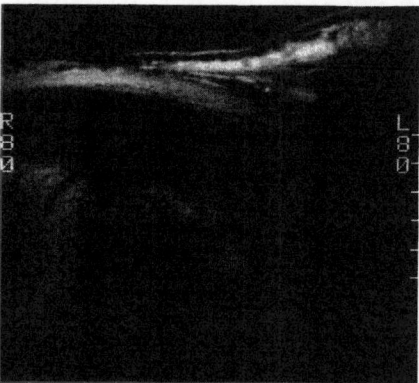

a   b

Fig. 19.3. Sagittal images through the capitate bone: **a** with the wrist in wrist neutral position, **b** with the wrist in extension. Note the shape of the median nerve is changing in its course through the carpal tunnel, with flattening at the distal level (*arrows*). This flattening of the nerve is less important in extension

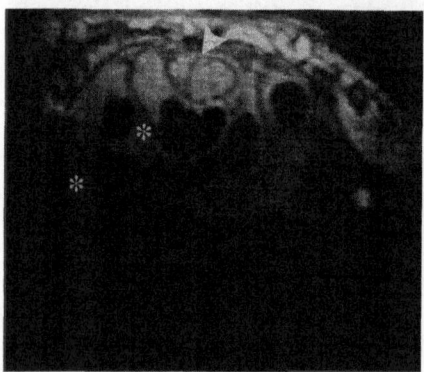

Fig. 19.4. Gradient echo axial image through the proximal carpal tunnel. Normal anatomic variant: note the distal position of the musculotendinous junctions of the flexor digitorum superficialis and profundus muscles (*asterisks*). The median nerve division (palmocutaneous branch, *arrowhead*) is usually seen more proximally

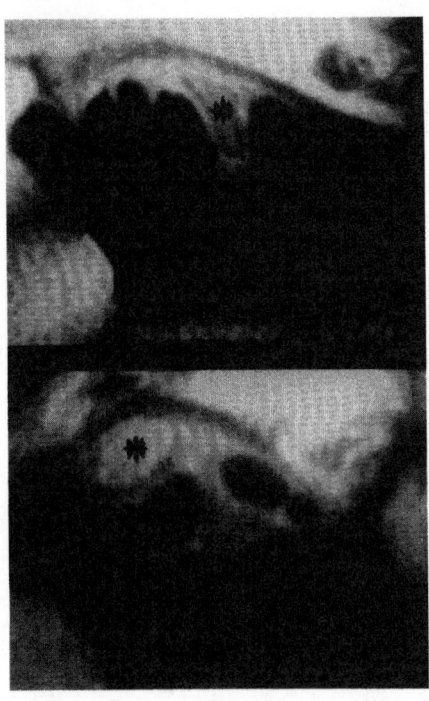

Fig. 19.5. Normal variants of the median nerve shape are numerous, as demonstrated by these aspects seen at the same level (level of the pisiform) in two normal subjects. Median nerve section can appear larger in the case of slightly oblique sections or lateral or medial inclinations

Table 19.1. Carpal tunnel cross-sectional area (cm^2) in normal subjects and patients with carpal tunnel syndrome (*CTS*)

Proximal level		Narrowest level		Authors
Normal subjects	Patients with CTS	Normal subjects	Patients with CTS	
2.53±0.06 (*n*=3)	1.90±0.22 (*n*=7)	2.20±0.19 (*n*=3)	1.75±0.29 (*n*=7)	Bleecker et al. [18] (CT evaluation)
3.82±0.78 (men, *n*=10) 3.33±0.61 (women, *n*=15)	3.48±0.36 (*n*=14)	2.92±0.56 (men, *n*=10) 2.37±0.31 (women, *n*=15)	2.43±0.26 (*n*=14)	Monagle et al. [5]
1.78±0.13 (*n*=20)	1.68±0.8 (*n*=20)	–	–	Allman et al. [3]

In wrist extension, the median nerve is seen anteriorly, deep to the flexor retinaculum and superficial to the flexor digitorum superficialis tendon of the index finger.

In dorsiflexion and palmarflexion of the wrist, the median nerve is forced against the transverse carpal ligament [1] due to friction forces between median nerve tendons and the flexor retinaculum. The median nerve deviation is up to 20 mm during flexion and extension [15].

The shape of the median nerve is most altered in the flexed position, where it is flattened compared with its elliptical shape in the neutral and extended position

Table 19.2. Meta-analysis of carpal tunnel measurements using MRI in normal subjects (*ns*) and patients with carpal tunnel syndrome (*CTS*). *P* values refer to the comparison between patients with CTS and normal subjects

	Distal radius Normal subjects	Distal radius Patients with CTS	Proximal level pisiform scaphoid Normal subjects	Proximal level pisiform scaphoid Patients with CTS	Distal level trapezium hamate Normal subjects	Distal level trapezium hamate Patients with CTS	Authors
Median nerve cross-sectional area (mm^2) (MNCS)	9±1.3	10±1.0 (NS)	8.2±1.4	15.4±4.7 (P<0.001)	8±0.9. (P<0.05)	11±2.2	Allman et al. [3] (CTS, n=20; ns, n=20)
	10.07±1.7	16.69±4.7 (P<0.01)	10.20±1.84	17.83±5.9 (P<0.01)	9.72±2.49	13.85±4.32 (P<0.1)	Monagle et al. [5] (CTS, n=14 women; ns, n=15 women)
	8±2	–	8.5±2.5	–	8±2	–	Buchberger [16]
	–	–	7.0±1.4	–	8±1.9	–	Middelton et al. [38] (CTS, n=18)
Median nerve flattening ratio	2.5±1.0	1.8±0.6 (P<0.05)	3.3±1.1	3.4±1.5 (P<0.25)	2.9±0.9	3.8±1.2 (P<0.05)	Mesgarzadeh et al. [37] (CTS, n=9; ns, n=17)
	–	–	3.2±0.5	3±0.6 (NS)	3.4±0.4	5.1±0.5 (P<0.001)	Allman et al. [3]. (CTS, n=20; ns, n=20)
	1.86±0.66	2.06±0.36 (NS)	2.09±0.72	2.51±0.57 (NS)	2.68±1.04	2.50±047 (NS)	Monagle et al. [5] (CTS, n=14 women; ns, n=15 women)
	–	–	3.0±1.0	–	3.2±1.0	–	Buchberger [16]
Volar bowing of the flexor retinaculum	–	–	–	–	5.8±4.7	18.1±5.6 (P<0.005)	Mesgarzadeh et al. [17]
	–	–	2.5±0.7	4.5±1.2 (P<0.05)	1.9±0.6	3.5±1.0 (P<0.05)	Allman et al. [3]
	–	–	–	–	2.48±1.25	3.78±1.06 (P<0.005)	Monagle et al. [5]
	–	–	–	–	2±2.0	–	Buchberger [16]
Median nerve swelling ratio MNCS/MNCS distal radius	–	–	1.1±0.2	2.4±0.6 (P<0.0005)	1.1±0.3	2.1±0.7 (P<0.0005)	Mesgarzadeh et al. [17]

of the wrist (Stoller [1]) and the anteroposterior diameter and the cross-sectional area decrease [3] (Fig. 19.3).

19.3   Pathophysiology

The median nerve supplies the abductor pollicis brevis and opponens pollicis muscles, the caput superficiale of the flexor pollicis brevis muscle and the two radial lumbrical muscles, and it sends a sensory branch to the volar side of the wrist [11, 16, 17].

Bleecker et al. [18] correlated the carpal canal size (measured with CT) with anthropometric parameters (height, weight and wrist circumference) in primary carpal tunnel syndrome (Table 19.1) and stressed the importance of the canal size in carpal tunnel syndrome. The cross-sectional areas of the carpal tunnel in women are described by Deker to be smaller by 25% than the corresponding areas in men [19, 20].

Pressure measured by catheter is 2.5 mmHg in asymptomatic patients compared with 32 mmHg in patients with carpal tunnel syndrome. Pressures may also varies in extremes of dorsiflexion and palmarflexion [21, 22].

Nerve entrapment with chronic compression may induce interference with the intraneural microvascular supply and an inflammatory reaction, first affecting the epineurium. Venous congestion may produce epineurial edema and increased endoneurial fluid pressure.

In the early stages, symptoms are mainly related to local disturbances in the microvasculature and may be intermittent or even relieved after exercise, parallel to recovery of the intraneural circulation or drainage of intraneural edema [23]. As the disease progresses, inflammation of the epineurium may turn into fibrotic changes, further contributing to a chronic constriction of the nerve. Longstanding compression leads to damage to the myelin sheath and axonal degeneration induced by fibrosis, with permanent loss of nerve function and atrophy of the innervated muscles [8, 11, 24–26].

19.4   Differential Diagnosis

The median nerve and its palmocutaneous branch can be damaged at a proximal level, proximal to the carpal tunnel; the flexor muscles of the forearm and in particular the flexor pollicis longus are then weakened, whereas in carpal tunnel syndrome the terminal phalanx of the thumb has no motor impairment [4].

The ulnar tunnel, or Guyon's canal, contains the ulnar nerve and artery and vein and is located between the pisiform and the hook of the hamate. Causes of nerve entrapment include ganglia, repeated local trauma, vascular diseases, anomalous muscles in the canal or a fibromuscular arch at the origin of the flexor digitorum brevis muscle [1, 8]. Compression of the ulnar nerve may result in changes in diameter of the cross-section of the nerve (normal diameter 3 mm). Enlargement of Guyon's canal has been described following carpal tunnel release [1].

19.5   MR Imaging Technique

19.5.1   Positioning

As shown before, positional variations are important and precise positioning is very helpful in carpal tunnel and compression evaluation.

Images are acquired using a surface coil with the arm at the side of the patient. Larger patients may need to have the arm extended over the head. Spatial resolution depends on the choice of the field of view, the matrix and the slice thickness. A good compromise should be found between resolution and signal-to noise-ratio [27]. A field of view of 8–12 cm with a matrix of 256+256 and a slice thickness of 3 mm at 1.5 T gives satisfactory results [28]. Three-dimensional acquisitions give thin adjacent slices minimizing the partial volume effect [29]. In-plane resolution up to 70 μm can been obtained at the carpal tunnel using specific coils and modified sequences [9, 30–32].

19.5.2   Sequences

Spin echo T1-weighted, T2-weighted sequence and at least one sequence among T2-weighted, STIR and gradient echo sequences, with special care regarding the choice of flip angle and TE to avoid the magic angle phenomenon [33, 34], should be performed in the axial plane. The coronal plane is useful in the depiction of the flexor tendons. Morphometric measurements can easily be done on the T1-weighted sequences with a good anatomic depiction. Comparison with the contralateral wrist often is helpful but may be misleading because involvement is bilateral in at least half of the patients [35].

19.6   Carpal Tunnel and Median Nerve Measurements

Several authors have made quantitative MR measurements to express changes in the carpal tunnel and the median nerve [10, 29, 35] (Tables 19.1, 19.2).

Changes in the median nerve include flattening or deformity at the level of the hamate and bulbous swelling at the level of the pisiform or the distal radius [8]. Measurements have been proposed by different authors [3, 5, 17, 36, 38].

- The cross-sectional area of the median nerve is significantly higher at the proximal (pisiform) level in patients with carpal tunnel syndrome than in volunteers [3, 5].

- The swelling ratio is calculated by dividing the cross-sectional area of the nerve at the pisiform level by that at the distal radius; this ratio is also significantly higher in patients with carpal tunnel syndrome compared with normal volunteers [37].
- The median nerve flattening ratio (the ratio of the length of the major axis of the nerve to that of its minor axis) is significantly higher in patients with carpal tunnel syndrome than in volunteers (Fig. 19.6) at the distal level (hamate) [3, 37]. The median nerve may display enlargement at the level of the pisiform and compression with flattening at the level of the hook of the hamate [3].
- Volar bowing of the flexor retinaculum is determined by drawing a straight line between its attachments (Fig. 19.7) to the pisiform and scaphoid bone at the proximal level (proximal volar bowing) and its attachment to the beak of the trapezium and the hook of the hamate at the distal level (distal volar bowing), and measuring the distance from this line to the palmar apex of the flexor retinaculum. Mesgarzadeh et al. [37] proposed the bowing ratio (bowing distance divided by the distance between the hook of the hamate and the beak of the trapezium) in order to eliminate the effects of magnification and wrist size. The bowing measurements are significantly higher in patients with carpal tunnel syndrome than in volunteers at the level of the hook of the hamate.

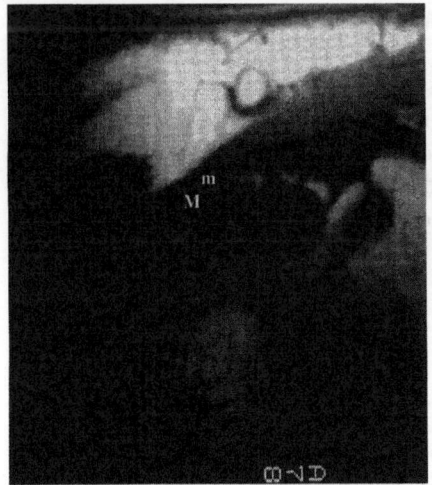

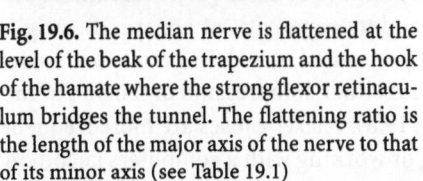

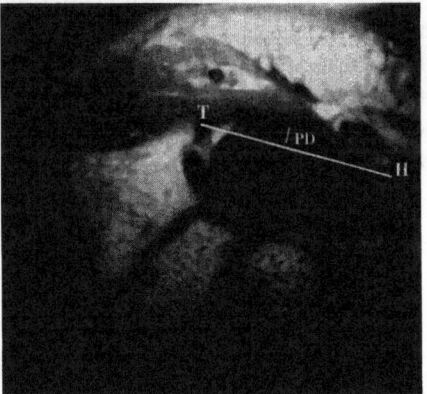

Fig. 19.6. The median nerve is flattened at the level of the beak of the trapezium and the hook of the hamate where the strong flexor retinaculum bridges the tunnel. The flattening ratio is the length of the major axis of the nerve to that of its minor axis (see Table 19.1)

Fig. 19.7. The bowing measurement expresses the volar displacement of the flexor retinaculum in the case of carpal tunnel syndrome. PD/TH relates to the trapezium-hamate distance and is called bowing ratio (see Table 19.1)

The mean cross-sectional area of the carpal tunnel was shown to be smaller in patients with carpal tunnel syndrome than in volunteers at both proximal and distal levels in the neutral position [3], but no significant difference was observed in recent studies [5, 18, 39] (Table 19.2).

Attempts to use MR imaging to measure the diameter or area of the median nerve require a good spatial resolution and MR imaging is probably of secondary use in the diagnosis of carpal tunnel syndrome. Identifying the cause of median nerve alteration has more effect on the therapeutic decision.

Recently a study by Radack et al. [40] compared the measurements in 165 patients referred for wrist MR imaging, a subset of whom (22 patients) were referred for carpal tunnel syndrome. The study demonstrated that none of the usual signs was sensitive for the diagnosis of carpal tunnel syndrome. Specificity was high for flexor retinaculum bowing, median nerve flattening and the presence of tenosynovitis [40].

Dynamic contrast-enhanced MR imaging has shown that vascular phenomena are probably of interest in the genesis of a certain type of carpal tunnel syndrome. Two patterns of abnormal enhancement have been described: marked enhancement attributed to nerve edema or lack of enhancement attributed to nerve ischemia. Wrist flexion or extension are associated with variation in enhancement of the nerve and exacerbation of clinical symptoms [11]. Contrast injection could help in the diagnosis of intraneural processes such as schwannoma and neurinoma, and more generally to identify the cause of compression.

19.7   T2 Signal Intensity of the Median Nerve

Compression of the median nerve results in an increased signal intensity of the nerve on T2-weighted sequences. This signal modification is not specific and can be seen in nerve abnormalities such as edema or demyelination within neural fibers. Moreover high signal intensity of the median nerve has been described in normal volunteers. Signal intensity of the median nerve can be low in cases of fibrosis in advanced or old compression [1, 17, 28, 38].

19.8   Etiology

Tenosynovitis of the flexor tendons or more likely fibrous thickening of the flexor tendons has been observed intraoperatively in 85% of cases [16]. More than 50% have no identifiable etiologic reason [15] and tenosynovitis of nonspecific origin represent a major cause of carpal tunnel syndrome [20, 41]. In predisposed subjects, overuse or recurrent microtrauma with either compression or tension of the nerve may result in nerve damage [8] (Fig. 19.8). Theses causes are more frequent as the number of jobs that requires typing or working with a computers keyboard

a

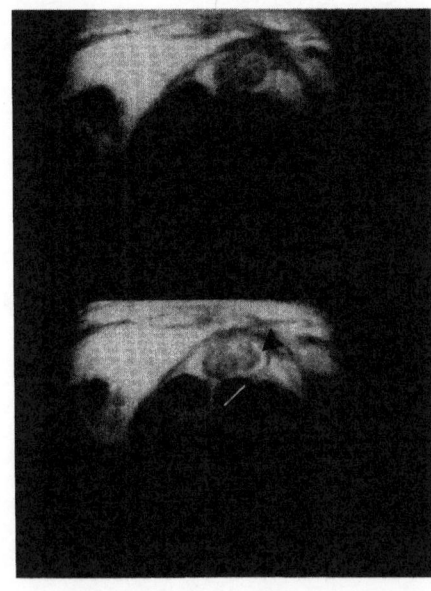

b

Fig. 19.8a, b. Tenosynovitis in a typist with bilateral carpal tunnel syndrome. Axial SE T1-weighted image (b) shows a slight enlargement of the space between the flexor tendons with contrast enhancement on the post-gadolinium image (b) of the tendon sheaths (*arrowhead*) and the median nerve sheath (*arrow*)

increases [16]. In the so-called dynamic carpal syndrome symptoms are bought on by repetitive wrist motion. These symptoms subside with rest but return when the repetitive motion resumes. In those patients with inconclusive physical and electrodiagnostic examinations the diagnosis of carpal tunnel syndrome may be apparent on pre-exercise MR imaging but abnormalities appear or are worsened on MR imaging following provocative wrist exercise [42].

Traumatic conditions such as Colles' fracture, fracture of the carpal bones or carpometacarpal joints, and post-traumatic conditions such as carpal instability, hypertrophic bony callus and fibrosis may cause a narrowing of the carpal tunnel [16, 28] (Fig. 19.9).

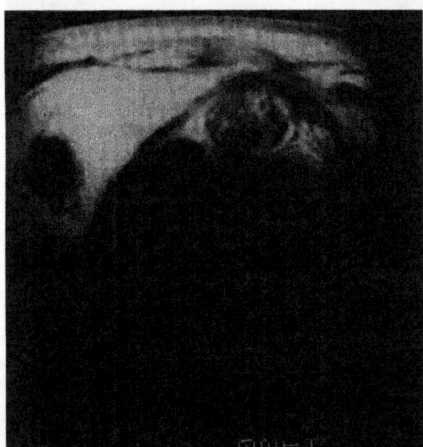

Fig. 19.9. SE T1-weighted image: fat infiltration and enlargement of the median nerve in a patient with chronic carpal tunnel syndrome due to reduction of the cross-sectional area of the tunnel by hypertrophic callus of a distal radius fracture

Osteoarthritis of the carpus with consequent modification of the bony structures may lead to encroachment of the tendon sheaths and the nerve and reduction of the cross-sectional area of the carpal tunnel.

Inflammatory processes can cause an increase in the volume of synovium in the carpal bone joints or the tendon sheath. Rheumatoid arthritis is the most frequent of those inflammatory processes; gout, pseudogout, amyloid deposition (frequent in patients with renal failure)and granulomatous infectious processes such as tuberculosis have also been described [22] (Figs. 19.10, 19.11, 19.12).

Tumor of peripheral nerve can be located in the carpal tunnel. Signal intensity is usually intermediate on T1-weighted images and high on T2-weighted images, with variable inhomogeneity on both sequences. The morphologic appearance may help

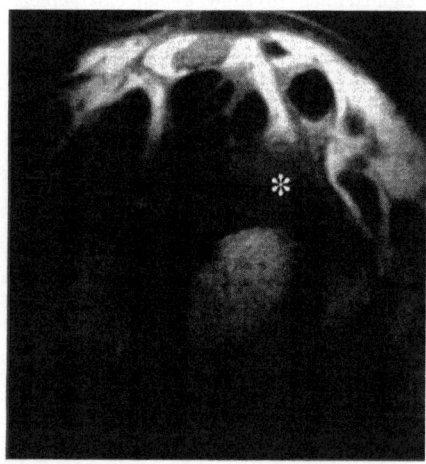

Fig. 19.10. SE T1-weighted image through the proximal section of the carpal tunnel: carpal joint synovitis (*asterisk*) in a patient with rheumatoid arthritis

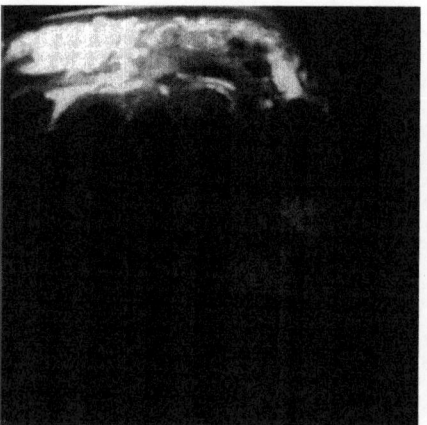
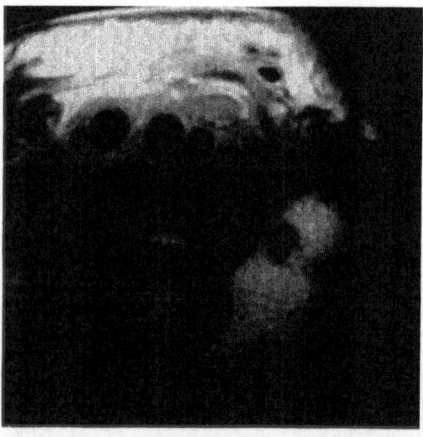

a   b

Fig. 19.11. SE T1-weighted pre- (a) and post-contrast (b) images in a patient with chronic renal failure. Tenosynovitis is well depicted after contrast injection. Carpal erosions are also present. Pathological analysis demonstrated amyloid deposition

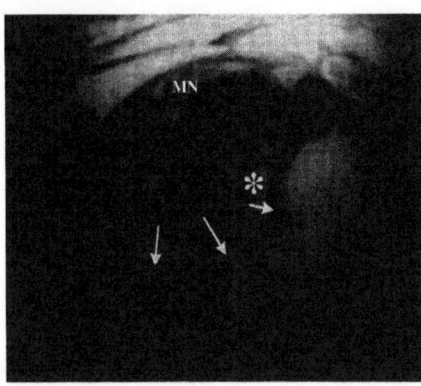

Fig. 19.12. Postcontrast SE T1-weighted axial image in a patient with primitive osteochondromatosis of the wrist. Enhanced synovium (*asterisk*) pushes forward the tendinous elements and the median nerve (*MN*). The carpal bones are severely eroded (*arrows*)

the differential diagnosis among tumors [43]. Schwannoma (also called neurilemmoma, neurinoma, perineural fibroblastoma or peripheral glioma) appears as a globoid mass separated from the intact nerve fibers by a fibrous capsule, the nerve of origin being stretched over the capsule. Neurofibroma, in the solitary form or associated with neurofibromatosis, is a fusiform unencapsulated mass (Fig. 19.13). The tumor spreads within the fascicles and the nerve is entangled irretrievably within the tumor mass [8]. Visualization of the relationship with nearby structures is improved by contrast injection and may help in the etiologic diagnosis and therapeutic decision-making [44]. Malignant peripheral nerve sheath tumor (also called malignant schwannoma, neurogenic sarcoma, neurofibrosarcoma) accounts for about 10% of all soft tissue sarcomas. Tumor margins are partially indistinct, sometimes with infiltration of the nearby structures [43]. Hamartomas, ganglia, arborizing lipomas and hemangiomas may also be encountered in the carpal tunnel [1, 16, 45] (Figs. 19.14, 19.15).

Carpal tunnel syndrome is frequent in patients with acromegaly and is due to bone and ligament hypertrophy and water retention [46–48]. Carpal tunnel syndrome is also diagnosed in about 80% of patients with hypothyroidism [49] and about 15% of patients with diabetes mellitus [50]. The diagnosis of compressive

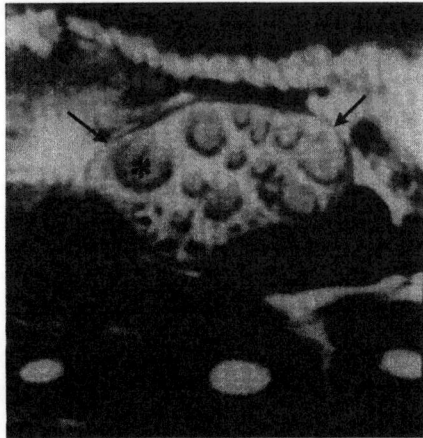

Fig. 19.13. SE T1-weighted image through the metacarpophalangeal joints: neurofibroma of the median nerve (*arrows*). The bundles (*asterisk*) of the nerve as well as interstitial tissue of the nerve are enlarged.

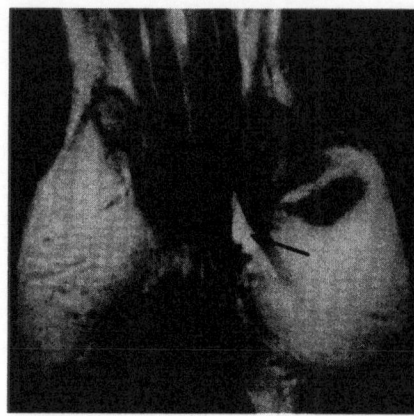

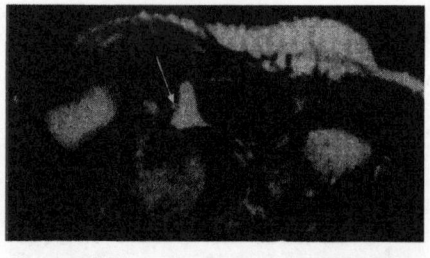

Fig. 19.14. Spin echo T2-weighted images in the coronal (**a**) and axial (**b**) planes: a high-signal, fluid-containing synovial cyst of the carpal joint extends into the carpal tunnel (*arrows*). (Courtesy of Dr. Didier Godefroy)

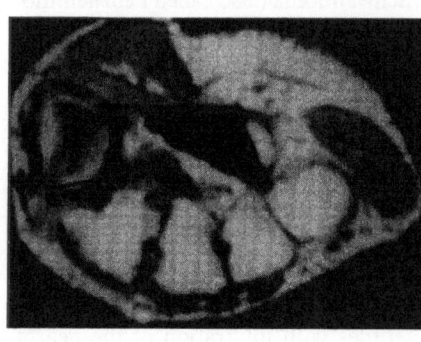

Fig. 19.15. Axial T1-weighted-image showing an unusual location of giant cell tumor of the carpus (*arrow*). The space occupied by the flexor tendons and the nerve is markedly reduced. (Courtesy of Dr. Didier Godefroy)

tunnel syndrome versus mononeuropathy of the median nerve is sometimes unclear [51]. Deposits of calcium, uric acid crystals or amyloid have been described. Systemic conditions such as pregnancy, postmenopausal condition and lupus erythematosus have also been implicated [15].

Traumatic section of the nerve with a wide gap or delayed reconstruction may lead to hypertrophic scarring and may form bulbous neuromas (Fig. 19.16).

Patients with an arteriovenous shunt in the forearm for dialysis are vulnerable to carpal tunnel syndrome. The increased vascularity, venous hypertension and associated edema have been proposed as possible mechanisms [4].

Developmental etiologies include persistent median artery, hypertrophy of the lumbrical muscles, anomalous muscles and a distal position of the flexor digitorum superficialis muscle [1, 14].

19.9   Treatment

Initial treatment for carpal tunnel syndrome includes various combinations of splints, nonsteroidal anti-inflammatory drugs, corticosteroids and local injection of steroids. Surgical treatment is recommended when there is a diminution of

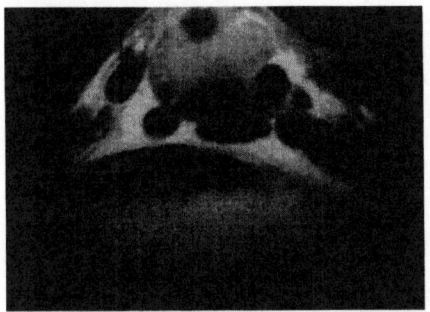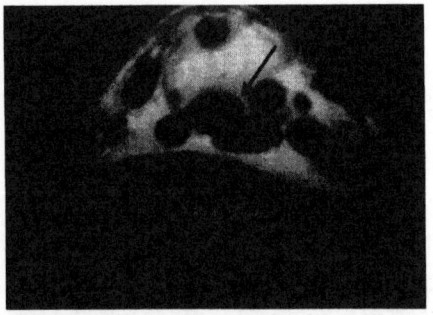

a   b

Fig. 19.16. SE T1-weighted pre- (a) and post-contrast (b) images through the proximal level of the carpal tunnel. Bulbous neuroma of the median nerve corresponding to hypertrophic and inflammatory scar several months following traumatic section of the nerve. The scar is in contact and between the flexor tendons (*arrow*)

muscle strength. Surgical decompression consists in a large section of the flexor retinaculum that may extend proximally into the volar carpal ligament.

Endoscopic carpal tunnel release is a new technique that gives good clinical results. However, this procedure may be complicated by incomplete release, laceration of the ulnar artery, median nerve or flexor tendons, and fracture of the hook of the hamate [52, 53]. Preoperative assessment of the carpal tunnel is useful in patients scheduled for endoscopic retinacular release. Epineurotomy is indicated in the case of thickened or scarred epineurium.

Complications of surgical treatment are reflex sympathetic dystrophy, hypertrophic scar formation, scarring involving the nerve, damage to the branches of the median ulnar nerve, flexor tendon adhesions and bow-stringing of tendons [1].

19.10   Postoperative Studies

Nerve conduction is improved by surgery in about 40% of patients [3, 48] (Fig. 19.17). Release of the transverse carpal ligament may cause the flexor tendons or contents of the carpal tunnel to demonstrate a volar convexity because of the loss of the normal roof support. Several authors mentioned the modification of the carpal arch and particularly the increase in the distance between the hook of the hamate and the beak of the trapezium after flexor retinaculum release [29, 54] Altogether carpal tunnel volume increases by up to 24% [13] Widening of the fat stripe posterior to the flexor digitorum profundus tendons is a normal postoperative finding. Two studies that investigated recurrent carpal tunnel syndrome reported visible flexor retinaculum after surgery. Their conclusions are not clear concerning whether it was an incomplete release or a postoperative recurrence [29, 55].

Significant clinical recovery is correlated with a decreased distal flattening ratio [3, 37], whereas swelling persists in the majority of cases. T2 signal intensity of the median nerve decreased by more than 10% [3].

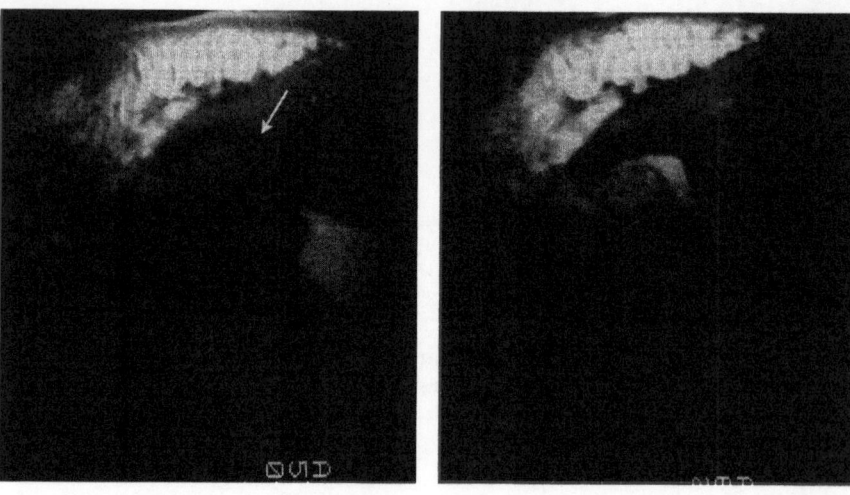

a   b

Fig. 19.17. Axial SE T1- (**a**) and fast SE T2-weighted (**b**) images through the hamate in a patient treated for carpal tunnel syndrome. Five days after surgery the flexor retinaculum is widely open. The space between the flexor tendons is enlarged. The median nerve and the interstitial space show a slightly hyperintense signal corresponding to post-release edema

However, not all patients respond well after surgical treatment. In these cases, exact determination of the underlying pathology is necessary for selecting treatment, especially for indicating surgical re-exploration [16]. Unsuccessful surgical release or recurrence after a short interval are usually caused by insufficient release [29, 54, 56], chronic neuritis in delayed surgery, persistence of a known cause of compression (i.e., fracture, osteophyte) or nerve tumors.

Acknowledgements. I thank Sylvie Urban for assistance in preparing the manuscript, and Pascal Gennerat for the illustrations. Many thanks go also to the team at the CIERM, in particular Jacques Bittoun and Ilana Idy Peretti, where most of the images were acquired.

References

1. Stoller DW, Brody GA (1997) Carpal tunnel syndrome The wrist and hand. In: Stoller DW (ed) Magnetic resonance imaging in orthopaedics and sports medicine, 2nd edn. Lippincot-Raven, Philadelphia
2. Phalen GS (1972) The carpal-tunnel syndrome. Clinical evaluation of 598 hands. Clin Orthop 83:29–40
3. Allmann KH, Horch R, Uhl M, Gufler H, Altehoefer C, Stark GB, Langer M (1997) MR imaging of the carpal tunnel. Eur J Radiol 25:141–145
4. Spinner RJ, Bachman JW, Amadio PC (1989) The many faces of carpal tunnel syndrome. Mayo Clin Proc 64:829–836
5. Monagle K, Dai G, Chu A, Burnham R, Snyder RE (1999) Quantitative MR imaging of carpal tunnel syndrome. AJR 172:1581–1586

6. Grundberg AB (1993) Carpal tunnel decompression in spite of normal electromyography. J Hand Surg 8:348–349
7. Jacobson JA (1999) Musculoskeletal sonography and MR imaging. Radiol Clin North Am 37:713–719
8. Martinoli C, Serafini G, Bianchi S, et al (1996) Ultrasonography of peripheral nerves. J Periph Nerv Syst 1:169
9. Bruhn H, Michael L, Gyngell MI, Hänicke W, Merboldt KD, Frahm J (1991) High-resolution fast low-angle shot magnetic resonance imaging of the normal hand. Skeletal Radiol 20:259–265
10. Healy C, Watson JD, Longstaff A, Campbell MJ (1990) Magnetic resonance imaging of the carpal tunnel. J Hand Surg [Br] 15:243–247
11. Sugimoto H, Miyaji N, Ohsawa T (1994) Carpal tunnel syndrome: evaluation of median nerve circulation with dynamic contrast-enhanced MR imaging. Radiology 190:439–466
12. Robbins H (1963) Anatomical study of the median nerve in the carpal tunnel and etiologies of the carpal tunnel syndrome. J Bone Joint Surg 45:953–965
13. Zeiss J, Skie M, Ebraheim N, Jackson WT (1989) Anatomic relations between the median nerve and flexor tendons in the carpal tunnel: MR evaluation in normal volunteers. AJR 153:533–536
14. Binkovitz LA, Cahill DR, Ehmen RL, Berquist TH (1988) Magnetic resonance imaging of the wrist: normal cross sectional imaging and selected abnormal cases. Radiographics 8:1171–1202
15. Arminio JA (1986) Etiology of carpal: tunnel syndrome. Del Med J 58:189–192
16. Buchberger W (1997) Radiologic imaging of the carpal tunnel. Eur J Radiol 25:112–117
17. Mesgarzadeh M, Schneck CD, Bonakdarpour A, Mitra A, Conaway D (1989) Carpal tunnel: MR imaging. I. Normal anatomy. Radiology 171:743–748
18. Bleecker ML, Bohlman M, Moreland R, Tipton A (1985) Carpal tunnel syndrome: role of carpal canal size. Neurology 35:1599–1604
19. Dekel S, Papaioannou T, Rushworth G, Coates R (1980) Idiopathic carpal tunnel syndrome caused by carpal stenosis. BMJ 280:1297–1299
20. Neal NC, McManners J, Stirling GA (1987) Pathology of the flexor tendon sheath in the spontaneous carpal tunnel syndrome. J Hand Surg [Br] 12:229–232
21. Lundborg G, Gelberman RH, Minteer-Convery M, Lee YF, Hargens AR (1982) Median nerve compression in the carpal tunnel: functional response to experimentally induced controlled pressure. J Hand Surg 7:252–258
22. Gelberman RH, Eaton R, Urbaniak JR (1993) Peripheral nerve compression. J Bone Joint Surg Am 75:1854
23. Shon LC (1994) Nerve entrapment neuropathy, and nerve dysfunction in athletes. Orthop Clin North Am 25:25–47
24. Said G (1976) Fusiform enlargement of mechanic origin of a peripheral nerve. Acta Neuropath (Berl) 35:47–54
25. Bodne D, Quinn SF, Kloss J, et al (1988) Reactive perineurial fibroblastic proliferation of the median nerve: MR characteristics. J Comput Assist Tomogr 12:532–534
26. Jolesz FA, Polak JF, Ruenzel PW, Adams DF (1984) Wallerian degeneration demonstrated by magnetic resonance: spectroscopic measurements on peripheral nerve. Radiology 152:85–87
27. Bittoun J, Saint-Jalmes H, Querleux B et al (1990) In vivo high-resolution MR imaging of the skin in a whole-body system at 1.5 T. Radiology 176:457–460
28. Weiss KL, Beltran J, Shamam OM, Stilla RF, Levey M (1986) High-field MR surface-coil imaging of the hand and wrist. I. Normal anatomy. Radiology 160:143–146
29. Richman JA, Gelberman RH, Rydevick BL, Hajek PC, Braun RM, Gylys-Morin VM (1989) Carpal tunnel syndrome: morphologic changes after release of the transverse carpal ligament. J Hand Surg [Am] 14:852–857
30. Dion E, Oberlin C, Codanda, Idy-Peretti I, Jolivet O, Dauge MC, Grellet J (1992) IRM en haute résolution du canal carpien. Corrélations anatomiques. J Radiol 73:293–301
31. Wong EC, Jesmanowicz A, Hyde JS (1991) High-resolution, short echo time MR imaging of the fingers and wrist with a local gradient coil. Radiology 181:393–397

32. Foo TFK, Shellock FG, Hayes CE, Schenck JF, Slayman BE (1992) High-resolution MR imaging of the wrist and eye with short TR, short TE and partial echo acquisition. Radiology 183:277–281

33. Erickson Scott, Cox IH, Hyde JS, Carrera GF, Strandt JA, Estkowski LD (1991) Effect of tendon orientation on MR imaging signal intensity: a manifestation of the "Magic Angle" phenomenon. Radiology 181:389–392

34. Fullerton GD, Cameron IL, Ord VA (1985) Orientation of tendons in the magnetic field and its effect on T2 relaxation times. Radiology 155:433–435

35. Beltran J, Noto AM, Herman LJ, Lubbers LM (1987) Tendons: high-field-strength, surface coil MR imaging. Radiology 162:735–739

36. Richman JA, Gelberman R, Rydevik BL, Gylys-Morin VM, Hajek PC, Sartoris DJ (1987) Carpal tunnel volume determination by magnetic resonance imaging three-dimensional reconstruction. J Hand Surg [Am] 12:712–717

37. Mesgarzadeh M, Schneck CD, Bonakdarpour A, Mitra A, Conaway D (1989) Carpal tunnel: MR imaging. II. Carpal tunnel syndrome. Radiology 171:749–754

38. Middelton WD, Kneeland JB, Kellman GM et al (1987) MR imaging of the carpal tunnel: normal anatomy and preliminary findings in the carpal tunnel syndrome. AJR 148:307–316

39. Pierre-Jerome C, Bekkelund SI, Meligren-S, Nordstrom R (1997) Quantitative MR imaging and electrophysiology of preoperative carpal tunnel syndrome in a female population. Ergonomics 40:642–649

40. Radack DM, Schweitzer ME, Taras J (1997) Carpal tunnel syndrome are the MR findings a result of population selection bias? AJR 169:1649–1653

41. Inglis AE, Straub LR, Williams CS (1972) Median nerve neuropathy at the wrist. Clin Orthop 83:48–54

42. Brahme SK, Hodler J, Braun RM, Sebrechts C, Jackson W, Resnick D (1997) Dynamic MR imaging of carpal tunnel syndrome. Skeletal Radiol 26:482–487

43. Stull MA, Moser RP, Kransdorf MJ, Bogumill GP, Nelson MC (1991) Magnetic resonance appearance of peripheral nerve sheath tumors. Skeletal Radiol 20:9–14

44. Dion E, Idy-Peretti I, Bellin MF, Codanda R, Grellet J, Bittoun J (1991) MR imaging of the carpal tunnel using a specific high resolution gradient coil (abstract). Radiologic Society of North America, Chicago

45. Enziger FM, Weiss SW (1983) Soft tissue tumors. Mosby, St Louis

46. O'Duffy JD, Randall RV, MacCarty CS (1973) Median neuropathy (carpal tunnel syndrome) in acromegaly. A sign of endocrine overactivity. Ann Intern Med 78:379–383

47. Baum H, Ludecke DK, Hermann HD (1986) Carpal tunnel syndrome and acromegaly. Acta Neurochir (Wien) 83:54–55

48. Fléchaire A, Flocard F, Vincent E, Bady B (1991) Syndrome du canal carpien et endocrinopathies. Sem Hop Paris 67:1781–1784

49. Sanders V (1962) Neurologic manifestations of myxoedema. N Engl J Med 266:547–552

50. Yamagushi DM, Lipscomb PR, Soule EM (1965) Carpal tunnel syndrome. Minn Med 48:22–23

51. Fraser DM, Cambell PW, Ewing DJ, Clarke BF (1979) Mononeuropathy in diabetes mellitus. Diabetes 28:96–101

52. Menon J (1994) Endoscopic carpal tunnel release: preliminary report. Arthroscopy 10:31

53. Rowland EB, Kleinert JM (1993) Endoscopic carpal-tunnel release in cadavers: an investigation of the results of 12 surgeons with this training model. J Bone Joint Surg Am 75:1854

54. Gartsman GM, Kovvach JC, Crouch CC, Noble PC, Bennett JB (1986) Carpal arch alteration after carpal tunnel release. J Hand Surg [Am] 11:372–374

55. Langloh ND, Linscheid RL (1972) Recurrent and unrelieved carpal-tunnel syndrome. Clin Orthop 83:41–47

56. Silver MA, Gelberman RH, Gellman H, Rhoades CE (1985) Carpal tunnel syndrome: associated abnormalities in ulnar nerve function and the effect of carpal tunnel release on these abnormalities. J Hand Surg 10:710–713

20   Angiography and Vascular Disorders of the Hand

FRANCESCO FLORIO, SILVERIO BALZANO, MICHELE NARDELLA,
VINCENZO STRIZZI, MARIO CAMMISA

20.1   Introduction

The study of the anatomy and vascular pathology of the hand appears problematic due to the hand's anatomical complexity, and the variety of clinical-pathological situations involving the hand. Currently, the use of diagnostic angiographic methods (arteriography and venography) has to be considered in the context of a multidisciplinary approach to vascular pathology, which gives increasing importance to noninvasive techniques (echo-color Doppler, magnetic resonance angiography). Furthermore, a diagnostic angiographic approach cannot be considered separately from the possibility of using interventional radiology treatments, directly connected to the angiographic technique.

20.2   Anatomy

The main blood flow to the hand arises from the radial and ulnar arteries, both of which are branches of the brachial artery. Occasionally, the axillary artery divides into the radial and ulnar artery without giving rise to a brachial artery. Sometimes, the brachial artery branches off into the two arteries precociously. These anatomical variants become important when it is necessary to insert a needle directly into the axillary or brachial artery. Sometimes both the radial and ulnar artery are absent; in these cases they are substituted by an interosseous artery and its branches. Normally, the radial artery starts from the neck of the radius and goes to the palm of the hand, anastomosing itself with the deep branch of the ulnar artery giving rise to the deep palmar arc. Along its course, the recurrent radial artery, the muscular artery and other small branches arise. In addition, at the level of the wrist, the radial artery gives rise to the posterior carpal arc before ending in the principal artery of the thumb and in the deep palmar arc. The recurrent ulnar artery, the common artery, the interosseous artery and muscular branches start from the ulnar artery; at the end, it forms the superficial palmar arc. Both palmar arcs receive an arterial branch from the contralateral artery. Finally, the metacarpal palmar arteries begin from the deep palmar arc while the digital palmar arteries begin from the superficial palmar arc. Generally, the radial artery supplies blood to the thumb and the radial side of the forefinger while the ulnar artery supplies blood to the remaining fingers. In 40% of cases the metacarpal palmar circle and the anastomosis of the digital arteries at the base of the fingers supply a double flow to the phalanges (Fig. 20.1).

The venous system of the upper limb is divided into the superficial venous circle and the deep venous circle; the two systems are connected at different levels by thin intercommunicating vessels. With respect to the superficial venous circle, the blood flow at the level of the hand goes through the veins of the dorsal net which drain into the two superficial main veins of the forearm: the basilic vein, situated internally, and the cephalic vein, situated laterally. An antecubital vein links these two at the level of the anterior side of the elbow. The deep veins of the palm of the hand drain blood into the ulnar and radial veins, which follow the course of the homonymous arteries and join at the level of the elbow. Here they form the two omeral veins. The basilic vein, situated internally, flows into the omeral vein, just before the latter becomes the axillary vein. The cephalic vein, instead, goes up again sideways and on to the humerus, flowing into the axillary vein [8, 17, 19].

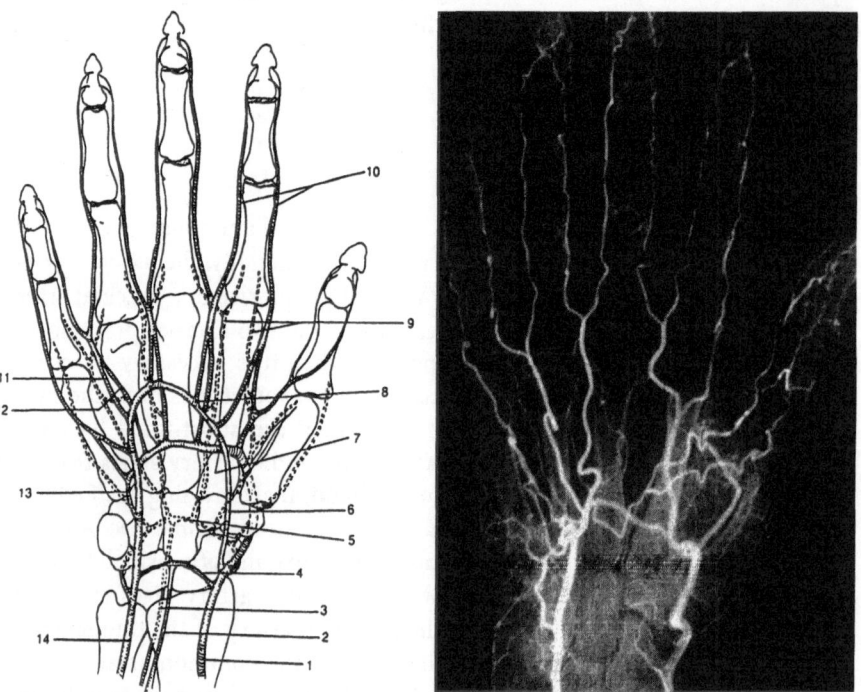

a   b

Fig. 20.1a, b. Classic arterial anatomy of the hand. *1* radial artery, *2* anterior interosseous artery, *3* posterior interosseous artery, *4* palmar carpal branch, *5* dorsal carpal branch forming the dorsal carpal rete, *6* superficial palmar branch of the radial artery, *7* deep palmar arch, *8* superficial palmar arch, *9* dorsal metacarpal arteries, *10* proper palmar digital arteries, *11* common palmar digital arteries, *12* palmar metacarpal, *13* deep palmar branch of the ulnar artery, *14* ulnar artery. (From Rose and Kadir [17], p 86)

20.3 Imaging and Interventional Techniques

Nowadays, any angiographic investigation is easier, safer and more effective because of the availability of digital angiography, which allows for a reduction in both radiation exposure and the quantity of contrast medium. Digital angiography provides better spatial and contrast resolution compared with traditional angiography. Any kind of interventional procedure is much easier, thanks to the possibilities of taking electronic measurements of vessel diameter and techniques such as "road-mapping".

20.3.1 Arteriography

For arteriography of the hand the percutaneous transfemoral approach is generally preferred. Direct needle insertion in the axillary or brachial artery is used less often as it is more difficult and potentially prone to more complications. Today small-caliber catheters are available which allow an increased flow of contrast medium. Generally, selective catheterization of the omeral artery (through the subclavian and the axillary artery) is necessary. The use of hydrophilic guidewires and of small-caliber catheters made from soft and antitraumatic material, makes any procedure of arterial catheterization very safe.

Usually, in order to obtain adequate visualization of the more peripheral arterial branches of the hand, a small quantity of contrast medium (8–12 ml) has to be injected. The flow of injection is regulated case by case (4–6 ml/s). It is preferable to use non-ionic contrast medium, with a low concentration of iodine, to reduce the sensation of heat and pain to the extremities. When imaging children or uncooperative patients it is helpful to use some type of sedation. The visualization of the more peripheral branches of the arterial tree of the hand is improved by an intra-arterial injection, before injecting the contrast medium, of a vasodilator (usually 100–200 µg of nitroglycerin and sometimes 12–25 mg of tolazoline). This can also be useful in the differential diagnosis between vasal spasm and peripheral stenoses. The same effect can be obtained by immersing the hand in hot water or inducing artificially a post-ischemic hyperemia. For the latter technique a pressure band is placed at the base of the arm for 3 or 4 min, while buflomedyl (100 mg) in injected intra-arterially. The injection of contrast medium is done at the moment the pressure is released, when post-ischemic vasodilatation is at a maximum.

Complications are very rare; they can occur at the access point (hematoma, dissection) or in the catheterized arterial district (dissection of the arterial wall, distal embolism) [3, 8, 16, 19].

20.3.2 Venography

Upper limb venography is performed with the patient in a supine position studying both the superficial and deep veins, even if investigation is more frequently carried out on deep veins. The opacification of the omeral, axillary and subclavian veins is obtained by inserting a no. 20–22 needle into the basilic vein of the arm or forearm. Generally, for good visualization of the veins, 20–30 cm³ of contrast medium is injected with a flow of 3–4 cm³/s. To opacify distant deep veins, it is necessary to insert a needle into a vein of the wrist and to inject contrast medium at this point, applying a tourniquet in the proximity of the elbow, to facilitate the passage of contrast medium from the superficial veins to the deep veins, through small intercommunicating vessels which link the two systems.

20.3.3 Fibrinolysis

Fibrinolysis is an extremely useful technique in emergency situations. It is used for the treatment of acute thrombosis within 48 h of onset. Selective catheterization of the thrombosed arterial branches is necessary, with the end of the catheter as close as possible to the thrombus. Often the treatment is more effective by performing mechanical thrombolysis with an angiographic guide. A (partial) fragmentation of the thrombus is induced and so better adhesion of the molecules of the fibrinolytic agent to the thrombus is acquired. Currently, multi-sidehole small catheters are available that are connected to electric pumps automatically injecting the fibrinolytic agent. It is preferable to use a bolus-injection technique followed by continuous infusion for 24–48 h. The fibrinolytic agents used are urokinase and recombinant tissue plasminogen activator (rTPA). The technique of local fibrinolytic therapy has shown a significant improvement in the percentage of immediate technical success compared with systemic fibrinolytic therapy. At the same time, it allows for a reduction in bleeding complications, which is related to the smaller quantity of drugs injected [1, 2, 7, 9].

20.3.4 Embolization

Embolization is an interventional radiology procedure that can be useful both in emergency situations (acute bleeding) and in elective conditions (preoperative or definitive treatment of vascular malformations). A large-lumen catheter is pushed up as far as the omeral artery; a microcatheter is inserted inside this, which can selectively reach even the smallest peripheral branches of the artery. The use of such a coaxial system has two substantial advantages: First, it provides for a variation in the choice of microcatheter according to the particular situation, which allows ever more selective catheterization and embolization without having to further apply a catheter to the principal arterial branch. Secondly, it allows contrast medium injection into the space between the carrying catheter and the microcatheter. This allows a panoramic study and is used to check the effects of the embolization in real time. In this way, two safe routes are created: the microcatheter for the injection of embolic agents, and the carrying catheter for the confirmation of embolization.

There are two types of microcatheter: flux-driven, very thin extremely soft ones, whose end is pushed by the blood flow in the vessel lumen; and non-flux-driven larger ones which require the help of a micro-guide to be pushed into the vessel lumen.

In the embolization phase, two factors are very important: the kind of embolic material used and the method of injection. Regarding the embolic agent, the choice is influenced by the type of embolization performed (temporary or permanent), the target organ, the type of catheter used, and the state of the blood flow in the target organ. Embolic agents can be divided into two categories: reabsorbable (or temporary) materials and non-reabsorbable (or permanent) materials. Among the first (for temporary occlusions) the most commonly used are autologous materials and Gelfoam; among the second (for permanent occlusions) are Ivalon, bucrylate, absolute ethanol, stainless-steel coils, and detachable balloons.

Bucrylate is the liquid embolizing agent most commonly used. It has to be injected with a coaxial system by a microcatheter. Metallic coils, which induce vessel occlusion by thrombosis, are especially used to obstruct large arteriovenous fistulas or large vessels, particularly for preoperative embolization of tumor masses and embolization of aneurysms.

A disadvantage of the use of coils is the potential for wrong placement or displacement as well as the wrong choice of the dimensions of the coils. Detachable balloons, released in the arteries with the help of coaxial systems, have the disadvantage of high cost and the risk of the progressive loss of strain with the possibility of migration and/ or recanalization of the vessel.

With regard to the method of injection, in order to guarantee optimal embolization and maximum safety, the embolic agents (mechanical devices or particulate materials) generally require extreme caution in their use and low speed of injection, to avoid both iatrogenic damage to the vessel wall and, above all, unintentional back flow (reflux) of the embolic agent. In some cases, a "jam flow" technique may be needed, whereby a balloon catheter is set at the mouth of the vessel creating an obstruction, in order to avoid any risk of reflux of embolic agents while at the same time obtaining complete filling of the distal branches [14, 15, 21].

20.3.5 Angioplasty

It is extremely rare to use angioplasty for the treatment of focal stenosis at the level of distal arteries of the wrist or hand. This is due to the very small size of these vessels. Angioplasty is frequently used for the treatment of proximal vascular stenoses causing ischemia at the level of the hand. Arteriosclerotic fibromuscular dysplasic stenoses can be successfully treated by angioplasty, with or without an endovascular stent, at the level of both subclavian and omeral arteries. The technique for this kind of treatment, for the subclavian-brachial district, is not substantially different from that used for the treatment of stenosis of other arterial districts. It is obvious that the caliber of the catheters used and the diameter of the angioplasty balloon have to be suited to the caliber of the vessels being treated.

Also in this arterial district, angioplasty shows a good percentage of success (90%) with a 3–4 year patency of 80–95%. The risk of complications is minimal (0.5–4.8%); included in this percentage are the complications caused by vascular access procedures, usually femoral [4, 10].

20.4   Clinical Applications of Angiographic Techniques

The use of angiographic techniques (both for diagnostic and for interventional procedures) is diverse and can be required in non-emergency and in emergency situations.

20.4.1   Emergency Procedures

20.4.1.1   Acute Ischemia

Acute ischemia of the upper limbs is the clinical condition that most frequently requires the use of the angiographic technique. Acute ischemia of the hand can be due to either arterial or venous thrombosis. From the clinical point of view, in the case of acute ischemia it is usually straightforward to distinguish between venous and arterial thrombosis. In the first case, as well as ischemia, there is also edema and cyanosis.

Arterial thrombotic ischemia can be linked to pathological conditions situated along the proximal (stenosis or thrombosis of the subclavian-axillary and omeral axis) or distal arterial tree. In the latter case, the most frequent condition is peripheral embolism. Among the most common clinical causes of peripheral embolism of the hand are proximal arteriosclerotic lesions and cardiac arrhythmia. Traumatic vascular arterial lesion is the most common cause of acute ischemia of the hand. The pathogenetic mechanism is usually a disruption of the vessel wall or dissection with acute thrombosis (Fig. 20.2).

Echocolor Doppler is able to document the point of vascular thrombosis with sufficient accuracy. However, in this clinical situation an angiographic procedure is almost always required in order to achieve more accurate topographical localization of the vascular thrombosis as well as for the correct planning of treatment, which may include interventional radiology. In the case of arterial thrombosis, the angiographic procedure should be as detailed as possible, including the evaluation of the patency of the complete arterial tree, from the subclavian artery to the more peripheral branches. In the case of embolism, the angiographic examination reveals the typical sign of defects in the vascular lumen.

In the case of venous thrombosis the venography examination must be a detailed study of all venous systems. The evaluation of the patency of the superficial and deep vascular systems is essential.

In the case of acute thrombosis, local thrombolysis is usually successful, especially if linked to subsequent treatment of the local occlusion by angioplasty or stenting. Even a post-traumatic dissection can be treated by stenting. Stenosis of vessels is

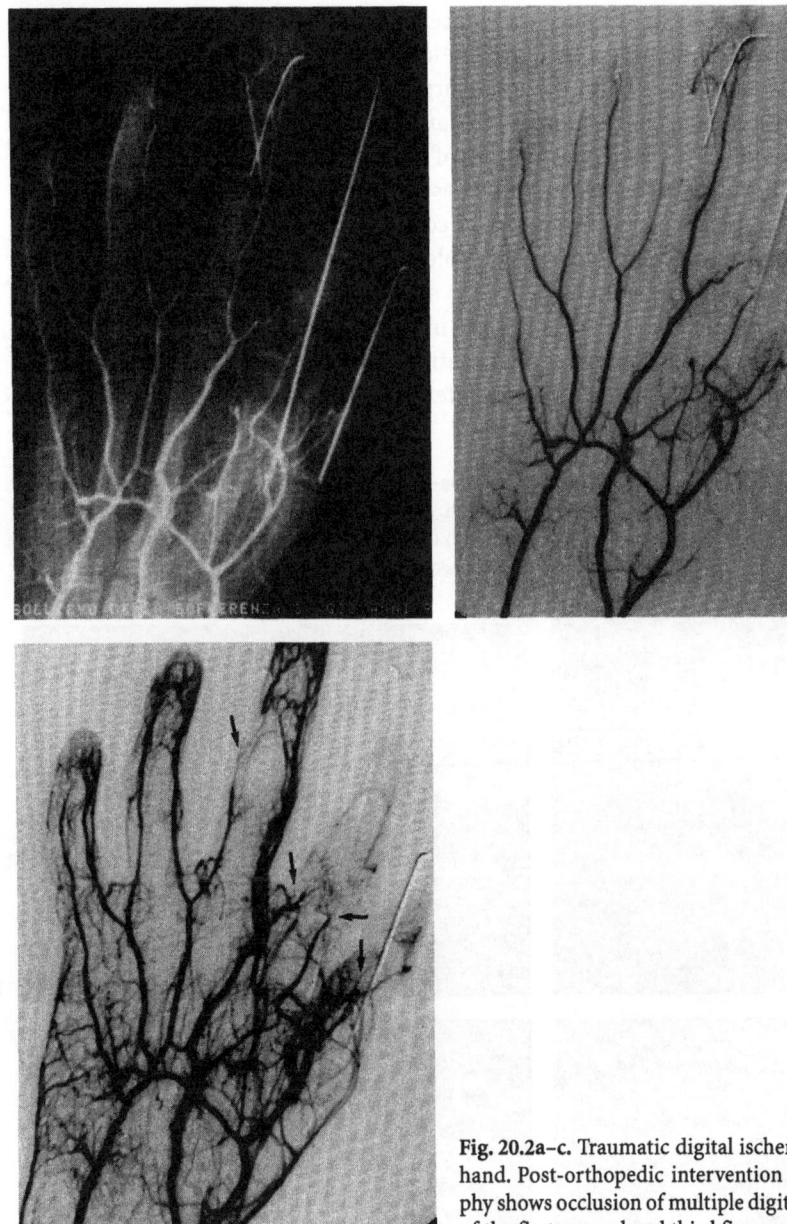

Fig. 20.2a–c. Traumatic digital ischemia of the hand. Post-orthopedic intervention angiography shows occlusion of multiple digital arteries of the first, second and third fingers (*arrows*)

often detected after fibrinolytic treatment of arterial thrombosis. Also in these situations, with or without stent, angioplasty can be applied successfully [6, 11].

20.4.1.2 Hemorrhage

Acute traumatic lesions are the most frequent causes of hemorrhage; hemorrhage can also occur as a result of spontaneous or traumatic rupture of pre-existing vascular lesions such as aneurysms or pseudo-aneurysms (Fig. 20.3) and arterio-venous malformations. In case of traumatic hemorrhage it is unusual to use embolization to stop the bleeding, because surgical intervention is generally the only therapeutic choice. The angiographic examination can show the exact site of the bleeding and can evaluate the integrity of the arterial tree, in order to give to the surgeon the most precise preoperative vascular map possible, for use in intervention planning. The use of embolization could become necessary in situations in which surgical intervention is not possible due to particular pathological or anatomical conditions.

Embolization is more frequently used in the case of hemorrhage resulting from rupture of peripheral vascular malformations. In these cases embolization can be a preparation for a successive surgical intervention to eradicate the malformation.

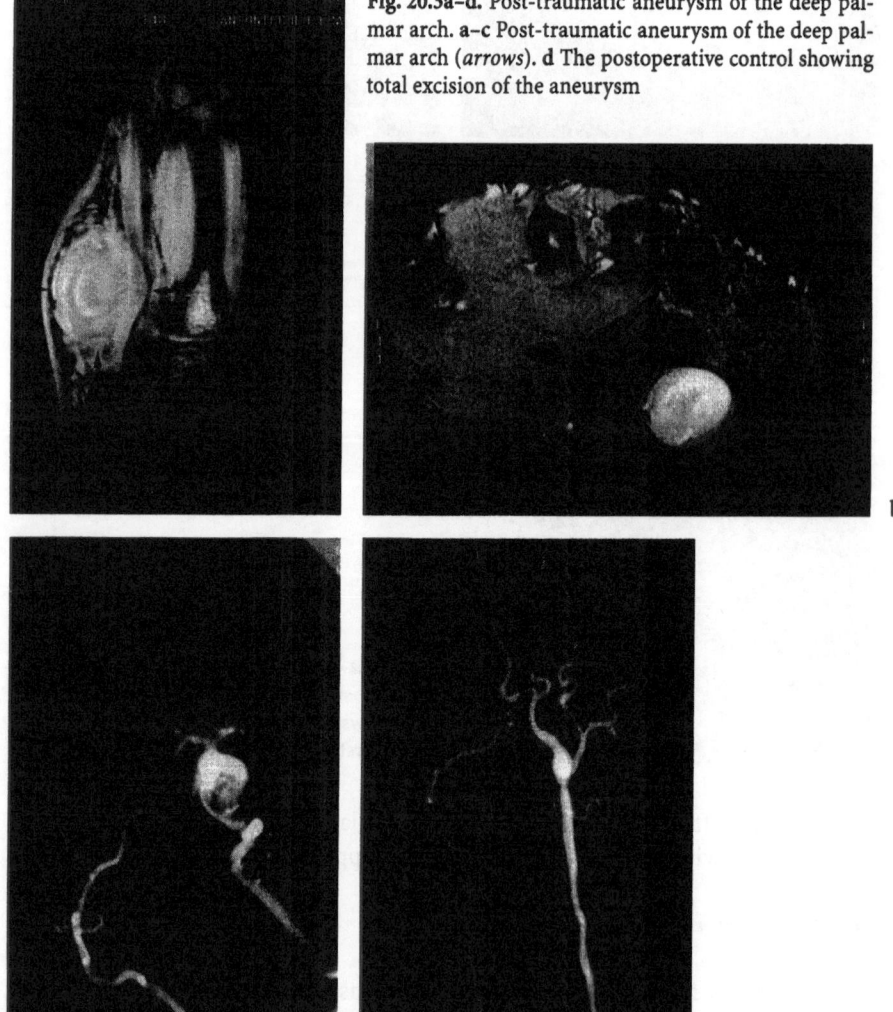

Fig. 20.3a–d. Post-traumatic aneurysm of the deep palmar arch. **a–c** Post-traumatic aneurysm of the deep palmar arch (*arrows*). **d** The postoperative control showing total excision of the aneurysm

20.4.2   Elective Procedures

20.4.2.1   Chronic Ischemia

Chronic ischemia can be caused by various pathological conditions. Arteriosclerotic vascular lesions are usually located at the proximal site of the arterial tree (subclavian and/or axillary artery), whereas, diabetic arteriopathy involves the peripheral arterial branches. Chronic trauma after particular types of work, activities and hobbies is among the most frequent causes of chronic ischemia of the hand. In this case, the lesions are usually located in the peripheral palmar and digital branches. The lesions are caused by repetitive and progressive endothelial damage followed by platelet deposition and subsequent occlusion of the vessel. Classical syndromes from chronic trauma are *hypothenar hammer syndrome* and *thenar hammer syndrome*. In the former, the ulnar artery is involved at the hypothenar eminence. The ulnar artery lies superficial, and so unprotected, where it crosses the surface of the hamate. In the latter, the radial artery is damaged by trauma occurring at the level of the second metacarpal; the causes are identical to those of hypothenar hammer syndrome. A traumatic action, even of modest severity but repetitive, at the level of the palm or of the back of the hand can cause these syndromes. These repetitive actions occur in some manual occupations or in some sports (pounding motions, use of vibrator tools, tennis, handball) and cause traumatic lesions of arteries resulting in obliteration of arteries of the palmar arches and/or of digital arteries (Fig. 20.4). Congenital malformation of the palmar arches can be a predisposing factor. In both syndromes, arteriography shows, at the level of the arteries, the presence of vasospasm, occlusion, formation of pseudoaneurysm or distal embolization. The severity of the ischemic symptoms increases if the palmar arch is incomplete. Freezing and electric shock are other causes of multiple and extensive arterial occlusions.

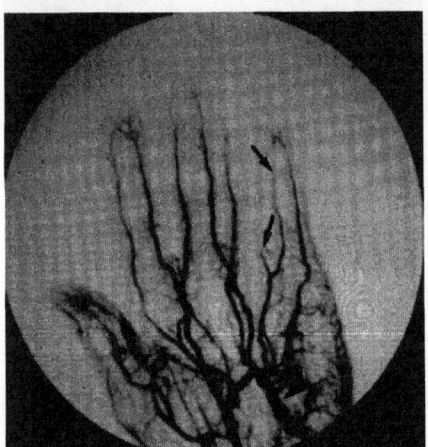
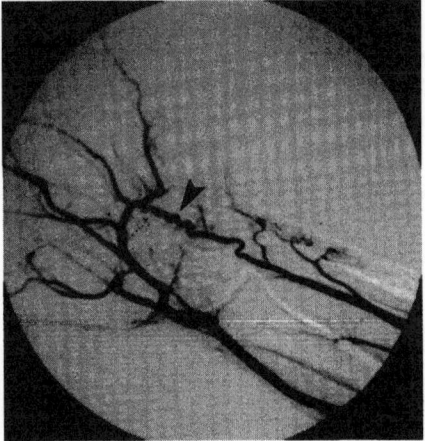

a   b

Fig. 20.4a, b. Hammer syndrome. There is discontinuity of the ulnar artery (corkscrew sign) (*arrowhead*), with occlusion of the fourth and fifth (radial side) finger digital arteries (*arrows*)

Chronic ischemia can also be adjunct to vasomotor phenomena (*Raynaud's syndrome*) or to collagen vascular disease. Raynaud's syndrome is characterized by the constriction of the small arteries of the extremities in response to pain, cold and emotional stimuli. It manifests itself in three phases: ischemic, cyanotic and erythematous. It is much more frequent in the hand, being limited to the fingers, excluding the thumb. The symptoms are typically linked to the winter season and are especially seen in young women. At the angiography examination, the arteries appear to be normal especially in the purely vasomotor phase. When arteriolar disease is established, the examination can identify arterial-venular hyperemia in the fingers. The injection of tolazoline can be useful to differentiate vasospasm from stenoses of other types.

In connective tissue diseases (dermatomyositis, scleroderma, rheumatoid arthritis, systemic lupus erythematosus) the pathophysiological mechanism of vascular damage is represented by concentric intimal thickening, causing obliteration of the lumen. This occurs especially in small vessels. The angiograms in such diseases are not specific. In general, the true digital arteries are involved, with absence of collateral circles. In addition, a complete or relative reduction of the radial artery diameter and of the deep palmar arch has been reported. Bilateral involvement is also typical of those diseases (Figs. 20.5, 20.6).

Finally, there are other ischemic lesions of an inflammatory type or idiopathic, such as *Burger disease* or *Takayasu's arteritis.*

Burger disease, affecting young male smokers, is an inflammatory process that involves the arteries and the veins, with a medium-sized or small lumen, of the extremities. The vessels show diffuse intimal thickening, and adventitial fibrosis without lesions of the tunica media. Multiple stenoses and occlusions at the level of the forearm and of the hand can be seen with angiography; also some collateral circles and some saccular aneurysms can develop. The arterial vessels show a rectilinear course, and an evenly reduced lumen, with regular contours. The collat-

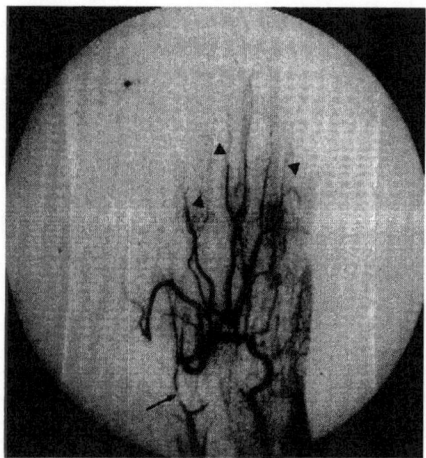 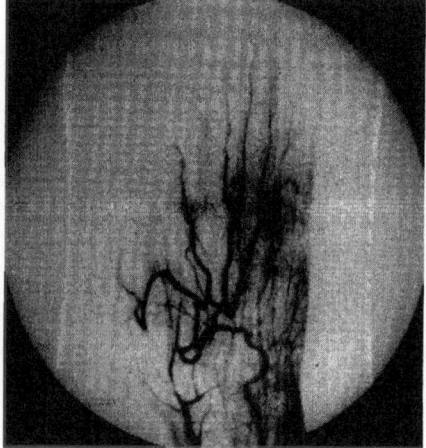

a   b

Fig. 20.5a, b. Scleroderma. There is occlusion of multiple digital arteries (*arrowheads*) and superficial palmar arch (*arrows*)

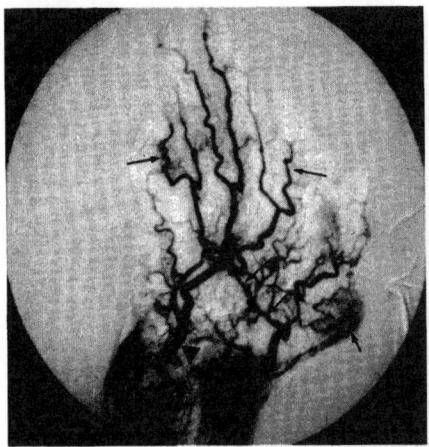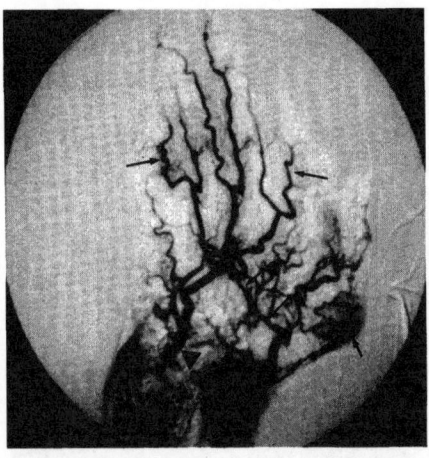

a   b

Fig. 20.6a, b. Rheumatoid arthritis. There is sparing and interruption of the superficial palmar arch (*arrowheads*) and a vasculitic disorder of the digital arteries (*arrows*)

eral branches are few and particularly thin. All arterial segments show insufficient opacification, like a "bare tree".

Takayasu's arteritis appears in the second decade of life and affects predominantly women. It is characterized by an inflammatory process which causes intimal thickening with connective tissue proliferation. The aorta and its principal branches are primarily affected and the left subclavian artery is also affected in 75% of cases. The angiographic manifestation of a smooth, tapered stenosis, involving the proximal part of the vessel, is characteristic of this condition.

Fibromuscolar dysplasia of the upper limbs is uncommon, but when it is present it has the characteristic appearance of a "string of pearls".

In such situations of chronic ischemia, the possibilities of interventional radiology are almost exclusively restricted to endovascular treatment with angioplasty and/or stenting of the proximal stenosis (Fig. 20.7). Arteriography can also be helpful in the diagnosis of these pathologies, which, however, are usually diagnosable from the symptomatology and anamnesis.

Chronic ischemia can also be caused by the "steal phenomenon". This can develop after hemodialysis access graft construction or post-traumatic arteriovenous fistula (Fig. 20.8), due to elevated shunt flow. The ischemic symptomatology, in the arterial tree distal to the point of the access graft, can be severe.

20.4.2.2 Preoperative Vascular Map

Arteriography plays an important role in preoperative anatomical evaluation. It is especially useful in reconstructive surgery. An accurate evaluation of the patency of the peripheral arterial tree of the hand is essential in order to achieve successful surgery of vascular anastomosis.

Similar problems exist when surgical intervention for the removal of arteriovenous malformations is necessary. In these cases it is absolutely essential to know

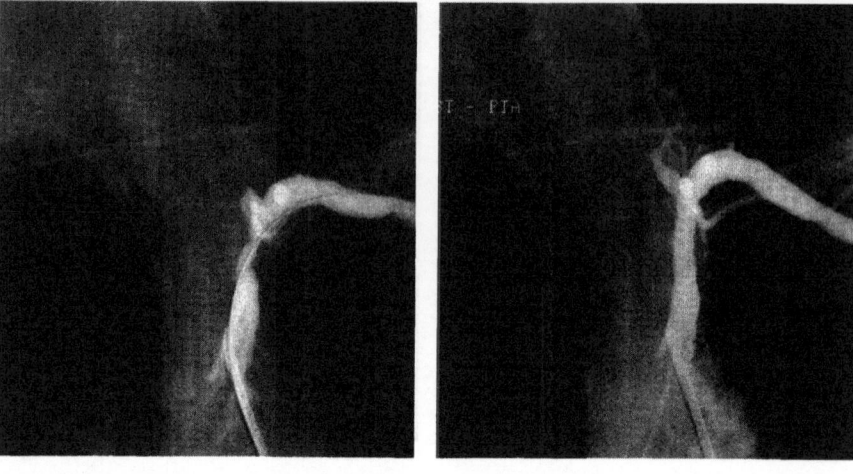

a   b

Fig. 20.7A, B. Stenosis of the subclavian artery. High-grade stenosis of the subclavian artery is seen (**A**); after angioplasty there is total resolution of the stenosis (**B**)

precisely the complex anatomy of the arterial feeding vessels as well as of the draining veins.

As has already been pointed out, in such situations angiography has a dual function: diagnostic and, when possible, curative by means of embolization. The latter can be, in the case of the arteriovenous malformations, considered either definitive treatment, or as often happens, a preparative treatment for an eventual surgical intervention. It is evident that an embolization, even if partial, of the arteries feeding the fistula is a much less risky than direct surgical intervention [5, 8, 12, 13, 16, 18–20].

20.5   Conclusions

As in the study of other vascular districts, noninvasive imaging techniques (color Doppler and magnetic resonance imaging) have progressively reduced the field of application of angiography. But the situations in which angiography is essential or useful are still numerous. The reduction in angiographic diagnostic examinations is largely compensated for by the increased use of interventional radiology procedures. These procedures are increasingly sophisticated and have improved during recent years. Their therapeutic purposes have been extended to the vascular pathology of the hand.

Fig. 20.8a–f. Traumatic arteriovenous fistula (AVF). There is enlargement of the radial artery and large feeding arteries shunting flow into an AVF of the first finger (**a, b**), with large draining veins (**c**). Following embolization (**d–f**) there is total occlusion of the AVF (microcatheter tip: *arrowhead*)

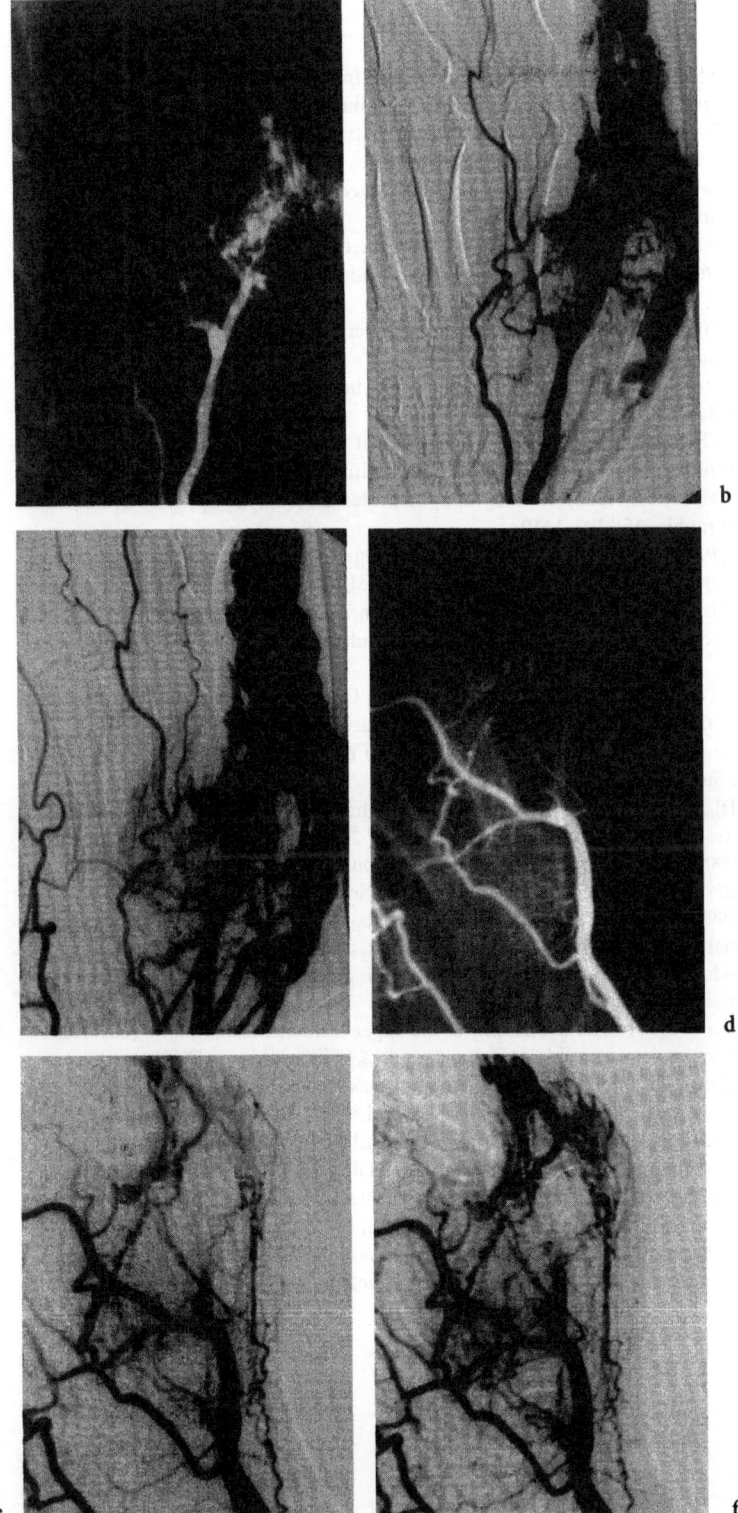

References

1. Becker GJ, Holden RW (1992) Fibrinolytic therapy. In: Castaneda-Zuniga WR, Tadavarthy SM (eds) Interventional radiology. Williams and Wilkins, Baltimore, pp 599–634
2. Belkin M, Belkin B, Bucknam CA, et al (1986) Intra-arterial fibrinolytic therapy. Efficacy of streptokinase vs urokinase. Arch Surg 121:769–773
3. Cercueil JP, Becker F, Holtzmann P et al (1997) Arteriographie de la main. Aspects techniques. J Radiol 78:677–679
4. Henry M, Amor M, Henry I et al (1999) Percutaneous transluminal angioplasty of the subclavian arteries. In: ETC 99, 10th international course book of peripheral vascular intervention. Paris, Europa Edition, pp 617–627
5. Jackson JE, Mitchell A (1997) Advanced vascular interventional techniques in the management of trauma. Semin Interv Radiol 14:139–150
6. Jones NF (1991) Acute and chronic ischemia of the hand: pathophysiology, treatment and prognosis. J Hand Surg [Am] 16:1074–1083
7. Kaufman JA, Bettmann MA (1992) Thrombolyis of peripheral vascular occlusions with urokinase. A review of the clinical literature. Semin Interv Radiol 9:159–165
8. Loring LA, Hallisey MJ (1995) Arteriography and interventional therapy for diseases of the hand. Radiographics 15:1299–1310
9. Lupattelli L (1994) Il trattamento fibrinolitico locoregionale. In: Corso monotematico: radiologia interventistica. XXXVI Congresso Nazionale SIRM, 21–25 March, Milan, pp 147–165
10. Mathias K, Jager H (1999) Pta proximal subclavian artery obstruction. In: ETC 99, 10th international course book of peripheral vascular intervention. Paris, Europa Edition, pp 607–616
11. McLafferty RB, Edwards JM, Taylor LM, et al (1995) Diagnosis and long-term clinical outcome in patients diagnosed with hand ischemia. J Vasc Surg 22:361–369
12. Nehler MR, Dalman RL, Harris EJ, et al (1992) Upper extremity arterial bypass distal to the wrist. J Vasc Surg 16:633–642
13. Neill-Cage DJ, Rechnic M, Braun M (1997) Bilateral thenar Hammer syndrome as a result of cumulative trauma: a case report. J Hand Surg [Am] 22:1081–1083
14. Novak D (1990) Complication of arterial embolization. In: Dondelinger RF, Rossi P, Kurdziel JC (eds) Interventional radiology. Thieme Medical, New York, pp 314–324
15. Novak D (1990) Embolization materials. In: Dondelinger RF, Rossi P, Kurdziel JC (eds) Interventional radiology. Thieme Medical, New York, pp 295–313
16. Reid SC, Kirchner TM, Pagan-Marin H (1997) Arteriography and intervention in extremity trauma. Semin Interv Radiol 14:193–204
17. Rose SC, Kadir S (1991) Arterial anatomy of the upper extremities. In: Kadir S (eds) Atlas of normal and variant angiographic anatomy. Saunders, Philadelphia, pp 55–95
18. Spittell PC, Spittell JA (1993) Occlusive arterial disease of the hand due to repetitive blunt trauma: a review with illustrative cases. Int J Cardiol 38:281–292
19. Sutton D (1983) Arteriography of the upper extremities. In: Abrams HL (ed) Abrams' angiography (vascular and interventional radiology). Little Brown, Boston, pp 1923–1936
20. Valji K, Hye RJ, Roberts AC, et al (1995) Hand ischemia in patients with hemodialysis access grafts: angiographic diagnosis and treatment. Radiology 196:697–701
21. Young AT, Tadavarthy SM, Yedlicka JW, et al (1992) Vascular embolotherapy. In: Castaneda-ZunigaWR, Tadavarthy SM (eds) Interventional radiology. William and Wilkins, Baltimore, pp 9–73

21   Osteonecrosis of the Carpal Bones

PETER G. BRACKE, JAN E. VANDEVENNE, LUDO F. COENEN,
PHILIPP K. LANG

21.1   Introduction

Avascular necrosis and aseptic necrosis are terms describing a wide spectrum of ischemic disease in bone tissue. Definitions of these and related terms are discussed followed by an overview of the pathophysiology. Imaging findings on conventional radiographs, computed tomography (CT), magnetic resonance (MR) imaging and bone scintigraphy are described for the different stages of avascular necrosis. Finally, this chapter emphasizes the specific locations of the wrist that are most frequently involved, such as the lunate and the scaphoid bone, and less frequently the capitate and the hamulus of the hamate bone.

21.2   Overview and Definitions

The terms osteonecrosis and aseptic necrosis are, although often found in radiologic reports, in fact terms defined by anatomopathologists. Radiologists have borrowed these terms to describe different pathologic conditions varying from bone ischemia to cortical bone and marrow cell death, fracture and irreversible bone deformation and/or fragmentation.

Osteonecrosis, bone infarct and osteochondrosis have a common origin although their definition and presentation are slightly different. A *bone infarct* is a localized area of ischemic necrosis resulting from reduction of the arterial blood supply or obstruction of the venous outflow and is often, though not exclusively, diaphyseal.

Osteochondrosis may be defined as a form of osteonecrosis due to vascular impairment with ischemia of one or more of the growth centers in children, followed by regeneration and calcification. The terms osteochondrosis and osteonecrosis have been used interchangeably.

Osteonecrosis is the sum of morphologic changes that result from cell death. Osteonecrosis is most often epiphyseal. Avascular necrosis or osteonecrosis presents with a spectrum of reversible and often, mainly irreversible, changes to the bony elements depending on the degree of ischemia, the localization, and the size and the number of possible repair mechanisms. The natural course and multifactorial etiology of avascular necrosis is further explained in the next section on pathophysiology.

The most important factor among the different etiologies seems to be a blockage of the vascular structures resulting in reversible or irreversible damage to the osteocytes. Various investigators have studied the blood supply of the carpus employing different techniques. Although controversy exists about the flow patterns, a consensus prevails that poor vascularization of the carpus is a major prognostic factor in carpal fracture healing and the development of osteonecrosis. The small bones of the carpus have a limited vascular supply and venous outflow, because much of their surface is covered by cartilage. This creates a relatively poor circulation particularly in the proximal two thirds of the scaphoid, the proximal capitate, the entire lunate bone and the base of the hook of the hamate. Therefore, these bones are vulnerable to ischemia and avascular necrosis after injury.

Another consequence of the large proportion of bone covered by cartilage is the relatively limited amount of nerve endings. This explains why the initial stages of avascular necrosis are often insidious, with only vague nonspecific clinical findings. The clinical spectrum of avascular necrosis ranges from totally asymptomatic to accelerated osteoarthritis with painful carpal instability leading to arthrodesis. The radioclinical diagnosis of osteonecrosis has a high specificity but poor sensitivity because patients usually present with late-stage disease.

Radioisotope bone scans are sensitive but only establish that some pathology is present without providing any information about the bone morphology or pathology characteristics. MR imaging has proven useful in the evaluation of osteonecrosis by depicting radiographically and clinically occult forms of avascular necrosis and by allowing follow-up through different stages due to specific signal intensity changes depending on the degree of the disease process. The treatment modalities are not uniform, often controversial and differ according to the initial presentation, clinical picture and radiographic and MR imaging findings.

21.3   Pathophysiology

Osteonecrosis is cell death in the different components of bone: hematopoietic fat marrow (marrow cells) and mineralized tissue (osteocytes). Osteonecrosis is not a specific disease entity. It is the final common pathway of a number of conditions, most of which lead to impairment of the blood supply to the involved bone segment, which explains the frequently used terms of "avascular necrosis" or "aseptic necrosis".

The different physiopathologic models are based on obstruction of the arteries, veins, capillaries and extravascular compression. The most probable etiology is obstruction of the veins. This can be accentuated or provoked by various well-known factors (Table 21.1).

Osteonecrosis presents as a continuous spectrum of reversible and irreversible changes in the cortical bone and the bone marrow. These findings are most often described at the level of the hip but are applicable to other anatomic sites.

Table 21.1. Etiological factors inducing osteonecrosis

Trauma
    Carpal fracture – dislocation
    Barotrauma
    Radiation
Idiopathic
    Arteriosclerosis
    Alcoholism
    Pancreatitis
    Osteomyelitis
Metabolic – endocrine disorders
    Cushing's disease
    Hyperlipidemia
Systemic disease
    Gout
    Systemic lupus erythematosus
    Rheumatoid arthritis
    Collagen (vascular) diseases
    Lymphoproliferative disorders
Coagulation disorders
    Pregnancy
    Hemoglobinopathies (sickle cell anemia)
Renal transplantation

21.3.1 Reversible Phase

Cellular ischemia may lead to cell death of osteocytes and hematopoietic marrow cells. Six hours of anoxia is considered sufficient to result in death of the hematopoietic marrow cells. Osteocytes, osteoblasts and osteoclasts may survive approximately 6–48 h [1]. Marrow fat cells survive anoxia for 2–5 days. In the presence of adequate circulation, breakdown products invoke an inflammatory response characterized by initial hyperemia with dilation of the vascular channels towards the zone of bone necrosis. Inflammatory cells are directed to the necrotic focus where they infiltrate the dead trabecular bone and start phagocytosis. This inflammatory response initiates the repair mechanism. These changes are also noted in patients with recurrent episodes of ischemia without bone necrosis. This process can develop and reoccur without apparent clinical symptoms. The hyperemia in combination with more pronounced phagocytosis can result in extensive localized porosis, seen on conventional radiographs. In these cases there is a more painful clinical presentation.

21.3.2 Irreversible Phase

Phagocytosis of the dead trabeculae creates a demarcation zone between the living and dead bone. This demarcation zone is called the reactive interface and signals the beginning of the irreversible phase of osteonecrosis. Further infiltration of the inflammatory, mesenchymal cells and capillaries leads to increasing morphologic degradation and the deposition of necrotic debris in the intertrabecular spaces. Subsequently mesenchymal cells differentiate to osteoblasts on the surface of the dead trabeculae. This repair process begins at the outer rim of the necrotic area and diffusely infiltrates the necrotic segment. The osteoblasts start to synthesize layers of new viable bone on top of the necrotic bone with resultant trabecular thickening. Osteoclastic activity leads to remodeling of repaired cancellous bone. During this phase, the bone is weak and can easily be deformed by excessive loading resulting in compression and collapse. During the repair process different stages of resorption, repair and remodeling can be present creating a mixed "pepper and salt" image displaying different stages of osteonecrosis in the same anatomic area.

In the late stages flattening of the articular surface can become apparent. Deformation is the result of subchondral fractures. Osteoclasts remove dead bone while new fibrous cartilage is formed bridging the microfractures. In many cases spontaneous healing is inadequate, with further deformation and flattening of the carpal bones, subchondral fractures, joint subluxation, instability, overload, further ischemia resulting in progressive disease and finally deteriorating end-stage destructive osteoarthritis.

21.4   Imaging of Osteonecrosis

After death of bone and marrow cells the bone matrix and fat cells remain initially unchanged. Therefore there are no specific changes shown on conventional radiographs (stage 1). After the death of the fat marrow cells, breakdown products induce vessel dilation with an influx of inflammatory cells accentuated by resorption of dead bone by osteoclasts. These findings lead to the development of apparent osteoporosis in the viable bone while the necrotic bone remains relatively dense, resulting in an apparent "paroxysmal" osteodensification (stage 2). This is particular evident in the case of waist fractures of the scaphoid, with relative osteoporosis of the distal pole and condensation of the proximal part that is undergoing avascular necrosis. Progressive disease demonstrates irregularity of the articular surface, subchondral cyst formation, collapse (stage 3) and fragmentation, and finally degenerative joint disease (stage 4).

MR imaging is nowadays considered the most useful modality for detection of osteonecrosis [2]. MR imaging has been reported to be as sensitive as scintigraphy in the detection of avascular necrosis and to possess even greater specificity in diagnosis. Most data on osteonecrosis are related to osteonecrosis of the hip: however, osteonecrosis in other sites has a similar MR appearance. In the carpal bones, signal intensity within the marrow depends on the stage of the lesion. The imaging protocol for avascular necrosis is listed in Table 21.2.

The application of MR imaging to the detection and evaluation of avascular necrosis is facilitated by the bright signal intensity generated from the normal

Table 21.2. MR imaging protocol for avascular necrosis

Sequence	sl	TR	TE	TI	FA	Slice thickness (cm)	Matrix	FOV	Acquisitions
1. Coronal SE T1-weighted sequence	12	452	20	0	90°	2–3	224×512	120	2
2. Coronal PD and SE T2-weighted sequence	19	3000	14	85	180°	2–3	110×256	125	3
3. Coronal SE T1-weighted sequence after intravenous contrast	12	452	20	0	90°	2–3	224×512	120	2
4. Axial TSE FS T2-weighted sequence	12	3000	96	85	180°	2	252×256	120	3
5. Sagittal SE T1-weighted sequence	12	671	20	0	90°	3	202×512	120	1

fatty marrow content of the carpal bones. Characteristically, decreased signal intensity of the bone marrow on T1-weighted images is evident in devascularized bone.

On T1-weighted imaging sequences, the sensitivity rate of MR imaging for the detection of decreased marrow signal associated with avascular necrosis of the carpal bones is 87.5%. With the addition of T2-weighted imaging sequences, specificity is reported to be 100%. Usually, the marrow has areas of focal or diffuse decreased signal intensity on T2-weighted images. Regions of increased signal intensity on T2-weighted images surround the hypointense areas and presumably represent the interface between nonviable, or dead, bone and reparative granulation tissue. T2-weighted images, however, seem to have a lower sensitivity in detecting carpal avascular necrosis due to the inherent low signal-to-noise ratio. Intravenous administration of contrast medium can provide further information regarding tissue viability. In the initial stages of cellular death there is normal fatty marrow or early marrow necrosis with mummified fat, in both cases presenting as an area of high signal intensity on T1-weighted images and intermediate signal intensity on T2-weighted images. Due to cellular death, cells are inert and there is no contrast uptake. In the subacute phase there is inflammatory response, and contrast produces enhancement of hyperemic tissue at the necrotic site and adjacent subchondral bone marrow. The enhancement is assessed on T1-weighted or proton density fat-suppressed images. The vascular supply of the carpal bones is usually from proximal to distal (see below). Absence of proximal pole bone marrow enhancement indicates lack of vascular perfusion in the development of avascular necrosis.

The degree of vascular enhancement relates to the viability of the necrotic segment. The viability of the necrotic bone is evaluated by comparing the rate of postenhancement increase in the signal of the proximal versus the distal fragment.

Discrete enhancement means that there are mesenchymal cells present and that reparation is going on. Moderate enhancement means that there is a high cellular content of mesenchymal tissue, which has a more favorable prognosis. If marked enhancement is present, there is viable mesenchymal tissue with prominent hyperemia, dilated vessels and edema reflecting the presence of a number of repair agents that are consistent with the best possible prognosis.

In the case of accompanying fracture, fracture healing demonstrates hyperemia at the fracture site and adjacent marrow. Non-union is characterized by persistent low signal intensity on T1-, T2-, and post-contrast fat-suppressed T1-weighted images. High signal intensity fluid may be seen separating fracture fragments. Callus or fibrous union may also demonstrate low signal intensity on T1- or T2-weighted images. Routine radiographs are sufficient to differentiate between these two possibilities.

21.5   Specific Locations of Osteonecrosis

As far as we know, there are no reports on avascular necrosis of the phalanges or metacarpals.

The two most common sites of avascular necrosis in the wrist are the proximal pole of the scaphoid and the lunate bone.

21.5.1   Scaphoid Bone (Preiser's Disease)

Idiopathic vascular necrosis of the scaphoid was described in 1910 by Preiser. Whenever the signs of avascular necrosis present without documented trauma the diagnosis of Preiser's disease is made.

Avascular necrosis of the scaphoid usually has a traumatic origin [3–6] and today there is discussion whether the so-called idiopathic form of avascular necrosis is not secondary to chronic mechanical trauma inducing small trabecular stress fractures that block the vascular blood supply. The vascular supply of the scaphoid bone is disrupted by fractures of the middle (the waist) and proximal thirds of the bone.

The major blood supply of the scaphoid arises from the radial artery and enters principally the waist at the dorsoradial side of the scaphoid (Fig. 21.1) [7]. The distal scaphoid receives nutritional elements through the synovial fluid. The proximal two thirds of the bone rely on intraosseous "diffusion". This relatively poorly vascularized region may predispose the proximal fragment to osteonecrosis in approximately 10–15% of scaphoid waist (middle) fractures (Fig. 21.2) and nearly all proximal third to proximal fifth fractures [8, 9]. This percentage increases to 30–40% in the case of fracture non-union. Evidence of this complication most frequently becomes apparent 4–6 months after the initial trauma when there is an increase in bone density (Fig. 21.3).

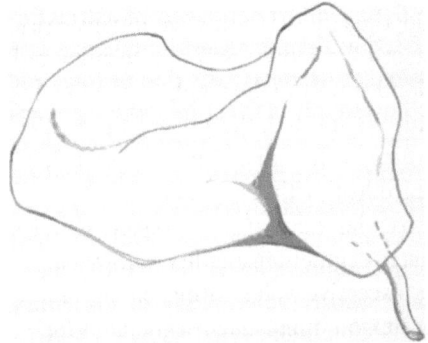

Fig. 21.1. Frontal view of the scaphoid. The major blood supply of the scaphoid arises from the radial artery and enters the waist or the dorsoradial ridge of the bone. Because of relatively poor vascular supply, the proximal two thirds of the scaphoid is vulnerable to ischemia

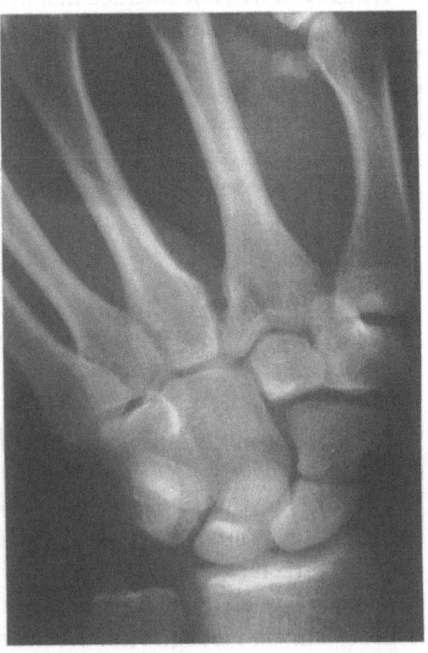

Fig. 21.2. Scaphoid waist fracture with displacement, prone to develop delayed healing, non-union, wrist instability and avascular necrosis

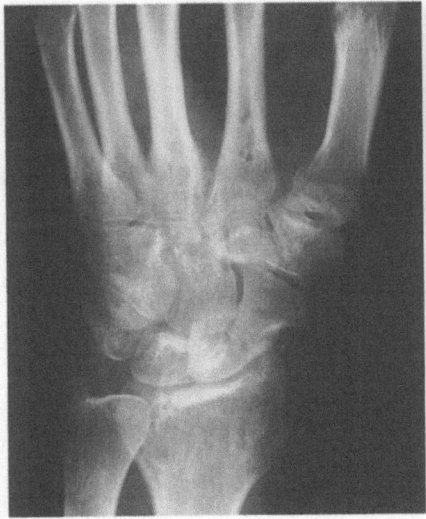

a

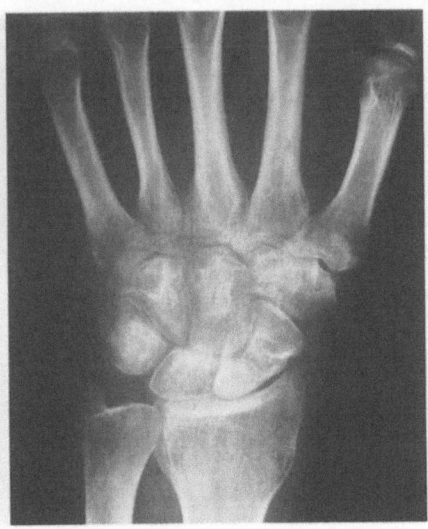

b

Fig. 21.3a, b. Control radiographs after scaphoid waist fracture. **a** Two months after initial trauma with external fixation and immobilization. **b** After 4 months there is apparent densification of the proximal pole of the scaphoid due to non-union and developing avascular necrosis

It has been well documented that nearly 80% of all wrist fractures occur in this vulnerable proximal portion of the scaphoid; thus there is always an intrinsic risk in delayed fracture healing and development of osteonecrosis due to impaired blood supply. Because there is retrograde blood supply in the scaphoid the general rule is that the more proximally the fracture is located, the greater the risk of osteonecrosis developing. In contrast, fractures of the tuberculum generally heal within 6 weeks and fractures of the distal third heal within 8 weeks.

A scaphoid fracture with secondary avascular necrosis may result in wrist shortening and present with dorsal intercalated segment instability (DISI). Due to destabilization of the triquetrum, there is excessive volar tilting of the lunate giving way to complete collapse into a volar flexion intercalated segment (VISI).

Because fracture of the proximal (vascular vulnerable) pole of the scaphoid is a relatively frequent carpal injury, there is a need for rational fracture management. The management of this type of wrist fracture largely depends on the ability to distinguish fracture ischemia from true avascular necrosis. All fractures at the level of the proximal pole of the scaphoid are at risk of developing ischemia. Ischemia is a transient phenomenon (Fig. 21.4) and is an essential component of the initial fracture healing by inducing hyperemic ingrowth and establishing an inflammatory response. The critical distinction in fracture vascularity is essential in the treatment management. Green advocated the direct visualization of punctate hemorrhages in cancellous bone found at surgery as the best determinant of true avascular necrosis. In his experience with 45 scaphoid non-unions treated by "Russe" bone grafting, union was achieved when bleeding was clearly visualized in the proximal pole. Conversely, with a paucity of punctate bleeding, successful union considerably decreased. In all cases with a total absence of bleeding, non-union was the rule [8].

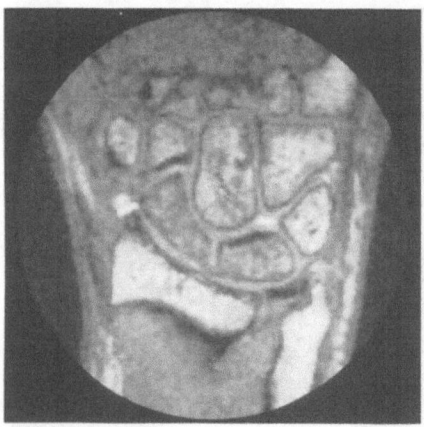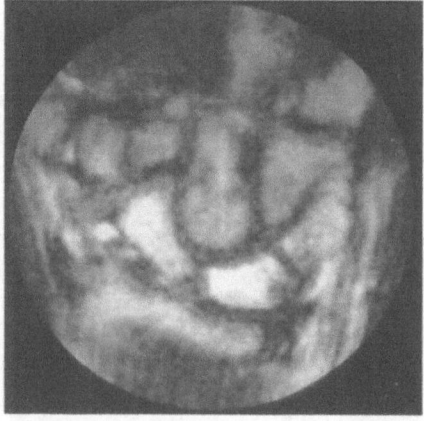

a   b

Fig. 21.4a, b. Three weeks after trauma, bone edema and hyperemia are the result of an inflammatory healing response. **a** Coronal DESS-3D sequence shows hypointensity of the lunate and scaphoid bone due to contusion and edema. **b** Coronal TSE T2-weighted image with corresponding endomedullary hyperintensity

Can MR imaging be of any help in resolving this problem prior to surgery [10–12]? Reactive marrow hyperemia of the distal pole may be confused with diffuse or extensive necrosis (Fig. 21.5) on T1- and T2-weighted images. Short time-to-invert (TI) inversion recovery (STIR) images can be used to document increased hyperemia of the distal pole marrow, which may not be appreciated on the T1-, T2- or T2*-weighted images. But the preceding sequences do not allow distinction between hyperemia and edema in the case of osteonecrosis (Fig. 21.6). In diffuse marrow necrosis, signal intensity changes may not be restricted to the proximal pole.

However, enhancement on T1- or proton density-weighted images with fat suppression after intravenous contrast administration is in favor of hyperemia, whereas necrotic tissue will not enhance (Fig. 21.7). The enhancement thus means that the normal repair mechanism is functioning. If there is no enhancement, the patient is more likely to undergo avascular necrosis. Enhancement may be shown more clearly using subtraction techniques. In the later stages, a return to normal signal intensity will occur after 3–4 months if hyperemia was present. In the case of fibrosis or sclerotic healing, the signal intensities will continue to be decreased on all imaging sequences (Fig. 21.8).

CT can be used during the healing process to document the extent of bone bridging spatially in a three-dimensional rendering [13] or to exclude non-union (Fig. 21.9).

If a patient is considered at risk of developing aseptic necrosis, due to the location of the fracture, careful follow-up is required during the immobilization period, which lasts up to 3 months. In the initial stages of aseptic necrosis internal fixation with a Herbert screw is often considered (Fig. 21.10). In the later stages,

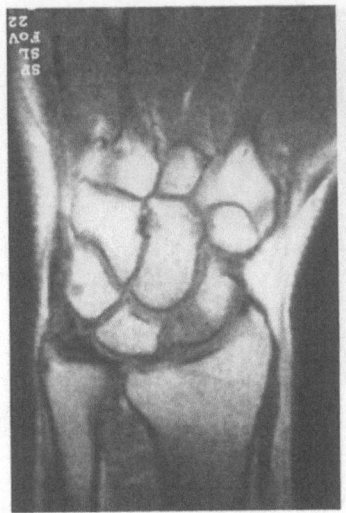 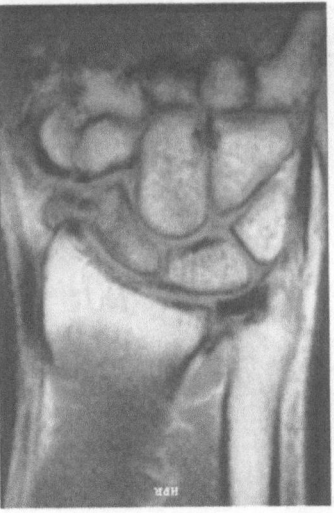

a   b

Fig. 21.5. a Coronal SE T1-weighted image. One-week-old waist fracture with edema of the distal pole. **b** Coronal SE T1-weighted image. One-week-old distal pole fracture with distal edema presenting as a hypointense homogeneous band sharply outlined against the fracture site

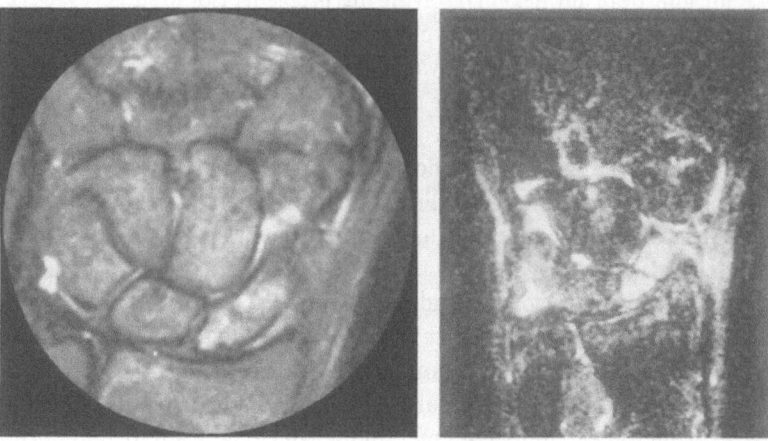

Fig. 21.6. a Coronal TSE FS T2-weighted image. Mild diffuse edema in the proximal and distal poles outlining the fracture. The hyperintensity of the signal is comparable between the two poles and probably due to diffuse edema. **b** Coronal STIR sequence. Radiocarpal and mediocarpal synovitis with hypointense fluid in both joint compartments. There is markedly hyperintense signal at both proximal and distal poles. The signal of the proximal pole is higher than that of the distal part of the scaphoid. A possible explanation here is that there is edema of the distal pole and that there is the beginning of necrosis at the proximal pole

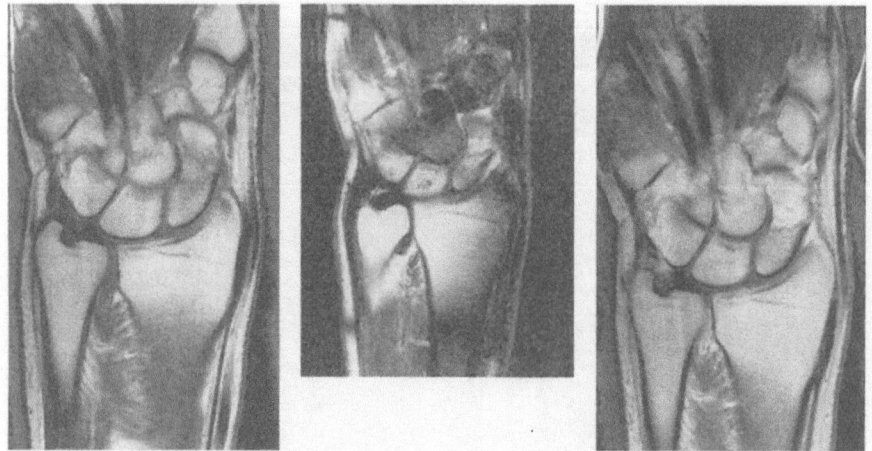

Fig. 21.7a–c. Four weeks after trauma. **a** Coronal SE T1-weighted image. Scaphoid waist fracture with edema at the proximal pole. **b** Coronal PD FS-weighted image. Diffuse mild edema of the proximal pole. **c** Coronal SE T1-weighted image after intravenous gadolinium. Diffuse strong enhancement shows the viability of the proximal pole. The diffuse contrast enhancement means that there is still viable bone and that the normal repair mechanisms are acting

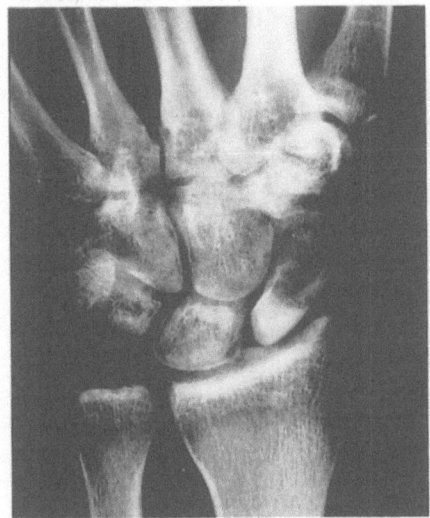

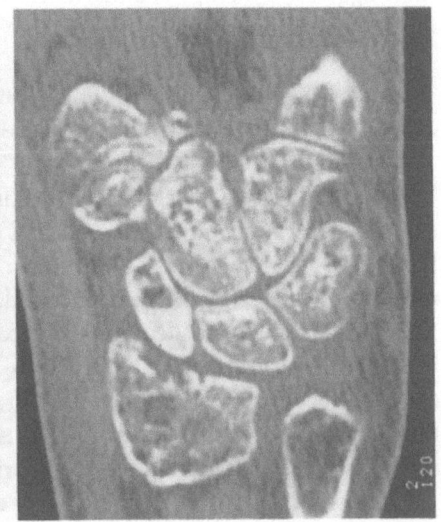

a

b

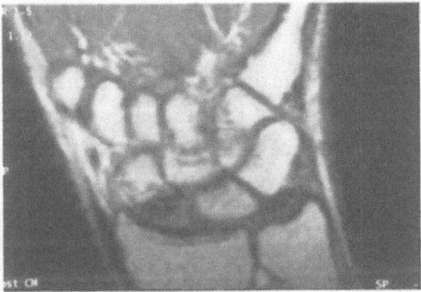

c

Fig. 21.8. a Diffuse avascular necrosis of the proximal pole with sclerosis. **b** Proximal pole densification on coronal CT due to avascular necrosis with secondary radioscaphoidal arthrosis. **c** Coronal SE T1-weighted image. In the final stages of avascular necrosis the signal intensity will decrease on all imaging sequences

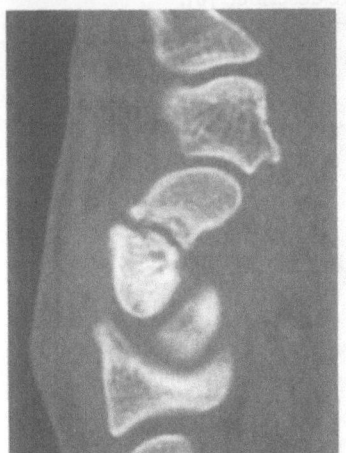

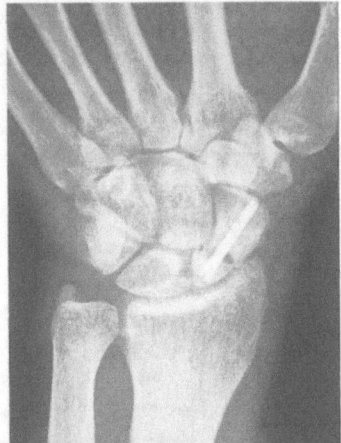

Fig. 21.9. Parasagittal CT image. Non-union of a midscaphoid fracture with diffuse sclerosis of the proximal pole and development of degenerative subchondral cysts

Fig. 21.10. Waist fracture of the scaphoid internally fixated with a Herbert screw

more aggressive therapy is undertaken with resection of the scaphoid, placement of a prosthesis or arthrodesis.

21.5.2 Lunate Bone (Kienböck Disease)

The onset of avascular necrosis of the lunate bone, also known as Kienböck disease [14, 15], can be quite insidious and often develops spontaneously [16]. This type of avascular necrosis peaks between the ages of 20 and 40 years. There is a 2:1 male-to-female ratio. Although uncommon, bilateral disease does occur [17, 18]. Kienböck disease is most commonly encountered in young men involved in manual labor. The cause of Kienböck disease is unknown, although the blood supply can easily be interrupted in the case of fracture [19, 20]. This is caused by the fact that the blood supply of the lunate bone is provided in 8–26% of cases by only one artery [21], usually entering the volar surface of the bone (Fig 21.11).

Increased axial loading forces associated with a negative ulnar variant can be a predisposing factor. In most patients, the ulna and radius are relatively equal in length. Ulnar variance is an index of relative inequality in their lengths and can be positive, in which case the ulnar length exceeds that of the radius, or negative, in which case the ulna is shorter than the radius. Due to the discrepancy in radial and ulnar lengths, the lunate bone is subject to increased stress. In these cases, shearing forces in combination with an irregular articular surface induce repetitive trauma that sometimes leads to osteonecrosis. Occult disruption of a tenuous blood supply secondary to single or repeated trauma may predispose the lunate bone to osteonecrosis [22]. The series of events that take place in Kienböck disease start with lunate flattening and elongation, proximal migration of the capitate, scapholunate dissociation and finally end-stage osteoarthritis of the radiocarpal joint accompanied with wrist pain and instability. Classically, four stages are described [8].

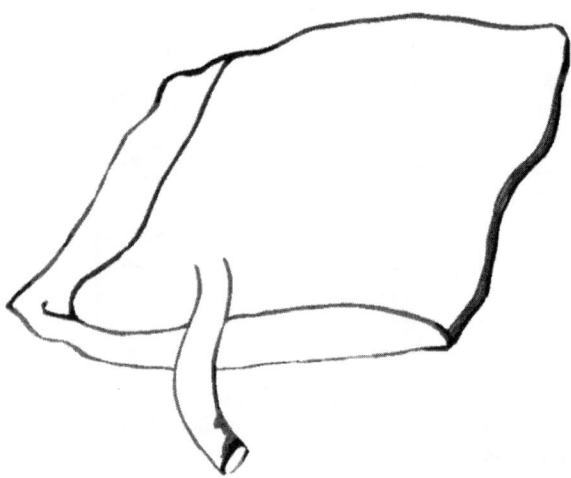

Fig. 21.11. Frontal view of the lunate. The volar arterial plexus is the dominant feeder of the lunate and is derived from branches of the ulnar, radial and anterior interosseous arteries. Especially the proximal part of the lunate shows poor intramedullary arborization of the arterial branches

21.5.2.1 Stage 1

Stage 1 of Kienböck disease is clinically indistinguishable from a wrist sprain [15]. Initially, patients note dorsal tenderness about the lunate and may develop stiffness due to synovitis. The synovitis and inflammation may affect surrounding structures. These findings are, however, also present in a variety of other carpal conditions and are nonspecific. One patient has been described with acute carpal tunnel syndrome as the first indication of Kienböck disease. Plain radiographs are normal although an associated fracture line or compression fracture may be present in specific cases. At this early stage, radiographs are both insensitive and nonspecific for the diagnosis of Kienböck disease.

CT imaging, with the wrist positioned in two orthogonal imaging planes (axial and paracoronal to the lunate bone), can sometimes illustrate a subtle linear (micro)fracture line.

Before MR imaging became available, the standard test was scintigraphy by means of a three-phase ^{99m}Tc-MDP study [23,24]. When there is an abnormal uptake of technetium, especially in the third or delayed phase, a CT scan should be performed to assess trabecular bone morphology and to identify fractures. The technetium scan is extremely sensitive, but does not provide detail about the physiologic changes in the marrow, which can be seen on MR imaging. Thus bone scintigraphy may be helpful but is poor in differentiating fractures, osteochondral lesions, erosions and the spectrum of degenerative changes that present as sclerosis.

Nowadays, MR imaging is the best imaging modality to be performed after routine radiographs. MR imaging not only allows assessment of the lunate, but also facilitates ruling out or adding other disorders in the differential diagnosis. MR studies may reveal occult ganglion cysts as well as inflammatory arthritides with synovitis.

Magnetic resonance findings in Kienböck disease can also be grouped according to the stage of disease [12, 25, 26]. MR imaging offers comparable or greater sensitivity and improved specificity compared with that available from radiographs and scintigraphy. Focal or decreased low signal intensity is seen on T1-weighted images in affected areas of marrow involvement. Coronal plane images best display the largest anterior to posterior surface area of involvement. The addition of sagittal or axial sequences provides more accurate assessment of the volume of the marrow involvement and should be performed to exclude the presence of an associated fracture line. On T2*-weighted images the lunate demonstrates uniformly low signal intensity.

In early Kienböck disease, T1-weighted images show unaffected marrow with the high signal intensity of fat, isointense with the other carpal bones of the wrist. The distribution of low signal intensity necrosis may be restricted to the volar or dorsal portion of the lunate bone with an eccentric or central distribution pattern. Radiocarpal joint effusions or more localized synovitis demonstrate bright signal intensity on T2-weighted images and fat-suppressed images and are sometimes noted as an accompanying nonspecific finding. Depending on the degree of the bone edema distinction can be made between grade 0 (Fig. 21.12) (less than 50% of the bone involved) and grade 1 (Fig. 21.13) (more than 50% of

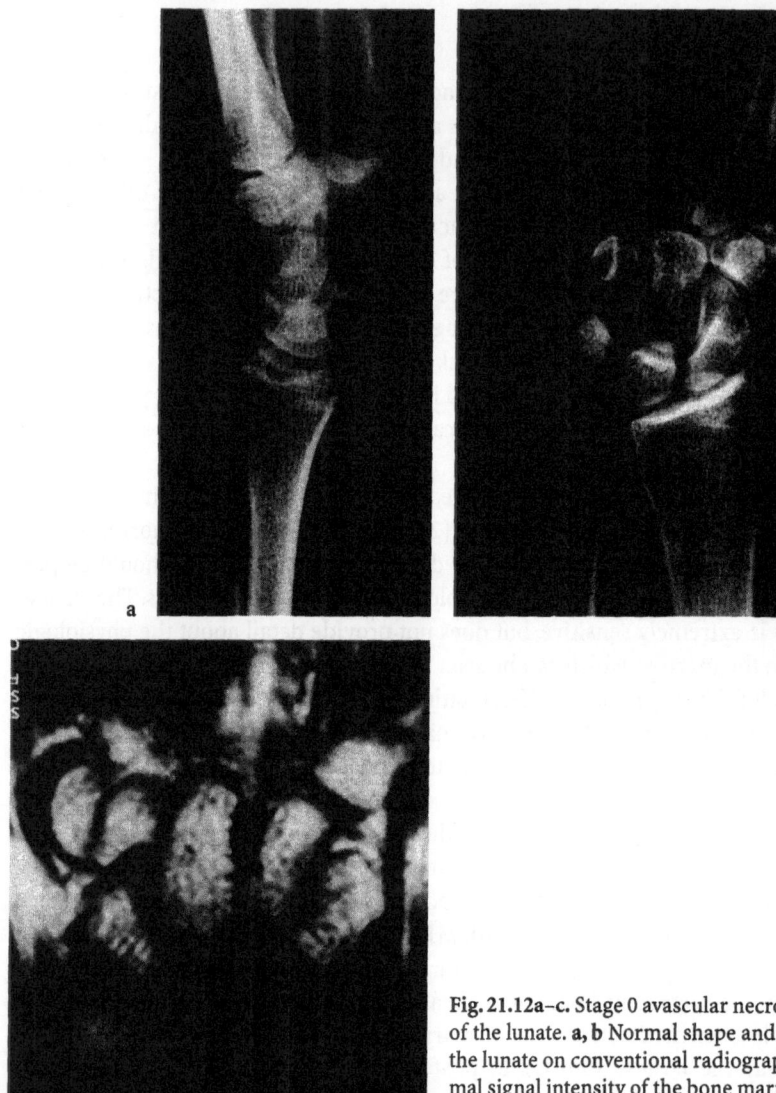

Fig. 21.12a–c. Stage 0 avascular necrosis (AVN) of the lunate. **a, b** Normal shape and density of the lunate on conventional radiographs. **c** Normal signal intensity of the bone marrow on the T1-weighted coronal image with hypointense lines due to trabecular microfractures

the bone). Grade 0 can then be considered as a precursor stage presenting with minimal edema sometimes accompanied by a horizontal low signal intensity stress fracture line in T1-weighted images [11].

21.5.2.2 Stage 2

As the condition progresses, plain film radiographs and (spiral) CT show increased density of the lunate as the result of sclerosis. In this stage bone flattening starts, usually more pronounced on the radial aspect of the bone, probably by

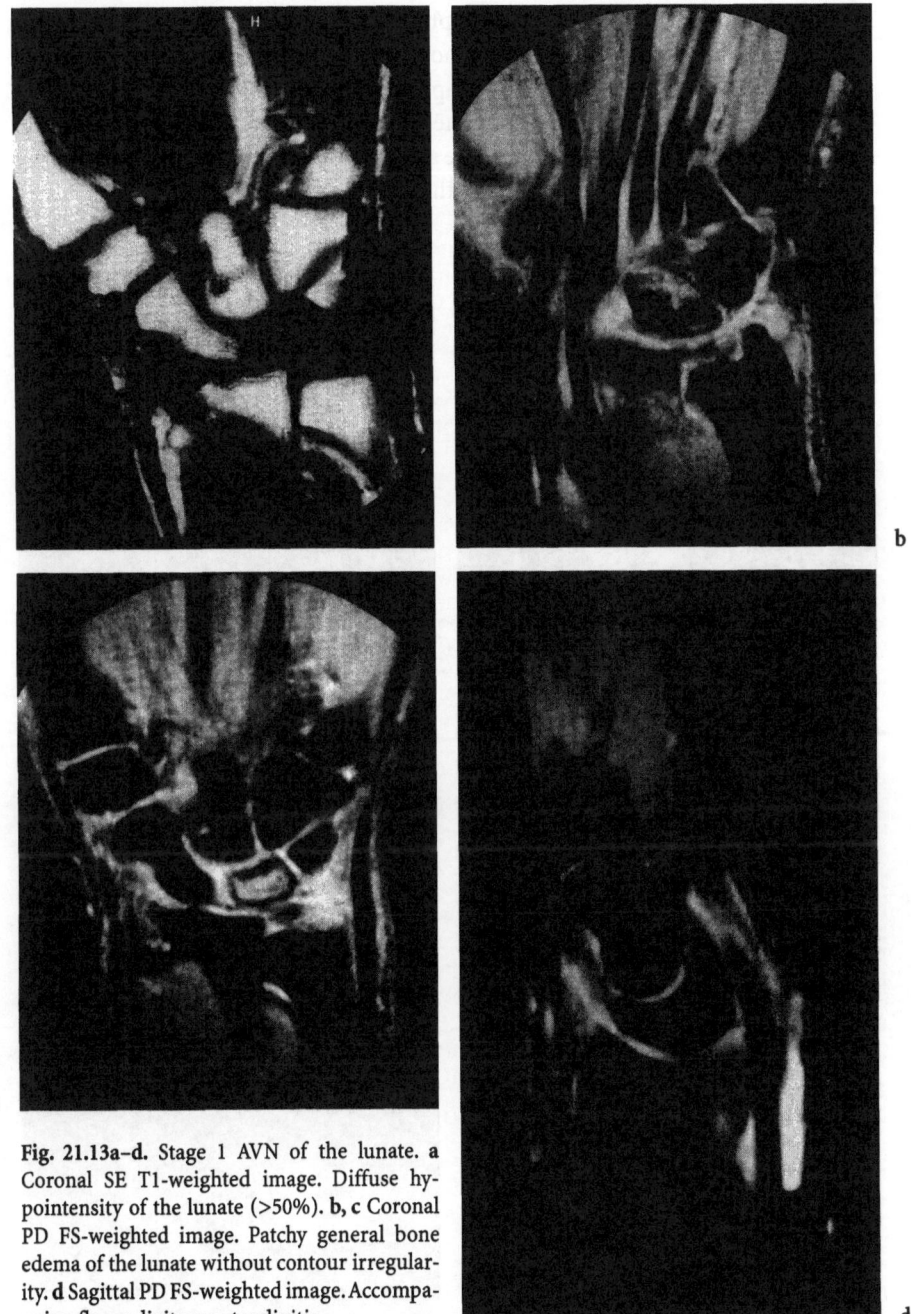

Fig. 21.13a–d. Stage 1 AVN of the lunate. **a** Coronal SE T1-weighted image. Diffuse hypointensity of the lunate (>50%). **b, c** Coronal PD FS-weighted image. Patchy general bone edema of the lunate without contour irregularity. **d** Sagittal PD FS-weighted image. Accompanying flexor digitorum tendinitis

increased loading of the scapholunate ligament. The global morphology and size remain unchanged, however, even in late stage 2 disease. Scintigraphy is invariably positive. Due to compression of the bone trabeculae there is a low signal intensity on T1-weighted images and a heterogeneous mixed signal intensity on T2-weighted images (Fig. 21.14). STIR or fat-suppressed images demonstrate areas of increased signal intensity with a patchy inhomogeneous distribution in patients who show sclerosis in corresponding radiographs. Intravenous contrast can be useful to differentiate between viable and dead bone segments and acts as a prognostic factor. If there is contrast enhancement there are still areas of viable bone, possibly leading to a better prognosis and less aggressive therapeutic measurements.

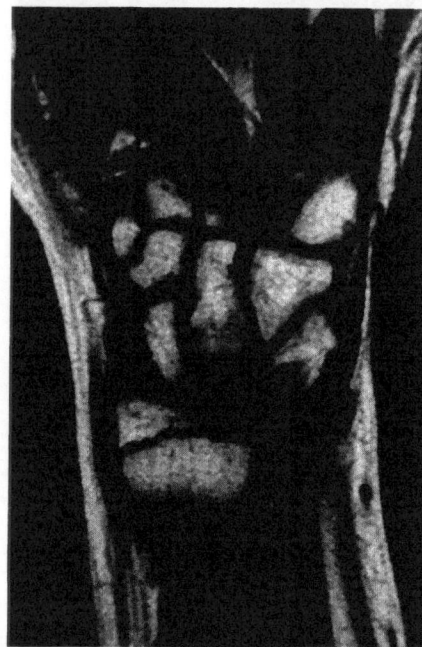

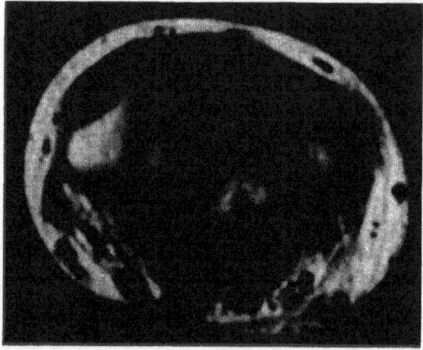

Fig. 21.14a–d. Stage 2 AVN of the lunate. a, b Coronal and axial SE T1-weighted images. Diffuse hypointense bone marrow abnormality. Linear separation line between necrotic and edematous bone marrow with contour irregularity (crescent sign). c Coronal PD FS-weighted image. Patchy areas of edema and granulation tissue with mixed signal intensities. d Sagittal PD FS-weighted image. Anteroposterior elongation of the lunate

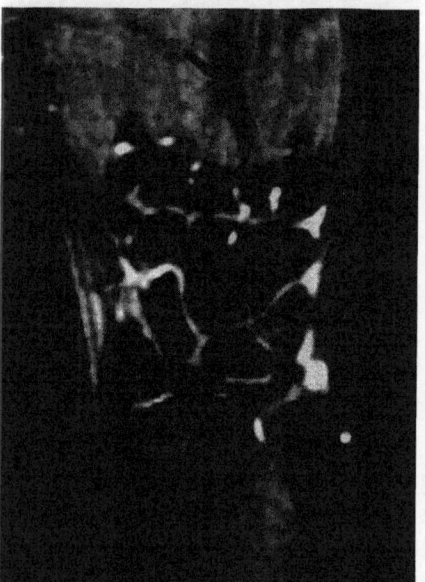

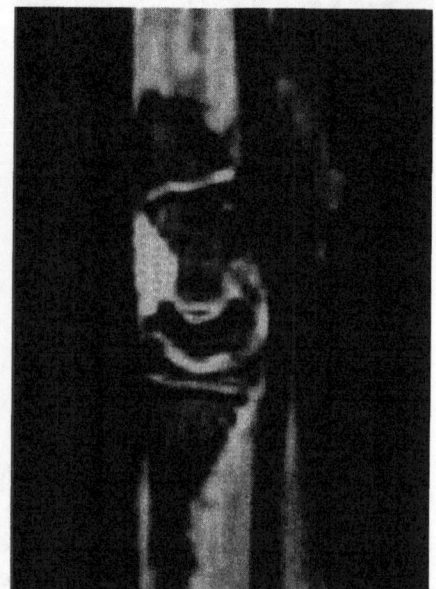

21.5.2.3   Stage 3

In stage 3 vascular necrosis the lunate undergoes distal to proximal collapse in the coronal plane and elongation in the axial and sagittal planes (Fig. 21.15). As a consequence, proximal migration of the capitate takes places inducing interruption of the distal carpal row. The absence or presence of scapholunate (SL) dissociation with rotatory subluxation of the scaphoid divides patients into stage 3A and 3B, respectively. Rotation of the scaphoid may be accompanied by ulnar deviation of the triquetrum. With scaphoid rotation, the inability to see the entire long axis of the scaphoid in a single coronal plane is the MR imaging equivalent of the radiographic "signet ring" sign (rotation of the scaphoid on its transverse axis, principally the result of the dorsal rotation of the proximal pole as described in tears of the interosseous ligaments) in conventional anteroposterior radiographic projections (Fig. 21.16). Necrotic and cystic changes due to the intercarpal friction forces develop and induce further fragmentation and collapse. These cystic changes are best appreciated on STIR or fat-suppressed images where they are depicted between areas of fibrosis and sclerosis.

21.5.2.4   Stage 4

Stage 4 is marked by degenerative arthrosis of the lunate and carpus leading to pronounced radiocarpal osteoarthritis. Fibrosis and sclerosis due to reinforcement of the bone trabeculae at the repair tissue interface predominate, resulting in low signal intensity on T1-weighted images. There are also no remaining regions of increased signal intensity on T2-weighted images (Fig. 21.17) or fat suppressed images in this end stage. The imaging findings are listed in Table 21.3.

21.5.2.5   Treatment

The treatment of Kienböck disease is a subject of great debate among hand surgeons. Because the condition is relatively rare, no single surgeon or center has been able to develop a large enough experience with all stages of the disease to provide truly definitive treatment recommendations. Besides, before MR imaging became available, the initial stages of Kienböck disease often passed undetected. As a result, many types of procedures are recommended in the literature. In general, treatment modalities depend on the stage of disease.

MR imaging is thus essential in describing the exact findings with respect to deformity of the bone, the residual capacity of viable bone and the presence of degenerative changes in combination with associated reasons for carpal instability. On the basis of the MR findings and staging the optimal therapeutic protocol can be determined. MR imaging also has the advantage that the postoperative results can be followed in terms of the signal intensity changes of the marrow. Early stages marked by the absence of changes in articular cartilage, minimal collapse of the lunate and permanent carpal instability patterns are usually treated with procedures designed to unload and revascularize the lunate (Fig. 21.18). This can be accompanied by

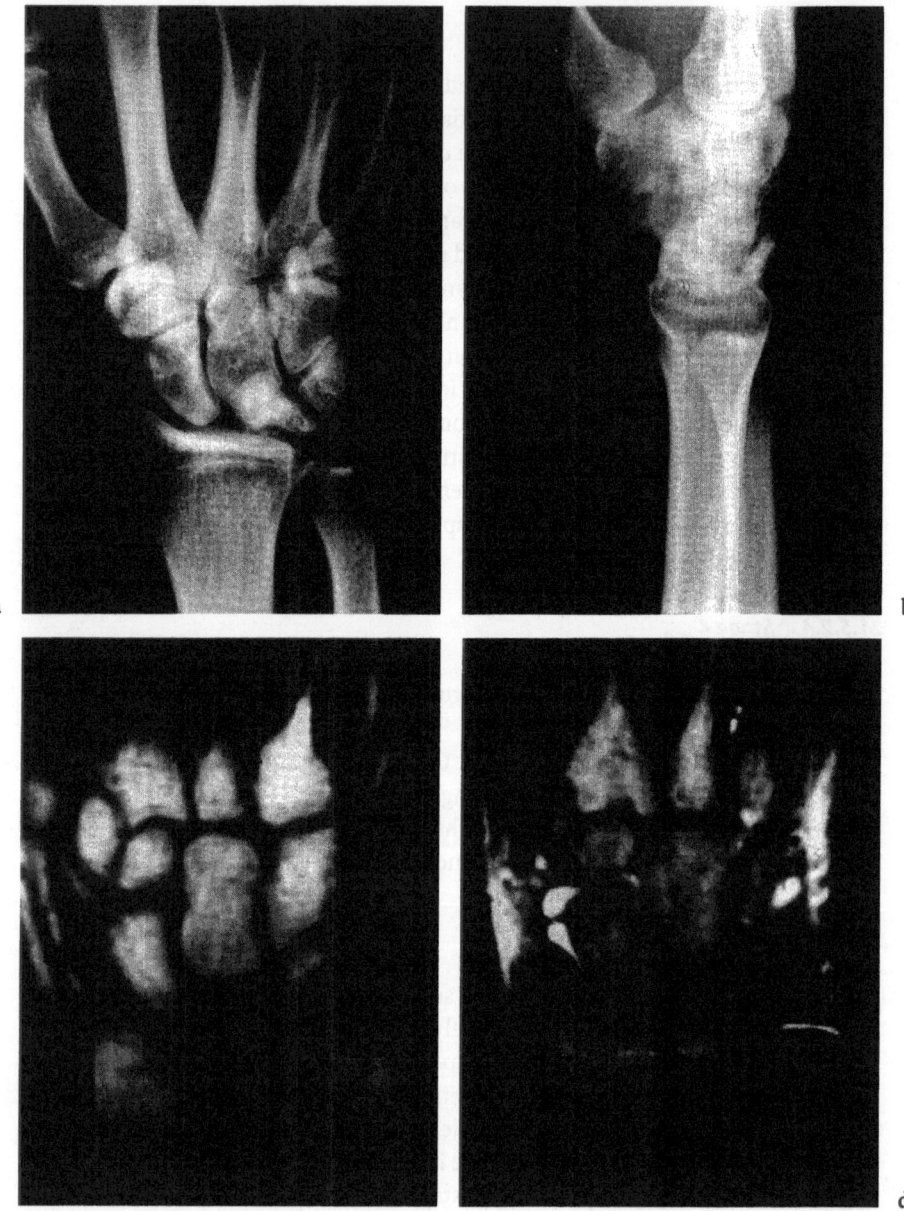

Fig. 21.15a–d. Stage 3A AVN of the lunate. **a, b** Structural deformation with flattening and fragmentation of the lunate with proximal migration of the scaphoid. **c** Coronal SE T1-weighted image. Low signal intensity on all imaging sequences. **d** Coronal SE T2-weighted image. Reactive synovitis due to excessive loading of the radiocarpal compartment

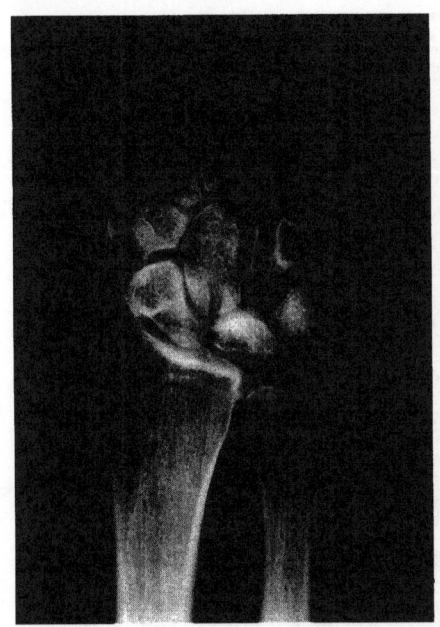
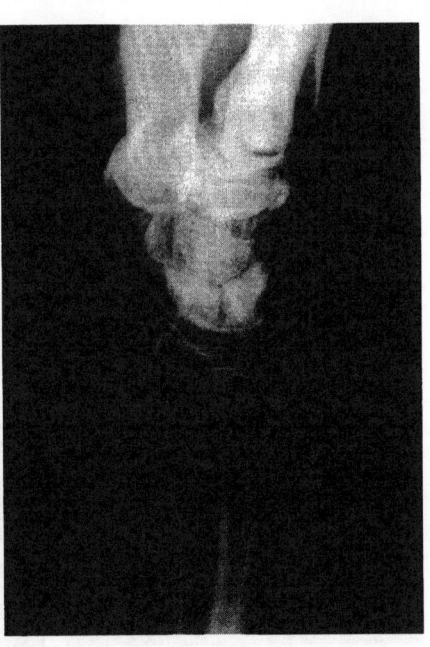

a   b

Fig. 21.16a, b. Stage 3B AVN of the lunate. **a, b** Deformation of the lunate, proximal migration of the capitate and associated rotation of the scaphoid: the "signet ring" sign

Table 21.3. Summary of stage classification of Kienböck disease

Stage	Radiography			MR imaging	
	Contour	Density		T1	T2
Stage 0	Normal	Normal		Normal; linear pattern (stress fracture)	–
Stage 1	Normal	Normal		Low	Low or patchy high Focal changes (<50%)
Stage 2	Normal	Increased		Low	Low or patchy high Focal changes (>50%)
Stage 3A	Collapse; carpal shift	Increased		Low	Low or inhomogeneous
Stage 3B	Collapse; carpal shift		Subluxation of scaphoid	Low	Low or inhomogeneous
Stage 4	Fragmentation		Radiocarpal degeneration	Low	Low cysts

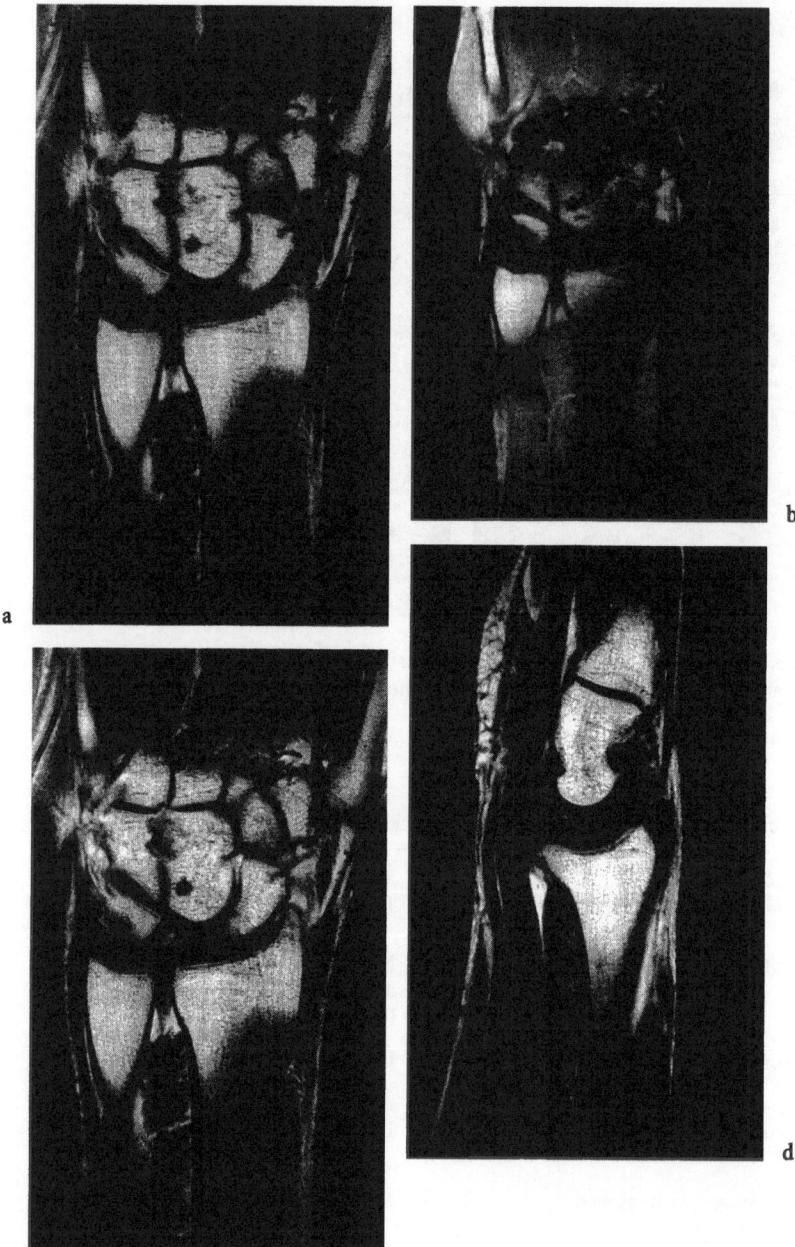

Fig. 21.17a–d. Stage 4 AVN of the lunate. **a, b** Coronal SE T1-weighted image and PD FS-weighted image. There is deformation and fragmentation of the lunate with diffuse low signal intensity on all imaging sequences. Osteolytic reaction with degeneration of the radiocarpal compartment. **c, d** Coronal and sagittal SE T1-weighted image with intravenous gadolinium. The arthrotic changes of the carpus and flattening of the lunate are best evaluated on sagittal images. Use of intravenous contrast shows that there is no viable residual bone. There is no contrast uptake

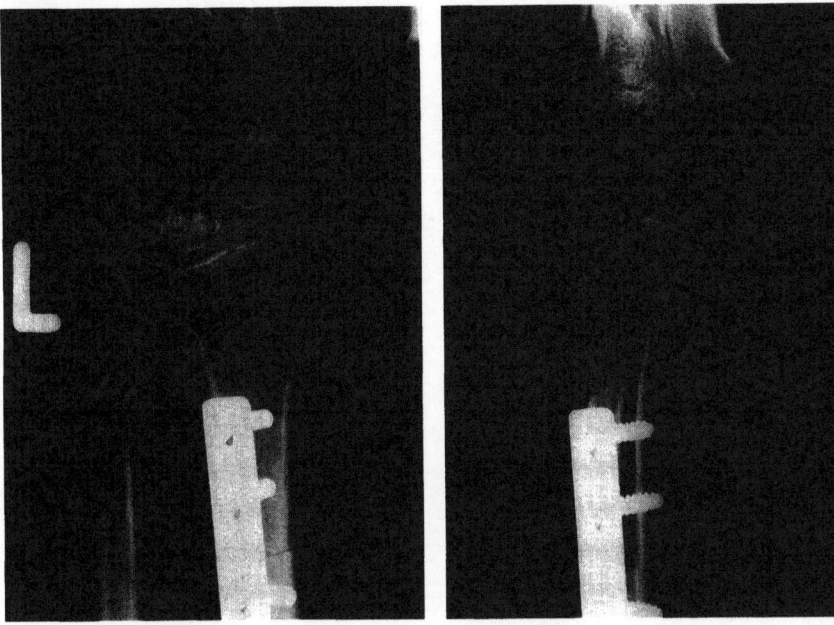

Fig. 21.18a, b. In the early stages of AVN conservative therapy is indicated. In stage 2 disease revascularization (bone grafting) and equalization (radial osteotomy) can be performed. The bone graft was initially removed from the distal radial diaphysis with subsequent transverse radial osteotomy in this case

procedures to reduce the radioulnar imbalance by radial osteotomy or ulnar lengthening [27]. Later stages, with established instability patterns and degenerative arthritis, must be treated with arthrodesis [28,29] and salvage procedures (Figs. 21.19, 21.20).

21.5.3   Hamulus of the Hamate Bone

Telfer et al. [9, 30] have defined the base of the hamulus of the hamate as another potential high risk-zone for developing ischemia after fracture. The major portion of the hook and the body derive their blood supply from separate sources that demonstrate few, if any, intraosseous connections. The base of the hook has no independent nutrient vessels.

Therefore the hamate hook is prone to develop ischemia after injury and delayed fracture healing subsequently resulting in osteonecrosis. The diagnosis can be made by observing sequential images with the typical hamate hook incidence, but is best depicted by means of CT examination. MR imaging has been helpful in differentiating viable from dead avulsed bone fragments and in determining whether internal fixation is advisable [11]. However, early excision of the hamulus is often considered due to the poor healing of the fragment and the risk of aseptic necrosis [8]. Therefore the role of MR imaging in the diagnosis is of only limited importance.

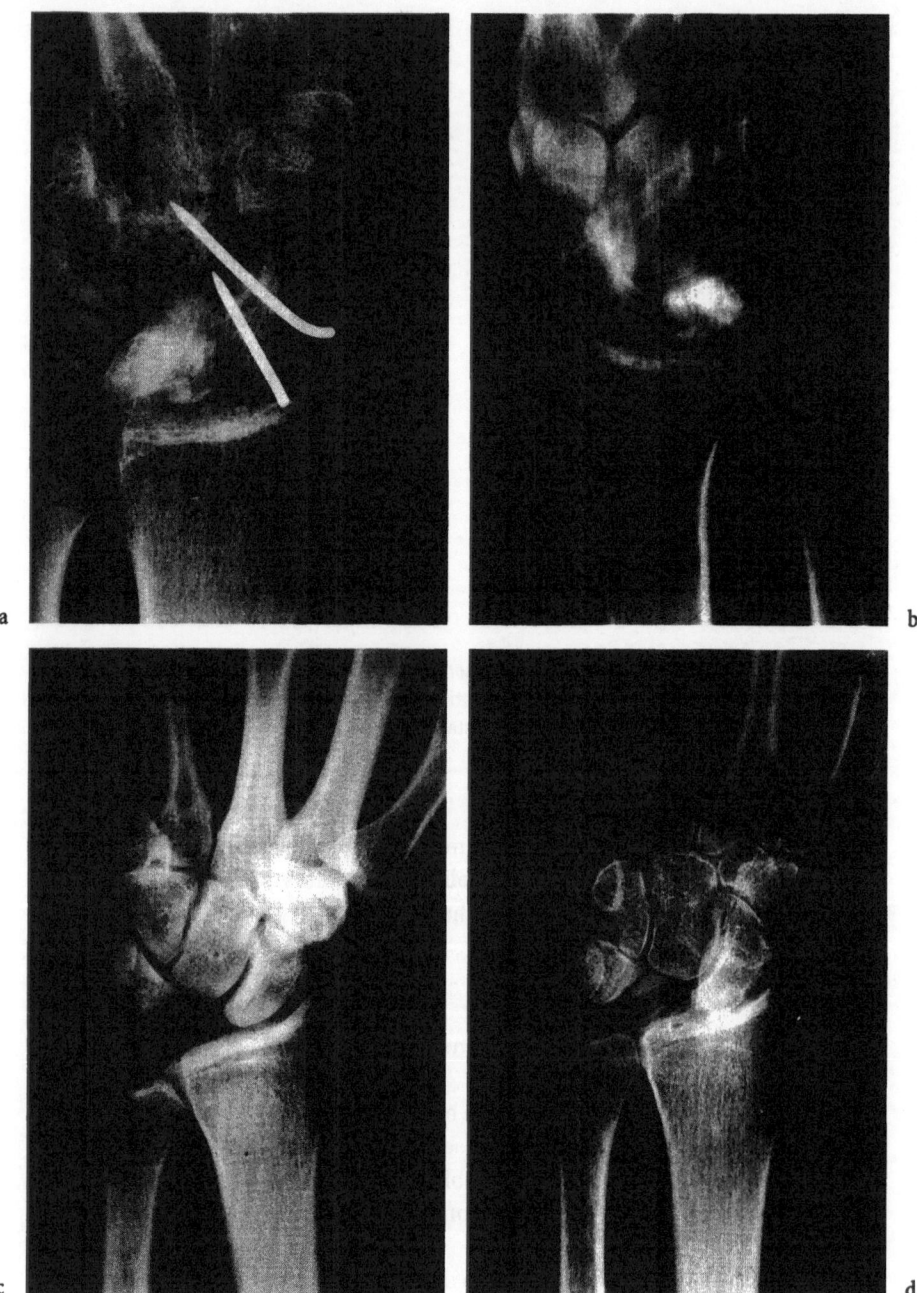

a

b

c

d

Fig. 21.19. a, b In stage 3 AVN fusion of the carpal bones (with the capitate) is performed to shift the axial loading forces away from the lunate. **c, d** In some cases surgical resection is performed to stop further fragmentation. Silicone rubber implants were used in the 1980s but this treatment has been abandoned because of the risk of silicone-related synovitis

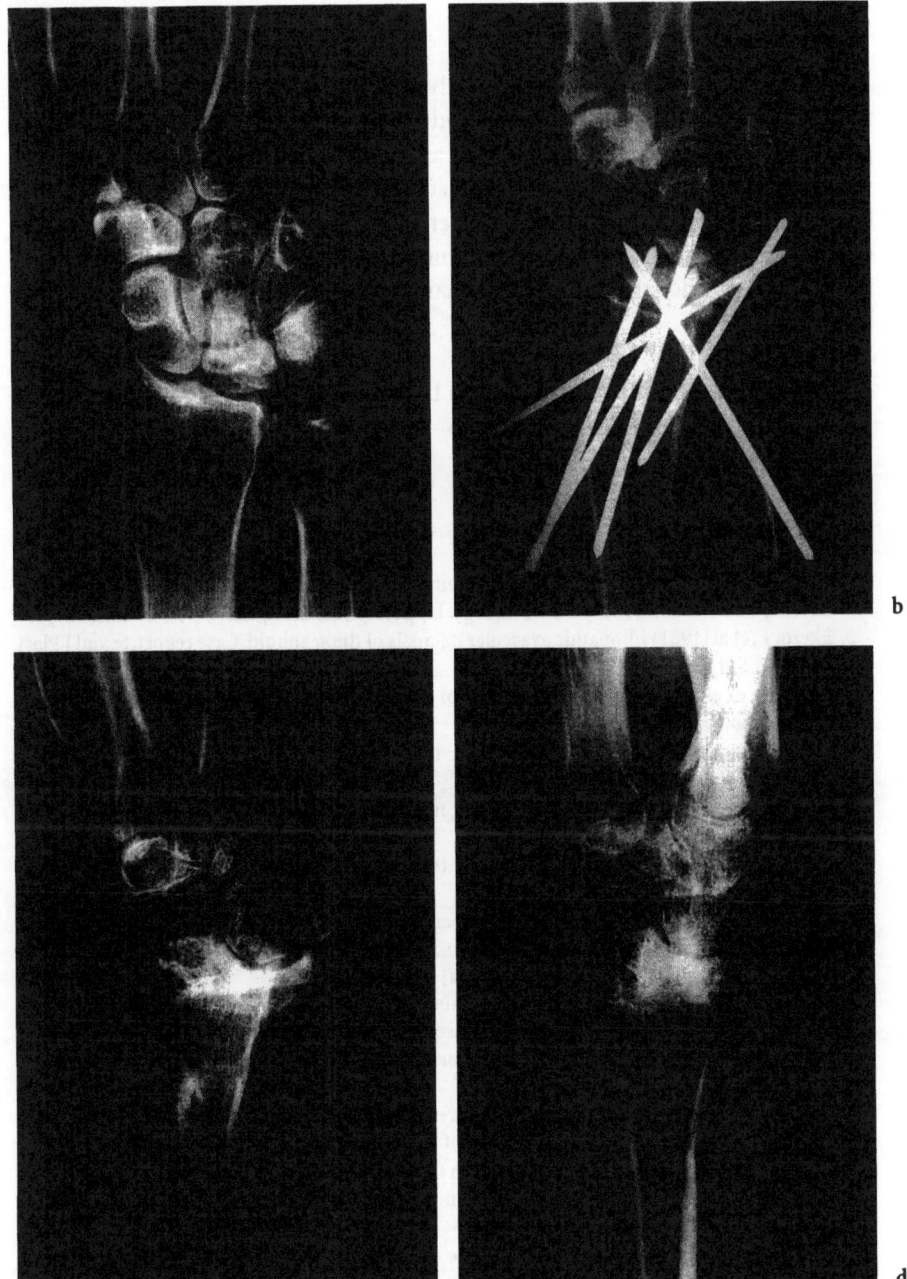

Fig. 21.20a–d. In stage 4 AVN, due to pain and deteriorating wrist instability, more aggressive carpal arthrodesis is performed with radiocarpal or pancarpal fusion. a Stage 4 AVN with fragmentation of the lunate, scaphoid rotation and radiocarpal arthrosis. b Arthrodesis of the radiocarpal compartment, proximal carpal row and ulnar osteotomy. c, d Normal postoperative results

21.5.4 Capitate

Avascular necrosis of the capitate is rarely seen [31]. Like the scaphoid, the proximal part of the capitate obtains its blood supply by means of diffusion or retrograde blood supply. Therefore, the head and neck of the capitate are subjected to major vascular disruption when fractured. The capitate is thus one of the carpal bones that can develop osteonecrosis after suffering isolated trauma or in the case of a scaphoid fracture with subsequent impingement of the capitate by the radius in a fork-like fashion. In the case of avascular necrosis midcarpal arthrodesis may be required.

Acknowledgements. Special thanks go to Luc Van Wynsberghe for the graphics.

References

1. Resnick D (1995) Diagnosis of bone and joint disorders. Saunders, Philadelphia
2. Greenspan A (2000) Orthopedic radiology. Lippincott, Philadelphia
3. Ekerot L, et al (1981) Idiopathic avascular necrosis of the scaphoid. Case report. Scand J Plast Reconstr Surg 15: 69–72
4. Filan SL, et al (1995) Avascular necrosis of the proximal scaphoid after fracture union. J Hand Surg [Br] 20:551–556
5. Jensen CH, et al (1995) Idiopathic avascular necrosis of the scaphoid in a child. Scand J Plast Surg Hand Surg 29:359–360
6. Martini G, et al (1995) Idiopathic avascular necrosis of the scaphoid. A case report. Rec Prog Med 86:238–240
7. Gelberman RH (1986) The vascularity of the wrist. Identification of vascular patterns at risk. Clin Orthop 202:40–49
8. Nicholas JA, Hershman EB (1995) The upper extremity in sports medicine. Mosby, St Louis
9. Van Demark R, et al (1992) Avascular necrosis of the hamate: a case report with reference to the hamate blood supply. J Hand Surg [Am] 17:1086–1090
10. Desser TS, et al (1990) Scaphoid fractures and Kienböck's disease of the lunate: MR imaging with histopathologic correlation. Magn Reson Imaging 8:357–361
11. Golimbu CN, et al (1995) Avascular necrosis of carpal bones. Magn Reson Imaging Clin North Am 3:284–303
12. Zlatkin MB, et al (1992) Magnetic resonance imaging of the wrist. Magn Reson Q 8:65–96
13. Friedman L, et al Computed tomography of wrist trauma. Can Assoc Radiol J 41:141–145
14. Almquist EE (1986) Kienböck disease. Clin Orthop 202:68–78
15. Szabo RM, et al (1993) Diagnosis and clinical findings of Kienböck's disease. Hand Clin 9:399–408
16. Irowa GO (1987) Avascular necrosis of the carpal lunate: a case report. J Manipul Physiol Ther 10:323–328
17. Kahn ML, et al (1986) Lunate osteomyelitis in a patient with bilateral Kienböck's disease. Orthop Rev 15:521–525
18. Mok CC et al (1997) Bilateral Kienböck disease in SLE. Scand J Rheumatol 26:485–487
19. Hocker K, et al (1995) Fracture of the lunate – a rare injury. Handchir Mikrochir Plast Chir 27:247–253
20. Minami A, et al (1992) Kienböck' disease in an eleven-year-old girl. A case report. Ital J Orthop Traumatol 18:547–550
21. Mestdagh H (1982) Arterial vascularization of the semilunar bone. Ann Chir Main 1:246–248

22. White RE Jr, et al (1984) Transient vascular compromise of the lunate after fracture-dislocation or dislocation of the carpus. J Hand Surg [Am] 9:181–184
23. Patel N, et al (1992) High-resolution bone scintigraphy of the adult wrist. Clin Nucl Med 17:449–453
24. Stuckey SL, et al (1997) Bone scan findings in Kienböck's disease. A case report with atypical findings and literature review. Clin Nucl Med 22:481–483
25. Jackson MD, et al (1990) Magnetic resonance imaging of avascular necrosis of the lunate. Arch Phys Med Rehabil 71:510–530
26. Viegas SF, et al (1989) Magnetic resonance imaging in the assessment of revascularization in Kienböck's disease. A preliminary report. Orthop Rev 18:1285–1288
27. Sundberg SB, et al (1984) Kienböck's disease. Results of treatment with ulnar lengthening. Clin Orthop 187:43–51
28. Kleinman WB, et al (1990) Scapho-trapezio-trapezoid arthrodesis for treatment of chronic static and dynamic scapho-lunate instability: a 10-year perspective on pitfalls and complications. J Hand Surg [Am] 15:408–414
29. Pardini AG (1984) Silastic arthroplast for avascular necrosis of the carpal lunate. Int Orthop 8:223–227
30. Telfer JR, et al (1994) Avascular necrosis of the hamate. J Hand Surg [Br] 19:389–392
31. Lapinsky AS, et al (1992) Avascular necrosis of the capitate: a case report. J Hand Surg [Am] 17:1090–1092
32. Acalis A, et al (1996) Idiopathic necrosis of the capitate. Acta Orthop Belg 62:46–48

22 Ungual and Subungual Disease

Jean-Luc Drapé, Alain Chevrot, Jacques Bittoun

22.1 Introduction

It may seem surprising to devote a chapter to the nail unit, as the imaging of this structure has developed poorly over time. However, high-frequency transducers have recently allowed accurate imaging of the fingertips with ultrasonography. Now magnetic resonance (MR) imaging of the nail unit is also available thanks to small dedicated surface coils. These new resources could modify the imaging strategy of ungual and subungual diseases. The main indication is the investigation of nail tumors. Neoplasia of the nail area may be benign, but is sometimes aggressive or malignant. A history of trauma, an associated infection or the interposed nail plate may mislead the physician. Deep tumors located under the matrix or the nail bed exert pressure upward and may cause ridging or even anonychia or onycholysis. Thus every suspicious tumor of the nail unit should undergo radiography and a biopsy. An additional imaging modality such as ultrasonography or MR imaging should help in doubtful cases by confirming and accurately locating an ungual or subungual tumor.

22.2 Imaging Modalities

22.2.1 Plain Films

Plain films remain the main complementary imaging modality for the nail unit. The bony structure of the distal phalanx and the joint space of the distal interphalangeal joint are best explored with radiographs. However, radiographs do not adequately image the soft tissues of the fingertip, as only thickening or calcifications can be shown. The technique to study the soft tissues must be optimized with low-voltage radiographs. High-resolution one-layer breast films have gradually replaced films without a screen. Digital films with small fields of view provide better contrast resolution but also a lower spatial resolution. The basic views include posteroanterior and lateral plain films of the involved finger. In some cases, subtle erosions of the distal phalanx may only be highlighted on oblique views. A certain amount of magnification can optimize the readability.

Most of the isolated ungual dystrophies should undergo radiography before surgery. This can depict abnormalities of the soft tissues such as a thickening of the posterior nail fold in the case of mucoid cyst or an asymmetry of the subungual space on comparative lateral radiographs when a mass is located in the nail bed (Fig. 22.1) [11, 26]. A careful study of the soft parts may show phleboliths suggesting a hemangioma or the mottled calcifications of a parosteal chondroma or exceptional epidermoid cyst (Fig. 22.2). Primary subungual calcifications in the normal nail bed may be seen in the elderly, especially women (Fig. 22.3). Similar subungual calcifications of the toes are combined in 10% [6]. Seven percent of adults present soft tissue calcifications close to the distal phalanges of the fingers. These are due to mechanical injuries of the collagen fibers close to their bony insertion. They are also particularly common in the toenail bed of elderly women. The detection of radio-opaque foreign bodies (metal, glass) is possible with plain films, but CT is more sensitive and can depict tiny radiolucent fragments of glass.

Above all, radiographs are accurate for imaging the distal phalanx and the distal interphalangeal joint. They provide decisive information regarding a subungual exostosis with pedicled ossifications which may lift up the nail plate (Fig. 22.4), or a glomus tumor or an epidermoid cyst with a clear-cut dorsal bone erosion (Fig. 22.5). Radiologic features of an enchondroma of the distal phalanx are characteristic with a well-circumscribed lobulated expansile lytic lesion with mottled calcifications. A pathologic fracture may justify the indication of plain films (Fig. 22.6). Radiographs may also depict bone erosions or cysts, isolated or associated with abnormalities of the soft tissues. An erosion of the distal phalanx may seem aggressive in the case of a metastasis, an invasive squamous carcinoma or a keratoacanthoma (Fig. 22.7). Radiographs can also detect dense bone abnormalities, as with an osteoid osteoma or psoriatic arthropathy with periosteitis. Osteoarthritis of the distal interphalangeal joint may develop dorsal osteophytes impinging the distal band of the extensor tendon. The lateral view is accurate to show these osteophytes and may reveal a thickening of the posterior nail fold due to a mucoid pseudocyst (Fig. 22.1).

In the case of acute trauma, the presence of an extensive hematoma involving more than 25% of the visible nail plate must suggest a severe injury of the nail bed

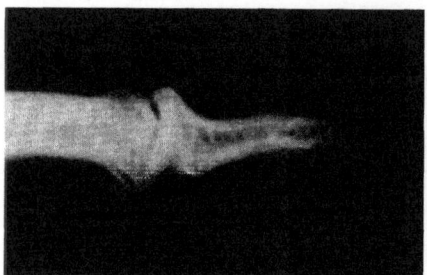 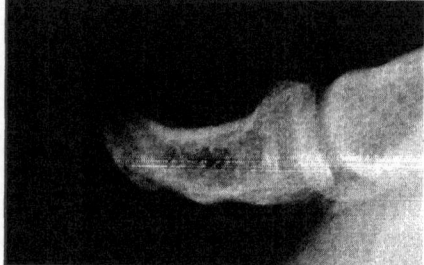

Fig. 22.1. Mucoid pseudocyst of the second finger. There is osteoarthritis of the distal interphalangeal joint with joint space narrowing and osteophytes of the head of the middle phalanx. Thickening of the posterior nail fold and clear-cut bone erosion of the dorsal cortex of the distal phalanx is seen

Fig. 22.2. Epidermoid cyst of the thumb in a 27-year-old man. The posterior nail fold is thickened and presents mottled calcifications. There is bone erosion of the dorsal cortex of the distal phalanx

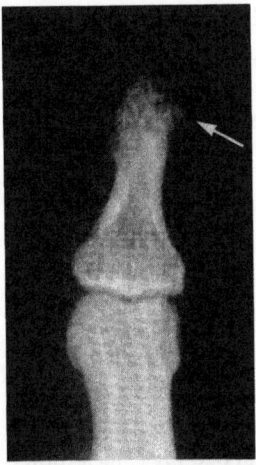

Fig. 22.3. Primary subungual calcification (*arrow*) of the nail bed in a 66-year-old woman

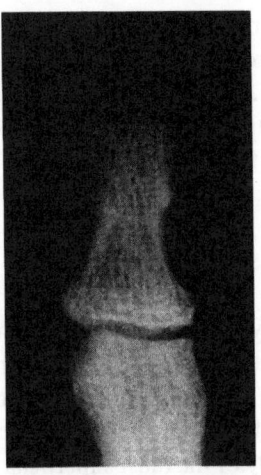

Fig. 22.4. Subungual exostosis of the third finger

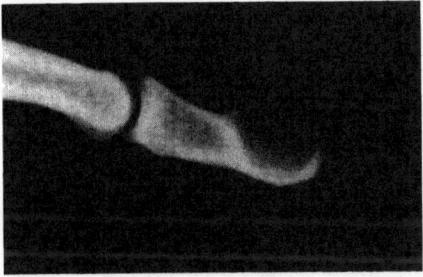

Fig. 22.5. Epidermoid cyst of the third finger in a 22-year-old man

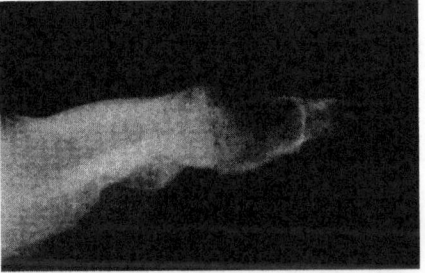

Fig. 22.6. Enchondroma of the distal phalanx of the thumb. There is pathologic fracture of this enchondroma

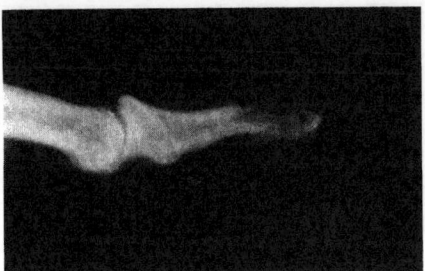

Fig. 22.7. Keratoacanthoma of the second finger. Aggressive osteolysis of the tuft of the distal phalanx is seen

or a fracture of the distal phalanx. A radiograph is then indicated to image the distal phalanx. Nearly 50% of injuries of the nail bed are associated with a fracture [50]. Crushing of the tuft must be distinguished from fractures of the shaft, which carry a worse prognosis. Plain films must differentiate simple transverse fractures with mild lesions of the tuft from complex fractures with two or more shaft fragments and extensive tuft lesions.

In post-traumatic dystrophies, radiographs can show clear-cut bone erosion of the distal phalanx due to an epidermoid cyst developing upon an epidermal inclusion (Fig. 22.5). A hook deformity may be secondary to retraction on a volar scar or to a lack of support by a shortened distal phalanx; the amount of bone loss must be assessed on the radiographs [44].

22.2.2   Ultrasonography

Ultrasonography should be more widely used in imaging the nail unit. However, its operator-dependent characteristic and the poor experience of radiologists in this anatomic region are limiting factors. High-frequency 7.5–20 MHz probes dedicated to musculoskeletal or skin imaging are suitable. An interposition material is necessary for the study of the most superficial structures. The nail bed presents a rather homogeneous hypoechoic appearance, included between the high-intensity echoes of the dorsal cortex of the phalanx and of the nail plate. The nail plate may produce two parallel high-signal echoes (Fig. 22.8). Imaging the matrix area is possible with 30 MHz B-mode imaging but is tricky due to the overlying echoes of the proximal and lateral nail folds [27]. Furthermore axial slices suffer from artifacts caused by the convexity of the nail plate. Ultrasonography has been proposed for detecting glomus tumors of the fingertips. Tumors less than 3 mm are hardly visible but tumors located in the pulp are more accessible [25, 41]. Doppler imaging may reveal the vascular features of the lesion in some cases (Fig. 22.9). Ultrasonography is also appropriate to highlight radiotransparent foreign bodies, such as thorns. A combined granulomatous reaction may be revealed with imaging.

Very high resolution ultrasonographic studies remain in the field of research and began with skin imaging in 1979 [2]. Ultrasonography appeared as an effec-

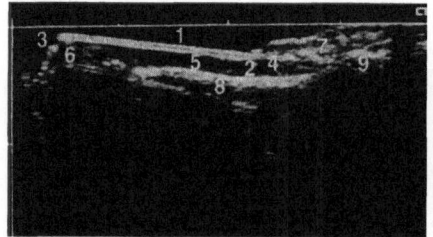
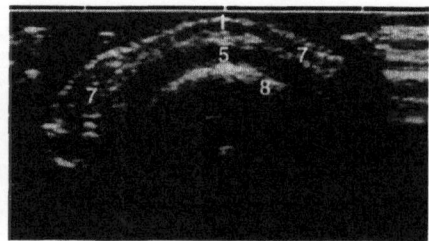

a   b

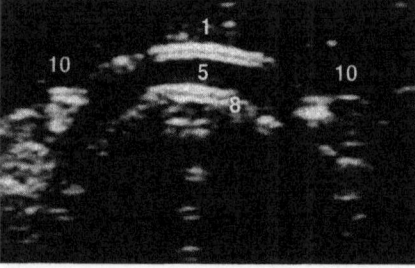

c

Fig. 22.8a–c. Ultrasonography of the normal nail unit. a Sagittal view, b proximal axial view, c distal axial view. 1 Nail plate, 2 nail root, 3 free edge of the nail plate, 4 matrix, 5 nail bed, 6 hyponychium, 7 proximal nail fold, 8 dorsal cortex of the distal phalanx, 9 distal interphalangeal joint, 10 lateral nail fold

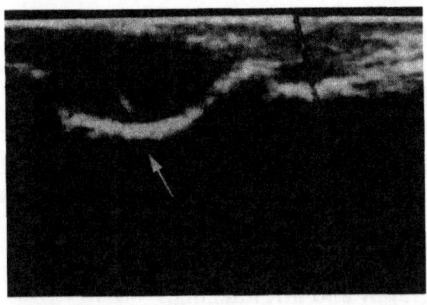

Fig. 22.9. Doppler imaging of a glomus subungual tumor. Sagittal view shows clear-cut erosion of the dorsal cortex (*arrow*). The limits of this vascularized subungual tumor with the nail bed are ill defined

tive and noninvasive method of measuring the thickness of the dermis [47]. A- and B-mode ultrasonographs dedicated to skin imaging have been developed as research and clinical tools, mainly for tumoral and inflammatory diseases [46]. M-mode, high-frequency Doppler and three-dimensional (3D) investigations remain works in progress. Twenty-megahertz probes provide the best compromise between a high spatial resolution and sufficient depth. Fifty-megahertz or higher probes only allow imaging of the epidermis, with an axial resolution of about 37.5 μm and a lateral resolution of about 125 μm [21]. Paradoxically, studies of the nail unit are few. A.Y. Finlay introduced ultrasonography for the assessment of the thickness of the nail plate with a 20 MHz A-mode probe [22, 23]. The distal conduction speeds (mean of 2470 m/s) were well correlated with the measurements of the free edge of the nail plate with a micrometer. The distal reduction of about 8.8% in the ultrasound transmission time compared with the proximal measurements should be due to a the greater thickness and hydration of the nail plate at the level of the lunula. J.B.E. Jemec also studied the A-mode ultrasound structure of the nail plates of post-mortem thumbs in situ and after resection [31]. The spatial resolution was about 75 μm with a 20 MHz probe. Contrary to Finlay, he noted compartments of different echo speeds, a superficial dry layer (ultrasound velocity of 3103 m/s) and a deep hydrated layer (ultrasound velocity of 2125 m/s). On the other hand, he could not differentiate the different layers of the nail bed. T. Hirai proposed 30 MHz B-mode to image nail matrix abnormalities in the case of nail plate deformities [27].

22.2.3 Xeroradiography

Xeroradiography, another imaging modality for soft tissues, is no longer used.

22.2.4 Angiography

Arteriography was once proposed for the diagnosis of glomus tumors and osteoid osteomas [11, 13], but it does not seem justified any longer given the availability of CT and MR imaging [17, 28, 30].

22.2.5 Computed Tomography

Despite recent technological advances in computed tomography (CT) with helical acquisitions, its indications remain limited in imaging the pathologies of the fingertip. The irradiation remains insignificant at this level with a volumetric acquisition of 0.5–1 mm thick slices. High-quality multiplanar and 3D reformatted views of the phalanx may be calculated. CT images are adequate to detect the tiny nidus of an osteoid osteoma (Fig. 22.10). However, evaluation of the soft tissues remains poor and is inferior to ultrasonography and MR imaging.

22.2.6 Magnetic Resonance Imaging

MR imaging has proved its striking abilities in contrast resolution for the soft tissues and yet studies of the nail unit are rare. Only a few cases of subungual tumors, mainly glomus tumors, have been reported in the literature [17, 18, 28, 29, 30, 35, 39, 45].

22.2.6.1 Technique

The restrictions of MR imaging of the nail unit are very specific. The spatial resolution must be high with a pixel size of about 100–150 μm in the axis perpendicular to the nail plate, in order to discriminate the different layers of the nail bed (epithelium and dermis). The ability to obtain high-resolution images has been known since 1986 [1, 32]. At the same time, high-resolution modules were developed on whole-body MR units by several teams and the first clinical applications were for skin imaging [7, 43]. The next studies extended to the wrist, the fingers [8, 16, 24, 49] and the eye [24]. Imaging was based either on dedicated local gradient

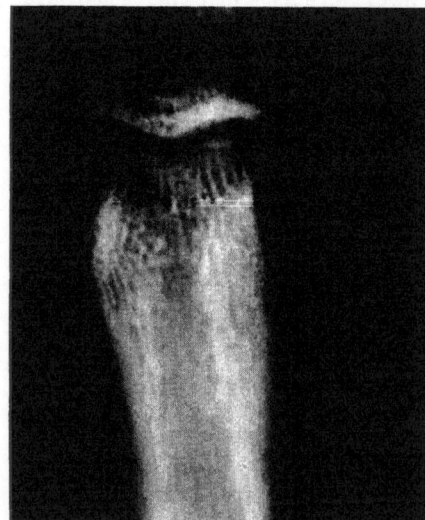

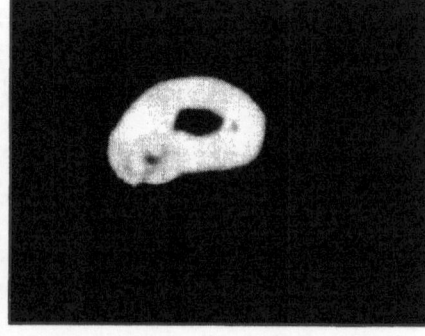

b

Fig. 22.10a, b. Osteoid osteoma of the neck of the middle phalanx of the third finger. a Radiograph depicts periosteal and endosteal thickening of the ulnar cortex. b Axial CT slice highlights a tiny calcified nidus in the palmo-ulnar cortex

a

coils or on specific acquisition sequences, not available on standard MR units. However, very small surface phased-array or flexible coils dedicated to the imaging of the wrist or the fingers have recently become available. When they are used with high-field MR units with strong gradients (higher than 20 mT/m), such high spatial resolutions are reached with acceptable acquisition times. Thus MR imaging of the nail unit is now possible with the newest MR units.

A 3 cm field of view is the most suitable, because it provides imaging of the whole unit with a high signal-to-noise ratio. For the small fingers (fifth finger) a 2 cm field of view is often necessary. The nail plate must be placed on the surface coil to provide the maximum signal. Good patient cooperation and efficient immobilization with adhesive strips are necessary to avoid movement artifacts, which are very disturbing at such resolutions. The positioning of the arm is variable, either elevated or close to the body. The position is more comfortable for toe imaging. The patient may be in procubitus with the feet first, the dorsal aspect of the toes against the coil. The basic examination includes axial T1- and T2 weighted images, and T1 or T2 sagittal images, or even 3D gradient echo images in the axial or sagittal planes according to the pathology. Three-dimensional slices are essential for detecting tiny lesions of 1–2-mm, in order to compensate for the overly thick spin echo slices (about 2–3 mm). The injection of 0.1 mmol/kg gadoterate is at request. The addition of a fat saturation sequence optimizes the enhancement.

22.2.6.2 *MRI of the Normal Nail Unit*

The nail plate itself provides no signal on all sequences. This lack of signal is probably due to the strongly organized structure of keratin. Like collagen, this scleroprotein leads to major shortening of the relaxation times [42]. If the inferior surface of the nail plate is underlined by the high signal of the epithelium of the matrix and the nail bed, the upper surface of the nail plate is not visible. Its interface with the air, also without signal, is not detectable. Applying Vaseline to the nail plate provides excellent delineation of the upper surface of the nail plate whatever the sequence used (Fig. 22.11A). The presence of fat results in the chemical shift artifact and can significantly disturb the measurements of the nail plate thickness (up to 40%). On sagittal slices, the nail root is very thin and surrounded by the high signal of the matrix cul-de-sac. The nail plate progressively thickens towards the free edge of the plate, but *faster* at the level of the distal matrix (in the lunula area). This fact is consistent with direct measurements [33,34]. On the other hand, MR imaging is not able to discriminate the different histologic layers or the two ultrasound layers of the nail plate [31].

Proximal axial slices depict the posterior nail fold, the extensor and flexor tendons, the collateral ligaments of the distal interphalangeal joint, the matricophalangeal ligaments and the volar plate. The proximal and distal matrix surround the nail root (Fig. 22.11B). A slice at the level of the distal matrix clearly shows the thickening of the epithelium along the median line, although the crests are not directly visible. The lateral nail folds are well visible, as are the lateral interosseous ligaments which delineate the rima ungualum (Fig. 22.11C). The submatrix dermis

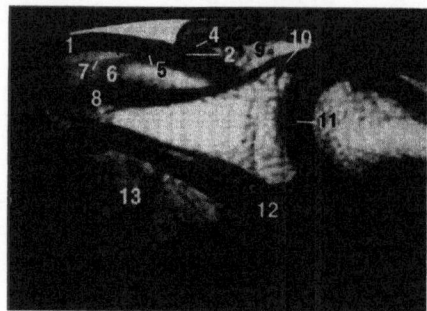

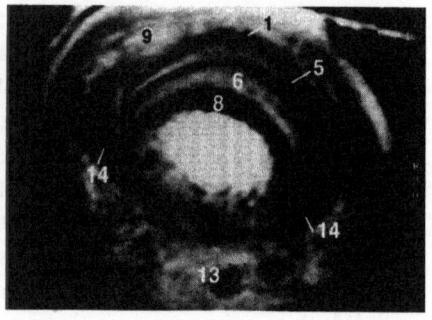

a   b

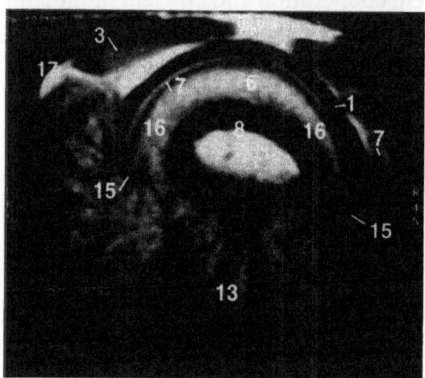

Fig. 22.11. a Sagittal T1 weighted spin echo image of the normal nail unit of the thumb. **b** Proximal axial proton density-weighted spin echo image. **c** Distal axial T1-weighted spin echo image. *1* Nail plate, *2* nail root, *3* Vaseline, *4* proximal matrix, *5* distal matrix, *6* nail bed, *7* epidermis of the nail bed, *8* dorsal cortex of the distal phalanx, *9* proximal nail fold, *10* terminal band of the extensor tendon, *11* distal interphalangeal joint, *12* flexor tendon, *13* pulp, *14* matricophalangeal ligament, *15* lateral interosseous ligament, *16* rima ungualum, *17* lateral nail fold

c

appears with a rather homogeneous and intense signal. On an axial slice of the nail bed, the thin epithelium has a high signal while the underlying dermis presents a thin superficial layer of low signal and a deep layer of heterogeneous signal. This heterogeneity is reinforced by the injection of gadoterate, which enhances numerous glomus bodies. These capsulated round organs 300 μm in diameter appear as very intense nodes on T2-weighted and postenhanced images (Fig. 22.12).

Sagittal slices are adapted to the analysis of the distal interphalangeal joint with the insertion of the distal band of the extensor tendon at the base of the distal phalanx, the cartilage of the joint and the volar plate. The nail root and the matrix cul-de-sac are well depicted only on these slices (Fig. 22.11A). A magnetic susceptibility artifact can disturb the analysis of the free edge of the nail plate, especially

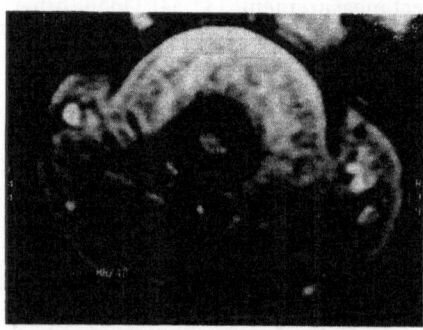

Fig. 22.12. Post-enhanced 3D gradient echo image of the distal nail bed. Note the numerous enhanced dots of the glomus bodies

on the 3D gradient echo images (Fig. 22.13). There is no difference in signal in any sequence between the nail matrix and the epithelium of the nail bed or the volar aspect of the proximal nail fold. However, in this plane the matrix seems thinner than the epithelium of the nail bed, which is in contradiction to the histologic findings of a thick ruffled epithelium. In any case. the transition between the matrix and the nail bed is marked by a dramatic increase in thickness of the epithelium. Another matrix pattern is the particular magnetic behavior of the submatrix dermis. The submatrix dermis appears as an oval area of high signal on T2-weighted images with a strong and homogeneous enhancement after injection of gadoterate. This highly intense submatrix area is strongly correlated with the lunula (Fig. 22.14) [19]. This area is small and covered with the proximal nail fold in fingers devoid of lunula. Histologic examinations show a loose dermis area with less developed collagen bundles than in the nail bed. The study of the microvascularization reveals a more regular angioarchitecture in this area than in the distal nail bed. Therefore, the lunula appears linked to a well-circumscribed area of the underlying dermis with specific histologic and vascular patterns. The significance and function of this area remain to be clarified. According to H.P. Baden, the fact that matrix keratinocytes produce "soft" keratins in vitro, is in favor of the in vivo synthesis of nail proteins under the influence of this dermis [3, 4]. This could explain the tendency of the nail to renew itself after superficial destruction of the matrix. The adjacent epidermis grows again, covering the matrix, and could be reprogrammed for synthesis of the nail plate [4].

The distal epithelium thickens at the level of the hyponychium. The lack of fat tissue in the nail bed, except for a thin layer under the nail root, means there is no susceptibility to a chemical shift artifact.

Coronal slices are disappointing because they depend on finger positioning. A slight rotation leads to hardly interpretable slices. Double obliquity slices can eliminate this inconvenience. However, the conformation of the nail unit is poorly

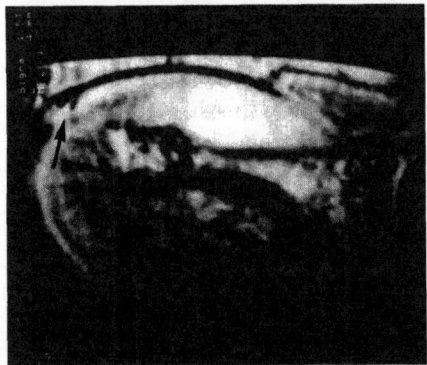
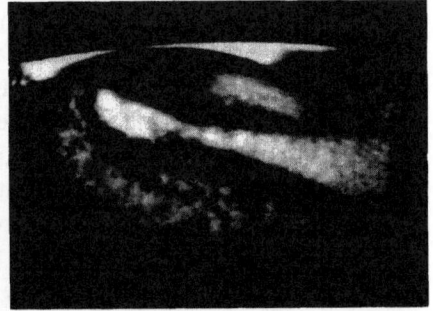

Fig. 22.13. Magnetic susceptibility artifact on a sagittal gradient echo image. Dark dots beneath the free edge of the nail plate are due to magnetic susceptibility artifacts (*arrow*)

Fig. 22.14. Submatrix area on a sagittal T2-weighted image. Note the oval high signal area in the dermis beneath the matrix

adapted to the coronal plane: its different components are tangential to it and thus prone to partial volume artifacts.

22.2.6.3   Clinical Applications

The MR imaging indications in pathologies of the nail unit remain works in progress. MR imaging may be of interest for the investigation of post-traumatic nail dystrophies (Fig. 22.15) and of the ligamentous apparatus, but actually the investigation of a subungual tumor is the main indication. Tumors of the nail unit may be difficult to diagnose compared with skin tumors. The lesions implanted in the matrix area are covered by the proximal nail fold and the nail root, and can sometimes be revealed only by a nail dystrophy. Deformities of the nail plate are often benign, while partial or complete onycholysis is evocative of a malignant lesion. MR imaging could be an intermediate procedure between plain films and a surgical biopsy. Negative MR findings should mean a biopsy is not necessary.

The search for glomus tumors is the most common indication for MR imaging. Glomus tumors result from hyperplasia of one or several glomus bodies and may be assimilated to hamartomas [12]. The clinical interest is significant. The classic triad of pain, painful point and cold sensitivity is strongly evocative but rather uncommon. The mean diagnostic delay ranges from 4 to 7 years in the literature [12, 26, 39, 42]. MR imaging has an excellent sensitivity and must be used in preference to arteriography. Some interpretation difficulties may be due to histologic variations, revealed in 1924 by P. Masson [38]. These are not routinely noted in pathology reports because they have no prognostic value. However, they must be known because of their influence on the signal behavior of the tumor. This signal can indeed vary according to the dominant histologic component. Four types are then identified [17]:

- *a vascular type* with a large number of vessel lumina. There is very strong enhancement after gadoterate injection and rather high signal on T2-weighted images (Fig. 22.16).
- *a cellular or solid type* with a dominant proliferation of epithelioid cells (glomus cells) and a relative poverty of vascular lumina. This type is particularly difficult to diagnose, because its signal is quite close to that of the nail bed dermis on T1- and T2-weighted images (Fig. 22.17). The injection of gadoterate can be useful to increase the contrast. The thin contiguous 3D slices are also helpful to identify a peripheral capsule.
- *a mucoid type* with mucoid degeneration of the stroma. The enhancement is low after injection, while the signal is very high on T2-weighted images because of the mucoid component (Fig. 22.18).
- *a mixed type* combining the different elementary components (Fig. 22.19).

The vascular and the mixed types are by far the most common lesions.

The tumor margins are most often well defined, with the lesion confined by a pseudocapsule due to reactive peripheral tissue. This capsule presents a very low signal on all sequences and is better visualized on T2-weighted images (Fig. 22.16).

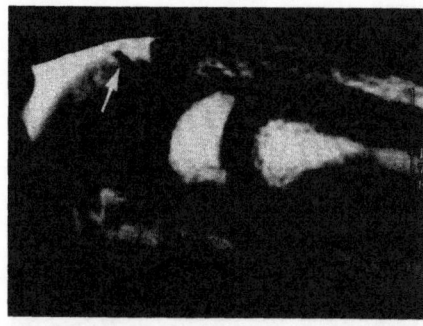

Fig. 22.15. Post-traumatic hook deformity of the nail plate. The sagittal image shows the fibrous replacement of the bone defect and the deformity of the distal nail matrix (*arrow*)

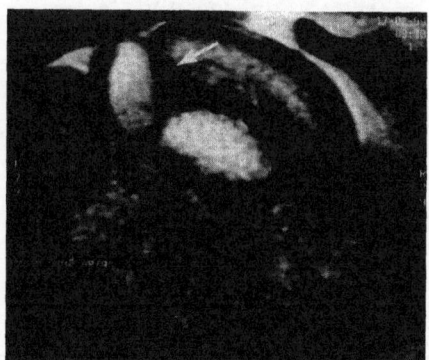

b

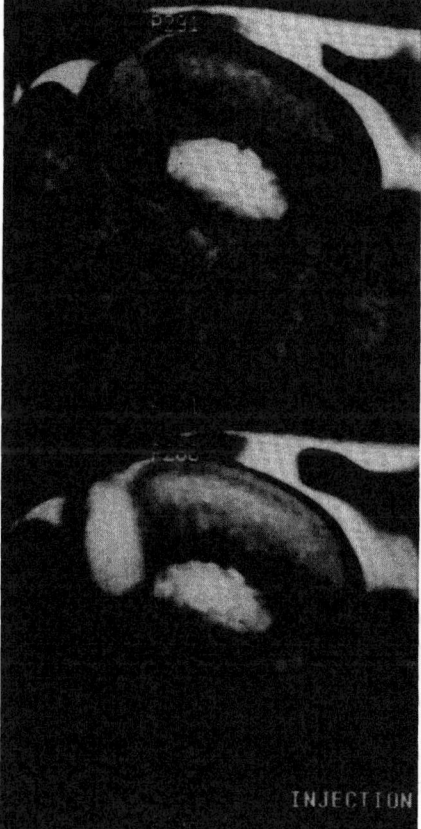

a

Fig. 22.16a, b. Vascular type of glomus tumor. The patient had a history of digital pain for 5 years. **a** Axial T1-weighted image before (*top*) and after (*bottom*) injection of gadoterate. **b** Axial T2-weighted image. Note the strong homogeneous enhancement and the high signal. A low signal peripheral capsule is more visible on the T2-weighted image (*arrow*)

Its accurate analysis is facilitated by the injection of gadoterate. In 25% of cases the capsule is partially or completely absent with ill-defined tumor margins [18]. Peroperative adhesions with the nail bed are often noted in these cases (Fig. 22.20). The local invasion of the capsule is debated and has been reported on histologic findings in 1–2% of cases by E. Kohout but was not found by R.E. Carroll [12, 37]. The risk of leaving in situ some tumor tissue after surgery is higher in ill-defined lesions. The

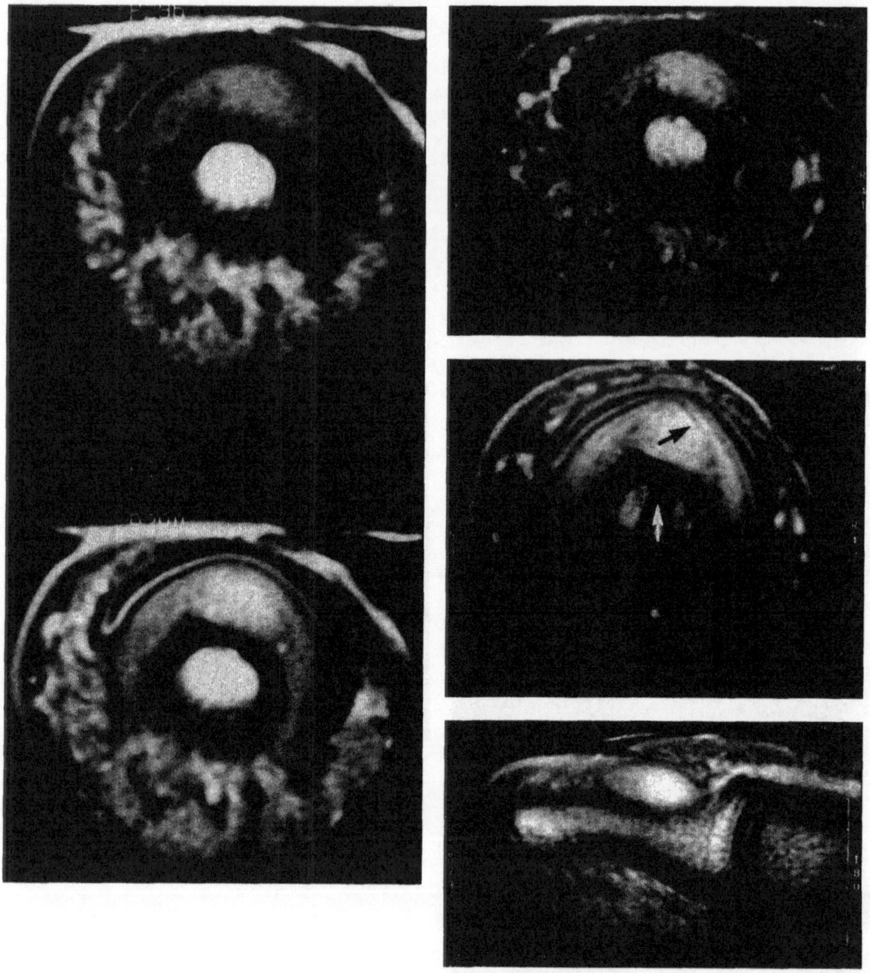

Fig. 22.17a–d. Solid type of glomus tumor. This tumor of the third finger was not detected with ultrasound and Doppler imaging. a Axial T1-weighted images before (*top*) and after (*bottom*) injection of gadoterate. Note the faint enhancement of the tumor. b Axial T2-weighted image shows an ill-defined lesion of slightly high signal. c Axial 3D postenhanced gradient echo image depicts a peripheral capsule (*black arrow*) and the deformity of the nail matrix (*arrowhead*) and of the underlying dorsal cortex (*white arrow*). d Sagittal postenhanced T1-weighted image shows the submatrix location of the tumor in the center of the oval submatrix area

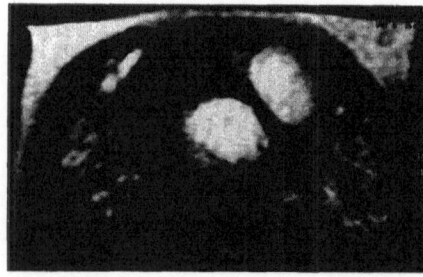

Fig. 22.18. Mucoid type of glomus tumor. Axial T2-weighted image shows very high signal of the tumor despite a low enhancement after injection of gadoterate

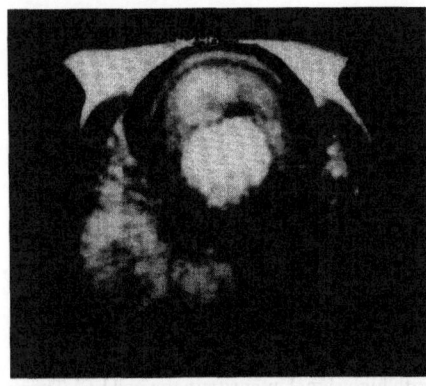

Fig. 22.19. Mixed type of glomus tumor. Axial postenhanced T1-weighted image depicts heterogeneous enhancement with a central low signal area

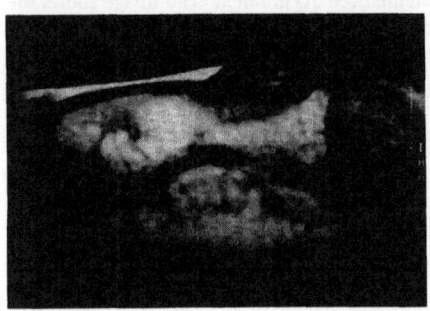

a

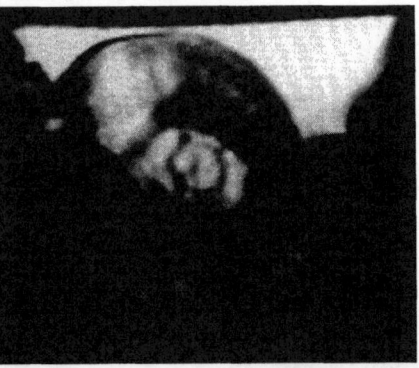

b

Fig. 22.20a, b. Adhesive glomus tumor. **a** Sagittal and **b** axial postenhanced T1-weighted images depict an ill-defined vascularized tumor of the distal nail bed. The medial aspect of the tumor has a blurred boundary with the nail bed

recurrence rate ranges from 12% to 24% in the literature [12, 15, 42, 48]. MR imaging is certainly useful in these cases with a high risk of recurrence, as well as for multiple lesions involving the same finger. MR imaging may be disturbed by scar tissue in the case of recurrent pain after surgery, but is highly accurate for detecting a residual or recurrent tumor (Fig. 22.21) [14].

MR imaging accurately depicts the location of the tumor, most often beneath the nail plate in the dermal tissue of the nail bed. These locations may be difficult to detect with ultrasound, because of artifacts produced by the nail plate curvature [25]. The lesion is close to the periosteum of the distal phalanx and bone erosions are commonly highlighted on axial MR images, while they are occult on plain radiographs (Fig. 22.17). Axial slices are essential for determining the median or lateral location of the lesion in the nail bed, and for assessing an invasion of the rima ungualum and the pulp (Fig. 22.22). The surgical approach can be influenced by the MR findings, which help to choose between a lateral or a transungual approach. Sagittal slices are necessary to assess the relationship of the tumor with the matrix.

Less commonly, the lesions may involve the pulp or the posterior nail fold. There is good contrast between healthy tissue and the tumor because of the pres-

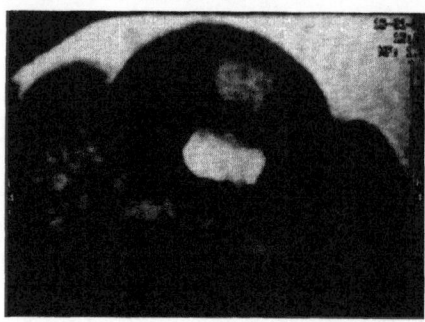 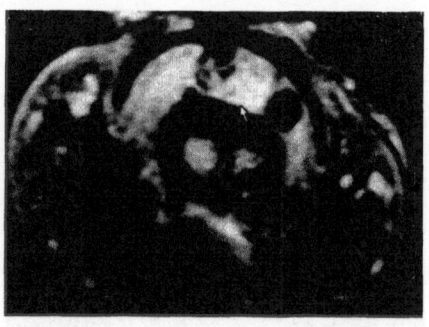

a   b

Fig. 22.21a, b. Recurrent glomus tumor 3 years after previous surgery. a Axial spin echo T2-weighted image depicts a round recurrent tumor with high signal intensity in the nail bed. There are no visible artifacts or scar tissue. b Axial postenhanced 3D gradient echo image shows the enhanced tumor (*arrow*) surrounded by dark artifacts due to the previous surgery

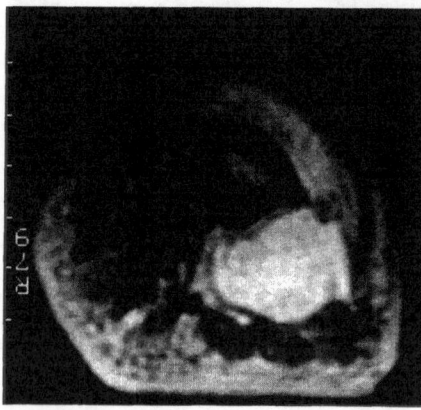

Fig. 22.22. Lateral glomus tumor of the thumb. Axial postenhanced 3D gradient echo image shows well-defined enhanced tumor in the rima ungualum. The dorsal aspect of the lesion invades the nail bed while the volar aspect extends toward the pulp. There is bone erosion of the volar cortex of the distal phalanx

ence of fat tissue in the hypodermis. The tumor is spontaneously visible on T1-weighted images, surrounded by the high signal of the fatty hypodermis. On the other hand, the injection of gadoterate will erase the tumor limits by leveling out the signals (Fig. 22.23). Its interest is in detecting an extension toward the nail bed.

Among the other vascular tumors, *hemangiomas* are one of the most common soft tissue tumors and locations on the fingers are not rare [36]. Although some hemangiomas regress completely (e.g., juvenile hemangioma), most persist if untreated but possess a limited growth potential. The histologic classification of hemangiomas has a poor prognostic value. There is therefore no evidence of malignant transformation except for hemangioendotheliomas, for which carcinologic resection is debated [9]. Hemangiomas can invade the eponychium (Fig. 22.24), or the nail bed and the pulp via the rima ungualum. They displace the lateral interosseous ligaments, but bony erosions are rare even with large lesions. The signal behavior may be quite different from that of deep intramuscular hemangiomas [10]. On T1-weighted images, the high signal of fatty overgrowth tissue is uncommon. When the tumor is small, it can appear solid and homogeneous like a glomus

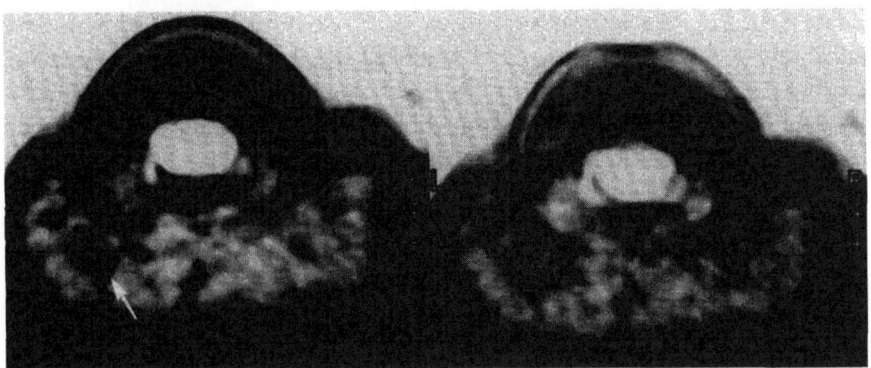

Fig. 22.23. Glomus tumor of the pulp. Axial T1-weighted images before (*left*) and after (*right*) injection of gadoterate. A 2 mm tumor with low signal intensity (*arrow*) is spontaneously depicted within the surrounding high signal fatty tissue. After injection of gadoterate the contrast of the lesion decreases. A postenhanced fat saturation image would be preferable

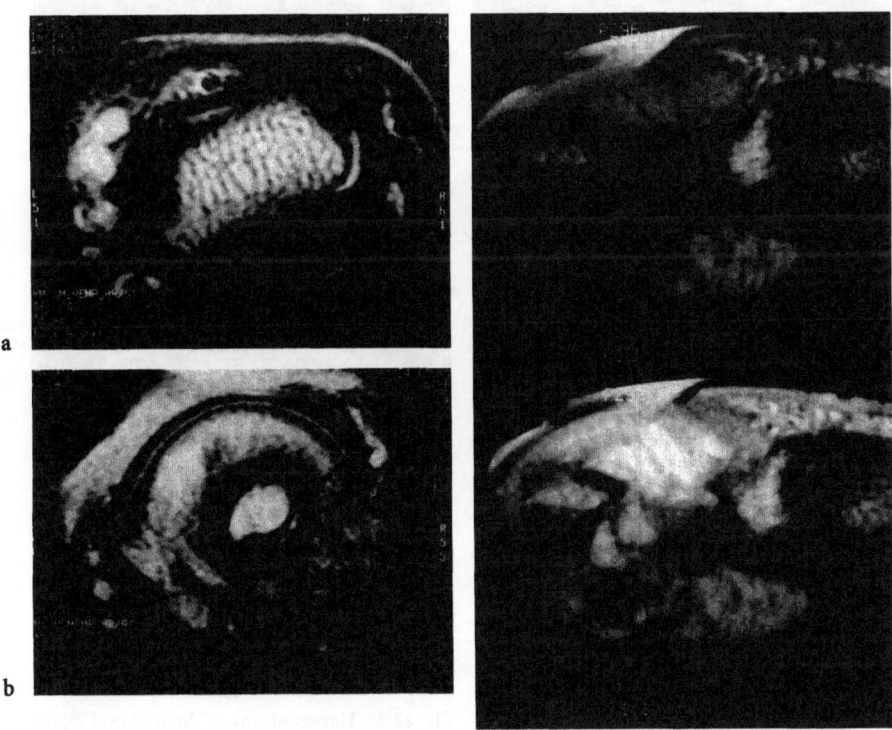

Fig. 22.24a–c. Hemangioma of the third finger. **a** Axial T2-weighted image at the level of the distal interphalangeal joint depicts a multinodular very high signal lesion in the posterior nail fold. **b** Axial T2-weighted image at the level of the nail bed shows the extension of the lesion in the lateral part of the nail bed, the rima ungualum and the pulp. **c** Sagittal T1-weighted image before (*top*) and after (*bottom*) injection of gadoterate depicts serpentine vascular enhancement in the nail bed and the pulp

tumor (Fig. 22.25) or without high signal on T2-weighted images and with faint enhancement (Fig. 22.26). In all cases, small circular, linear or serpentine vascular spaces must be carefully looked for. The injection of gadoterate and gradient echo images may be helpful to highlight flow artifacts (Fig. 22.27). The enhancement may be only peripheral due to thrombosis. Axial and sagittal slices may depict fluid/fluid levels in the vascular spaces (Fig. 22.28). The differential diagnosis with traumatic hematomas or digital varix may be difficult on MR slices as well as histologically.

Numerous other tumors of the nail unit can benefit from MR imaging. The most common and most characteristic lesions are:

- Among the epithelial tumors, *inclusion or epidermoid cysts* of the distal phalanx are rare, usually secondary to trauma with the inclusion of epidermal tissue in the subcutaneous tissues, or even in the bone. An old trauma may go unnoticed. Scar tissue can lead to a cyst in a postoperative setting [6]. In osseous locations, the distal phalanx expands progressively and the bowing

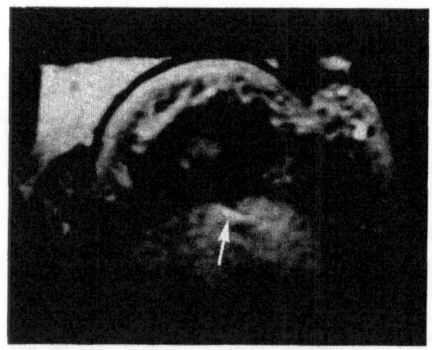

Fig. 22.25. Hemangioma of the pulp similar to a glomus tumor. Axial postenhanced 3D gradient image depicts a homogeneous enhanced tumor of the pulp similar to a glomus tumor. Note the flow artifacts of small vessels on the dorsal aspect of the tumor (*arrow*)

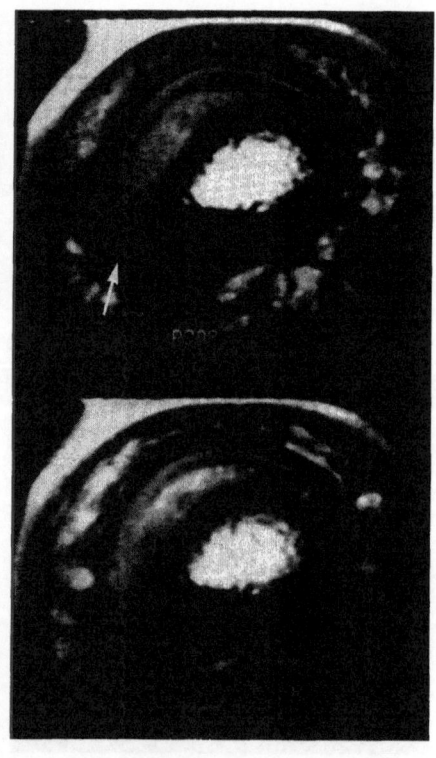

Fig. 22.26. Hemangioma of the nail bed. Axial T1-weighted images before (*top*) and after (*bottom*) injection of gadoterate. Note the enlargement of the lateral part of the nail bed and of the rima ungualum. The matricophalangeal ligament is displaced (*arrow*). Note the faint enhancement due to thrombosis of the hemangioma

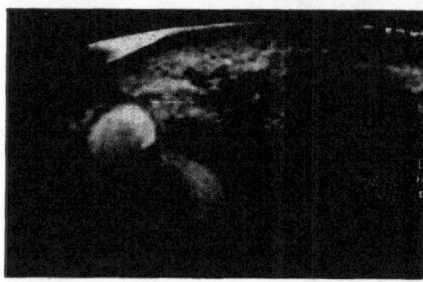

Fig. 22.27. Hemangioendothelioma of the pulp. Sagittal postenhanced 3D gradient echo shows a bilobulated tumor of the pulp with a central dark flow artifact

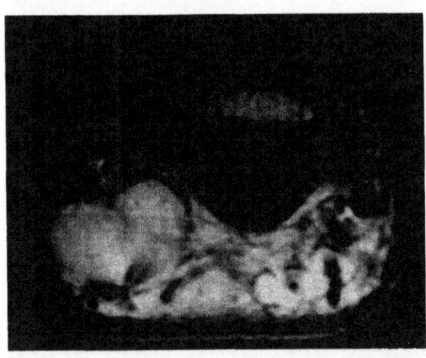

Fig. 22.28. Hemangioma of the volar aspect of the middle and distal phalanx of the third finger. Axial postenhanced T1-weighted image shows several blood-filled vascular cavities with a fluid/fluid level

becomes obvious. Pain appears late, sometimes due to a pathologic fracture. Radiographs depict a clear-cut round erosion with thin peripheral sclerosis (Fig. 22.5). On MR images, the signal behavior is heterogeneous and varies from a slight to a very high signal on T2-weighted images, depending on the amount of orthokeratin. The enhancement is also variable and heterogeneous, but is seldom strong (Fig. 22.29). A thin epidermal shell may be depicted as a thin peripheral layer of signal similar to that of normal epidermis. Small bony erosions are often more visible on axial slices. Artifacts, especially on gradient images, may indicate the area of the initial penetrating injury.

- *Onychomatricomas* (filamentous tumor of the matrix with a fan-like nail plate) can be suspected when one is confronted with four patterns [5]: a yellowish color along the whole length and a variable width of the nail plate; a prominent nail plate; an increased transverse curvature of the nail plate; and matrix tumor depicted after resection of the nail plate. The nail plate is like a flattened tunnel in which filamentous digits penetrate. Sagittal MR images are essential to highlight the tumor core in the matrix area and the tumor digitations penetrating in the fan-like nail plate. The distal part of these filaments presents a high signal on T2-weighted images, due to a mucoid stroma. Axial slices depict holes in the nail plate, filled with these filaments (Fig. 22.30).

- MR imaging is of little value for imaging *fibrous tumors*, although they have rather specific patterns. Numerous types of fibrous tumors can have a sub- or periungual location. These tumors, ranging from dermatofibromas to fibrokeratomas, have variable clinical symptoms although they present a rather uniform histology. In fact, Koenen's tumor, acquired fibrokeratoma and dermatofibroma present a certain "clinical continuity". In the case of acquired periungual fibrokeratoma, MR imaging depicts the proximal part originating from the posterior nail fold and lying in a groove of the nail plate. Above all, MR images show the deep implantation close to the nail root (Fig. 22.31). The signal depends on the histologic composition: very low signal on all sequences with large amount of collagen fibers, high signal on T2-weighted images with edematous stroma. The lesion may present septa. The acanthotic shell has a signal similar to that of normal epithelium. MR imaging can depict lesions of the volar aspect of the posterior nail fold with

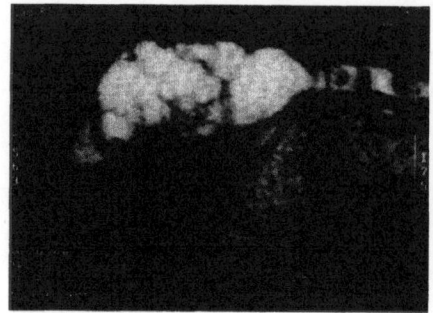

Fig. 22.29a, b. Epidermoid cyst of the posterior nail fold. a Sagittal T2-weighted image depicts a high signal tumor of the posterior nail fold with numerous septa. b Axial T1-weighted images before (*top*) and after injection (*bottom*) of gadolinium depict the deformity of the nail plate and the nail matrix underlying the tumor. Note the heterogeneous enhancement of the lesion

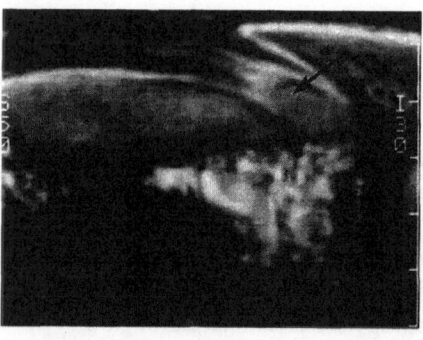
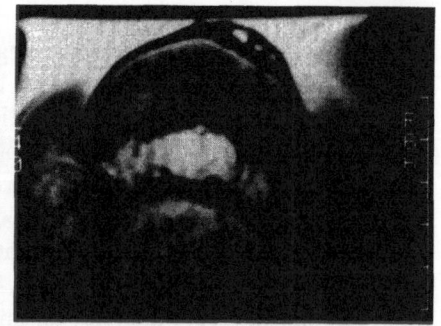

Fig. 22.30a, b. Onychomatricoma. a Sagittal 3D gradient echo image shows the core of the tumor (*arrow*) in the nail matrix. Filamentous expansions invade the fan-like nail plate. b Axial T2-weighted image depicts high signal filaments in the nail plate

an epithelial invagination. This invagination acts as an accessory matrix and produces a keratotic pseudonail.

- *Giant cell tumors* develop from the tendon sheaths or from the articular synovium. They are the second most common tumor of the soft tissues of the hand. They are located mainly on the dorsal aspect of the interphalangeal joints of the fingers and are solitary. These lesions seldom involve the nail unit. There are no calcifications, unlike in synovialosarcomas. The tumors can extend toward the distal phalanx with a cortical defect depicted on radiographs and MR images

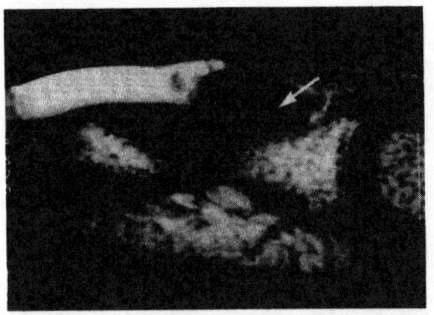

a

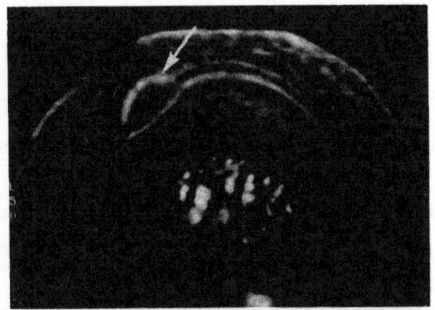

b

Fig. 22.31a–c. Digital acquired fibrokeratoma. **a** Sagittal T1-weighted image depicts the implantation of the tumor (*arrow*) in the matrix area. **b** Axial proximal gradient echo image shows the tumor lifting up the proximal nail matrix (*arrow*). **c** Axial distal gradient echo image depicts the distal expansion of the tumor lying in a groove of the nail plate. Note the high signal of the peripheral epidermal shell of the lesion

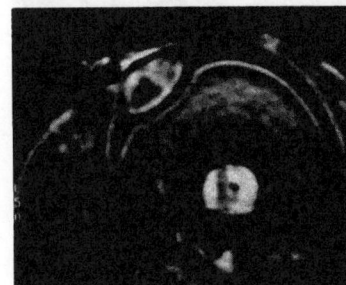

c

(Fig. 22.32). The isolated bony involvement of a finger is exceptional, but is easily associated with other bony locations. The bony tumor is expansile and may induce a pathologic fracture. The histologic patterns of pigmented villonodular synovitis are present. Hemosiderin deposits lead to a brownish color and characteristic artifacts are depicted on MR slices (Fig. 22.33). These artifacts are often less obvious than for the knee locations. In the other cases, the signal is not specific with a rather intermediate signal on T2-weighted images and a strong enhancement on postcontrast images (Fig. 22.34).

- *Mucoid pseudocysts* of the fingers are easily diagnosed, but often present recurrences. MR imaging can explain some cases of therapeutic failure, despite the numerous treatments available. Most of the cysts are isolated and involve the posterior nail fold. Their MR imaging patterns are specific with smooth walls, low signal on T1-weighted images, and very high signal on T2-weighted images. Intracystic septa are highlighted on T2-weighted images (Fig. 22.35). The injection of gadoterate shows only faint peripheral enhancement. MR imaging is essentially helpful when it detects satellite cysts, or even an extension beneath the nail matrix, which are clinically occult (Fig. 22.36) [20]. This location beneath the matrix is seldom reported in the literature. In the rare painful cases, the symptoms can mimic a glomus tumor. A bony erosion may be depicted on the radiographs when the cyst is huge. The compression of the matrix produces a fissure of the nail plate with a claw dystrophy. The location beneath the matrix is often occult and can lead to recurrence. In most cases MR imaging depicts a pedicle between the cyst and the distal interphalangeal joint. In all cases, the pedicle is lateral beneath the

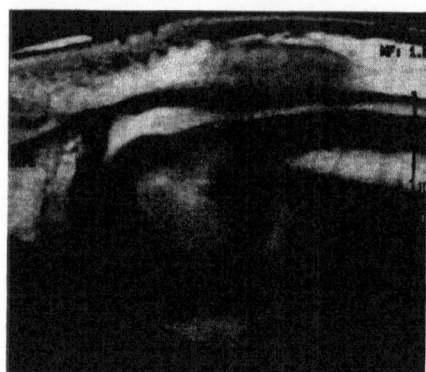

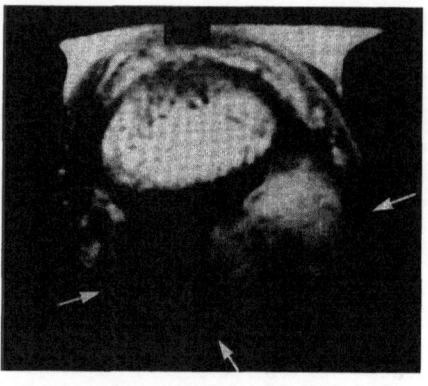

Fig. 22.32. Giant cell tumor of the tendon sheaths and the distal interphalangeal joint. Sagittal postenhanced T1-weighted image depicts an enhanced volar tumor invading the distal interphalangeal joint with bone erosions of the basis of the distal phalanx and of the head of the middle phalanx. Note the dorsal node developing from the extensor tendon

Fig. 22.33. Giant cell tumor of the flexor tendon sheath. Axial postenhanced T1-weighted image shows a volar tumor located at the distal insertion of the flexor tendon. Note the dark signal of peripheral hemosiderin deposits (*arrows*)

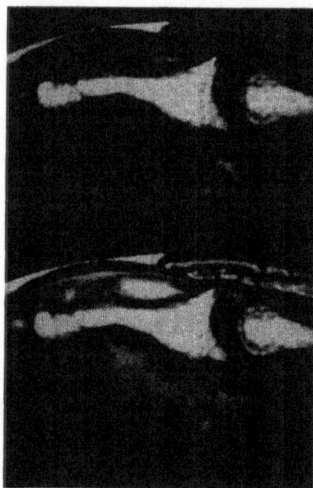

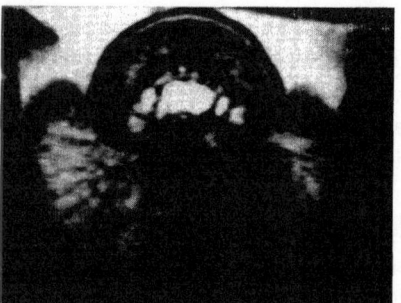

b

a

Fig. 22.34a, b. Giant cell tumor of the flexor tendon sheath. a Axial T1-weighted images before (*top*) and after (*bottom*) injection of gadoterate show nonspecific strong enhancement of the volar tumor. b Axial T2-weighted image does not highlight hemosiderin deposits but shows an unusual homogeneous low signal of the lesion

insertion of the distal band of the extensor tendon on the basis of the distal phalanx (Fig. 22.37). The pedicle must be resected during surgery in order to avoid a recurrence. The injection of oxygenated methylene blue in the volar aspect of the distal interphalangeal joint during surgery can highlight this pedicle, although the interpretation of this test is difficult [40]. The detection of a pedicle is even more essential for locations beneath the matrix, because the isolated tying of the pedicle may be sufficient. Therefore, a surgical approach of the matrix is not necessary and avoids a secondary nail dystrophy. Axial T2-weighted MR images are accurate for depicting such a pedicle. In most cases,

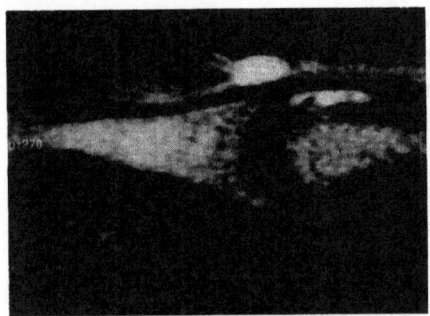
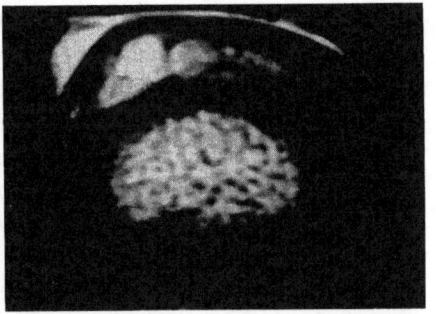

Fig. 22.35ab. Mucoid pseudocyst of the posterior nail fold. **a** Sagittal T2-weighted image shows the high signal cyst implanted in the posterior nail fold, close to the distal insertion of the terminal band of the extensor tendon and close to the nail root. **b** Axial T2-weighted image depicts a lateral high signal cyst with septa

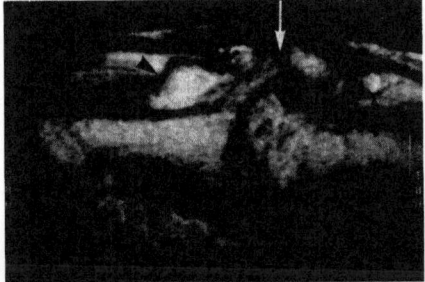

Fig. 22.36. Mucoid pseudocyst of the posterior nail fold with submatrix extension. Sagittal T2-weighted image shows multiple cysts in the posterior nail fold (*arrows*) and an expansion beneath the matrix (*arrowhead*). Note the severe osteoarthritis of the distal interphalangeal joint. Huge dorsal osteophytes lift up the extensor tendon (*white arrow*)

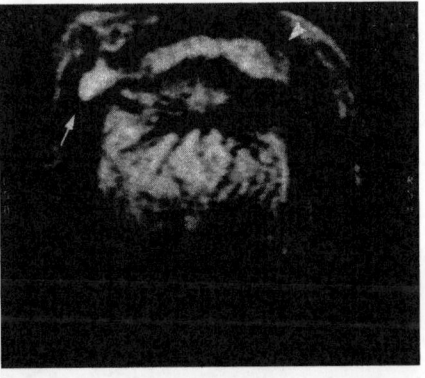

Fig. 22.37. Pedicled mucoid pseudocyst of the posterior nail fold. Axial T2-weighted image shows a high signal lateral pedicle (*arrow*) beneath the lifted extensor tendon (*arrowhead*)

plain films show osteoarthritis of the distal interphalangeal joint with dorsal osteophytes of the head of the middle phalanx, lifting up and wounding the extensor tendon (Figs. 22.36, 22.37). The dorsal osteophytes must also be resected with the cyst and the pedicle, in order to avoid a recurrence.

- MR imaging is not useful for the diagnosis of common chondromas or subungual exostosis (Fig. 22.38). On the other hand, it can depict unusual sites of chondromas, such as periosteal or soft tissue chondromas (nail bed) (Fig. 22.39). The signal behavior is characteristic of cartilage, with a very high signal on T2-weighted images and faint peripheral enhancement. Enhanced septa can be also depicted. In the exceptional cases of sarcomatous degeneration, MR imaging provides additional information, with an unusual mottled enhancement for the low-grade lesions, and a more diffuse enhancement for the less differentiated lesions. If the detection of the nidus of an osteoid osteoma must be obtained with CT, eventually after a bone scan, MR imaging is superior for detecting the associated abnormalities (Fig. 22.40). Nearly 8% of osteoid osteomas occur in the phalanges, but the distal phalanx is seldom involved [6]. The soft tissues are often swollen with bowing of the nail plate. As in other locations, the nidus can be intramedullary, cortical or periosteal. The osteoid tissue appears with a high signal intensity on the gradient echo images (Fig. 22.40). The large inflammatory reactions are difficult to depict on CT images, while they are obvious on MR images at the level of the nail bed and of the trabecular bone.

22.3 Conclusion

Imaging of the nail unit remains basic and mostly restricted to radiographs. We must not forget ultrasonography in the detection of tumors or foreign bodies in the soft parts. Recent advances in high-resolution MR images allow further investigation of the nail unit. An accurate assessment of the extension of subungual tumors, such as glomus tumors, is now available preoperatively.

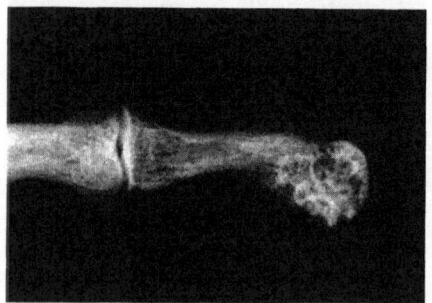 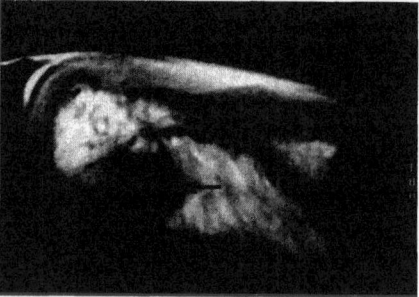

a   b

Fig. 22.38a, b. Subungual exostosis. **a** Lateral radiograph shows a pedicled osteochondroma developing from the tuft. **b** Sagittal T1-weighted image depicts the high signal of the trabecular bone of the osteochondroma. Note the thick low signal fibrocartilaginous cap (*arrow*)

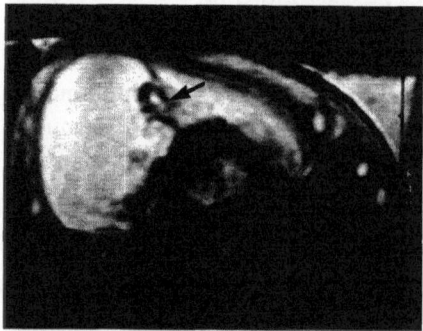

Fig. 22.39. Parosteal chondroma. Axial 3D gradient echo image depicts a homogeneous lesion of the bone surface with high signal intensity. Peripheral calcifications surrounding the implantation appear with low signal (*arrows*). Note the lack of bony invasion

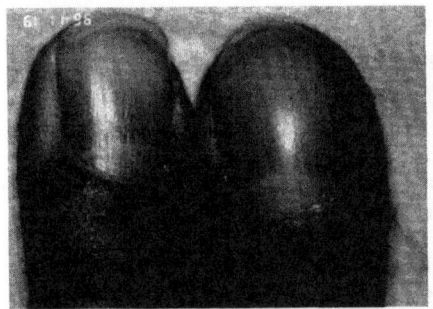

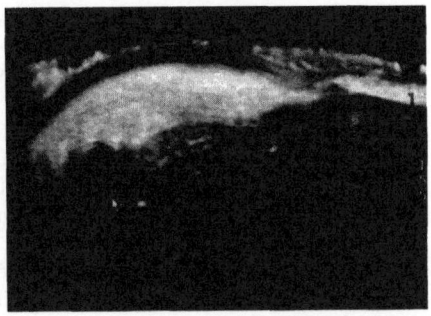

a

b

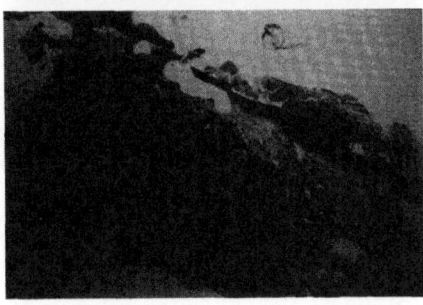

c

Fig. 22.40a–c. Osteoid osteoma of the distal phalanx (by courtesy of Dr. Robert Baran, Cannes, France). a Clubbing of the fingertip. b Sagittal postenhanced 3D gradient echo image depicts the enhanced inflammatory reaction of a thickened nail bed. Note the hypercurvature of the nail plate. The calcified nidus (*arrow*) is well depicted due to susceptibility artifacts. c Histologic view with osteoid tissue

References

1. Aguayo JB, Blackband SJ, Schoeniger J, Mattingly MA, Hintermann M (1986) Nuclear magnetic resonance imaging of a single cell. Nature 322:190–191
2. Alexander H, Miller DL (1979) Determining skin thickness with pulsed ultrasound. J Invest Dermatol 72:17–19
3. Baden HP, Kubilus J (1983) Fibrous proteins of bovine hoff. J Invest Dermatol 81:220–224
4. Baden HP (1987) Structure composition, and physiology of nails. In: Baden HP (ed) Diseases of the hair and nails. Year Book, Chicago, pp 3–11
5. Baran R, Klint A (1992) Onychomatrixoma. Br J Dermatol 126:510–515
6. Baran R, Haneke E (1994) Tumours of the nail apparatus and adjacent tissues. In: Baran R, Dawber (eds) Diseases of the nails and their management. Blackwell, London, pp 417–497
7. Bittoun J, Saint-Jalmes H, Querleux B, Darrasse L, Jolivet O, Idy-Peretti I, Wartski M, Richard S, Leveque JL (1990) In vivo high resolution MR imaging of the skin a whole body system at 1.5 T. Radiology 176:457–460
8. Blackband SJ, Chakrabarti I, Gibbs P, Buckley DL, Horsman A (1994) Fingers: three-dimensional MR imaging and angiography with a local gradient coil. Radiology 190:895–899
9. Bourekas EC, Mark LC (1996) Malignant hemangioendothelioma (angiosarcoma) of the skull: plain film, CT and MR appearance. Am J Neuroradiol 17:1946–1948
10. Buetow PC, Kransdorf MJ (1990) Radiologic appearance of intramuscular hemangioma with emphasis on MR imaging. AJR 154:563–567
11. Camirand P, Giroud JM (1970) Subungual glomus tumour. Radiological manifestations. Arch Dermatol 102:677–679
12. Carroll RE, Berman AT (1972) Glomus tumors of the hand: review of the literature and report of 28 cases. J Bone Joint Surg 54:691–703
13. Chevrot A, d'Izarn JJ, Pallardy G (1976) Tumeurs glomiques et kystes épidermoïdes des phalanges: aspect radiologique avec étude angiographique des tumeurs glomiques. J Radiol 57:645–647

14. Dailiana ZH, Drapé JL, Le Viet D (1999) A glomus tumour with four recurrences. J Hand Surg [Br] 24:131–132
15. Davis TS, Graham WP III, Blomain EW (1981) A ten-year experience with glomus tumors. Ann Plast Surg 6:297–299
16. Dion E, Idy-Peretti I, Bellin MF, Oberlin C, Grellet J, Bittoun J (1991) MR imaging of the carpal tunnel with a specific high-resolution coil. Radiology 181:106
17. Drapé JL, Idy-Peretti I, Goettmann S, Wolfram-Gabel R, Dion E, Grossin M, Benacerraf R, Guérin-Surville H, Bittoun J (1995) Subungual glomus tumors: evaluation with MR imaging. Radiology 195:507–515
18. Drapé JL, Idy-Peretti I, Goettmann S, Guérin-Surville H, Bittoun J (1996a) Standard and high-resolution magnetic resonance imaging of glomus tumors of toes and fingertips. J Am Acad Dermatol 35:550–555
19. Drapé JL, Wolfram-Gabel R, Idy-Peretti I, Baran R, Goettmann S, Sick H, Guerin-Surville H, Bittoun J (1996b) The lunula: a magnetic resonance imaging approach to the subnail matrix area. J Invest Dermatol 106:1081–1085
20. Drapé JL, Idy-peretti I, Goettmann S, Salon A, Abimelec P, Guerin-Surville H, Bittoun J (1996) MR imaging of digital mucoid cysts. Radiology 200:531–536
21. El-Gammal S, Hoffmann K, Auer T, Korten M, Altmeyer P, Höss A, Ermert H (1991) A 50-MHz high-resolution ultrasound imaging system for dermatology. In: Altemeyer P, El-Gammal S, Hoffmann K (eds) Ultrasound in dermatology. Springer, Berlin Heidelberg New York, pp 41–54
22. Finlay AY, Moseley H, Duggan TC (1987) Ultrasound transmission time: an in vivo guide to nail thickness. Br J Dermatol 117:765–770
23. Finlay AY, Western B, Edwards C (1990) Ultrasound velocity in human fingernail and effects of hydratation: validation of in vivo nail thickness measurement techniques. Br J Dermatol 123:365–373
24. Foo TK, Shellock FG, Hayes CE, Schenck JF, Slayman BE (1992) High resolution MR imaging of the wrist and eye with short TR, short TE, and partial echo acquisition. Radiology 183:277–281
25. Fornage BD (1988) Glomus tumours in the fingers: diagnosis with ultrasound. Radiology 167:183–185
26. Gandon F, Legaillard P, Brueton R, Le Viet D, Foucher G (1992) Forty-eight glomus tumors of the hand: retrospective study and four-year follow-up. Ann Hand Surg 11:401–405
27. Hirai T, Fumiiri M (1995) Ultrasonic observation of the nail matrix. Dermatol Surg 21:158–161
28. Holzberg M (1992) Glomus tumor of the nail: a "red herring" clarified by magnetic resonance imaging. Arch Dermatol 128:160–162
29. Hou SM, Shih TTF, Lin MC (1993) Magnetic resonance imaging of an obscure glomus tumour in the fingertip. J Hand Surg [Br] 18:482–483
30. Jablon M, Horowitz, Bernstein DA (1990) Magnetic resonance imaging of a glomus tumor of the finger tip. J Hand Surg [Am] 15:507–509
31. Jemec GBE, Serup J (1989) Ultrasound structure of the nail plate. Arch Dermatol 125:643–646
32. Johnson GA, Thomson MB, Gewalt SL, Hayes CE (1986) Nuclear magnetic resonance imaging at microscopic resolution. J Magn Reson 68:129–137
33. Johnson M, Comaish JS, Shuster S (1991) Nail is produced by the normal bed: a controversy resolved. Br J Dermatol 125:27–29
34. Johnson M, Shuster S (1993) Continuous formation of nail along the bed. Br J Dermatol 128:277–280
35. Kneeland JB, Middleton WD, Matloub HS, Jesmanowicz A, Froncisz W, Hyde JS (1987) High resolution MR imaging of glomus tumor. J Comput Assist Tomogr 11:351–352
36. Kodachi K, Kojima T (1990) Hemangioma of the finger. Handchir Mikrochir Plast Chir 22:49–52
37. Kohout E, Stout AP (1961) The glomus tumor in children. Cancer 14:555–556

38. Masson P (1924) Le glomus neuromyo-artériel des régions tactiles et ses tumeurs. Lyon Chir 21:256–280

39. Matloub HS, Muoneke VN, Prevel CD, Sanger JR, Yousif NJ (1992) Glomus tumor imaging: use of MRI for localization of occult lesions. J Hand Surg [Am] 17:472–475

40. Newmeyer WL, Kilgore ES, Graham WP (1974) Mucous cyst: the dorsal distal interphalangeal joint ganglion. Plast Reconstr Surg 53:313–315

41. Ogino T, Ohnishi N (1993) Ultrasonography of a subungual glomus tumour. J Hand Surg [Br] 18:746–747

42. Rettig AC, Strickland JW (1977) Glomus tumor of the digits. J Hand Surg 2:261–265

43. Richard S, Querleux B, Bittoun J, Idy-Peretti I, Jolivet O, Cermacova E. Lévêque JL (1991) In vivo proton relaxation times analysis of the skin layers by magnetic resonance imaging. J Invest Dermatol 97:120–125

44. Rosenthal EA (1983) Treatment of finger tip and nail bed injuries. Orthop Clin North Am 14:675–697

45. Schneider LH, Bachow TB (1991) Magnetic resonance imaging of glomus tumor. Orthop Rev 20:255–256

46. Serup J (1991) Ten year's experience with high-frequency ultrasound examination of the skin: development and refinement of technique and equipment. In: Altmeyer P, El-Gammal S, Hoffmann K (eds) Ultrasound in dermatology. Springer, Berlin Heidelberg New York, pp 41–54

47. Tan CY, Marks R, Payne P (1981) Comparison of xeroradiographic and ultrasound detection of corticosteroid induced dermal thinning. J Invest Dermatol 76:126–128

48. Varian J, Cleak DK (1980) Glomus tumors in the hand. Hand 12:293–299

49. Wong EC, Jesmanowicz A, Hyde JC (1991) High-resolution short echo time MR imaging of the fingers and wrists with a local gradient coil. Radiology 181:393–397

50. Zook EG (1988) The perionychium. In: Green DP (ed) Operative hand surgery. Churchill Livingstone, New York, pp 1331–1375

Subject Index

List of Contributors

S. Balzano, MD
IRCCS Hospital "Casa Sollievo della Sofferenza"
Viale Cappuccini
71013 San Giovanni Rotondo
Italy

A. Barile, MD
Department of Radiology
Ospedale "S. Salvatore"
University of L'Aquila
67100 L'Aquila
Italy

L. H. L. De Beuckeleer, MD
Department of Radiology
Universitair Ziekenhuis Antwerpen
Wilrijkstraat 10
2650 Edegem
Belgium

J. Bittoun, MD
CIERM, CHU de Bicêtre
Université Paris-Sud
75, rue du Général-Leclerc
94275 Le Kremlin-Bicêtre Cedex
France

J. L. Bloem, MD, PhD
Department of Radiology
Leiden University Medical Center
P.O. Box 9600
2300 RC Leiden
The Netherlands

H. M. Bonél, MD
Department of Diagnostic Radiology
Ludwig-Maximilians-University
Marchioninistrasse 15
81377 Munich
Germany

O. Bottinelli, MD
Department of Radiology
IRCCS Policlinico S. Matteo
27100 Pavia
Italy

P. G. Bracke, MD
Department of Musculoskeletal Radiology
Universitair Ziekenhuis Antwerpen
Wilrijkstraat 10
2650 Edegem
Belgium

M. Cammisa, MD
IRCCS Hospital "Casa Sollievo della Sofferenza"
Viale Cappuccini
71013 San Giovanni Rotondo
Italy

R. Campani, MD
Department of Radiology
IRCCS Policlinico S. Matteo
27100 Pavia
Italy

A. Castriota Scanderbeg, MD
Department of Radiology
IRCCS "S. Lucia"
Via Ardeatina 306
00179 Rome
Italy

A. Catalucci, MD
Department of Radiology
Ospedale "S. Salvatore"
University of L'Aquila
67100 L'Aquila
Italy

A. Chevrot, MD
Department of Radiology
Groupe Hospitalier Cochin
2, rue du Faubourg Saint-Jacques
75679 Paris Cedex 14
France

L. F. Coenen, MD
Department of Orthopedic Surgery
Universitair Ziekenhuis Antwerpen
Wilrijkstraat 10
2650 Edegem
Belgium

B. Dallapiccola, MD
Institute of Medical Genetics
University "La Sapienza" and CSS-Mendel
Institute
Rome
Italy

A. M. Davies, MD
MRI Centre
Royal Orthopaedic Hospital
Birmingham B31 2AP
United Kingdom

E. Dion, MD
Department of Radiology
Groupe Hospitalier Pitié-Salpêtrière
47–83 Boulevard de l'Hôpital
75651 Paris Cedex 13
France

J.-L. Drapé, MD
Department of Radiology
Groupe Hospitalier Cochin
27, rue du Faubourg Saint-Jacques
75679 Paris Cedex 14
France

A. M. Dupont, MD
Department of Radiology
Groupe Hospitalier Cochin
27, rue du Faubourg Saint-Jacques
75679 Paris Cedex 14
France

J. Dutton, MD
Department of Nuclear Medicine
Addenbrooke's Hospital
Hills Road
Cambridge CB2 2QQ
United Kingdom

J. M. Elliott, MD
Department of Radiology
Nuffield Orthopaedic Centre
Windmill Road
Headington
Oxford OX3 7LD
United Kingdom

C. Faletti, MD
Department of Radiology
CTO Hospital
Turin
Italy

A. Feydy, MD
Department of Radiology
Groupe Hospitalier Cochin
27, rue du Faubourg Saint-Jacques
75679 Paris Cedex 14
France

F. Florio, MD
IRCCS Hospital "Casa Sollievo della Sofferenza"
Viale Cappuccini
71013 San Giovanni Rotondo
Italy

I. Fogelman, MD
Department of Nuclear Medicine
Guy's Hospital
St. Thomas Street
London SE1 9RT
United Kingdom

M. Fuchsjäger, MD
Department of Radiology
University of Vienna
Währinger Gürtel 18–20
1090 Vienna
Austria

H. K. Genant, MD
Department of Radiology
University of California San Francisco
505 Parnassus Avenue
San Francisco
CA 94143-0628
USA

D. Godefroy, MD
Department of Radiology
Groupe Hospitalier Cochin
27, rue du Faubourg Saint-Jacques
75679 Paris Cedex 14
France

A. J. Grainger, FRCR
Department of Radiology
Freeman Hospital
High Heaton
Newcastle upon Tyne NE7 7DN
UK

G. Guglielmi, MD
IRCCS Hospital "Casa Sollievo della Sofferenza"
Viale Cappuccini
71013 San Giovanni Rotondo
Italy

H. Imhof, MD
Department of Radiology
University of Vienna
Währinger Gürtel 18–20
1090 Vienna
Austria

F. Kainberger, MD
Department of Radiology
University of Vienna
Währinger Gürtel 18–20
1090 Vienna
Austria

D. de la Kethulle de Ryhove, MD
Department of Radiology
Universitair Ziekenhuis Antwerpen
Wilrijkstraat 10
2650 Edegem
Belgium

C. van Kuijk, MD, PhD
Department of Radiology
Academic Medical Centre
University of Amsterdam
Meibergdreef 9
1105 AZ Amsterdam
The Netherlands

P. K. Lang, MD
Department of Radiology
Stanford University Medical School
Stanford
CA 94305-5105
USA

M. Maas, MD
Department of Radiology
Academic Medical Center
University of Amsterdam
Meibergdreef 9
1105 AZ Amsterdam
The Netherlands

C. Masciocchi MD
Department of Radiology
Ospedale "S. Salvatore"
University of L'Aquila
67100 L'Aquila
Italy

M. Mastantuono, MD
Department of Radiology
Policlinico Umberto I
Viale Regina Elena 324
00161 Rome
Italy

V. M. Metz, MD
Department of Radiology
University of Vienna
Währinger Gürtel 18–20
1090 Vienna
Austria

S. M. Metz-Schimmerl, MD
Department of Radiology
University of Vienna
Währinger Gürtel 18–20
A-1090 Vienna
Austria

M. Nardella, MD
IRCCS Hospital "Casa Sollievo della Sofferenza"
Viale Cappuccini
71013 San Giovanni Rotondo
Italy

H. Nishimura, MD
Department of Radiology
Kurume University School of Medicine
67 Asahi-Machi
Kurume 830-0011
Japan

W. R. Obermann, MD, PhD
Department of Radiology
C2-S
Leiden University Medical Center
Albinusdreef 2
2333 ZA Leiden
The Netherlands

R. Passariello, MD
Department of Radiology
Policlinico Umberto I
Viale Regina Elena 324
00161 Rome
Italy

E. Pessis, MD
Department of Radiology
Groupe Hospitalier Cochin
27, rue du Faubourg Saint-Jacques
75679 Paris Cedex 14
France

T. Rand, MD
Department of Radiology
University of Vienna
Währinger Gürtel 18–20
A-1090 Vienna
Austria

M. F. Reiser, MD
Department of Diagnostic Radiology
Ludwig-Maximilians-University
Marchioninistrasse 15
81377 Munich
Germany

D. Resnick, MD
Department of Radiology
Veterans Affairs Medical Center
University of California at San Diego
3350 La Jolla Village Drive
San Diego, CA 92161
USA

R. R. van Rijn, MD PhD
Department of Radiology
University Hospital Rotterdam
Dr. Molewaterplein 40
3015 GD Rotterdam
The Netherlands

M. P. J. F. Ritt, MD, PhD
Department of Plastic
Reconstructive and Hand Surgery
Academic Medical Center
University of Amsterdam
Meibergdreef 9
1105 AZ Amsterdam
The Netherlands

L. Satragno, MD
Department of Radiology
Policlinico Umberto I
Viale Regina Elena 324
00161 Rome
Italy

A. M. De Schepper, MD
Department of Radiology
Universitair Ziekenhuis Antwerpen
Wilrijkstraat 10
2650 Edegem
Belgium

A. De Serio, MD
IRCCS Hospital "Casa Sollievo della Sofferenza"
Viale Cappuccini
71013 San Giovanni Rotondo
Italy

V. Strizzi, MD
IRCCS Hospital "Casa Sollievo della Sofferenza"
Viale Cappuccini
71013 San Giovanni Rotondo
Italy

I. Sulzbacher, MD
Clinical Institute for Pathology
Allgemeines Krankenhaus
Waehringer Guertel 18–20
1090 Vienna
Austria

D. J. Theodorou, MD
Department of Radiology
Veterans Affairs Medical Center
University of California at San Diego
3350 La Jolla Village Drive
San Diego, CA 92161
USA

S. J. Theodorou, MD
Department of Radiology
Veterans Affairs Medical Center
University of California at San Diego
3350 La Jolla Village Drive
San Diego, CA 92161
USA

J. E. Vandevenne, MD
Department of Musculoskeletal Radiology
Universitair Ziekenhuis Antwerpen
Wilrijkstraat 10
2650 Edegem
Belgium

H.-J. van der Woude, MD
Department of Radiology
Leiden University Medical Center
P.O. Box 9600
2300 RC Leiden
The Netherlands